Disulfiram and its
Metabolite, Diethyldithiocarbamate

Disulfiram and its Metabolite, Diethyldithiocarbamate

Pharmacology and status in the treatment of alcoholism, HIV infections, AIDS and heavy metal toxicity

Peter K. Gessner

Professor of Pharmacology and Therapeutics
School of Medicine and Biomedical Sciences
State University of New York at Buffalo
Buffalo, New York

Teresa Gessner

Research Professor of Pharmacology
Roswell Park Graduate Division
State University of New York at Buffalo
Roswell Park Cancer Institute
Buffalo, New York

 SPRINGER-SCIENCE+BUSINESS MEDIA, B.V.

First edition 1992

© 1992 Peter K. Gessner and Teresa Gessner
Originally published by Chapman & Hall in1992
Typeset in 10½/12pt Garamond by Interprint Ltd, Malta
by TJ Press, Padstow, Cornwall

ISBN 978-0-412-36010-7

A catalogue record for this book is available from the British Library

Library of Congress Cataloging-in-Publication data

Gessner, Peter K, 1931–
    Disulfiram and its metabolite diethyldithiocarbamate pharmacology and
    status in the treatment of alcoholism, HIV infections, AIDS and heavy
    metal toxicity / Peter K. Gessner, Teresa Gessner.
        p. cm.
    Includes bibliographical references and index.
    ISBN 978-94-010-5028-9   ISBN 978-94-011-2328-0 (eBook)
    DOI 10.1007/978-94-011-2328-0
    1. Disulfiram — Physiological effect. 2. Diethyldithiocarbamate–
    Physiological effect. 3. Diethyldithiocarbamate — Therapeutic use –
    Testing. I. Gessner, Teresa, 1933– II. Title.
    RM666.D583G47 1991
    616.86'1061 — dc20   91-19580
                                                                    CIP

Contents

Figure acknowledgements   *xi*
Preface   *xiii*
Glossary   *xv*

1   INTRODUCTION AND SCOPE OF MONOGRAPH   1
   1.1   Introduction   1
   1.2   Scope of monograph   3
   1.3   Earlier reviews   5

2   RELEVANT PHYSICAL AND CHEMICAL PROPERTIES   7
   2.1   Introduction and general properties   7
   2.2   Acid-catalyzed decomposition   8
   2.3   Formation of metal complexes   9

**3   REACTIONS OF DISULFIRAM AND DIETHYLDITHIO-
     CARBAMATE WITH BLOOD CONSTITUENTS**   13
   3.1   Introduction   13
   3.2   Formation of copper complexes   14
   3.3   Formation of mixed disulfides   15
   3.4   Uptake of disulfiram by blood cells   17
   3.5   Summary   19

**4   ASSAY METHODS FOR DISULFIRAM AND METABOLITES
     IN BIOLOGICAL MATERIALS**   21
   4.1   Introduction   21
   4.2   General considerations   22
   4.3   Specific methods   25
   4.4   Other methods   26

5 METABOLISM OF DISULFIRAM AND DIETHYLDITHIO-CARBAMATE   29
   5.1   Introduction   29
   5.2   Formation of mixed disulfides with generation of
          diethyldithiocarbamate   30
   5.3   Formation of disulfiram from diethyldithiocarbamate   32
   5.4   Formation of the copper complex   34
   5.5   *S*-glucuronide of diethyldithiocarbamic acid   34
   5.6   Formation of carbon disulfide and diethylamine   36
   5.7   Metabolism of carbon disulfide and formation of
          carbonyl sulfide   37
   5.8   The methyl ester of diethyldithiocarbamic acid   38
   5.9   The methyl ester of diethylmonothiocarbamic acid   40
   5.10   Other metabolites   41

6 PHARMACOKINETIC ASPECTS OF THE DISPOSITION OF DISULFIRAM AND METABOLITES   43
   6.1   Introduction   44
   6.2   Methods   44
   6.3   Urinary excretion of disulfiram metabolites   51
   6.4   Pulmonary excretion of disulfiram metabolites   54
   6.5   Plasma disulfiram and metabolites following its
          administration   56
   6.6   Diethyldithiocarbamate and metabolites following its
          administration   60

7 HEAVY METALS: EFFECTS OF DIETHYLDITHIOCARBAMATE AND DISULFIRAM ADMINISTRATION   65
   7.1   Introduction   65
   7.2   Thallium   69
   7.3   Zinc   71
   7.4   Cadmium   73
   7.5   Lead   79
   7.6   Nickel   81
   7.7   Copper   85
   7.8   Mercury   88
   7.9   Platinum   90
   7.10   Polonium   93

8 DISULFIRAM AND DIETHYLDITHIOCARBAMATE AS ENZYME INHIBITORS   95
   8.1   Introduction   96
   8.2   Inhibition of drug metabolizing enzymes   102

8.3	Inhibition of dopamine β-hydroxylase	120
8.4	Inhibition of superoxide dismutase	126
8.5	Inactivation of glutathione peroxidase	133
8.6	Effect of catalase	135

9 INHIBITION OF ALDEHYDE DEHYDROGENASE — **137**

9.1	Introduction	137
9.2	Phenomenology of the inhibition by disulfiram	145
9.3	Mechanism of the inhibition	150
9.4	Role of disulfiram metabolites	154
9.5	Inhibition of aldehyde dehydrogenases in blood	158
9.6	Inhibition of metabolism of endogenous aldehydes	162
9.7	Aldehyde and xanthine oxidases	166

10 THE DISULFIRAM–ETHANOL REACTION — **167**

10.1	Introduction	167
10.2	Discovery and therapeutic application	168
10.3	Pharmacological characteristics	171
10.4	Blood acetaldehyde determination	177
10.5	The acetaldehyde hypothesis	178
10.6	Quest for animal models of the reaction	184
10.7	Effect of disulfiram on ethanol metabolism	191
10.8	The dopamine β-hydroxylase hypothesis	193
10.9	Effect of ethanol in animals pretreated with disulfiram metabolites	199
10.10	Treatment of the disulfiram–ethanol reaction	201

11 DISULFIRAM THERAPY OF ALCOHOL ABUSE — **205**

11.1	Introduction	205
11.2	Goals of disulfiram therapy	209
11.3	Disulfiram treatment components correlated with reduction of drinking days	209
11.4	Disulfiram therapy paradigms	214
11.5	Election of and continuation in treatment	223
11.6	Characteristics of disulfiram's therapeutic effects	224
11.7	Side effects of disulfiram therapy	232
11.8	Chemical compliance monitoring	244
11.9	Disulfiram implants	245

12 IMMUNOMODULATORY EFFECTS OF DIETHYLDITHIOCARBAMATE — **247**

12.1	Introduction	248
12.2	Stimulation of antibody response to sheep red blood cells	249

12.3   Enhancement of mitogen-induced
        lymphoproliferation   251
12.4   Effect on lymphoproliferative response to alloantigens 255
12.5   Interaction with asymmetrical neocortical lesions   256
12.6   Effects on cell-mediated cytotoxicity   257
12.7   Effect on delayed-type hypersensitivity reaction   261
12.8   Induction of T-cell differentiation   261
12.9   Effect on lymphocyte populations *in vivo*   267
12.10   Effects on mononuclear phagocytic cells   272
12.11   Experimental therapeutics   273
12.12   Immunomodulatory effects of related compounds   275
12.13   Conclusions   275

13   CLINICAL STATUS OF DIETHYLDITHIOCARBAMATE AS AN
     IMMUNOSTIMULANT   279
13.1   Introduction   279
13.2   In the treatment of HIV infections and AIDS   280
13.3   In gastrointestinal surgery patients   290
13.4   As a therapeutic agent in autoimmune disease   290
13.5   In patients with neoplastic disease   291
13.6   As an adjuvant for influenza vaccination   292
13.7   Summary   292

14   MODULATION OF VARIOUS BIOLOGICAL PHENOMENA   295
14.1   Cytotoxicity   295
14.2   Modulation of the effects of oxidative stress   301
14.3   Modulation of the effects of radiation and
        hyperthermia   306

15   MODULATION OF CANCER CHEMOTHERAPY   313
15.1   Introduction   313
15.2   Preclinical studies   315
15.3   Clinical studies   328
15.4   Conclusions   334

16   TOXICOLOGY   335
16.1   Introduction   335
16.2   Acute toxicity   336
16.3   Chronic toxicity   341
16.4   Effects on liver   342
16.5   Testing for mutagenicity   343
16.6   Testing for carcinogenicity   344
16.7   Testing for teratogenic and reproductive toxicity   345

Appendix – The road to Anatabuse – *Professor Erick Jacobsen*   347
References   353
Author and citation index   413
Subject index

Figure
acknowledgements

Figure 7.2 Dr. A. Oskarsson, Toxicology Laboratory, National Food Administration, Sweden and Dr. H. Lindahl. Redrawn with permission from, *Toxicology Letters*, **49**, 87 (1989). © Elsevier Science Publishers, The Netherlands.

Figure 8.1 Dr. F. Green, Department of Pharmacology, Pennsylvania State University College of Medicine and Dr. G.E Miller. Adapted with permission from, *Biochemical Pharmacology*, **32**, 2433 (1983), Pergamon Press plc.

Figure 10.1a Dr. R. Preisig, Institut für klinische Pharmakologie, Universität Bern and Dr. Ch. Beyeler. Adapted with permission from *Alcoholism, Clinical and Experimental Research*, **9**, 118–24 (1985). © The Research Society on Alcoholism and *Schweizerische Medizinische Wochenschrift*, **117**, 52–60 (1987) © Schwabe & Co. A.G.

Figure 10.2 Dr. K.O. Lindros, Research Laboratories of the State Alcohol Monopoly, Finland. Reprinted with permission from, *Alcoholism, Clinical and Experimental Research*, **5**, 528–30 (1981). © The Research Society on Alcoholism.

Figure 13.2 Dr. E.M. Hersh, Arizona Cancer Center, Reprinted with permission from *Journal of the American Medical Association*, **265**, 1538–44. © 1991 American Medical Association.

Figure 14.1 Dr. D. Rigas, School of Medicine, University of Oregon

Health Sciences Centre, Redrawn with permission from *Biochemical and Biophysical Research Communications*, **88**, 373–9. © Academic Press.

Figure 14.2 Dr. R.G. Evans, Fricke Radiobiology Research Laboratories, Rochester, Maine. Adapted with permission from *International Journal of Radiation Oncology, Biology and Physics*, 9, 1635 (1983), Pergamon Press plc.

Appendix *The Road to Antabuse* by E. Jacobsen. Reprinted with permission. Dr. A. Konar, *A/S Dumex Ltd., Copenhagen*.

Preface

This book is aimed at those in the biomedical community that are interested in the therapeutic applications, pharmacology, biochemistry, toxicology and pharmacokinetics of the title compounds. Recent findings regarding the ability of diethyldithiocarbamate (ditiocarb, Imuthiol®) to delay the progression of HIV infections and AIDS, the discovery of its potential as a rescue agent in cancer chemotherapy, and the identification of disulfiram (Antabuse®) regimens that allow alcoholics to achieve abstinence of many months' duration have made writing this book an exciting experience. At the same time the fact that the two drugs differ substantially in their pharmacological effects in spite of their easy interconvertibility has rendered the writing intellectually challenging.

Diethyldithiocarbamate, an agent seemingly less toxic than aspirin, rivals it in the multiplicity and diversity of its pharmacological properties. Notable among these are the manyfold potent immunostimulant effects, and though most of these involve effects on T-cells, the mechanism of diethyldithiocarbamate's action remains far from clear. The drug is also a potent chelator of heavy metals and this has led to a number of clinical applications. As might be expected, it inhibits several important enzymes. Further, it is one of the most effective radioprotective agents; it also protects organisms against a variety of toxic agents.

Disulfiram, long employed in the treatment of alcoholism, has proven over the last thirty years notably free of side-effects. Its adoption as the treatment of choice for alcoholism by some public health authorities and the resultant decrease in alcohol-linked hospital admissions have rendered a critical in-depth review of its clinical literature timely. This book answers the need and should prove a useful reference source for clinicians and therapists in the field as well as for research scientists.

We offer in this book both an analysis of published data and a conceptual synthesis of diverse information gleaned from different disciplines (pharmacology, therapeutics, biochemistry and chemistry).

Wherever possible, we have attempted to integrate published findings into a narrative that includes critical discussion, novel conclusions and summaries of large bodies of information in tabular form. Many of the values we list in the tables were newly computed for this book from data in the literature.

Finally, the book is unusual, indeed to our knowledge unique, in that the author index is also a citation index. That is, under the name of each first author are listed chronologically all of that author's cited references and the pages on which each is cited in the book.

We would like to acknowledge the colleagues, many of whom are expert in the relevant fields, who helped us by reading and criticizing sections of the monograph or by discussing with us aspects of the subject. These include, alphabetically: Richard F. Borch, M.D., Colin Brewer, M.D., Janusz Z. Byczkowski, Ph.D., Richard K. Fuller, M.D., Donald Gallant, M.D., Robert McIsaac, Ph.D., Erling Petersen, Ph.D. Michael Phillips, M.D., Regina Pietruszko, Ph.D., Per Rønsted, M.D.; Robert Whitney, M.D., and Marek Zaleski, M.D. We would also like to thank the many workers in the field who responded to our request and provided us with updated information regarding their investigations. Additionally, we would like to thank the ever helpful staff of the SUNY at Buffalo Health Sciences Library, an excellent facility. Lastly, we appreciate the patience shown by our editors at Chapman and Hall.

Glossary of acronyms and abbreviations

The pages given are those where the first or primary definition can be found

ATCs: Alcoholism Treatment Centers   220
ADCC: antibody-dependent cellular cytotoxicity   257
ADH: alcohol dehydrogenase   98
AIDS: acquired immune deficiency syndrome   279
ALA: δ-aminolevulinic acid   80
ALAD: δ-aminolevulinic acid dehydratase   80
ALDH: aldehyde dehydrogenase   137
AP: alkaline phosphatase   240
AR: aldehyde reductase   163
ARC: AIDS-related-complex   285
AST: aspartate aminotransferase   240
ATP: adenosine triphosphate
AUC: area under the curve   59
AZT: azidothymidine; zidovudine   288
BAL: British antilewisite; 2,3-dimercaptopropanol; dimercaprol   76
BCNU: 1,3-bis(2-chloroethyl)-1-nitrosourea, carmustine   323
BUN: blood urea nitrogen   317
CCER: calcium carbimide-ethanol reaction   182
Cd: cadmium   73
CDC: Centers for Disease Control   281
CFU: colony forming units   321
Co: cobat   100
COMT: catechol-O-methyltransferase   163
Con A: concanavalin A   248
COS: carbonyl sulfide   37
CRBC: chicken red blood cells   260
CRBT: Community-Reinforcement Behavioral Therapy   217
CS_2: carbon disulfide   36

CST: colony stimulating factors   320
Cu: copper   85
Cu(DS)$_2$: bis(diethyldithiocarbamato)copper complex   14
CuZn-SOD: copper-zinc-containing superoxide dismutase   126
DA: dopamine   163
DBH: dopamine β-hydroxylase   120
DCH: delayed cutaneous hypersensitivity   261
DER: disulfiram-ethanol reaction   138
DHMA: 3,4-dihydroxymandelic acid   163
DHMAL: 3,4-dihydroxymandelicaldehyde   163
DHPG: 3,4-dihydroxyphenyl glycol   163
DMF: dose modifying factor   307
DmSEt: diethylmonothiocarbamic acid ethyl ester   26
DmSH: diethylmonothiocarbamate   41
DmSMe: diethylmonothiocarbamic acid methyl ester   40
DOPAC: 3,4-dihydroxyphenylacetic acid   163
DOPAL: 3,4-dihydroxyphenylacetaldehyde   163
DOPET: 3,4-dihydroxyphenylethanol   163
DPTA: diethylenetriaminepentaacetic acid   19
DSEt: diethyldithiocarbamic acid ethyl ester   25
DSGa: S-glucuronide of diethyldithiocarbamic acid   34
DSH: diethyldithiocarbamate   1
DSMe: diethyldithiocarbamic acid methyl ester   38
DSSD: disulfiram   1
DSSMe: N,N-diethyldithiocarbamyl-S-methyl disulfide   32
DTH: Delayed-type hypersensitivity   261
E-RFC: erythrocyte-rosette-forming cells   281
E: epinephrine   196
E$_1$: human hepatic cytosolic ALDH   139
E$_2$: human hepatic mitochondrial ALDH   139
EC-SOD: extracellular copper-zinc-containing superoxide   126
EC-SOD C: C isozyme of EC-SOD   133
EDTA: ethylenediaminetetraacetic acid   14
Et$_2$NH: diethylamine   36
F1: equine hepatic cytosolic ALDH   142
F2: equine hepatic mitochondrial ALDH   142
FCS: fetal calf serum   310
FDA: Food and Drug Administration   288
Fe-SOD: iron-containing superoxide dismutase   126
FSH: follicle-stimulating hormone   243
FTS: Facteur Thymique Serique   265
G3P: glyceraldehyde-3-phosphate   164
GGTP: γ-glutamyltranspeptidase   92

GLC: gas-liquid chromatography   27
GM-CFC: granulocyte-macrophage colony forming cells   321
GM-CSF: granulocyte/monocyte colony stimulating factor   272
GSH: glutathione   1
GSHPx: glutathione peroxidase   133
GSSG: oxidized glutathione   1
GST: glutathione-*S*-transferase   133
HBSS: Hank's balanced salt solution   311
Hg: mercury   88
HgAc: mercuric acetate   88
hGH: human gowth hormone   243
5-HIAA: 5-hydroxyindole acetic acid   163
5-HIAL: 5-hydroxyindoleacetaldehyde   163
HIV: human immunodeficiency virus   279
HIV$^+$: HIV-positive   280
HN$_2$: nitrogen mustard, mechlorethamine   323
HPLC: high pressure liquid chromatography   24
hProl: human prolactin   243
5-HT: 5-hydroxytryptamine   163
5-HTOL: 5-hydroxytryptophol   163
hTSH: human thyroid-stimulating hormone   243
HVA: homovanillic acid; 3-methoxy-4-hydroxyphenylacetic
  acid   163
i.m.: intramuscular
i.p.: intraperitoneal
i.v.: intravenous
IAL: indole-3-acetaldehyde   145
IFN: interferon   258
IgG: immunoglobulin G   249
IgM: immunoglobulin M   249
IL-1: interleukin-1   287
IL-2: interleukin-2   287
IL-3: interleukin-3   327
LCBF: local cerebral blood flow   70
LD$_{50}$: dose lethal to 50% of tested organisms
LDH: lactate dehydrogenase   240
LH: luteinizing hormone   243
LPS: lipopolysaccharide   251
LTBMC: long-term bone marrow cultures   327
MAO: monoamineoxidase   162
MC: 3-methylcholanthrene   115
2-ME: 2-mercaptoethanol   255
MeHg: methyl mercury   88

MEM: Eagle's minimum essential medium   311
MeSH: methanethiol   32
MFO: mixed function oxygenases   241
MHC: major histocompatibility complex   251
MHPG: 3-methoxy-4-hydroxyphenylglycol   163
MLC: mixed lymphocyte culture   256
Mn-SOD: manganese-containing superoxide dismutase   126
NADH: nicotinamide adenine dinucleotide, reduced form
NADPH: nicotinamide adenine dinucleotide phosphate,
  reduced form
NE: norepinephrine   163
NER: nitrefazol-ethanol reaction   182
Ni: nickel   81
Ni(CO)$_4$: nickel carbonyl   84
Ni$_3$S$_2$: nickel subsulfide   84
NIAAA: National Institute of Alcohol Abuse and Alcoholism   220
NK: natural killer (NK) cells   257
O$_2^-$: superoxide anion radical   126
OA: octopamine   197
P-420: cytochrome P-420   117
P-450: cytochrome P-450   120
p.o.: per os; oral
P5C: 1-pyrroline-5-carboxylate   165
PAI-1: plasminogen activator inhibitor   243
Pb: lead   79
PB: phenobarbital   115
PBL: peripheral blood lymphocytes   248
PBMC: peripheral blood mononuclear cells   248
PBMC-LPR: PBMC lymphoproliferaive response   254
PF4: Platelet Factor 4   243
PFC: plaque-forming cells   249
PGE$_2$: prostaglandin E$_2$ 272
PHA: phytohemagglutinin   248
PMN: polymorphonuclear granulocytes   295
Po: polonium   93
PrSSD: mixed disulfides of proteins with DS residues   17
PrSH: protein sulfhydryl groups   30
PSH: 2-thiopyridone   153
PSSMe: 2-thiopyridylmethyl disulfide   154
PSSP: 2,2'-dithiodipyridine   153
Pt: platinum   90
PWM: pokeweed mitogen   251
R$_a$: accumulation ratio   76

ROS: reactive oxygen species   126
S-LPR: splenic lymphoproliferaive response   251
s.c.: subcutaneous
SCN⁻: thiocyanate   117
Se-GSHPx: selenium-containing glutathione peroxidase   133
SF: surviving fraction   321
SGOT: serum glutamic oxaloacetic transaminase   240
SOD: superoxide dismutase   126
SPECT: single-photon emission computed tomography   70
SRBC: sheep red blood cells   248
αSRBC: anti-srbc   249
SSA: succinic semialdehyde   164
T_3: triiodothyronine   243
T_4: thyroxin   243
$T_{50\%}$: time required for 50% inactivation   129
TA: tyramine   197
T_C: cytotoxic T cells   257
TCDD: 2,3,7,8-tetrachlorodibenzo-*p*-dioxin   142
THO: tritiated water   124
Tl: thallium   69
TRH: thyrotropin-releasing factor   243
VMA: vanillylmandelic acid; 3-methoxy-4-hydroxymandelic acid   163
WR-2721: ethofos   312
Zn: zinc   71

1

Introduction and scope of monograph

1.1 INTRODUCTION   1
1.2 SCOPE OF MONOGRAPH   3
1.3 EARLIER REVIEWS   5

1.1 INTRODUCTION

Disulfiram (DSSD), widely known under the trade name, Antabuse®, is a symmetrical disulfide which can be reduced to two molecules of the thiol (DSH) which, at physiological pH is better than 99% ionized to diethyldithiocarbamate and so referred to in this book. The sodium salt of diethydithiocarbamic acid is available both in an anhydrous form and as a trihydrate. It was earlier given the appellation dithiocarb (West and Sunderman, 1958; Sunderman and Sunderman, 1958; Merck Index, 1968). More recently it has been assigned the International Nonproprietary Name ditiocarb sodium (Merck Index, 1989; USAN, 1990).

Suppliers of reagent grade chemicals (Aldrich, Baker, Fisher, ICN, Kodak, Merck, Sigma, Waco) stock, as a rule, the trihydrate and this has been the material used by most investigators in preclinical studies of the pharmacological properties of DSH. On the other hand, Imuthiol®, the brand of DSH produced by the French pharmaceutical company, Institut Mérieux and the form usually used in the study of the immunomodulatory and clinical effects of DSH, is the anhydrous salt. Accordingly, the DSH doses and concentrations are reported in this book in terms of the trihydrate except in Chapters 12, 13 and section 15.3 of Chapter 15 where, as noted therein, this information is given in terms of the anhydrous salt.

DSSD is best known for its ability to inhibit acetaldehyde oxidation *in vivo* and for causing, thereby, the disulfiram–ethanol reaction, an unpleasant syndrome which follows the consumption of even relatively small amounts of ethanol by individuals taking DSSD. This property of DSSD has led to its widespread clinical use as an aversive drug in the treatment of alcohol abuse. The formulations in which dispensable DSSD is marketed in different countries vary. Thus, in Scandinavia and much of Western Europe, but not the United Kingdom, United States or Australia, it is available in the form of effervescent tablets containing a wetting agent which speeds the dissolution of the DSSD. This can result in major differences in its bioavailability (section 6.5.7) and should be kept in mind when evaluating clinical studies from different countries.

The reduction of disulfiram to diethyldithiocarbamate occurs readily *in vivo* as well as *in vitro* and the thiol is the primary metabolite of disulfiram. The thiol, in turn, can be readily oxidized to the disulfide. Systems capable of bringing about this oxidation exist *in vivo*.

The easy interconvertibility of these two agents affects their chemical and biological properties. To emphasize the disulfide–thiol, oxidation–reduction, dimer–monomer relationship between them, we have adopted in this book the abbreviations DSSD for disulfiram and DSH for diethyldithiocarbamate. This usage is similar to that of Strömme (1963a) who used ASSA and ASH, the A presumably being an allusion to Antabuse. It is analogous to that of GSSG and GSH for the oxidized and reduced forms of glutathione, respectively. It has the advantage of serving as a clear reminder of the relationship between the two agents, a characteristic not shared with the other frequently used abbreviations for disulfiram (viz. DSF, TETD, TTD) and diethyldithiocarbamate (viz. DDC, DEDC, DDTC).

DSH has long been known for its avid chelation of heavy metals. This has led to interest in its antidotal effects in heavy metal poisoning. In that context it has been at times referred to under the generic name, dithiocarb. In particular it is recognized as the agent of choice in the treatment of nickel carbonyl intoxication. Also, it has been found to act as a rescue agent, preventing renal damage from cisplatin, an important chemotherapeutic agent.

More recently, the potent immunostimulant properties of DSH have been recognized and much excitement has been generated by the results of several controlled trials which indicate that it slows the progression of HIV infection.

To some extent the *in vivo* pharmacological activities of DSSD and DSH overlap, suggesting that the mutual interconvertibility of these agents occurs to a pharmacologically significant extent. Thus, as in the case of DSSD, administration of DSH can cause inhibition of acetaldehyde metabolism. Conversely, DSSD administration, like that of DSH, results in the chelation of heavy metals and in alterations in their distribution and excretion patterns.

1.2 SCOPE OF MONOGRAPH

DSSD and DSH have a large number of diverse effects on biological systems and no unitary explanation can be given for all of them at this time. These effects are subject to investigation and discussion in a large number of fields and citations to relevant work are mostly field-oriented. No review of their various actions has been written hitherto that is to any degree comprehensive. This vast literature can be subsumed under two headings. Firstly, the direct actions of these agents on biological systems and secondly, their interactions with other agents and drugs. In this monograph we strive to present as fully as possible the basic knowledge about these compounds and the underlying principles of their actions, illuminated by selected important examples that are discussed critically. A complete cataloguing of their actions is, however, beyond the scope of the book. We limit ourselves, therefore, to those interactions which are of clinical importance or potentially so, thus the interactions with ethanol, heavy metals, and chemotherapeutic agents.

Knowledge of the physical and chemical properties of DSSD and DSH, particularly regarding the easy reducibility of DSSD, the formation of metal complexes by DSH and its acid-catalyzed decomposition (Chapter 2) is required for any discussion of their biological actions.

The difficulty experienced by many investigators in accounting for DSSD *in vivo*, or even following its addition to blood *in vitro*, has been a source of confusion and controversy. Some find it possible to detect DSSD in blood, but only after special stabilizing procedures. Even when such procedures are used, more than a week of therapy is required before measurable amounts can be detected in the blood samples of patients. Others report that, following a single administration of DSSD, they are able to measure its levels in blood over periods of hours, or even days, and give half-lives for its disappearance. Consequently, emphasis has been given in this book to the reactions of DSSD and DSH with blood constituents (Chapter 3), and a critical discussion of the available analytical methods for the determination of these entities in a biological matrix (Chapter 4).

The metabolism of DSSD, DSH and that of the products of their biotransformations is considered in two parts; first (Chapter 5) the qualitative aspects of this metabolism are discussed. Next, a concerted effort is made to address the quantitative aspects of such metabolism (Chapter 6) by collating reported pharmacokinetic parameters with additional ones computed for this book using published data.

DSH is a therapeutically important avid chelator of heavy metals, from cadmium and nickel to platinum and polonium (Chapter 7).

Added to blood, DSSD is reduced stoichiometrically with the formation of the copper chelate of DSH. Accordingly, chelation is considered in close apposition to chapters on the disposition of these agents.

Many enzymes are inhibited by DSSD and DSH *in vitro*; in some instances this is mediated by the chelation of the metal at the active center of the enzyme. This and other mechanisms are discussed in section 8.1. *In vivo*, these agents are potent inhibitors of drug metabolizing enzymes of the hepatic endoplasmic reticulum. The extent and mechanism of such inhibition is reviewed in section 8.2. In somewhat larger doses they bring about an inhibition of dopamine β-hydroxylase, an enzyme which catalyzes the last step in the biosynthesis of norepinephrine (section 8.3). Given in very large doses to experimental animals, DSH and DSSD also cause the *in vivo* inactivation of some of the enzymes responsible for protecting the organism against reactive oxygen species, particularly superoxide dismutase (section 8.4).

The therapeutically important interaction between DSSD and ethanol is discussed under four parts. First, the inhibition of aldehyde dehydrogenase that follows DSSD administration, a subject which has been extensively investigated, is reviewed (Chapter 9). Next, the phenomenology and toxicology of the disulfiram–ethanol reaction (DER) is discussed. In this context the aldehyde and the dopamine β-hydroxylase hypotheses regarding the mechanism of the DER are considered and evaluated (Chapter 10). This is followed by a consideration of the DSSD therapy of alcoholism (Chapter 11). The therapy is a very effective one, given that the patient remains compliant. Accordingly, special attention is given to a comparison of the efficiency of various treatment paradigms in motivating patient compliance and reducing the number of days on which ethanol is imbibed. The time course of action, the side-effects, and other related matters are also discussed.

Chapter 12 is devoted to the potent immunostimulatory effects of DSH. These actions of DSH have attracted a great deal of research activity, initially almost exclusively among French investigators. The immunostimulant properties of DSH appear to be mediated by its action on T cells. This has led to clinical trials of its effectiveness in retarding the progression of HIV infection (Chapter 13), its experimental employment in patients with such autoimmune diseases as rheumatoid arthritis, as an adjuvant for influenza vaccinations, and in the stimulation of the immune system in patients undergoing gastrointestinal surgery.

The modulation by DSH and DSSD of various biological phenomena is discussed in Chapter 14. First, is collated the information regarding the biphasic cytotoxicity frequently reported to be caused by these agents seen in cell culture (section 14.1) and a hypothesis is advanced regarding the mechanism of this phenomenon. Next, we review the available information regarding the modulation of oxidative stress by these agents (section 14.2). Finally, since DSH is one of the more effective *in vitro* and *in vivo* radioprotective agents, the relevant phenomenology is considered in section 14.3.

The use of DSH as a rescue agent safeguarding against the development of renal toxicity during treatment with the important chemotherapeutic agent, cisplatin, is discussed in Chapter 15. Also presented therein are the more recent findings that DSH protects experimental animals against the myeloid toxicity of this and other chemotherapeutic agents.

Finally, the toxicology of these agents is discussed in Chapter 16. Both agents are relatively non-toxic, are not carcinogenic or mutagenic and do not cause teratogenic effects.

1.3 EARLIER REVIEWS

The chemical properties of dithiocarbamates and their disulfide derivatives were reviewed extensively by Thorn and Ludwig (1962). These authors also reviewed the biochemical and pharmacological properties of these agents, with particular emphasis on their fungicidal actions. Hulanicki (1967) reviewed the chelation of metals by DSH, and a shorter review of the chemical properties of DSH was published by Halls (1969). Physical and spectral properties of DSSD have been reviewed by Nash and Daley (1975). The analytical methods available for the determination of DSSD and its metabolites were reviewed comprehensively by Brien and Loomis (1983a). Eneanya *et al.* (1981) reviewed the metabolic disposition of DSSD as known at the time; its pharmacokinetic aspects were discussed by Brien and Loomis (1983b). Beauchamp *et al.* (1983) reviewed the disposition of a metabolite of DSSD and DSH, carbon disulfide. Fiala (1981) and Bertram (1988) have reviewed the effect of DSSD on the metabolism and activity of carcinogens. The antifungal activity of DSH has been discussed by Allerberger *et al.* (1991).

Truitt and Walsh (1971) undertook a critical analysis of the role of acetaldehyde and inhibition of dopamine β-hydroxylase in the manifestations of the DER. Various factors in the DER were reviewed subsequently by Kitson (1977) and by Peachey and Sellers (1981). The pharmacology and clinical employment of DSSD were reviewed by Faiman (1979). Haley (1979) considered various aspects of DSSD action, focusing in particular on toxic reactions and effects on the metabolism of other drugs. Side-effects of DSSD therapy were reviewed by Wise (1981). Rainey (1977) focused on the similarities between some toxic effects of DSSD and those of carbon disulfide.

Peachey *et al.* (1981b) have discussed the pharmacology and toxic complications of DSSD therapy in the context of a comparison with the parallel properties of calcium carbimide. A review of the toxicity of DSSD, with particular reference to the DER reaction, is to be found in Gosselin *et al.* (1984). A shorter overview of the subject of alcohol-sensitizing drugs was published by Brien and Loomis (1985).

A review of the clinical employment of DSSD, focusing on CNS involvement, was written by Kwentus and Major (1979). The early treatment literature has been reviewed by Lundwall and Baekeland (1971) and by Etzioni and Remp (1973). Cavanagh and Barnes (1973) have reviewed the induction of peripheral neuropathy by DSSD. A good clinical primer is to be found in the *Medical Letter* (1980); also noteworthy is article written by Sellers *et al.* (1981). A short discussion of the clinical employment of DSH is given by Gale (1981). The annotated bibliography on disulfiram in the treatment of alcoholism is a useful document (Busse *et al.*, 1978). Peachey and Naranjo (1983) have written an excellent review of the pharmacology, efficacy and clinical use of alcohol sensitizing drugs. A short monograph by McNichol *et al.* (1987) reviews some aspects of the clinical use and pharmacology of disulfiram. More recently the use of disulfiram in the treatment of alcoholism has been reviewed by Liskow and Goodwin (1987) and by Wright and Moore (1989; 1990).

Aldehyde dehydrogenase isozymes and the inhibitory effects of DSSD were reviewed by Pietruszko (1983, 1989). The mechanism of the inhibition of this enzyme by DSSD was reviewed by Kitson (1988), The relationship between the polymorphism of these isozymes and sensitivity to alcohol was reviewed by Agarwal and Goedde (1986, 1987, 1989) and Goedde and Agarwal (1990), and the pharmacology of acetaldehyde, with a discussion of the DER, by Brien and Loomis (1983c).

2

Relevant physical and chemical properties

2.1 INTRODUCTION AND GENERAL PROPERTIES   7
2.2 ACID CATALYZED DECOMPOSITION   8
2.3 FORMATION OF METAL COMPLEXES   9

2.1 INTRODUCTION AND GENERAL PROPERTIES

Chemically, disulfiram (DSSD; trade name Antabuse®), is tetraethyl-thiuram disulfide, or tetraethyl thioperoxydicarbonic diamide (Chemical Abstracts designation), or bis (*N*,*N*-diethylthiocarbamyl) disulfide. As the last name implies, it is a dimeric molecule wherein two diethyl-dithiocarbamate moieties are linked through sulfur atoms forming a disulfide bond. Its structure is given below:

$$
\begin{array}{ccc}
CH_3CH_2 & S \quad S & CH_2CH_3 \\
\diagdown \quad \| \quad \| \quad \diagup \\
N-C \qquad C-N \\
\diagup \qquad \diagdown \quad \diagup \qquad \diagdown \\
CH_3CH_2 & S-S & CH_2CH_3
\end{array}
$$

DSSD (molecular weight 296.54) is sparingly soluble in water and saturation occurs at about 40–100 µM. To obtain aqueous solutions higher than 15 µM it is necessary to use solvents such as ethanol (Kitson, 1975). Solutions up to 50 µM can be obtained by adding 50 µl of a 10 mM DSSD solution in ethanol to 10 ml buffer (Strömme, 1965a; Agarwal, R.P. *et al.*, 1986). The partition coefficient for DSSD between octanol and water is 646, giving a log P value of 2.81 (Johansson, 1990b).

Diethyldithiocarbamic acid (molecular weight 149.23; Chemical Abstracts designation, diethyl carbamodithioic acid) has a pK_a of 4.04. The unionized acid is lipid-soluble, consequently the distribution of diethyl-dithiocarbamate (DSH) between lipid solvents and water is a function of pH. Several investigators have determined $pH_{1/2}$, that is, the pH at which DSH is distributed equally between the aqueous and organic phases. The values reported have been 6.21 (Bode, 1954; Starý and Kratzer, 1968), 6.72 (Still, 1964 quoted by Yeh *et al.*, 1980), 7.0 (Aspila *et al.*, 1975). The sodium salt is available both in an anhydrous form (molecular weight 171.21) and as a trihydrate (molecular weight 225.26).

The disulfide bond of DSSD is rather unstable; the compound can be dissociated into two dithiocarbamate radicals by heating (Klebanskii and Fomina, 1960). In solution, DSSD is readily reduced to DSH by ascorbic acid (Goldstein, M. *et al.*, 1964) and by compounds with free sulfhydryls, as for instance by 0.14 mM reduced glutathione (Johnston, 1953), or 1 mM mercaptoethanol (Agarwal, R.P. *et al.*, 1986) as well as by free sulfhydryl groups of proteins. Such reactions result in the formation of mixed disulfides wherein the sulfur of the thiol becomes linked with the DS moiety; concurrently, half of the molecule of DSSD is released in the form of DSH (Strömme, 1965a; Neims et al., 1966b). DSSD is also reduced by cuprous ions to yield the cupric ion complex, $Cu(DS)_2$ (Akerstrom, 1956).

Just as DSSD is easily reduced to DSH, so the latter is readily oxidized to DSSD, for instance, by cytochrome c (Keilin and Hartee, 1940) and by hydrogen peroxide (Thorn and Ludwig, 1962).

2.2 ACID CATALYZED DECOMPOSITION

In acid solution DSH is protonated and the subsequent decomposition to form carbon disulfide and diethylamine proceeds through the dipolar ion as follows (Hulanicki, 1967):

Bode (1954) studied the half-life of DSH in water at various pH values; Hallaway (1959) did so in a phosphate–citrate buffer. From their results, obtained at 20° and 15°C, respectively, it is apparent (Fig. 2.1) that the DSH half-life is a linear function of pH. Specifically the least squares solution for the regression of Bode's half-life values on pH is given by the relationship $\log t_{1/2} = -2.53 + 1.00 \, pH$ while the regression of Hallaway's half-lives on pH is given by the relationship $\log t_{1/2} = -1.825 + 0.979 \, pH$. Hallaway (1959) also reported that there is an 8-fold increase in the rate of breakdown between 7° and 30°C.

Bubbling of air or oxygen through a solution of DSH does not change the rate of its acid-catalyzed decomposition, although it removes the very

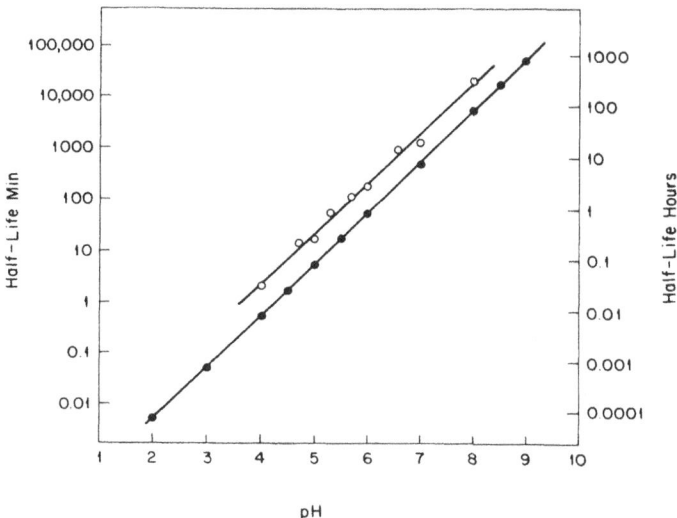

Figure 2.1 Plot of the half-life of diethyldithiocarbamate in water as a function of pH. Solid circles data of Bode (1954); open circles data of Hallaway (1959).

volatile carbon disulfide that is formed and precludes the reverse reaction sequence. Conversely, at highly alkaline pH, the equilibrium for the reaction sequence is very far to the left and, in the presence of diethylamine, carbon disulfide is quantitatively converted to DSH. Accordingly, such trapping of carbon disulfide in an alkaline alcoholic solution of diethylamine is the basis for a sensitive method for determination of carbon disulfide in breath. The DSH formed in this manner gives, in the presence of cupric ions, a deep yellow copper complex the concentration of which can be determined spectrophotometrically. Since carbon disulfide is a pulmonary metabolite of DSSD (section 5.6), the method is used in testing compliance of patients with DSSD therapy (section 11.8).

Even in the solid state, DSH slowly breaks down (Hallaway, 1959). Hence analytical grade samples of DSH have a half-life of about seven years under ordinary laboratory storage conditions.

2.3 FORMATION OF METAL COMPLEXES

Extraction of a metal (M) with ionic charge n from aqueous phase into a solution of DSH in an organic solvent can be viewed (Starý and Kratzer, 1968) as

$$[M^{n+}]_{aq} + n[DSH]_{org} \rightleftharpoons [M(DS)_n]_{org} + n[H^+]_{aq} \qquad (2.1)$$

The equilibrium, or extraction, constant for this equation will be

$$K = \frac{[M(DS)_n]_{org}[H^+]^n_{aq}}{[M^{n+}]_{aq}[DSH]^n_{org}} \qquad (2.2)$$

The extraction constant for the reaction of cupric ions with DSH to form the $Cu(DS)_2$ complex is very much larger than the parallel one for the formation of $Zn(DS)_2$. Accordingly $Zn(DS)_2$ will react quantitatively with copper to give $Cu(DS)_2$ via ligand exchange. Determination of extraction constants for a large number of DSH metal complexes has allowed the formulation of displacement series (Table 2.1). Given any two metals in this series, that on the right will displace the one on the left from its DSH complex via ligand exchange with the formation of the DSH complex of the metal on the right. Below the symbols for the metal in Table 2.1 is the value of $(1/n)\log K$ for the specified oxidation state of the metal.

The efficiency with which, in the presence of DSH, organic solvents will extract metals as their DS complexes is given by the two phase stability constant of the complex

$$\beta = \frac{[M(DS)_n]_{org}}{[M^{n+}][DS^-]^n} \qquad (2.3)$$

The value of β can be calculated from that of K by virtue of the relationship

$$(1/n)\log \beta = (1/n)\log K + pH_{1/2} \qquad (2.4)$$

where $pH_{1/2}$ is the pH at which 50% of the DSH is in the organic phase.

For $Cu(DS)_2$, β has a value of $10^{26.8}$. For $Zn(DS)_2$ that value is $10^{15.9}$ (Yeh *et al.*, 1980). From these figures it is clear that DSH is a very powerful ligand of metal ions. DSSD also chelates metal ions avidly; with copper, at least, the same metal complex appears to be formed whether the reaction is with DSSD or DSH.

The high lipophilicity of the metal complexes of DSH contributes to their tendency to undergo irreversible adsorption on surfaces such as glass, Teflon (Häring and Ballschmiter, 1980) and Sephadex gel (Strömme, 1965a). Some investigators working with DSSD and DSH seek to avoid such problems by taking special steps to remove traces of complexing metal ions from solutions they use. Thus, Strömme (1965a) used buffers 0.01 M with respect to EDTA and extracted them twice with 0.1 diphenylthiocarbazone in chloroform. Agarwal, R.P. *et al.* (1986) dialyzed albumin solutions, to be used in DSSD experiments, against Tris–EDTA. It should be noted, however, that the

Table 2.1 Order of extractability of metal diethyldithiocarbamates

Eckert (1957)	Mn				Zn As^{3+}	Sn^{2+} Fe^{3+}	Cd		Pb	Bi	Ni	Cu	Ag	Hg	
Stary and Kratzer (1968)	Mn^{2+} −2.21	Tl^{+} −0.53	Fe^{2+} 0.60	Co^{2+} 1.16	Zn^{2+} 1.48		Cd^{2+} 2.70	In^{3+} 3.45	Pb^{2+} 3.88	Bi^{2+} 5.60	Ni^{2+} 5.79	Cu^{2+} 6.85	Ag^{2+} 11.90	Hg^{2+} 15.97	Pd^{2+} >16
Ooms et al. (1977)					Zn^{2+} 1.15	Pb^{2+} 2.50	Cd^{2+} 2.75		In^{3+} 3.32	Bi^{3+} 5.23		Cu^{2+} 6.41		Hg^{2+} 13.46	
Yeh et al. (1980)			Fe^{2+} 0.98		As^{3+} 1.42		Cd^{2+} 2.73			Bi^{3+} 7.08				Hg^{2+} 13.58	

Values given in the table are those of $(1/n)$ log K, where K is the extraction constant in the system chloroform/water [except for Starý and Kratzer (1968) where the system was carbon tetrachloride/water] and n is the valency state of the metal.

complexation with metal ions, particularly copper, may be of considerable physiological significance. Thus, upon addition of DSSD to blood in a 5 µM concentration, the DSSD is quantitatively converted to $Cu(DS)_2$ (Johansson and Stankiewicz, 1985).

3

Reactions of disulfiram and diethyldithio-carbamate with blood constituents

3.1 INTRODUCTION 13
3.2 FORMATION OF COPPER COMPLEXES 14
3.3 FORMATION OF MIXED DISULFIDES 15
3.4 UPTAKE OF DISULFIRAM BY BLOOD CELLS 17
3.5 SUMMARY 19

3.1 INTRODUCTION

Disulfiram (DSSD) and diethyldithiocarbamate (DSH) interact with blood constituents in a variety of ways which are still poorly understood. Nevertheless these interactions are central to the design and evaluation of analytical procedures, as well as to the interpretation of experimental results and their biological consequences. Many investigators have reported on the difficulties experienced when seeking to recover DSSD added to blood, plasma or serum, and on their inability to detect DSSD in the plasma of animals or humans dosed with it. Conditions have now been described under which it is possible to stabilize DSSD added to blood *in vitro* and to recover it (Johansson, 1988). Using these conditions it is possible to detect DSSD in the blood of individuals dosed with it. The conditions that have to be used are, however, highly unphysiological and therefore underscore our poor understanding of how the interactions of DSSD with blood constituents permit its survival in blood *in vivo*.

The reactions of DSSD and DSH with blood constituents are best discussed under three headings. Firstly, the interaction of plasma copper with these agents to form the copper chelate of DSH (section 3.2). Secondly, the interaction of DSSD, in the absence of metal ions, with plasma proteins that results in the formation of mixed disulfides (section 3.3). Thirdly, the interaction of DSSD with the cellular elements of blood, particularly the erythrocytes (section 3.4).

3.2 FORMATION OF COPPER COMPLEXES

DSSD and DSH have a very high affinity for heavy metal ions, particularly those of copper, with which they form complexes. Divatia *et al.* (1952) observed that the inability to recover (by extraction with ethylene dichloride) DSSD added to blood, or plasma, could be overcome by equilibrating the sample first with copper sulfate. Quantitative recoveries ($100 \pm 5\%$) over a DSSD concentration range of 17–670 µM could be effected, the DSSD being present in the extract as its copper complex, $Cu(DS)_2$. Strömme (1965a) observed in his work on the interaction of DSSD with plasma proteins, the formation of heavy metal complexes and their adsorption at the top of the Sephadex column. Consequently, he took pains to remove heavy metal ions and complexes from his solutions and subsequently used EDTA buffers, as did Agarwal, R.P. *et al.* (1983, 1986). Under more physiological conditions, the heavy metals in blood and other tissues would be expected to play an important role in the fate of DSSD and DSH in such tissues. DSSD added to blood, or plasma, in an amount calculated to give a 5 µM concentration, is all reduced stoichiometrically to $Cu(DS)_2$ within 5 min (Johansson and Stankiewicz, 1985). The same complex is obtained upon the reaction of copper with either DSSD or DSH (Sauter *et al.*, 1976; Johansson and Stankiewicz, 1985).

The formation of the complex is a mass action reaction, the equilibrium of which very much favors the formation of the complex (section 2.3). In the presence of other compounds with a high affinity for copper, dissociation of the complex is to be expected. An illustration of these principles is provided by the fate of $Cu(DS)_2$ in the spiked plasma *in vitro*, wherein its levels decrease quite slowly (half-life > 20 h). Its disappearance is much more rapid, however, when ethylenediaminetetraacetic acid (EDTA) is present (Johansson and Stankiewicz, 1985). This is attributable to the fact that EDTA and DSH have similar affinities for cupric ions and compete for them. The two DS moieties of the $Cu(DS)_2$ complex in plasma are able to undergo decomposition with the stoichiometric formation of diethyldithiocarbamic acid ethyl ester (DSEt) under the conditions used analytically to ethylate DSH (Johansson and Stankiewicz, 1985), that is, following addition of mercaptoethanol and ethyl iodide.

The formation of ternary complexes between plasma proteins, copper and DSH has been suggested (Johansson and Stankiewicz, 1985). Formation of complexes of the form below:

$$
\text{protein}
\begin{array}{c}
\diagup S \diagdown \\
\quad\quad\quad Cu \\
\diagdown S \diagup
\end{array}
\begin{array}{c}
S \diagdown \\
\quad\quad C - N \\
S \diagup
\end{array}
\begin{array}{c}
CH_2CH_3 \\
\\
CH_2CH_3
\end{array}
$$

need not be limited to plasma. Morpurgo *et al.* (1983) have presented evidence that DSH forms such ternary complexes with copper-substituted carbonic anhydrase.

3.3 FORMATION OF MIXED DISULFIDES

Strömme (1965a), who was the first to address rigorously the question of the interaction of DSSD and DSH with serum proteins, developed a method for the separation of DSSD, DSH and serum proteins on a Sephadex column. Using a 15 min incubation period, he observed that ^{35}S-DSSD, added to human serum diluted with pH 8.5 EDTA buffer, reacts with serum proteins with the formation of a stoichiometric quantity of DSH and retention of 50% of the label bound to the protein. In human serum, almost all the reactive -SH groups are associated with albumin and the ^{35}S-labeled protein formed in the reaction of serum proteins with ^{35}S-DSSD has the same electrophoretic mobility as albumin. Suspecting the albumin complex formed to be a mixed disulfide, Strömme (1965a) used glutathione (GSH) [previously shown by Johnston (1953) to reduce DSSD in virtually stoichiometric fashion] and found it to liberate a stoichiometric quantity of DSH from the albumin complex. The observed phenomena can be represented, therefore, by two thiol–disulfide exchange reactions as follows:

$$\text{albumin–SH} + \text{DSSD} \rightarrow \text{albumin–S–SD} + \text{DSH}$$

$$\text{albumin–S–SD} + \text{GSH} \rightarrow \text{albumin–S–SG} + \text{DSH}$$

Strömme (1965a) also noted that a complete blockage of the albumin -SH groups could be obtained with a slight excess of DSSD, indicating the equilibrium of the first reaction above was displaced far towards the right side. The study of analogous reactions of ^{35}S-DSSD with a variety of native and denatured proteins (Neims *et al.*, 1966a) indicates that the amount of ^{35}S-DSH liberated in such reactions corresponds closely to the number of available sulfhydryls on the object proteins. For instance, native hemoglobin is known to possess 2 reactive thiol groups and 4 latent sulfhydryls per mole of protein. Upon reaction of hemoglobin with ^{35}S-DSSD, two mole equivalents of ^{35}S-DSH are liberated. However, if the hemoglobin is first denatured with sodium dodecyl sulfate, reaction with ^{35}S-DSSD liberates 5.6 moles equivalents of ^{35}S-DSH. Moreover, all the radioactivity is rapidly released from the ^{35}S-labeled hemoglobin upon addition of an excess of GSH, or, alternatively, cysteine (Neims *et al.*, 1966b).

In contrast to DSSD, DSH, when added to human serum diluted with pH 8.5 EDTA buffer, forms only a loosely bound adduct with serum proteins (Strömme, 1965a). The extent to which such adduct formation occurs is a function of the DSH concentration and, unlike the reaction of DSSD with albumin, it is readily reversible upon dilution with buffer.

The kinetics of the reduction of DSSD by serum albumin have been studied by Agarwal, R.P. *et al.* (1986), who followed the time-dependent changes in the ultraviolet difference spectrum of a mixture of these entities in Tris–EDTA buffer. They found that the reaction proceeds by a first-order mechanism, independent of the concentration of both initial reactants. This finding led them to propose that the first step in the reaction is a very rapid formation of a non-covalent DSSD–albumin adduct, which precedes a slower unimolecular reduction of DSSD with the liberation of DSH.

$$
\text{albumin–SH} + \text{DSSD} \rightarrow
\begin{bmatrix}
\text{albumin} - \text{S} \text{---} \text{S-D} \\
\quad\quad\quad\quad | \quad\quad | \\
\quad\quad\quad\quad \text{H} \quad\quad \text{S-D}
\end{bmatrix}
\rightarrow \text{albumin–SSD} + \text{DSH}
$$

At pH 7.4, the overall rate for the reaction is $0.0052\,\text{s}^{-1}$, which represents a half-life of 133 s.

Interestingly, in an earlier study Agarwal, R.P. *et al.* (1983) had pursued the interaction of DSSD with plasma proteins using an analytical method based on a multistep extractive procedure and HPLC analysis of the resulting heptane extracts. The sample was diluted with an equal part of pH 9.5 phosphate–EDTA buffer. The first extract, used to assay DSSD, was secured without any other pretreatment of the sample; the second, used to assay free DSH, was made following alkylation of the sample with methyl sulfate; the third, employed to assay for protein-bound DSH, was obtained following addition of cysteine and methyl sulfate. Under these circumstances, about 58% of the DSSD reacted with plasma components within 1 or 2 min with the formation of almost equal concentrations of free and protein-bound DSH; very similar results were obtained with albumin. Over the period of the next hour, or two, DSSD levels declined slowly with concomitant increase in protein-bound DSH and little or no change in the free DSH. The results were tantalizingly similar, yet rather different from those reported by Strömme (1965a), in that (a) the conversion was not complete within 15 min and (b) following the first couple of minutes, continued conversion of DSSD to protein-bound DSH occurred without the expected stoichiometric release of free DSH. Agarwal, R.P. *et al.* (1983) considered the possibility of the slow formation of a non-covalent adduct between DSH and the protein, but when exogenous DSH was incubated with plasma proteins *in vitro* no such adduct could be detected. As complex as the interaction between proteins and the DSSD–DSH system is in aqueous buffers, the introduction by Agarwal, R.P. *et al.* (1983) of lipophilic solvents and the perturbing effects these may have on the tertiary structure of plasma proteins, renders the situation substantially more complex.

3.4 UPTAKE OF DISULFIRAM BY BLOOD CELLS

Divatia *et al.* (1952) noted that upon a 10-min equilibration of whole blood with DSSD, added in a quantity calculated to give a *ca* 350 μM concentration of DSSD, there was an almost equal distribution of the DS moiety between plasma and the cells.

Pedersen (1980), following addition of ^{35}S-DSSD to plasma in a 1.7–13.5 μM concentration, could account for 80% of the label in terms of DSSD and total (free and cysteine-releasable) DSH. Furthermore, he found that upon addition of the DSSD to whole blood only 58% of the label could be thus accounted for in plasma, 24% of the label having been taken up into the erythrocytes. An observation by Pedersen (1980), left unexplained, is the large difference in the ratio of protein-bound to free DSH recoverable immediately following addition of DSSD to serum and whole blood (4.5 and 0.11, respectively). Interpretation of these findings is complicated by the use by Pedersen (1980) of the extractive procedures involving lipophilic solvents later used by Agarwal, R.P. *et al.* (1983), as described in section 3.2 (his phosphate buffer, however, contained no EDTA).

Pedersen (1980) found that, following p.o. ^{35}S-DSSD administration (to rats, in a 40 mg/kg dose), the distribution of the label in plasma changed yet again: virtually all of the ^{35}S was present as either protein disulfide-bound dithiocarbamate (PrSSD) or diethyldithiocarbamic acid methyl ester (DSMe), only threshold values of free DSH being detectable. The PrSSD/DSH ratio in plasma was similar to that previously reported by Strömme (1965b) following i.p. administration of ^{35}S-DSSD (to rats in a 10 mg/kg dose). The actual PrSSD levels, however, were markedly different. Thus while Strömme had found these to be 2.4, 2.2 and 0.82 μg/ml at 1, 2 and 4 h post administration, respectively, Pedersen reported values of only 0.025, 0.083 and 0.081 μg/ml at the corresponding time points. Pedersen (1980) did not advance any explanation for these results, though he did warn that some of the protein-bound DSH might originate from *ex vivo* conversion of DSH or DSSD.

Added to blood *in vitro*, DSSD is rapidly reduced and converted stoichiometrically to $Cu(DS)_2$. In this, the behavior of blood is similar to that of plasma. $Cu(DS)_2$ disappears, however, more rapidly from whole blood (down to 50% in *ca* 2 h at 23°C) than from plasma wherein its half-life exceeds 20 hrs (Johansson and Stankiewicz, 1985). This difference is attributable to the redistribution of the DS moiety from plasma to cells. This redistribution has been studied by incubating blood with either ^{14}C-DSSD or ^{14}C-Cu(DS)$_2$ for 30 min at 37°C. It is found that the uptake of label into the erythrocyte cell membrane is linearly proportional to the amount of the compound added to blood, but that the amount taken up into the cytosol of the erythrocyte is a hyperbolic function of this quantity (Johansson, 1990a). This hyperbolic relationship led Johansson (1990a) to postulate the involvement of a saturable transport mechanism. A replot of the ^{35}S-DSSD uptake

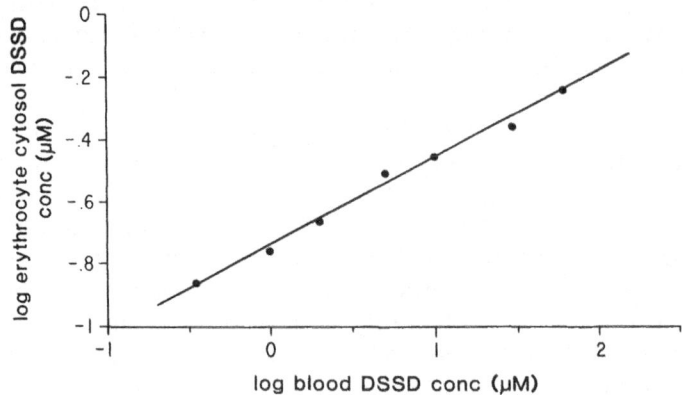

Figure 3.1 Plot of the logarithmic metameter of the uptake of disulfiram (DSSD) into the cytosol of the erythrocyte during a 30-min incubation at 37°C as a function of the logarithmic metameter of disulfiram blood concentration. Data of Johansson (1990a).

data (Fig. 3.1) shows, however, that rather than tending to approach some constant value, the amount found in the cytosol is a log–log linear function of the blood concentration of DSSD. This behavior is analogous to that observed for the adsorption of solutes on activated charcoal (Gessner and Hasan, 1987) and suggests that as the free DSSD concentration increases, DSSD interacts with -SH groups of progressively lower reactivity.

The recovery of added DSSD in the form of DSSD, be it from blood or plasma, has proved rather challenging. Both plasma and blood have considerable reductive power, that of blood being several times that of plasma. Much of this is due to the thiol content of blood being 40 times that of plasma. The ionization of thiols, and thus their reactivity towards disulfides, can be depressed by acidification. In the presence of diethylenetriaminepentaacetic acid (DPTA), a chelating agent, acidification of plasma to pH 4.5 with acetic acid stabilizes added DSSD and makes it possible to recover it quantitatively, if the analysis is carried out immediately. Using such methodology, Johansson (1988) was able to detect DSSD in the plasma of alcoholic patients in the second and third, though not the first week of DSSD therapy (400 mg every second day). He found that, 6 h after the latest dose, the plasma DSSD concentration in these patients was on average 0.16 µM. Clearly, given the rapidity with which DSSD disappears from blood *in vitro*, efficient processes must exist *in vivo* that either maintain it unreduced, or reoxidize the DSH that is formed from it. In this context, it should be noted that Johansson (1990a) has reported that addition of DSH to plasma spiked with DSSD increases the recovery of the latter by 20% (details not given), an observation that led him to conclude that DSH is oxidized to DSSD in fresh heparin plasma. Other evidence that DSH can be oxidized to DSSD in blood is discussed in section 6.3.

3.5 SUMMARY

In the presence of normal blood copper concentrations, added DSSD is stoichiometrically reduced with the formation of $Cu(DS)_2$. If the blood copper is chelated, DSSD is reduced with the formation of mixed disulfides. There is much evidence to suggest, however, that the DS moiety as such is relatively stable in blood, certainly in plasma. However, it may be present in a variety of forms, taxing the analytical abilities of investigators to discern them and quantitate them without materially affecting the distribution of the moiety between the different forms.

4

Assay methods for disulfiram and metabolites in biological materials

4.1 INTRODUCTION 21
4.2 GENERAL CONSIDERATIONS 22
    4.2.1 Diethyldithiocarbamate, free and bound 23
    4.2.2 Bis-(diethyldithiocarbamato) copper complex 23
    4.2.3 Carbon disulfide derivatives 24
4.3 SPECIFIC METHODS 25
    4.3.1 Method of Strömme 25
    4.3.2 Method of Johansson 25
4.4 OTHER METHODS 26

4.1 INTRODUCTION

Numerous methods have been published for the determination of disulfiram (DSSD) and its metabolites in biological material. The very multiplicity of published methods, most of which have been used subsequently only by their authors, if at all, is indicative of the difficulties inherent to the problem. Brien and Loomis (1983a) have written a comprehensive and detailed review of this subject. Accordingly, this chapter deals first with a discussion of overriding issues; secondly, with methods deemed noteworthy because of their inherent advantages, and thirdly with such other methods as were used in measuring the plasma levels of DSSD and metabolites, values from which the pharmacokinetic parameters listed in the tables of Chapter 7 were computed.

4.2 GENERAL CONSIDERATIONS

Following its *in vivo* administration, or its *in vitro* addition to blood, DSSD disappears so rapidly as to have frustrated the efforts of many investigators to detect it as such in this fluid (Cobby *et al.*, 1977b; Pedersen, 1980; Masso and Kramer, 1981; Agarwal, R.P. *et al.*, 1986; Johansson, 1986). This is due, to a large extent to the high reductive power of blood. As shown by Strömme (1965a), sulfhydryl groups of serum proteins reduce DSSD with the formation of mixed disulfides (section 3.3) and the release of stoichiometric amounts of diethyl-dithiocarbamate (DSH). Also, endogenous copper reacts with DSH, as well as with DSSD, to form the bis-(diethyldithiocarbamato) copper complex, $Cu(DS)_2$ (section 3.2). In none of these reactions is the DS moiety degraded, yet it is clear that it can exist in blood in a variety of interrelated forms. Accordingly, the analytical task is one which requires definition. Optimally, it would be desirable to identify and quantitate the amounts of all the different forms of the DS moiety present in the biological matrix. That, however, is a daunting analytical task yet to be achieved. Many of the extant efforts at measuring one or more of these forms involve procedures which are either known to bring an *ex vivo* redistribution of the DS moiety between the various forms, or are likely to do so.

Some investigators report being able to account, in terms of one or more analytical entities, for all of the DSSD added to either serum (Strömme, 1965a), plasma (Agarwal, R.P. *et al.*, 1983) or blood (Divatia *et al.*, 1952; Sauter and van Wartburg, 1977; Johansson and Stankiewicz, 1985; Johansson, 1986, 1988). The analytical entities assayed do not necessarily reflect those actually present in the sample. The work from the laboratory referenced last illustrates this well. Johansson (1986) reported that within 5 min of addition of DSSD, in a concentration range of 3.4–3400 nmol/ml, to fresh heparinized plasma no detectable amount of DSSD could be found. In the same time frame, all of the added DSSD was recoverable, however, as $Cu(DS)_2$ (Johansson and Stankiewicz, 1985). Alternatively, if the plasma was acidified to pH 5.5 with acetic acid and hematoporphyrin was added to it, the DSSD was stabilized and could be recovered as such (Johansson, 1988). Similarly, added DSSD can be recovered from blood that is acidified to pH 4.5 with acetic acid and treated with diethylenetriaminepentaacetic acid. The rationale behind this approach is that acidification represses the ionization of sulfhydryl groups, suppressing their nucleophilic character and decreasing their reactivity towards disulfides. Using this latter procedure, Johansson (1988) was able to detect DSSD in the blood of patients who had been on daily DSSD therapy for at least 1 week. An unresolved question is in what form was the DSSD present in the blood before it was 'stabilized' by this procedure.

4.2.1 Diethyldithiocarbamate, free and bound

DSH is considered an obligatory intermediate in DSSD metabolism, and many investigators aspire to measure its levels in blood or plasma. Because of the reaction of DSSD with sulfhydryls to form mixed disulfides, DSH can exist in blood in both 'bound' and free form. Upon reduction with reduced glutathione (GSH), for instance, the mixed disulfides release the bound DS moiety as one mole equivalent of DSH (Strömme, 1965a). This has relevance to the *in vivo* fate of DSSD, as shown by the fact that, following administration of ^{35}S-DSSD to rats, ^{35}S-DSH can be displaced from serum proteins *ex vivo* with GSH (Strömme, 1965b). Surprisingly, subsequently published analytical methods have seldom addressed empirically the question of the fate of such mixed disulfides. In assays that include addition of a reducing agent such as cysteine (Sauter *et al.*, 1976; Pedersen, 1980) or 2-mercaptoethanol (Johansson, 1986), liberation of DSH would be expected. It is of interest to note in this context that Sauter *et al.* (1976) and Sauter and van Wartburg (1977) found that all DSH and DSSD added to blood could be accounted for if 10 mg/ml cysteine was added to the blood sample, but not otherwise. It is less clear, however, what might be the effect of exposure to lipophilic solvents, or alkylating agents, on recoveries of the various forms of the DS moiety. Such solvents would be expected to cause some denaturation of the proteins of blood or plasma, exposing sulfhydryl groups able to react with DSSD. It is noteworthy that the majority of methods used for the assay of DSSD and its metabolites in blood and plasma involve extraction with lipophilic solvents (Divatia *et al.*, 1952; Cobby *et al.*, 1977b; Faiman *et al.*, 1977, 1978b; Davidson and Wilson, 1979; Jensen and Faiman, 1980; Pedersen, 1980; Masso and Kramer, 1981; Giles *et al.*, 1982; Agarwal, R.P. *et al.*, 1983). The degree to which the consequent denaturation results in additional reaction of protein sulfhydryls with DSSD has not been addressed. The work of Pedersen (1980) suggests (section 3.4) that there is a need to further explore possible *ex vivo* conversions, particularly as they may occur in methods using extractive fractionation procedure and alkylation steps.

4.2.2 Bis-(diethyldithiocarbamato) copper complex

The Cu(DS)$_2$ complex, formed by the reaction of DSSD and DSH with copper, is an intense yellow chromophore with absorption at 430 nm.

The use of exogenous copper to bring about formation of this complex and its subsequent spectrophotometric determination has been the basis for a number of methods for the analysis of the DS moiety in biological fluids (Domar *et al.*, 1949; Linderholm and Berg, 1951; Divatia *et al.*, 1952; Prickett and Johnston, 1953; Tompsett, 1964; Sauter *et al.*, 1976). Johansson (1986), using high pressure liquid chromatography (HPLC), also utilizes the absorption at 430 nm to estimate the levels of the complex formed from endogenous copper in blood or plasma. Irth *et al.* (1986, 1988) have developed an HPLC method which utilizes formation of the complex in a post-column derivatization system. The DSSD in the column effluent is exposed to finely divided metallic copper, obtained by the reduction of Cu(I)Cl, and the concentration of the resulting chromophore, $Cu(DS)_2$, is measured by a spectrophotometric detector. DSH on the other hand, is chromatographed following derivatization to $Pb(DS)_2$ by reaction with lead acetate. It is then converted to the $Cu(DS)_2$ chromophore by use of a post-column copper(II) phosphate reactor. The system is likely to be sensitive to other forms of the DS moiety, as well as to other dithiocarbamates and should allow analysis of complex mixtures with a minimum of precolumn clean-up.

Ironically, many of the methods developed to assay the various forms of the DS moiety in plasma incorporate the use of 10^{-2}M EDTA buffers (Faiman *et al.*, 1977, 1978b; Davidson and Wilson, 1979; Jensen and Faiman, 1980; Masso and Kramer, 1981; Agarwal, R.P. *et al.*, 1983), a measure likely to preclude the existence and thereby detection of the $Cu(DS)_2$ form. Johansson and Stankiewicz (1985) have reported that in blood, though not in plasma, $Cu(DS)_2$ levels decline rapidly and that at low plasma DSSD levels intermediate plasma protein–Cu–SD complex exists.

4.2.3 Carbon disulfide derivatives

Carbon disulfide (CS_2) is formed during DSSD and DSH metabolism (section 5.6). Following CS_2 administration, more than 90% of the free CS_2 found in blood is associated with erythrocytes, specifically with hemoglobin, although it also binds to other proteins, particularly albumin (Lam *et al.*, 1986). CS_2 reacts *in vivo* with amines and amino acids to form acid-labile metabolites, mostly dithiocarbamate derivatives (McKenna and DiStefano, 1977a, b) which chelate copper (Lam and DiStefano, 1986). It also binds to sulfhydryl groups with the formation of trithiocarbamates (Lam and DiStefano, 1986).

The possible presence of such CS_2-derived dithiocarbamates is a source of concern relative to assay methods for DSH and DSSD which rely on the acid-induced generation of CS_2 (Prickett and Johnston, 1953; Brown *et al.*, 1974; Sauter *et al.*, 1976; Sauter and von Wartburg, 1977).

4.3 SPECIFIC METHODS

Optimally, a method for the separation and quantitation of the various forms of the DS moiety in blood or plasma would not involve exposing the sample to non-aqueous media and would not subject it to derivatization procedures. The two methods that come closest to meeting this criterion are those of Strömme (1965a) and Johansson (1986); the method of Irth *et al.* (1986, 1988), though not yet applied to biological samples other than urine, holds significant promise.

4.3.1 Method of Strömme

Strömme (1965a,b) used radiometric assay in conjunction with gel filtration on a Sephadex G-25 column as a method of separation. DSSD and DS-protein mixed disulfides elute separately. DSH, the *S*-glucuronide of diethyldithiocarbamic acid (DSGa), and sulfate elute together. DSH is determined in an aliquot of the eluate by acidification with 2.5×10^{-2}M hydrochloric acid and trapping of the CS_2 formed, DSGa by trapping the CS_2 formed upon boiling with 7.3 M phosphoric acid for 3.5 h, a correction being made for the DSH, and the sulfate by measuring the radioactivity before and after precipitation of barium sulfate.

Using this method, Strömme (1965a,b) reported recoveries for DSSD ($n=9$) and DSH ($n=8$) of 94.2 and 95.5%, respectively. Recoveries for DSGa ($n=9$) were 83.3%. In the determination of sulfate by precipitation with $BaCl_2$, DSH was found to co-precipitate and was therefore removed from the sample by acidification prior to precipitation of the sulfate.

4.3.2 Method of Johansson

Johansson (1986) used a reverse phase HPLC system with direct injection of heparin plasma onto a precolumn for on-line enrichment and purification. To analyze for DSSD and $Cu(DS)_2$, plasma samples are injected onto the precolumn without any additions. To analyze for DSH (protein bound and free) and the methyl ester of diethyldithiocarbamic acid (DSMe), mercaptoethanol is added to assure reduction of DSH bound to plasma protein cupric ion; this is followed by addition of ethyl iodide to bring about ethylation of DSH to the ethyl ester of diethyldithiocarbamic acid (DSEt). In a modification of this method, Johansson *et al.* (1989) used direct injection of plasma, spiked with a diethyl-monothiocarbamic acid ethyl ester standard (DmSEt), for determination of its diethylmonothiocarbamic acid methyl ester (DmSMe), a metabolite of DSSD (section 5.9).

Using the same method, Johansson and Stankiewicz (1985) reported that upon addition of 5 nmol DSSD per ml of blood or plasma, all of it is reduced with the formation of $Cu(DS)_2$. Addition of the alkylating mixture of mercaptoethanol and ethyl iodide to plasma aliquots results in all of the DS moiety being ethylated to DSEt. Johansson (1986) reported recoveries from plasma of 95% and 100% for DSMe and DSH, respectively.

Because DSSD cannot be recovered from plasma when the latter is injected onto the precolumn without additions (Johansson, 1986), an alternative procedure was devised. It involves 'stabilization' of the plasma sample by acidification to pH 5.5 with lactic acid and addition of hematoporphyrin, a chelator of bivalent ions (Johansson, 1988). In the case of blood, acidification with acetic acid to pH 4.5 is used because lactic acid causes hemolysis, and diethylenetriaminepentaacetic acid is added as a chelating agent.

4.4 OTHER METHODS

Two criteria have been used in selecting assay methods considered in this section. The first of these is whether the method is applicable to either blood or plasma. The second is whether the method was used in generating data that were used in computing the pharmacokinetic parameters reported in the tables of Chapter 6. Five sets of methods, in addition to those of Strömme (1965a,b) and Johansson (1986) previously discussed, meet these criteria. Chronologically they are those of Prickett and Johnston (1953), Faiman *et al.* (1977), Cobby *et al.* (1977b), Jensen and Faiman (1980), Giles *et al.* (1982) and Lieder and Borch (1985). They are considered below.

In the method of Prickett and Johnston (1953) DSH is decomposed in the blood sample by addition of $6\,N\,H_2SO_4$. The CS_2 formed is trapped in a solution of diethylamine and copper chloride and the concentration of the $Cu(DS)_2$ complex formed is measured spectrophotometrically. Recoveries from whole blood were uniformly low (15–20%), though the data, obtained from six to nine animals per point, evidences orderly progression.

The method of Faiman *et al.* (1977) is based on a multistep extractive fractionation procedure and radiometric measurement. Blood is diluted with nine volumes 0.01 M EDTA buffer at pH 8.5 to which DSSD carrier has been added. A pentane extract of the sample is considered to contain DSSD and DSMe and is subjected to TLC to effect separation; the aqueous layer from the first extraction is alkylated with methyl iodide and again extracted with pentane; the latter is considered to contain DSMe derivatized from DSH. The aqueous layer from the second extraction is considered to contain protein-bound DSH, DSGa and sulfate. The first is defined as the fraction precipitable with trichloroacetic acid, the last as that which is precipitable with $BaCl_2$, and the balance of the activity is ascribed to DSGa. No information was published regarding recoveries. Cobby *et al.* (1978) have expressed concern regarding the adequacies of the separation procedures in the assay; the question is a legitimate one in view of the statement of Sauter *et al.* (1976) that their efforts to separate DSSD and DSH by lipophilic solvent extraction at pH 9 failed because the DSH was found to contaminate the DSSD by approximately 30%. Brien and Loomis (1983a) have expressed concern regarding equilibration between ^{35}S-DSH and carrier DSSD; Such an equilibrium is, according to Strömme (1965a), instantaneous at pH 3–4; its rate at higher pH values is not known. The results obtained using this method by Faiman *et al.* (1983) in rats administered ^{35}S-DSMe, raise additional concerns, since significant levels of DSSD and DSH were reported as present in the tissues, yet the rats failed to excrete any CS_2, a well established metabolite of both DSH and DSSD.

The method of Cobby *et al.* (1977b) as employed by Cobby *et al.* (1978) is limited in scope to the analysis of plasma for DSMe and administered DSH. The former is accomplished by gas–liquid chromatography (GLC) of a carbon tetrachloride extract of plasma. To assay DSH, the plasma is alkylated with methyl iodide prior to carbon tetrachloride extraction. Non-linear, but highly reproducible calibration curves for DSH in plasma were obtained. Recoveries for DSMe were $78 \pm 2\%$.

The method of Jensen and Faiman (1980) is based on a multistep extractive fractionation procedure parallel to that of Faiman *et al.* (1977), but chloroform rather than pentane is used. Also, an HPLC assay rather than a radiometric one is employed. The aqueous layer obtained following methylation of DSH and extraction is further analyzed for diethylamine (Et_2NH) and CS_2 (rather than DSGa, protein-bound DSH and sulfate) by addition of excess CS_2 to one aliquot and excess Et_2NH to another. Alkylation of the DSH thus formed is effected with methyl iodide. HPLC analyses are performed on the resultant chloroform extracts. Reported recoveries from plasma for DSSD, DSH, DSMe, Et_2NH and CS_2 were 51.0 ± 3.8, 85 ± 10.1, 91.0 ± 3.1, 52.0 ± 5.6 and 48.7 ± 10.5, respectively. The large standard deviations for some of the recoveries may have contributed to what Jensen (1984) terms 'the marked variability' of the data obtained using the method.

The method of Giles *et al.* (1982) is one for the determination of DSMe and DSH in plasma. DSMe is assayed by extraction into chloroform, concentration of the extract, and HPLC, using an acetonitrile–pH 4 acetate buffer mobile phase. The DSH assay is based on alkylation with methyl iodide prior to the extraction step and subtraction of the value obtained for DSMe. Reported recoveries for DSMe were 99.5%.

Lieder and Borch (1985) elaborated a very efficient and rapid method for the ethylation of DSH in plasma by applying triethyloxonium tetrafluoroborate (Meerwein's reagent) for the purpose. The ethylation occurs within seconds of the additions of 10 µl of the reagent to 0.5 ml of plasma and with an efficiency ranging from 70 to 100% depending on the origin and age of the ethylating agent. The ethyl ester is then quantitatively (95%) extracted into chloroform and analyzed by HPLC. The quantitation of DSH is subject to some of the ambiguities that were discussed above, that is, regarding possible redistribution of DSH due to the presence of the alkylating agent and the use of solvent extraction.

5

Metabolism of disulfiram and diethyldithiocarbamate

5.1 INTRODUCTION 29
5.2 FORMATION OF MIXED DISULFIDES WITH GENERATION OF
     DIETHYLDITHIOCARBAMATE 30
5.3 FORMATION OF DISULFIRAM FROM DIETHYLDITHIOCARBAMATE 32
5.4 FORMATION OF THE COPPER COMPLEX 34
5.5 S-GLUCURONIDE OF DIETHYLDITHIOCARBAMIC ACID 34
5.6 FORMATION OF CARBON DISULFIDE AND DIETHYLAMINE 36
5.7 METABOLISM OF CARBON DISULFIDE AND FORMATION OF
     CARBONYL SULFIDE 37
5.8 THE METHYL ESTER OF DIETHYLDITHIOCARBAMIC ACID 38
5.9 THE METHYL ESTER OF DIETHYLMONOTHIOCARBAMIC ACID . . 40
5.10 OTHER METABOLITES 41

5.1 INTRODUCTION

The first and rapid step in the metabolism of disulfiram (DSSD) is the reduction of its disulfide bond. This biotransformation can be effected by endogenous thiols, sulfhydryl groups of proteins (section 5.2), or reduced forms of redox cycling metal ions (section 5.4). Moreover, such reactions can occur in blood, liver and other tissues. The eventual end result of these reactions is the conversion of both the DS moieties of DSSD to diethyldithiocarbamic acid (DSH). The sulfhydryl groups of thiols and proteins react with DSSD to yield immediately one equivalent of DSH. The second equivalent of DSH becomes available when the DS residue-containing mixed disulfide is subsequently reduced. In the case of proteins the latter reduction can be brought about by a vicinal sulfhydryl group, if one is present. This results in the formation of an intramolecular disulfide bond between the protein's vicinal sulfhydryls while DSH is released (section 8.1). Reducing metal ions react with DSSD to form chelates from which DSH can be later displaced (section 5.4).

Conversely, DSH is easily oxidized back to DSSD by such endogenous oxidants as hydrogen peroxide and Fe^{3+}. That some oxidation of DSH to DSSD occurs *in vivo* and is likely to occur in various cellular or subcellular preparations *in vitro*, is indicated by what happens following administration of ^{35}S-labelled DSH (section 5.3). Thus the commonality of some of the pharmacological effects of DSSD and DSH derives from their, at least partial, interconvertibility.

Apart from thiol–disulfide exchanges and metal complex formation, the further metabolism of DSSD is considered to occur via DSH. The biotransformation of DSH proceeds either degradatively, or via conjugation to glucuronide or methyl ester. Rapid degradation of DSH to diethylamine and carbon disulfide occurs spontaneously at acidic pH (section 5.6) and it can take place in the stomach after an oral dose. Carbon disulfide is oxidatively desulfurated to carbonyl sulfide (section 5.7). DSH forms two conjugates. One of these, the glucuronide (section 5.5), is easily excreted as such. The other, the lipophilic methyl ester of DSH (section 5.8), is highly pharmacologically active *in vivo* (section 9.4.2). It undergoes further biotransformations, including desulfuration to the monothioester and degradation to the sulfate. The diethyl-monothiocarbamic acid methyl ester (section 5.9) is also active pharmacologically *in vivo* (section 9.4.3). The enzymes and the redox systems necessary for the biotransformation of DSSD and DSH are present in the blood, liver, and probably most other tissues, hence metabolism of these compounds is likely to occur, to a varying extent, at many sites.

5.2 FORMATION OF MIXED DISULFIDES WITH GENERATION OF DIETHYLDITHIOCARBAMATE

Many sulfhydryl containing proteins and endogenous thiols reduce DSSD with the liberation of one mole equivalent of DSH and formation of one mole equivalent of a DS-containing mixed disulfide. In blood, for instance, reduction of DSSD can occur via a thiol–disulfide exchange reaction with the protein sulfhydryl groups (PrSH in Fig. 5.1) of albumin (Strömme, 1965a; Agarwal, R.P. *et al.*, 1986) or hemoglobin, as well as with the sulfhydryls of cysteine or glutathione (Kelner and Alexander, 1986).

Albumin, in the native state, has one (effectively 0.7–0.8) reactive sulfhydryl group (Kolthoff and Tan, 1965; Strömme, 1965a) available for the protein thiol–disulfide exchange reaction; hemoglobin has two (Neims *et al.*, 1966b). The reaction between albumin and ^{35}S-DSSD results in the liberation of one mole of ^{35}S-DSH, per mole of albumin,

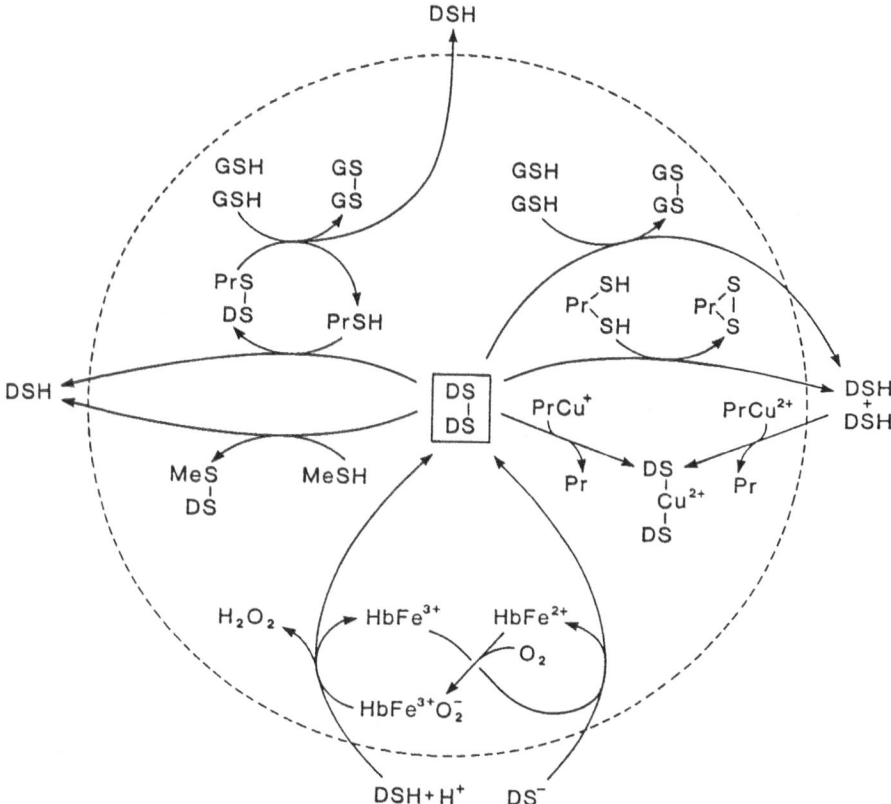

Figure 5.1 Schematic of the interconversions of disulfiram and diethyldithiocarbamate through interactions of disulfiram with sulfhydryl groups of proteins, endogenous thiols and metalloproteins. To guide the eye, disulfiram (DSSD) is shown at the center and diethyldithiocarbamate (DSH) is shown (multiple representations) beyond the periphery of a dashed circle. Other entities are represented as follows. GSH, reduced glutathione; GSSG, oxidized glutathione; MeSH, methanethiol; MeS-SD, *N*, *N*-diethyldithiocarbamyl-*S*-methyldisulfide; Pr, a protein, PrSH, a protein sulfhydryl; PrS-SD, a mixed disulfide with diethyldithiocarbamate; Pr-Cu, a copper–protein complex; DS-Cu-SD, bis (diethyldithiocarbamato) copper complex; HbFe^{2+}, deoxyhemoglobin; HbFe^{3+}, methemoglobin; HbFe^{3+}O$_2^-$, oxyhemoglobin. This schematic is based on reported interactions with albumin, hemoglobins, and aldehyde dehydrogenases.

and fixation of a second ^{35}S-DS residue (Strömme, 1965a); that between hemoglobin and ^{35}S-DSSD results in the liberation of two moles of ^{35}S-DSH, per mole of heme protein, and fixation of two ^{35}S-DS residues (Neims *et al.*, 1966b).

The kinetics of DSSD interaction with serum albumin in the presence of EDTA have been studied by Agarwal, R.P. *et al.* (1986). There is a rapid formation of an albumin-DSSD non-covalent adduct which has a half-life of 133 seconds and is reduced with the release of free DSH. The rapidity of the reaction and the fact that albumin is the major drug-binding plasma protein, puts it center stage at the first step in the metabolism of DSSD to DSH.

Turning to the possible roles of endogenous thiols, reduced glutathione (GSH) rapidly and non-enzymatically reduces DSSD to DSH (Johnston, 1953). GSH, moreover, also liberates DSH from some mixed disulfides of proteins with DS residues (PrS-SD in Fig. 5.1), e.g. those of albumin or oxyhemoglobin (Strömme, 1965a; Neims *et al.*, 1966b). Thus, GSH displaces, in the form of ^{35}S-DSH, about 80% of the label that becomes bound to the soluble proteins of the liver and serum follow-ing the administration of ^{35}S-DSSD to rats (Strömme, 1965b). Cysteine also can reduce DSSD to DSH (Neims *et al.*, 1966a). Quantitatively, however, the role of GSH is more important because it is much more abundant than cysteine, its levels in cells being 0.5–10 mM (Meister and Anderson, 1983). The oxidized disulfide form of glutathione, GSSG, is less abundant in cells because it is easily extruded and is found chiefly in extracellular fluids (Akerboom and Sies, 1981). Moreover, GSH is maintained in the reduced form by the activity of cellular glutathione reductase and the NADPH reducing equivalents derived from glucose metabolism. In erythrocytes, in particular, a very active hexose mono-phosphate shunt and the glutathione reductase are crucial to this purpose (Srivastava and Beutler, 1969). Already in 1963, it was pointed out that the glutathione–glutathione reductase system offers an effi-cient protection against DSSD poisoning in erythrocytes (Strömme, 1963b).

The reduction of DSSD by methanethiol (MeSH) is a special and potentially important instance of mixed disulfide formation, since the product, *N*,*N*-diethyldithiocarbamyl-S-methyl disulfide (DSSMe, Fig. 5.1), is a very potent *in vitro* inhibitor of E_2, the mitochondrial low-K_m aldehyde dehydrogenase (ALDH). Accordingly, since E_2 is quite resis-tant *in vitro* to inhibition by DSSD (section 9.2.2), it has been suggested that DSSMe might the active entity which is responsible for the *in vivo* inhibition of this enzyme following administration of DSSD (MacKerell *et al.*, 1985). To date, however, DSSMe has not been reported to be a metabolite of either DSSD or DSH.

5.3 FORMATION OF DISULFIRAM FROM DIETHYLDITHIOCARBAMATE

Following the i.p. administration of ^{35}S-DSH some of the label is found to be irreversibly bound to plasma proteins from which it is displaced by GSH yielding ^{35}S-DSH (Strömme, 1965b). *In vitro*, DSH does not become irreversibly bound to proteins (section 3.1). Accordingly, the occurrence of such binding *in vivo* is seen as an indication that some DSH is oxidized *in vivo* to the DSSD which then participates in thiol exchange reactions with the sulfhydryl groups of proteins to form mixed disulfides. Strömme (1965a) suggested a possible involvement of cytochrome c, or methemoglobin, in the oxidation of DSH.

In erythrocytes, oxyhemoglobin ($HbFe^{3+}O_2^-$) and methemoglobin ($HbFe^{3+}$) can each catalyze oxidation of DSH to DSSD (Fig. 5.1). Of the two, the reaction catalyzed by $HbFe^{3+}O_2^-$ is some five times faster than that catalyzed by $HbFe^{3+}$ (Kelner and Alexander, 1986). To a degree, the two reactions can be coupled in a cycling process involving consumption of oxygen and production of hydrogen peroxide. Erythrocytes have an efficient, glucose-dependent, GSH regenerating system. Since GSH readily reduces DSSD to DSH (section 5.2), in its presence no detectable accumulation of DSSD occurs (Kelner and Alexander, 1986). Hemoglobin ($HbFe^{2+}$) also effects the reduction of DSSD to DSH.

There is also evidence that heme-containing enzymes of the liver share oxyhemoglobin's ability to catalyze oxidation of DSH to DSSD. Thus, upon incubation with hepatic microsomes and NADPH under aerobic conditions, DSH is converted to DSSD (Masuda, 1988; Masuda and Nakamura, 1989). The conversion is inhibited by *n*-octylamine (Masuda and Nakamura, 1989), but not by heating of the microsomal fraction at 45 °C for 5 min (Masuda, 1988). This rules out the involvement of the microsomal flavin-containing monooxygenase, which is not inhibited by *n*-octylamine (Poulsen *et al.*, 1979), but is inactivated by the heat treatment (Ziegler, 1980). Instead, it suggests the involvement of P-450. This is further supported by the fact that the formation of DSSD from DSH parallels P-450 levels when the latter are manipulated. Thus, phenobarbital pretreatment of the animals results in both higher microsomal P-450 levels and greater DSSD formation. Carbon tetrachloride pretreatment of the animals has the opposite effect, as does exposure of the microsomes themselves to cumene hydroperoxide (Masuda and Nakamura, 1989). Appropriately, for a P-450 mediated reaction, no DSSD is formed in the absence of NADPH and it is markedly suppressed upon incubation under 100% nitrogen. Since it is not inhibited by carbon monoxide (Masuda, 1988), however, the reaction cannot involve the full monooxygenase cycle. By analogy with the reaction of DSH with oxyhemoglobin to yield DSSD and hydrogen peroxide (Kelner and Alexander, 1986), DSH might react with the superoxo–ferriheme complex of P-450 ($Fe^{3+}O_2^-$), and possibly also with a carbonyl–ferriheme complex, to give DSSD.

5.4 FORMATION OF THE COPPER COMPLEX

Johansson and Stankiewicz (1985) have observed that human blood catalyzes a complete reduction of DSSD to DSH, with simultaneous formation of a stoichiometric molar concentration of $Cu(DS)_2$ (Fig. 5.1). They suggested the complex is an important lipophilic metabolite of DSSD, which they detected in plasma of 10 of 11 alcoholics on DSSD therapy and four of four volunteers. The role of albumin in this reaction has not been defined. However, in addition to having a free sulfhydryl group, it also has associated with it some loosely bound copper which likely participates in the reduction of DSSD.

5.5 S-GLUCURONIDE OF DIETHYLDITHIOCARBAMIC ACID

The glucuronide of DSH, N,N-diethyldithiocarbamoyl-1-thio-β-D-glyco-pyranosiduronic acid (DSGa, compound **V** in Fig. 5.2) was first iso-lated by Kaslander (1963) from the urine of subjects administered DSSD. The structure of the derivatized DSGa (the triacetyl methyl ester) was confirmed by elemental analysis and by comparison of melting points and infra-red spectra with those of a synthetic sample of the compound. Strömme (1965b) showed DSGa is a urinary meta-bolite of ^{35}S-DSSD given i.p. to rats. He identified it by comparing its chromatographic and electrophoretic behavior to that of authentic DSGa. Gas chromatographic–mass spectroscopic confirmation of the structure of DSGa has been supplied by Eneanya *et al.* (1983) follow-ing its isolation from bile, obtained from a rat liver perfused *in vitro* with DSH.

Using a liver perfusion system, Masuda *et al.* (1988) found 60–70% of infused DSSD to be metabolized to DSH and its glucuronide. They observed, moreover that the fraction metabolized to DSGa can be enhanced by inducers of glucuronidation. It can be calculated, based on the areas under the concentration–time curves for the metabolites (Masuda *et al.*, 1988, their Fig. 6), that livers from normal rats convert 21% of infused DSSD to DSGa. In livers from rats pretreated with 3-methylcholanthrene (40 mg/kg/day for 3 days), or phenobarbital (0.1% in drinking water for 5–6 days), the DSGa production is increased markedly, that is, to 39 and 51% of the infused DSSD, respectively. Depending upon whether DSSD or DSH is administered, DSGa may account, respectively, for 2–11% or about 30% of the administered dose excreted in the urine (Strömme, 1965b; Gessner, T. and Jakubowski, 1972; Faiman *et al.*, 1984). DSGa is synthesized enzymatically by transfer of the glucuronic acid moiety of uridinediphosphoglucuronic acid to DSH (Dutton and Illing, 1972). The reaction is analogous to the

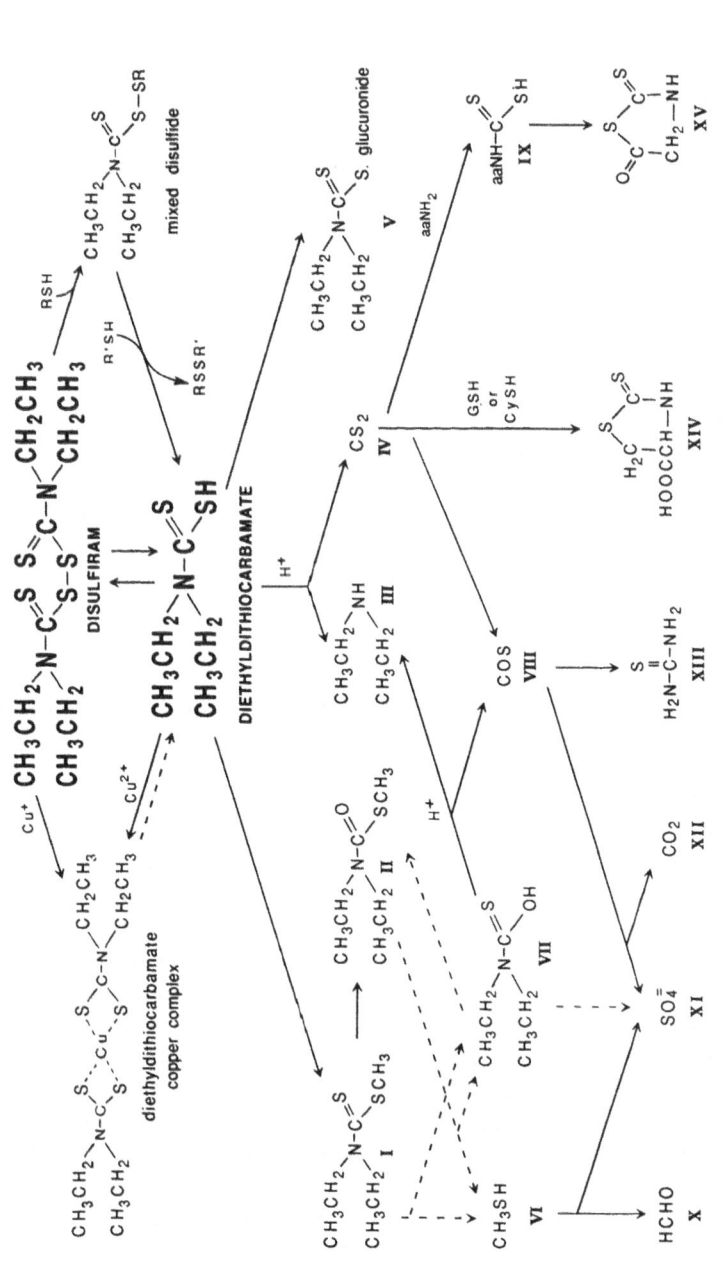

Figure 5.2 Pathways of disulfiram metabolism via diethyldithiocarbamate. **I**, diethyldithiocarbamate; **II**, diethylmonothiocarbamic acid methyl ester (DmSMe); **III**, diethylamine (Et₂NH); **IV**, carbon disulfide (CS₂); **V**, diethyldithiocarbamoyl-S-glucuronide (DSGa); **VI**, methanethiol (MeSH); **VII**, diethylmonothiocarbamate; **VIII**, diethylmonothiocarbamate; **IX**, amino acid dithiocarbamate; **X**, formaldehyde; **XI**, sulfate; **XII**, carbon dioxide; **XIII**, thiourea; **XIV**, thiazolidine-2-thione-4-carboxylic acid; **XV**, 2-thio-5-thiazolidinone.

formation of O-glucuronides and involves microsomal glucuronyltransferase. DSGa is stable in acetate buffer at pH 5.5, but it is hydrolyzed by β-glucuronidase (Dutton and Illing, 1972). By analogy with O-glucuronides, conversion of DSH to DSGa *in vivo* is most likely to be chiefly hepatic, since liver is a rich source of glucuronyltransferases.

5.6 FORMATION OF CARBON DISULFIDE AND DIETHYLAMINE

Johnston and Prickett (1952) first reported on the formation of carbon disulfide (CS_2, **IV**) from DSSD by rat liver homogenates. Later, they showed that CS_2 is also produced from DSSD in rats *in vivo* (Prickett and Johnston, 1953). *In vitro*, the process involves two steps, namely, the enzymatic reduction of DSSD to DSH followed by the spontaneous decomposition of the DSH to diethylamine (Et_2NH, **III**) and CS_2 (Johnston and Prickett, 1952). Non-enzymatic degradation of DSH to Et_2NH and CS_2 occurs through proton-catalyzed decomposition. The half-life of DSH becomes progressively shorter with decreasing pH and with increasing temperature; at room temperature the half-life is in the range of 19–73 h at pH 7.4, but only 30–120 s at pH 4 (section 2.2).

In humans, CS_2 is present in both the blood (Johansson, 1989b) and expired air (Merlevede and Casier, 1961) following administration of DSSD. Its presence in expired air is utilized in monitoring the compliance of patients with their DSSD therapy (section 11.8). The data of Merlevede and Casier (1961) indicate that in humans the $t_{1/2}$ for CS_2 as a metabolite of DSSD, administered per os, is about 12 h (section 6.5.1). In contrast, humans administered DSH orally, excrete CS_2 by a process with a half-life of only 20–30 min. This indicates that in the stomach there is considerable acid-catalyzed decomposition of DSH to CS_2 and Et_2NH, but very limited conversion of DSSD to DSH. Data obtained by Strömme (1965b) show that in rats administered DSSD or DSH i.p. (in doses of *ca* 37 and 93 mg/kg, respectively) the difference between the half-lives of CS_2 (63 vs 31 min, respectively), appears to be much less dramatic. The exposure of orally administered DSH to the acid environment of the stomach may be responsible for the rapid formation of CS_2, which is then quickly eliminated in breath as observed by Merlevede and Casier (1961).

The rate of ^{35}S-CS_2 production following oral administration of ^{35}S-DSSD in rats chronically pretreated with DSSD is significantly higher than in naive animals (Neiderhiser *et al.*, 1983). This suggests that DSSD can induce its own metabolism. However, since the total amount excreted as CS_2 does not change, the induction must involve an early step. Some suggestion that such induction may also occur in humans derives from the data of Rogers *et al.* (1978).

The formation from DSSD and DSH of Et$_2$NH (**III**), the complementary metabolite to CS$_2$, has been studied much less extensively (see tables 6.1–6.3), the emphasis having been often on the fate of the sulfur moiety of DSSD or DSH. Following p.o. administration of ^{14}C-DSSD to rats, 27% of the dose is excreted as ^{14}C-Et$_2$NH (Neiderhiser and Fuller, 1980). Most human studies of Et$_2$NH excretion following DSSD dosing have had compliance testing in alcoholics as a goal (section 11.8) and have not been quantitative (Neiderhiser *et al.*, 1976; Gordis and Peterson, 1977; Fuller and Neiderhiser, 1981). Faiman *et al.* (1984) have reported the urinary excretion of Et$_2$NH to be minuscule (1.6% of the dose), but the methods for urine collection and analysis were not described.

5.7 METABOLISM OF CARBON DISULFIDE AND FORMATION OF CARBONYL SULFIDE

Carbonyl sulfide (COS, **VIII**) is found in the blood of alcoholics chronically treated with DSSD (Johansson, 1989b). The levels of COS in the blood 4 h following DSSD administration show wide interindividual variations (range 20–540 nmol/l).

The metabolism and toxicology of CS$_2$ have been studied extensively, because occupational exposure to it occurs in viscose rayon industry (for review, see Beauchamp *et al.*, 1983). Briefly, inhaled CS$_2$ is metabolized chiefly by the cytochrome P-450 monooxygenase system to the more toxic metabolite, COS. Administration to rats of ^{14}C- and ^{35}S-CS$_2$ (19 mg/kg i.p.) indicates that more of the ^{35}S than ^{14}C derived activity is retained in tissues 3 h post administration (Snyderwine and Hunter, 1987). The amount which is biotransformed increases from 17% in 1-day-old animals to 42% in 40-day-old rats. This is in keeping with the general observation that young animals have a low monooxygenase capacity. Paradoxically, the tissue levels of covalently bound ^{35}S label at 3 h are higher in the younger than the older animals. This is in part due to the faster clearance of such label by the older animals (Snyderwine and Hunter, 1987). The above suggests that one may expect individual differences in the degree of desulfuration of CS$_2$ and its metabolites dependent upon the activity of the individual's cytochrome P-450 monooxygenase system. The mechanism of this desulfuration reaction involves the formation of atomic sulfur. It inactivates the cytochrome P-450 by attacking the cysteine residue that serves as the thiolate ligand of the cytochrome's heme iron (section 8.3.5). COS, in turn, is further metabolized to sulfate (**XI**) and carbon dioxide (**XII**), by a process mediated by cytosolic carbonic anhydrase (Chengelis and Neal, 1979).

CS_2 also undergoes anaerobic metabolism. Thus, it is known (Beauchamp *et al.*, 1983) that some CS_2 is metabolized to thiourea (**XIII**) and dithiocarbamate derivatives of amino acids (**IX**). The latter compounds in turn can give rise to 2-thio-5-thiazolidinone (**XV**). Both thiourea and 2-thio-5-thiazolidinone have been found in the urine of workers exposed to CS_2 (Van Doorn *et al.*, 1981, 1982; Beauchamp *et al.*, 1983). Conceivably, the dithiocarbamate derivatives of amino acids may also be metabolized to their methyl esters, since Jakubowski and Gessner (1972) found that such compounds can be methylated *in vitro* by a cytosolic methyltransferase. The reaction is less efficient, however, than the methylation of DSH by microsomal thiol-*S*-methyltransferase (Gessner, T. and Jakubowski, 1972). Thiazolidine-2-thione-4-carboxylic acid (**XIV**), which can be derived from dithiocarbamates of glutathione or cysteine, has been detected in the urine of alcoholics receiving DSSD therapy (Van Doorn *et al.*, 1982).

5.8 THE METHYL ESTER OF DIETHYLDITHIOCARBAMIC ACID

Diethyldithiocarbamic acid methyl ester (DSMe, I) was first identified as a metabolite of ^{35}S-DSSD in rats by Gessner, T. and Jakubowski (1972) by (a) chromatography against authentic DSMe (boiling point 112–114 °C at 4 mmHg) in four solvent systems and (b) isolation with purification to constant count of the isotopically diluted metabolite. Its formation from DSSD has also been observed in humans with confirmation of its identity by mass spectrometry (Cobby *et al.*, 1977a). It has also been observed to be formed from DSH in dogs (Cobby *et al.*, 1978) and from DSSD in mice (Jensen and Faiman, 1980). Guillaumin *et al.* (1986) found that upon administration of ^{35}S-DSH to mice the radioactivity which was taken up within 5 min by the liver, thymus and brain neocortex selectively persisted in these tissues for at least 45 min (section 6.6.5). When pentane extracts of the neocortex were analyzed by HPLC, they were found to contain ^{35}S-DSMe.

The methylation of DSH is effectively catalyzed by a liver microsomal methyl transferase (Gessner, T. and Jakubowski, 1972). This lipophilic thiol-S-methyltransferase has been purified from rat liver microsomes (see review by Weisiger and Jakoby, 1980) and DSH was found to be a very good substrate, its K_m value being 12 μM (Weisiger and Jakoby, 1979). The enzyme is ubiquitous in tissues. The highest specific activity of this enzyme is found in colonic mucosa; the specific activity of the cecal mucosa is comparable, but gastric mucosa is about 20% as active.

High activities are also found in the liver, lung and kidney. Erythrocytes have about 1/100th of the activity of the mucosa (Weisiger and Jakoby, 1980). On the basis of the above considerations a substantial amount of extrahepatic metabolism to DSMe should be expected, especially in the gut, lungs and kidneys.

Gessner, T. and Jakubowski (1972) reported that at 2 h following i.p. administration of ^{35}S-DSSD to mice, 15% of the ^{35}S in the liver is present in the form of DSMe. At 1, 3, and 6 h following administration of ^{35}S-DSSD substantial concentrations of DSMe are also found in the kidney as well as in the liver (Faiman *et al.*, 1978a, 1980). Nevertheless, no DSMe is excreted in the urine. Even after the i.p. administration of ^{35}S-DSMe itself to rats, there is no measurable urinary excretion of the unchanged compound (Gessner, T. and Jakubowski, 1972; Faiman *et al.*, 1983). Instead some 62–80% of the dose appears in the urine in the form of sulfate (Gessner, T. and Jakubowski, 1972; Faiman *et al.*, 1983). This contrasts with the much lower (20–40%) formation of sulfate when either DSH or DSSD is administered (Strömme, 1965b; Gessner, T. and Jakubowski, 1972). The fact that DSMe is so extensively metabolized to sulfate, led Gessner, T. and Jakubowski (1972) to propose that DSMe is a transient metabolite of DSSD on the chief pathway to sulfate formation (Fig. 5.2).

Once DSMe is formed there appears to be no substantial conversion of it back to DSH. Firstly, rats administered ^{35}S-DSMe fail to exhale any CS_2 in the breath (Faiman *et al.*, 1983). The same is true of dogs administered ^{35}S-DSMe (Jensen, 1984). Yet, CS_2 is a well-documented and substantial excretory product of DSH (section 5.6). Secondly, rats administered ^{35}S-DSMe do not excrete measurable amounts of DSGa, as shown by Gessner, T. and Jakubowski (1972) using specific analytical methods for DSGa, although, again, DSGa is a major excretory product of DSH (section 5.2). Subsequently, it has been reported that DSH can be detected in rat plasma 3–5 h following administration of DSMe in a 60–90 mg/kg dose (Johansson *et al.*, 1989). From the data presented by these authors, however, the formation of DSH from DSMe appears to be a minor pathway in comparison with the desulfuration route which yields the monothio ester (section 5.9).

DSMe is an important metabolite of DSSD because *in vivo* it is at least as potent and long lasting in inhibiting the low-K_m ALDH activity as DSSD (section 9.4.2), while its onset of action is significantly faster than that of DSSD (Yourick and Faiman, 1989). *In vitro*, DSMe does not inhibit the purified Class 1 or 2 ALDH of sheep liver (Kitson, 1976), or the low-K_m ALDH activity of rat hepatic mitochondria (Yourick and Faiman, 1987). However, it does inhibit the hepatic low-K_m ALDH activity following incubation with liver homogenate under aerobic conditions (Johansson *et al.*, 1989). Moreover, DSMe pretreated rats are sensitized to ethanol so that administration of the latter to such animals causes a marked elevation in blood acetaldehyde (section 9.4.2) and a significant fall in blood pressure (section 10.9).

5.9 THE METHYL ESTER OF DIETHYLMONOTHIOCARBAMIC ACID

Johansson *et al.* (1989) identified (by GLC–mass spectroscopy) a monodesulfurated metabolite of DSMe in the plasma of rats administered either DSSD or DSMe. This metabolite is referred to in this book as diethylmonothiocarbamic acid methyl ester (DmSMe, **II**), the inclusion of 'mono' in the name being adopted to avoid confusion with the parent dithio ester. DmSMe is highly lipid soluble, the log of its partition between octanol and water (Log P) is 1.85 (Johansson, 1990b). Its plasma levels, 3 to 5 hours after DSMe administration, exceed by 10- to 50-fold those of DSH. In rats, 5 h after the last dose of DSSD (30 mg/kg preceded 16 h earlier by 100 mg/kg) plasma levels of DmSMe exceed those of DSMe 25 fold (Johansson *et al.*, 1989). The value of DmSMe/DSMe ratio may be, however, a function of time of observation since in humans, for instance, DSMe plasma levels peak earlier than those of DmSMe (Johansson and Stankiewicz, 1989).

Johansson *et al.* (1989) have identified DmSMe in the plasma of alcoholics on DSSD therapy. In the majority (7/10) of patients receiving a single dose of DSSD (400 mg), however, the plasma levels of DmSMe were below the detection limit of the analytical method. In the remaining patients, the peak levels (278 ± 158 nM) were of the same magnitude as those of DSMe (312 ± 181 nM), the latter metabolite being detectable in 9 of 10 patients (Johansson and Stankiewicz, 1989). The times following DSSD administration at which the peak concentrations of DSMe and DmSMe were observed in these patients (1.8 and 3.3 h, respectively) suggest that DmSMe is formed from DSMe. In contrast, in volunteers maintained on various daily doses of DSSD for 2–4 weeks, the plasma DmSMe levels at 2 h after the final DSSD administration were generally detectable and as much as 10- to 20-fold higher than those of DSMe. On average, moreover, the DmSMe levels were higher the larger the daily DSSD dose and the longer the duration of daily DSSD dosing (Johansson and Stankiewicz, 1989).

In rat liver homogenates, DmSMe generation from DSMe was observed by Johansson *et al.* (1989) to require NADPH and aerobic conditions, analogously to monooxygenation. These observations led them to propose that the conversion of DSMe to DmSMe occurs via oxidative desulfuration of the thiocarbonyl group $>C=S$ to the carbonyl group $>C=O$. They reported that in homogenates in which such DmSMe formation has taken place, determination of the low-K_m ALDH activity reveals it to be depressed.

The importance of DmSMe as a metabolite of DSSD derives from the fact that, like DSMe, it is a potent and long-lasting *in vivo* inhibitor of the mitochondrial low K_m ALDH (section 9.4.3). Its onset of action is even faster than that of DSMe (Hart *et al.*, 1990). Although *in vitro* DmSMe behaves as a suicide inhibitor of the purified Class 2 ALDH of bovine liver, its potency is very low: a 25% inhibition of the enzyme is observed after a 24 h incubation with 2.76 mM DmSMe (Johansson, 1989c). This contrasts with the potent inhibitory effect of DmSMe on the low K_m ALDH activities in rat liver homogenate assays (Johansson *et al.*, 1989) where, following a 1-h incubation under aerobic conditions, 27.6 μM DmSMe causes a 75% inhibition of the low-K_m ALDH. Moreover, DmSMe is as potent as DSMe in sensitizing rats to the blood pressure lowering effects of subsequently administered ethanol (section 10.9).

Taken together the above observations strongly suggest that the ultimate. highly potent, inhibitor of the low-K_m ALDH is a further metabolite of DmSMe, rather than DmSMe itself. Such a metabolite may be generated by the enzyme(s) present in tissue homogenates, or in intact cells, when such preparations are used in the assays with either DmSMe or DSMe.

5.10 OTHER METABOLITES

Sulfate (**XI**) would be generated from the oxidative desulfuration of DSMe to DmSMe. Gessner, T. and Jakubowski (1972) suggested that sulfate might also be generated from DSMe via an esterase-catalyzed hydrolysis which could split off MeSH (**VI**) and generate diethyl-monothiocarbamate (DmSH, **VII**), initially in its tautomeric form (Fig. 5.2). It is also conceivable that DmSH may undergo methylation to form DmSMe. The latter, in turn, should also be cleavable by an esterase to MeSH and diethylcarbamate, thus providing an alternative route for the desulfuration of the dithiocarbamate moiety. Whether the proposed reaction occurs remains to be tested. Any MeSH formed would be readily converted to sulfate (Canellakis and Tarver, 1953; Derr and Draves, 1983, 1984). As for DmSH, it is known that monothiocar-bamates can be rapidly decomposed by acids (Ewing *et al.*, 1980) with the liberation of COS and the amine. It is therefore proposed here that some of the DmSH (**VII**) undergoes H^+ catalyzed metabolism to COS

(VIII) and Et$_2$NH (III). COS, in turn, is known to be extensively metabolized to sulfate and carbon dioxide (XII) (Beauchamp *et al.*, 1983).

Some of the metabolites of DSSD on the pathway to sulfate formation (see Fig. 5.2), that is, MeSH and DmSH, have not yet been identified as products of biotransformation of DSSD, DSH, DSMe or DmSMe in animals or humans. These pathways await further elucidation. Additionally, MeSH, whether a product of DSMe or DmSMe metabolism, or of endogenous origin (Kromhout *et al.*, 1980; McClain *et al.*, 1980; Cooper, 1983; Mardini *et al.*, 1984), may play an important role in the toxicity of DSSD. Thus MacKerell *et al.* (1985) proposed the mixed disulfide DSSMe, which could arise by a thiol–disulfide exchange reaction between DSSD and MeSH (Fig. 5.1), to be the potent active metabolite of DSSD, causing irreversible inhibition of the important mitochondrial low-K_m ALDH. Such a metabolite has not been found as yet, but is quite plausible.

NOTE ADDED IN PRESS

Hart and Faiman (*Bioch. Pharm.* **43**, 403–6, 1992) report the presence of (CH$_3$CH$_2$)$_2$NCO·SO·CH$_3$, S-methyl diethylmonothiocarbamate sulfoxide (DmSOMe), in the plasma of rats administered DSSD, DSH, DSMe or DmSMe. To-date the identification of DmSOMe as a metabolite of DSSD is based solely on the HPLC analysis of an evaporated chloroform extract of EDTA treated plasma. Incubation of synthetic DmSOMe with liver mitochondria for 60 min at 37°, caused a marked inhibition of the mitochondrial low-K_m ALDH activity (IC$_{50}$ 0.73 μM). Additionally, DmSOMe proved effective as an *in vivo* inhibitor of this activity (ID$_{50}$ 3.5 mg/kg). The latter inhibition was said to be unaffected by administration of an inhibitor of P-450 (unspecified), though administration of the P-450 inhibitor was stated to prevent both the DSSD-induced *in vivo* inhibition of the low-K_m ALDH activity and the appearance of DmSOMe in the plasma of rats treated with DSSD. Based on these results, Hart and Faiman (1992) suggest this metabolite as the most likely responsible for the *in vivo* inhibitory effects of DSSD on the low-K_m ALDH in the rat. No information is available at this time, however, regarding the *in vitro* effects of DmSOMe on the purified enzyme.

6

Pharmacokinetic aspects of the disposition of disulfiram and metabolites

6.1 INTRODUCTION 44
6.2 METHODS 44
6.3 URINARY EXCRETION OF DISULFIRAM METABOLITES 51
   6.3.1 Experimental animal data 51
   6.3.2 Human data 53
6.4 PULMONARY EXCRETION OF DISULFIRAM METABOLITES 54
   6.4.1 Human data 54
   6.4.2 Experimental animal data 55
6.5 PLASMA DISULFIRAM AND METABOLITES FOLLOWING
   ITS ADMINISTRATION 56
   6.5.1 Plasma disulfiram levels 56
   6.5.2 Plasma levels of free diethyldithiocarbamate 57
   6.5.3 Plasma levels of protein-bound diethyldithiocarbamate 58
   6.5.4 Plasma levels of diethyldithiocarbamic acid methyl ester 58
   6.5.5 Plasma levels of diethylmonothiocarbamic acid methyl ester . . . 59
   6.5.6 Plasma levels of the S-glucuronide of diethyl-
       dithiocarbamic acid 59
6.6 DIETHYLDITHIOCARBAMATE AND METABOLITES FOLLOWING
   ITS ADMINISTRATION 60
   6.6.1 Pulmonary carbon disulfide excretion 60
   6.6.2 Plasma diethyldithiocarbamate levels: free and bound 60
   6.6.3 Plasma levels of diethyldithiocarbamic acid methyl ester 61
   6.6.4 Excretion of sulfate and the S-glucuronide of diethyl-
       dithiocarbamic acid 62
   6.6.5 Tissue distribution 63

6.1 INTRODUCTION

The many investigations of the fate of disulfiram as a function of time have resulted in an accumulation of a wealth of information, little of which has been subjected to pharmacokinetic analysis. Continued lack of agreement regarding even such basic questions as whether disulfiram (DSSD) is detectable in the blood of patients or experimental animals dosed with it, may have inhibited a comparative discussion of the findings to date. In the context of this monograph, however, such a discussion is essential and accordingly the relevant pharmacokinetic parameters have been assembled or computed and are listed in Tables 6.1–6.3.

Normally, in considering the pharmacokinetics of a compound and its metabolites, it is usual to mingle information obtained from the administration of the parent compound and of its metabolites. There is little doubt that diethyldithiocarbamate (DSH) is a metabolite of DSSD *in vivo*. It is clear however, that, *in vivo*, DSSD can also form mixed disulfides and metal complexes. Under appropriate circumstance, these may disassociate to give DSH. Accordingly, the kinetics of DSH and its metabolites are discussed in two sections, the first of these (section 6.5) deals with kinetic events that follow DSH generation *in vivo* from DSSD, the second (section 6.6) with those that follow administration of exogenous DSH.

6.2 METHODS

Due to the infrequency with which pharmacokinetic parameters accompany the original studies, most of the listed values result from retrospective pharmacokinetic evaluations, some performed by Cobby *et al.* (1978), others computed for the purposes of this monograph. In performing these evaluations the published tabular or graphic data has been fitted by the non-linear least-squares computer program NLIN (Marquart, 1964) to either the first or second of the following two pharmacokinetic models, depending on whether the data represented plasma disappearance or cumulative excretion data, respectively. The two models are

$$c = c_0 e^{-Kt} \tag{6.1}$$

$$q = q_\infty (1 - e^{-Kt}) \tag{6.2}$$

where t is time elapsed, c and c_0 are the concentrations at times t and zero, respectively, q and q_∞ are the quantities excreted at times t and infinity, respectively, and K is the rate constant which is related to

Table 6.1 Half-lives for the disposition of disulfiram and its metabolic products

Line	Agent adm.	Dose (mg/kg)	Route	Entity measured	Half-life	Data: Base[a]	Data: Source	Source of calculations
MOUSE								
1	DSH	~625	i.p.	^{35}S/pl	24.2 min	2/4	Strömme and Eldjarn (1966, Figure 1)	This book
2	DSH	250	i.p.	DSH/pl	10 min		Bodenner et al. (1986a, Table 6)	Bodenner et al. (1986a)
3	DSH	250	s.c.	DSH/pl	11 min			
RAT								
4	DSSD	~4	i.p.	SO$_4$/ur	12.6 h	28/8	Eldjarn (1950a)	This book
5	DSH	60	i.v.	CS$_2$/br	24.9 min	5/4	Prickett and Johnston (1953, Table 1)	This book
6	DSH	600	i.v.	CS$_2$/br	10.3 min	12/4		This book
7	DSSD	30	i.v.	CS$_2$/br	20.1 min	6/4		This book
8	DSSD	60	i.v.	CS$_2$/br	17.1 min	7/4		This book
9	DSSD	60	i.v.	DSH/pl	10.2 min	3/3	Prickett and Johnston (1953, Table 3)	This book
10	DSH	200	i.v.	DSH/bl[b]	1.34 min	4/5	Prickett and Johnston (1953, Table 3)	Cobby et al. (1978)
11				DSMe/bl[b]	20.4 min			
12	DSSD	~37	i.p.	DSGa/ur	48.2 min	5/3	Strömme (1965b, Table 1)	This book
13	DSH	~93	i.p.	DSGa/ur	45.5 min	5/3		This book
14	DSH		i.p.	DSH/pl	5.21 min	12/3	Strömme (1965b, Tables 2 and 4)	This book
15				^{35}SPr/pl	134 min	2/5		
16				DSGa/pl	15.0 min	16/5		
17	DSSD	~37	i.p.	^{35}SPr/pl	117 min	2/3	Strömme (1965b, Tables 4 and 3)	This book
18				DSGa/pl	55.3 min	4/3		
19	DSH	~93	i.p.	DSH/pl[b]	7.97 min	4/3	Strömme (1965b, Table 2)	Cobby et al. (1978)
20				DSMe/pl[b]	76.2 min	3/5		
21	DSSD	~37	i.p.	CS$_2$/br	63.2 min	4/4	Strömme (1965b, Figure 2)	This book
22	DSH	~93	i.p.	CS$_2$/br	30.8 min	8/4		This book
23	DSMe	55	i.v.	SO$_4$/ur	2.71 h	18/4	Gessner and Jakubowski (1972, Table 3)	This book
24				^{35}S/ur	3.06 h	15/4		
25	DSSD	7	i.p.	^{35}S/ur	11.1 h	4/5	Faiman et al. (1980, Table 3)	This book
26	DSH	7	i.p.	CS$_2$/br	5.47 h	9/6		This book
27	DSSD	7	p.o.	CS$_2$/br	7.47 h	6/6	Faiman et al. (1980, Table 4)	This book

Table 6.1 —*Contd.*

Line	Agent adm.	Dose (mg/kg)	Route	Entity measured	Half-life	Base[a]	Data Source	Source of calculations
28	DSSD	~137	p.o.	^{14}C/ur	14.9 h	10/6	Neiderhiser and Fuller (1980, Figure 1)	This book
29	DSSD	40	p.o.	^{14}C/pl	7.41 h	13/4	Pedersen (1980, Table 11)	This book
30				^{14}C/ur	18h	5/8		Pedersen (1980)
31	DSSD	33	i.v.	DSH/pl	95.4 min	4/5	Giles et al. (1982)	Giles et al. (1982)
32	DSMe	7.7	i.p.	^{35}S/ur	3.96 h	12/8	Faiman et al. (1983, Table 2)	This book
33	DSSD	~146	p.o.	^{14}C-^{35}S/ur	15.9 h	9/5	Neiderhiser et al. (1983, Figure 1A)	This book
34	DSH	250	i.v.	DSH/pl	10 min	7/9	Bodenner et al. (1986a, Table 6)	Bodenner et al. (1986a)
35	DSH	250	i.p.	DSH/pl	20 min	5/12		
36	DSH	250	s.c.	DSH/pl	21 min	5/12		

DOG

Line	Agent adm.	Dose (mg/kg)	Route	Entity measured	Half-life	Base[a]	Data Source	Source of calculations
37	DSSD	20	i.v.	DSH/pl	30 min	2/7	Faiman et al. (1977, Figure 2)	Cobby et al. (1978)
38				DSMe/pl	22 min	3/8		
39	DSH	18	i.v. inf	DSH/pl	3.38 min	62/15	Cobby et al. (1978)	Cobby et al. (1978)
40	DSMe	19	i.v. inf	DSMe/pl	49.1 min	4/15		
41	DSSD	7	i.v.	DSSD/pl	19.1 min	17/7	Jensen (1984, Table 9)	Jensen (1984)
42	DSH	7	i.v.	DSH/pl	61.4 min	6/11		
43	DSMe	7.7	i.v.	DSMe/pl	56.5 min	6/14		
44	DSH	25	i.v.	DSH/pl	7.0 min	7/5	Lieder and Borch (1985)	Lieder and Borch (1985)
45	DSH	25	i.v.	DSH/pl	8.75 min		Bodenner et al. (1986a, Table 6)	Bodenner et al. (1986a)

HUMAN

Line	Agent adm.	Dose (mg)	Route	Entity measured	Half-life	Base[a]	Data Source	Source of calculations
46	DSSD	2000	p.o.	SO_4/ur	14.6 h	10/6	Eldjarn (1950b, Table 3)	This book
47				^{35}S/ur	13.9 h	10/6		Cobby et al. (1978)
48	DSSD	2000c	p.o.	DSH/ur	4.39 h	4/5	Linderholm and Berg	This book

No.	Compound	Dose	Unit	Route	Matrix	Half-life	[a]	Reference	Analysis
50	DSH	50		p.o.	CS_2/br	36.4 min	4/9	Merlevede and Casier (1961, Table 2)	This book
51	DSH	100		p.o.	CS_2/br	32.1 min	8/9		
52	DSH	250		p.o.	CS_2/br	46.3 min	13/14		
53	DSH	500		p.o.	CS_2/br	41.6 min	12/13		
54	DSSD	250		p.o.	^{35}S/ur	14.7 h[c]	5/3	Iber et al. (1977, Table 2)	This book
55	DSSD	250		p.o.	CS_2/br	4.70 h	8/16	Rogers et al. (1978, Figures 3 and 4)	This book
56						9.45 h	3/28		
57						10.7 h	6/25		
58	DSSD	800		p.o.	DSMe/pl	1.0 h	20/3	Pedersen (1980)	This book
59	DSSD	250		p.o.	DSSD/pl	7.3 h	10/10	Faiman et al. (1984)	Faiman et al. (1984)
60					DSH/pl	15.5 h	5/10		
61					DSMe/pl	22.1 h	3/10		
62					DEA/pl	13.9 h	5/10		
63					CS_2/pl	8.9 h	8/10		
64					CS_2/br	13.3 h	5/10		
65	DSSD	400	mg/kg	p.o.	DSMe/pl	6.44 h	3/5	Johansson (1986, Figure 1)	This book
66	DSH	75		i.v. inf.	DSH/pl	13.4 ± 0.7 min		Qazi et al. (1988)	Qazi et al. (1988)
67	DSH	150	mg	i.v. inf.	DSH/pl	13.1 ± 0.5 min		Qazi et al. (1988)	Qazi et al. (1988)
68	DSSD	400		p.o.	DSMe/pl	6.3 ± 1.5 h		Johansson and Stankiewicz (1989)	Johansson and Stankiewicz (1989)
69	DSSD	400		p.o.	DmSMe/pl	11.2 ± 3.0 h		Johansson and Stankiewicz (1989)	Johansson and Stankiewicz (1989)

[a] Total observation time as a multiple of calculated half-lives/number of time points available for analysis.
[b] only DSH measured; half-life for DSH measured.
[c] Two 1000 mg doses administered 4 h apart; for purposes of analysis both were treated as administered at the mid-point of this time interval.

DSSD, disulfiram; DSH, diethyldithiocarbamate; DSGa, diethyldithiocarbamate glucuronide; DSMe, diethyldithiocarbamate methyl ester; DmSMe, diethylmonothiocarbamate methyl ester; DEA, diethylamine; CS_2, carbon disulfide; SO_4 free sulfate; ^{35}SPr, protein-bound ^{35}S; i.d., intraduodenal; i.p. intraperitoneal; i.v., intravenous; p.o., per os; s.c., subcutaneous; bl, blood; br, breath; fe, faeces; pl, plasma; ur, urine.

Table 6.2 Fractional biotransformation and excretion of a disulfiram and its metabolic products

RAT

Line	Agent adm.	Dose (mg/kg)	Route	Metabolite measured	Time (h)	Fractional excretion (%)	Data source	Source of calculations
1	DSSD	~4	i.p.	SO_4/ur	∞	22.4	Eldjarn (1950a)	This book
2	DSH	60	i.v.	CS_2/br	∞	1.60 ± 0.71	Prickett and Johnston (1953, Table 1)	This book
3	DSH	600	i.v.	CS_2/br	∞	3.14 ± 0.56		This book
4	DSSD	30	i.v.	CS_2/br	∞	1.03 ± 0.19		This book
5	DSSD	60	i.v.	CS_2/br	∞	1.48 ± 0.24		
6	DSSD	~37	i.p.	DSGa/ur	∞	11.2	Strömme (1965b, Table 1)	This book
7	DSH	~93	i.p.	DSGa/ur	∞	33.8		
8	DSSD	~37	i.p.	SO_4/ur	4	8.1	Strömme (1965b, Table 1)	
9	DSH	~93	i.p.	SO_4/ur	4	10.1		
10	DSSD	~37	i.p.	CS_2/br	∞	2.5	Strömme Figure 2	This book
11	DSH	~93	i.p.	CS_2/br	∞	10.0	Gessner, T. and Jakubowski (1972, Table 3)	Gessner, T. and Jakubowski (1972)
12	DSH	114	i.v.	DSGa/ur	∞	30.0	Gessner, T. and Jakubowski (1972, Table 3)	
13				SO_4/ur	48	16.1		This book
14				^{35}S/ur	48	57.2	Gessner, T. and Jakubowski (1972, Table 3)	This book
15	DSMe	27	i.p.	SO_4/ur	48	79.4		
16	DSMe	55	i.p.	SO_4/ur	∞	62.3		
17	DSMe	27	i.p.	^{35}S/ur	48	87.0		
18	DSMe	55	i.p.	^{35}S/ur	∞	70.5		
19	DSSD	7	i.p.	^{35}S/ur	∞	67.2	Faiman et al. (1980, Table 3)	This book
20				^{35}S/fe	48	6.8		Faiman et al. (1980)
21			i.p.	CS_2/br	∞	12.4		This book
22	DSSD	7	p.o.	^{35}S/ur	48	66.8	Faiman et al. (1980, Table 4)	Faiman et al. (1980)
23				^{35}S/fe	48	6.5		
24				CS_2/br	∞	11.6		This book
25	DSSD	~137	p.o.	^{14}C/ur	∞	88.0	Neiderhiser and Fuller (1980, Figure 1 and Table 2)	This book
26				DEA/ur	24	27.8		This book
27	DSSD	40	p.o.	^{14}C/ur	96	90.6	Pedersen (1980, Tables 8 and 9)	Pedersen (1980)
28				^{14}C/fe	96	10.5		This book
29	DSSD	~146	p.o.	$^{14}C^{35}S$/ur	∞	77.5	Neiderhiser et al. (1983, Figure 1A)	This book
30	DSMe	7.7	i.p.	^{35}S/ur	∞	80.6	Faiman et al. (1983, Table 2)	This book
31				^{35}S/fe	48	15.3		Faiman et al. (1983)

No.	Compound	Dose (mg)	Route	Measurement	Time	Value	Reference	Reference
33				CS$_2$/br	48	8.5	Table 8	
34	DSSD	70	i.d.	^{35}S/ur	48	59.7	Jensen (1984, Table 8)	Jensen (1984)
35				CS$_2$/br	48	8.6	Jensen (1984, Table 8)	Jensen (1984)
36	DSSD	70	i.v.	^{35}S/ur	48	64.5	Jensen (1984, Table 8)	Jensen (1984)
37				CS$_2$/br	48	18.2	Jensen (1984, Table 8)	
38	DSSD	70	p.o.	^{35}S/ur	48	61.5	Jensen (1984, Table 8)	Jensen (1984)
39				CS$_2$/br	48	16.6		
DOG								
40	DSH	18	i.v. inf	DSMe/pl	Fr[a] 27.4±10.3		Cobby et al. (1978)	Cobby et al. (1978)
41	DSSD	7	i.v.	DSH/pl	Fr[a] 29.8±26.7		Cobby et al. (1978)	Jensen (1984)
42	DSH	7	i.v.	DSMe/pl	Fr[a] 46.6±11.3		Jensen (1984)	
HUMAN	mg							
43	DSSD	2000	p.o.	^{35}S/ur	144	73.7	Eldjarn (1950b, Table 3)	Eldjarn (1950b)
44				SO$_4$/ur	∞	63.4		This book
45	DSSD	2000[b]	p.o.	DSH/ur	∞	1.64	Linderholm and Berg (1951, Table 1)	This book
46	DSSD	250	p.o.	^{35}S/ur	∞	42.4±18.0	Iber et al. (1977, Table 2)	This book
47				^{35}S/fe	120	6.6±4.5		Iber et al. (1977)
48				CS$_2$/br	120	29.6±14.1		
49	DSSD	500	p.o.	CS$_2$/br	∞	44.5	Merlevede and Casier (1961)	Merlevede and Casier (1961)
50	DSSD	750	p.o.	CS$_2$/br	∞	37.8		
51	DSSD	1000	p.o.	CS$_2$/br	∞	58.7		
52	DSH	50	p.o.	CS$_2$/br	∞	28.2	Merlevede and Casier (1961, Table 2)	Merlevede and Casier (1961)
53	DSH	100	p.o.	CS$_2$/br	∞	34.0		
54	DSH	250	p.o.	CS$_2$/br	∞	62.3		
55	DSH	500	p.o.	CS$_2$/br	∞	81.9		
56	DSSD	250	p.o.	CS$_2$/br	∞	13.1±1.4	Rogers et al. (1978, Figure 4)	
57	DSSD	250	p.o.	DSCa/ur	∞	1.7±0.3	Faiman et al. (1984, Table 3)	Faiman et al. (1984)
58				DEA/ur	∞	1.6±0.8		
59				CS$_2$/br	∞	22.4±0.5		

[a] Fraction of parent compound transformed to metabolite.
[b] Two 1000 mg doses administered 4 h apart; for purposes of analysis both were treated as administered at mid-point of this time interval.

For abbreviations, see Table 6.1.

Table 6.3 Volumes of distribution of disulfiram and its metabolic products in experimental animals

Line	Agent adm.	Dose (mg/kg)	Route	Entity measured	Volume of distributions (l/kg)	Data source	Source of calculations
RAT							
1	DSH	~93	i.p.	DSH/pl	0.197	Strömme (1965b, Table 2)	This book
DOG							
2	DSH	18	i.v. inf.	DSH/pl	0.161±0.023	Cobby et al. (1978)	Cobby et al. (1978)
3	DSMe	19	i.v. inf.	DSMe/pl	2.53±0.95		
4	DSSD	7	i.v.	DSSD/pl	69.2±108.4	Jensen (1984)	Jensen (1984)
5	DSH	7	i.v.	DSH/pl	0.436±0.113		
6	DSMe	7.7	i.v.	DSMe/pl	0.606±0.351		
HUMAN							
7	DSH	75	i.v. inf.	DSH/pl	0.290±0.007	Qazi et al. (1988)	Qazi et al. (1988)
8	DSH	150	i.v. inf.	DSH/pl	0.275+0.006		

See Table 6.1 for abbreviations.

half-life by the relationship $t_{1/2} = 0.693/K$. Values of $t_{1/2}$ are listed in Table 6.1 and those of q_∞, the fractional excretion, in Table 6.2. The latter, being a prediction of the total amount of metabolite that would be eventually excreted, is based on the totality of the data. Thus, q_∞ may differ somewhat from the cumulated amount observed to have been excreted at the time of the last observation. In Table 6.3 are listed the values of the apparent volume of distribution in the few instances where these are available.

In fitting data to equation (6.1) a zero time shift was performed when necessary to insure that only the terminal exponential portion of the concentration–time curve was evaluated. Expiratory carbon disulfide (CS_2) excretion rate data were converted to cumulative excretion data by use of the trapezoidal rule. The CS_2 excretion data uniformly show a clear delay in the appearance, and thereby the onset of biotransformation, a delay occasioned, presumably, by phenomena related to absorption following oral administration. Accordingly, such data were fitted to the following model:

$$q = q_\infty(1 - e^{-K(t-T)}) \tag{6.3}$$

where T is an additional parameter relating to the absorption-induced delay.

The fitting of the simple models of equations (6.1)–(6.3) to metabolite data represents the use of simplifying working assumptions. Though the use of more complex models would have been appropriate, the numerical paucity of the data at hand precluded consideration of such models. Even so, as already noted by Cobby *et al.* (1978), it is necessary to recognize the limitations of kinetic analysis when the number of data points barely exceeds the number of unknown parameters; the resulting half-lives need to be viewed, therefore, as ball-park figures. To emphasize this, the values of these parameters, usually given to three significant figures in the tables, when cited in the text are generally rounded off to two significant figures. To give the reader some sense of the pharmacokinetic limitations of the database, we report, in Table 6.1, the total observation time (expressed in terms of half-lives) and the number of time points available for each analysis.

6.3 URINARY EXCRETION OF DISULFIRAM METABOLITES

6.3.1 Experimental animal data

The excretion of radioisotope label following administration of DSSD, synthesized from ^{14}C-labeled diethylamine and ^{35}S-labeled carbon disulfide, can be taken as a starting point for consideration of the pharmacokinetics of DSSD and its metabolites. Neiderhiser *et al.* (1983) administered this compound to rats p.o. and reported on the urinary excretion of the radioactivity; from their graph, computation yields an apparent half-life of 16 h for the radioisotope label (Table 6.1, line 33). Earlier, Neiderhiser and Fuller (1980) had reported on the urinary excretion of ^{14}C label following the p.o. administration of ^{14}C-DSSD to rats. Analysis of those data yields an apparent half-life of 15 h (Table 6.1, line 28). Pedersen (1980) has reported an apparent urinary excretion half-life of 18 h following p.o. administration of ^{14}C-DSSD to rats (Table 6.1, line 30), with 91% of the administered label being thus excreted by 96 h (Table 6.2, line 27); another 11% was excreted in the feces (Table 6.2, line 28).

The analysis of the data of Neiderhiser and Fuller (1980) indicates that eventually 88% of the administered ^{14}C label would be excreted in the urine (Table 6.2, line 25); at 24 h, when 40% of the label had been excreted, 4/7 of it was in a conjugated form, the remaining fraction (28%) was reported to be diethylamine (Et_2NH) (Table 6.2, line 26). This is a much higher proportion than the 1.6% of the administered DSSD reported by Faiman *et al.* (1984) to be excreted as Et_2NH by humans (Table 6.2, line 58). Neiderhiser and Fuller (1980) had, however, collected the urine in 1 N hydrochloric acid, while no such collection method was specified by Faiman *et al.* (1984). Not only is Et_2NH a volatile compound, while its hydrochloride is not, but also DSH is acid labile and any that might have been excreted would have been converted to Et_2NH. Conversely, under basic conditions Et_2NH and CS_2 combine to form DSH, and thus the report of Linderholm and Berg (1951) that, in individuals co-administered DSSD with 6–8 g sodium bicarbonate, 1.6% of the administered DSSD is excreted as DSH may be related (Table 6.2, line 45). Based on the data of Linderholm and Berg (1951), the apparent half-life derived from this excretion was calculated to be 4.4 h (Table 6.1, line 48). Strömme (1965b), who did not take similar measures to alkalinize the urine, reported no DSH to have been excreted following i.p. administration of ^{35}S-DSSD to rats.

As regards metabolites derived from the dithiocarboxyl portion of the DSSD molecule, the data of Faiman *et al.* (1980) yield, upon computation, a half-life of 11 h for the urinary excretion of the ^{35}S label (Table 6.1, line 25) following i.p. administration of ^{35}S-DSSD to rats. Faiman *et al.* (1980) also reported that in the 48 h post administration of ^{35}S-DSSD i.p. or p.o. to rats, 67% of the ^{35}S label was excreted in urine (Table 6.2, lines 19 and 22). In parallel experiments in the same species, Jensen (1984) reported values of 55, 62, 65, and 60% following i.p., i.v., p.o. and intraduodenal administration, respectively (Table 6.2, lines 32, 36, 38, and 34).

Following administration of ^{35}S-DSSD, Strömme (1965b) identified the S-glucuronide (DSGa) and sulfate as the main labelled urinary metabolites excreted by rats, with the glucuronide being excreted much more rapidly (calculated half-life 48 min; Table 6.1, line 12) than the sulfate. Though sulfate excretion was followed for too short a period to allow calculation of a half-life, that calculated from the data of Eldjarn (1950a) in the same species is 13 h (Table 6.1, line 4). Application of (6.2) to this information indicates that the fractional DSSD urinary excretions as DSGa and sulfate were 11 and 22%, respectively (Table 6.2, lines 6 and 1).

6.3.2 Human data

From data of Eldjarn (1950b) and Iber *et al.* (1977), respectively, quite similar values (14 and 15 h; Table 6.1, lines 47 and 54) are obtained for the apparent urinary excretion half-lives of label administered as ^{35}S-DSSD. The figure derived from the data of Iber *et al.* (1977) is especially interesting, being the mean of the half-lives for urinary excretion of label by 19 different subjects, all patients in an alcoholism treatment program. In general, as shown in Fig. 6.1, these half-lives are shorter in individuals receiving chronic disulfiram therapy. Also, no patient had a half-life of 15–19 h, suggesting a bimodality in their distribution. On average, the patients studied by Iber *et al.* (1977) excreted 42% of the administered label in urine, and 7% in feces (Table 6.2, lines 46 and 47). Although Eldjarn (1950b) reported a somewhat higher figure (74%; Table 6.2, line 43), it is within the range of those of Iber *et al.* (1977). Eldjarn (1950b) also determined the fraction eliminated as inorganic sulfate, and at 63% of the dose (Table 6.2, line 44), it is clearly the preeminent urinary metabolite derived from the dithiocarboxyl portion of the DSSD molecule.

There is little quantitative information regarding human urinary excretion of DSGa, the other major sulfur-containing DSSD metabolite found in rat urine. Kaslander (1963) recovered 0.75% of the DSSD dose from human urine as DSGa when isolating it for purposes of identification. Because of the many and laborious steps involved, he stressed this should be considered only as a minimum value. Faiman *et al.* (1984) reported 1.7% of the DSSD dose to be excreted as DSGa, however the assay method used was not specific for DSGa.

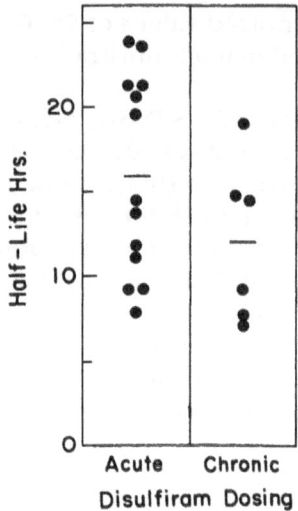

Figure 6.1 Plot of the apparent half-lives for urinary excretion of ^{35}S label by patients administered ^{35}S-disulfiram. (Left) Patients given a single dose of disulfiram. (Right) Patients who had been taking disulfiram for at least a month. Values computed from the data in Table 2 of Iber *et al.* (1977) by application of equation (6.2).

6.4 PULMONARY EXCRETION OF DISULFIRAM METABOLITES

6.4.1 Human data

The most detailed information regarding the pulmonary excretion of CS_2 following DSSD administration derives from human studies. Cobby *et al.* (1978) analyzed the data of Merlevede and Casier (1961) and reported that the terminal half-life for pulmonary CS_2 excretion following DSSD administration was 12 h (Table 6.1, line 49). The rates of pulmonary CS_2 excretion following DSSD administration to humans have also been the subject of a report by Rogers *et al.* (1978). One individual (Subject 1 in their Fig. 2) received 250 mg DSSD on two occasions: analysis of these data indicates half-lives of 9 and 11 h, respectively (Table 6.1, lines 56 and 57). Another individual had been taking DSSD chronically (their Fig. 1); analysis of the rate of pulmonary CS_2 output by this individual indicates a half-life of 5 h (Table 6.1, line 55). This much shorter value might be attributable to induction by DSSD of its own metabolism. [Such induction has been shown by Neiderhiser and Fuller (1980) to occur in rats, a 21-day pretreatment with DSSD lowering the apparent half-life for the urinary excretion of

^{14}C-DSSD label from 14.9 to 6.9 h.] From the report of Rogers *et al.* (1978) it is possible to calculate the fraction of the 250 mg DSSD dose exhaled as CS_2, on each of two occasions, by each of the two individuals studied (subjects 1 and 2 in their Fig. 4). This gives values of 15 and 13% for subject 1 and 12% on both occasions for subject 2 (overall mean for the two subjects 13%; Table 6.2, line 56). Merlevede and Casier (1961), on the other hand, reported that the CS_2 their subjects exhaled accounted for 45, 38 and 59%, respectively, of the 500, 750 and 1000 mg of DSSD doses administered (Table 6.2, lines 49, 50 and 51), while those of Iber *et al.* (1977) averaged 30% (Table 6.2, line 48). More recently, Faiman *et al.* (1984) reported 22% of 250 mg doses of DSSD administered orally to alcoholics to be excreted as CS_2 (Table 6.2, line 59); these authors also reported the half-lives for respiratory and blood CS_2 to be 13 and 9 h, respectively (Table 6.1, lines 64 and 63).

6.4.2 Experimental animal data

Prickett and Johnston (1953), Strömme (1965b) and Faiman *et al.* (1980) have reported on the time course of pulmonary CS_2 excretion following DSSD administration to rats. All agree that the fraction of the administered dose that can be accounted for as expiratory CS_2 in the first 2–4 h is quite low. Thus at 2 h they report 1.8% post 30 mg/kg and 2.5% post 60 mg/kg i.v. (Prickett and Johnston); 1.8% post 37 mg/kg i.p. (Strömme); 1.1 and 1.0% following 7 mg/kg i.p. and p.o., respectively (Faiman *et al.*, 1980). After the initial 2-h period, Prickett and Johnston (1953) and Strömme (1965b) both found the CS_2 excretion to taper and ceased collecting at 3 and 4 h, respectively. Faiman *et al.* (1980), who had not collected prior to the 2 h point, continued to collect for 48 h by which time they could account for 12–13% of the DSSD dose in this manner (Table 6.2, lines 21 and 24). Analysis of these data suggests half-lives of 5.5 and 7.5 h, respectively (Table 6.1, lines 26 and 27). The data of Prickett and Johnston (1953), and those of Strömme (1965b) indicate, however, a rapid initial CS_2 excretion (Table 6.1, lines 7, 8 and 22) which is not compatible with these long half-lives, raising the question of whether CS_2 formation from DSSD might reflect more than one process. Jensen (1984) has examined the effect of the route of administration on the fraction of ^{35}S-DSSD administered to rats that undergo pulmonary excretion as CS_2 during the first 48 h post adminis-tration. He reported the amount thus excreted after i.v. or p.o. administration (18 and 17%, respectively; Table 6.2, lines 37 and 39) to be markedly greater than after i.p. and intraduodenal administration (8.5 and 8.6%, respectively; Table 6.2, lines 33 and 35).

6.5 PLASMA DISULFIRAM AND METABOLITES FOLLOWING ITS ADMINISTRATION

6.5.1 Plasma disulfiram levels

A significant controversy exists whether it is possible, without very special stabilizing procedures, to detect DSSD in blood, plasma or serum following its administration, in quantities sufficient to allow its measurement (see Chapters 3 and 4). Most groups which have attempted to measure such levels have been unable to detect any measurable quantity of DSSD in these fluids at any time following its administration (Strömme, 1965b; Sauter *et al.*, 1977; Pedersen, 1980; Masso and Kramer, 1981; Johansson, 1986). Johansson (1988), using a DSSD-stabilizing procedure that involved acidification to pH 5.5 with acetic acid and addition of 10 mM diethylenetriaminepentaacetic acid, reported being able to detect DSSD in the blood of alcoholics administered 400 mg daily, but only after more than 7 days of therapy.

Two groups have reported finding DSSD in plasma at earlier times; Davidson and Wilson (1979) noted level in humans to vary 600-fold, a variation which could not be explained by differences in sampling times. In contrast, Faiman and co-workers have reported extensively on DSSD tissue levels following its administration to mice (Faiman *et al.*, 1977, 1978a), rats (Faiman *et al.*, 1980, Jensen, 1984), dogs (Faiman *et al.*, 1977, 1978a, Jensen, 1984) and humans (Jensen *et al.*, 1982; Faiman *et al.*, 1984). In mice administered 200 mg/kg ^{35}S-DSSD i.p., Faiman *et al.* (1978a) found the drug to disappear rapidly from plasma and to be undetectable after 45 min. Following administration of 200 mg/kg DSSD i.p. to rats, Faiman *et al.* (1978b) were unable to detect it in plasma after 45 min, though later Faiman *et al.* (1980) reported it as present in rat plasma at 1 and 5 h following administration of a 7 mg/kg dose and Jensen (1984) reported plasma concentrations of ^{35}S-DSSD to peak at 8 and 24 h following p.o. administration of a 70 mg/kg dose. In the dog, Faiman *et al.* (1978a) reported graphically that the disappearance of ^{35}S-DSSD, administered i.v. in polyethylene glycol, was rapid, no detectable levels being observed after 30 min; Jensen (1984) later reported the half-lives of DSSD, following its i.v. administration in dimethylsulfoxide to three dogs, to be 7.3, 9.3 and 40.8 min, respectively (average 19 min; Table 6.1, line 41). Finally, Faiman *et al.* (1984) have reported that, following its p.o. administration, the plasma half-life of DSSD in humans is 7 h (Table 6.1, line 59).

Jensen (1984) argues that, because he found 'marked variability' in plasma concentrations of DSSD and its metabolites following i.v. administration of DSSD, the variability observed after oral administration by

Davidson and Wilson (1979) and Jensen *et al.* (1982) cannot be fully ascribed to interindividual differences in absorption. However, he also reports that the infusion over a period of 90–120 s of 7 mg/kg DSSD in 2.7–3.4 ml dimethylsulfoxide was associated with a fall in heart rate from 90 to 30 beats/min in all three dogs, an effect not seen following injections of the dimethylsulfoxide vehicle alone. The hemodynamic consequences of such extreme bradycardia on drug distribution may have contributed to the observed variability in plasma levels. Additionally, interpretation of these results will be difficult as long as the analytical controversy remains unresolved (section 4.1).

6.5.2 Plasma levels of free diethyldithiocarbamate

DSH appears, at first sight, to present fewer difficulties of estimation. In keeping with this, a number of investigators have reported measurable quantities of it in blood following DSSD administration. There is a lack of unanimity in this regard, however, and the information regarding the kinetics of DSH disappearance when generated *in vivo* from DSSD are rather disparate. Prickett and Johnston (1953) reported that, in rats administered 60 mg/kg DSSD i.v., DSH disappeared from the blood quite quickly, only a trace being detectable at 60 min. Based on their data, DSH would appear to have had a half-life of just 10 min (Table 6.1, line 9). Pedersen (1980), following the administration of radiolabeled DSSD, found only a trace of DSH in the plasma of one of two rats at 0.5 h, and neither he nor Strömme (1965b) could detect any at 1 h. Cobby *et al.* (1978) analyzed the data of Faiman *et al.* (1977) for DSH levels in a dog administered 20 mg/kg ^{35}S-DSSD i.v. in polyethylene glycol and obtained a value of 30 min for the apparent half-life (Table 6.1, line 37). Giles *et al.* (1982) administered DSSD in 80% ethanol i.v. to rats; they reported a biphasic plasma DSH curve, with a terminal half-life of 95 min (Table 6.1, line 31).

In humans administered DSSD, some measure of DSH half-life can be gained from the data of Johansson (1986). The plasma levels he reported showed marked variability at a secondary peak, 8 h post administration, yet since they fell to baseline levels by 24 h, a half-life in excess of 6 h appears unlikely. In contrast, Faiman *et al.* (1984) have reported a half-life of 15.5 h for DSH in humans administered DSSD. The data from which that value is obtained are odd, in that the plasma levels of DSH, the metabolite, rose much more quickly and peaked well before those of DSSD, the parent compound, a phenomenon for which it is difficult to envisage a pharmacokinetic mechanism. The DSH blood levels observed by Jensen (1984) in two of three dogs administered

DSSD i.v. show minimal regression on time during the 6-h observation period. Likewise the DSH blood levels observed by Jensen (1984) in rats administered ^{35}S-DSSD i.p. and p.o., remained elevated for the 3-day duration of the experiment. The striking difference between the results of Pedersen (1980), Giles *et al.* (1982), Faiman *et al.* (1984) and Jensen (1984), all of whom used similar analytical methods, suggests that concerns raised by Pedersen (1980) regarding *ex vivo* conversions [between DSSD, DSH (free and bound) and diethyl-dithiocarbamic acid methyl ester (DSMe)] need to be further considered, particularly in assays employing solvent extraction. The concern regarding such *ex vivo* conversions is heightened by the fact that, following administration of ^{14}C-DSSD to rats (Pedersen, 1980), the sum of DSSD, DSH (free and bound) and DSMe in plasma accounts for only a small fraction of the radioactivity in blood. Thus Pedersen (1980) reported that from 1 to 48 h the sum of these entities accounted for 2–6% of the radioactivity in plasma and, in turn, at 48 h (data not available for earlier times) plasma radioactivity accounted for only 4.8% of that in whole blood.

6.5.3 Plasma levels of protein-bound diethyldithiocarbamate

Both Strömme (1965b) and Pedersen (1980) have reported significant plasma levels of protein-bound radioisotope label from which DSH was released upon treatment with a thiol. Strömme (1965b), sampling between 1 and 4 h post DSSD administration, was able to identify 14–24% of the plasma ^{35}S as protein-bound; Pedersen (1980), sampling between 0.5 and 96 h post administration, observed that only 1–8% of the plasma ^{14}C could be accounted for in this manner. From Strömme's data, the apparent half-life for the disappearance of protein-bound DSH from plasma was calculated to be 117 min (Table 6.1, line 17).

6.5.4 Plasma levels of diethyldithiocarbamic acid methyl ester

Plasma levels of DSMe have been followed in humans subsequent to DSSD administration by Pedersen (1980), Faiman *et al.* (1984), Johansson (1986), Johansson and Stankiewicz (1989), Johansson *et al.* (1991) and Andersen (1991). Pedersen's data from one subject suggest a terminal half-life of 60 min (Table 6.1, line 58). Johansson's very clean data from five alcoholics show a 6 h terminal half-life (Table 6.1, line 65). Johansson and Stankiewicz, who found the peak plasma concentration time in nine alcoholics administered 400 mg DSSD to be 1.8 ± 0.4 h, reported a mean half-life for DSMe of 6.3 ± 1.5 h (Table 6.1, line 68). Faiman *et al.* (1984) reported a half-life of 15 h (Table 6.1, line 60).

Faiman *et al.* (1977) have reported graphically (their Fig. 2) on the plasma DSMe levels in dogs following the i.v. administration of ^{35}S-DSSD. Cobby *et al.* (1978) calculated the half-life associated with these data to be 22 min, but have also questioned the separation procedures of the assay, noting that Faiman *et al.* (1977) reported the plasma levels of both DSH and DSMe to be 'declining virtually in parallel while exhibiting similar concentration magnitudes', a difficult phenomenon to envisage pharmacokinetically for a compound and its metabolite.

Andersen (1991) performed a comparative bioavailability study of the effervescent DSSD formulation marketed in Denmark by A/S Dumex and the non-effervescent DSSD formulation available in the United Kingdom from CP Pharmaceuticals. The cross-over study involved 24 volunteers each of whom received a single administration of 800 mg of each of the two DSSD formulations. Serum concentrations of DSMe were followed for 24 h after each administration. Relative bioavailability was deduced from a comparison of the areas under the curve (AUC) for serum DSMe. The mean AUC for the effervescent formulation was 2337 ± 1294 ng h/ml while that for the non-effervescent formulation was 855 ± 559 ng h/ml. On this basis Andersen estimated the bioavailability of the non-effervescent formulation to be 34% of the effervescent one. For both formulations the time corresponding to peak serum concentration were similar (3.8 ± 1.4 h for the effervescent formulation, 3.7 ± 1.0 h for the non-effervescent formulation) but the peak serum concentrations differed significantly ($P < 0.0001$) being 324 ± 168 ng/ml and 124 ± 63 ng/ml for the effervescent and non-effervescent formulations respectively.

6.5.5 Plasma levels of diethylmonothiocarbamic acid methyl ester

Johansson and Stankiewicz have reported the plasma half-life for the diethylmonothiocarbamic acid methyl ester (DmSMe) in three alcoholics administered DSSD to be 11.2 ± 3.0 h (Table 6.1, line 69) with peak concentration occurring at 3.3 ± 1.2 h. It should be noted, however that this metabolite could only be detected in the plasma of 3 of 10 alcoholics administered DSSD.

6.5.6 Plasma levels of the *S*-glucuronide of diethyldithiocarbamic acid

DSGa is another metabolite the plasma levels of which have been followed after DSSD administration (Strömme, 1965b). The apparent plasma half-life computed from these data is 55 min (Table 6.1, line 18), a value similar to the 48 min value obtained from the urinary DSGa excretion data of Strömme (1965b).

6.6 DIETHYLDITHIOCARBAMATE AND METABOLITES FOLLOWING ITS ADMINISTRATION

6.6.1 Pulmonary carbon disulfide excretion

Merlevede and Casier (1961) have reported that the excretion of CS_2 in breath following DSH administration is quite rapid. These workers administered DSH orally in doses of 50, 100, 250 and 500 mg p.o. to humans and collected CS_2 exhaled in the breath until the excretion ceased. Analysis of their data yields apparent half-lives of 36, 32, 46 and 41 min, respectively, for pulmonary CS_2 excretion (Table 6.1, lines 50–53). These half-lives are dramatically shorter than the corresponding ones observed following DSSD administration. As suggested by Strömme (1965b), this could be a reflection of acid-catalyzed decomposition of DSH, occasioned by its oral administration and exposure to the stomach environment. Merlevede and Casier (1961) also reported that as the dose of DSH increased so did the fraction of it that could be accounted for in terms of exhaled CS_2 (Table 6.2, lines 52–55). This suggests that pulmonary CS_2 excretion is less easily saturable than other pathways available for DSH or CS_2 disposition, or that some CS_2 in breath enters it via the esophagus. Even following the i.p. administration of ^{35}S-DSH, however, the apparent half-life for the pulmonary excretion of CS_2, as calculated from the data of Strömme (1965b), was only half as long (31 min; Table 6.1, line 22), as that following ^{35}S-DSSD administration (63 min; Table 6.1, line 21). Furthermore, Strömme reported that a greater fraction of the dose was excreted as CS_2 when rats were given ^{35}S-DSH (10%; Table 6.2, line 11) than when they were given ^{35}S-DSSD (2.5%; Table 6.2, line 10). Because different doses were used, it is not possible to determine whether this difference is a significant one.

6.6.2 Plasma diethyldithiocarbamate levels: free and bound

The AUC (area under the curve) figure obtained for plasma DSH by Bodenner *et al.* (1986b) following i.p. administration of DSH in a 250 mg/kg dose was only 54% of that obtained following i.v. administration of the same dose. This indicates that first-pass hepatic metabolism results in the degradation of almost 50% of DSH administered i.p.

The data from most studies suggest that the plasma half-life of DSH administered as such is quite short. A value of 5.2 min results from the data of Strömme (1965b) in rats following i.p. administration (Table 6.1, line 14); Cobby *et al.* (1978) reported a half-life of 3.4 min in dogs infused DSH i.v. (Table 6.1, line 39); Bodenner *et al.* (1986a) have published values of 10 and 11 min in mice administered DSH i.p. and s.c., respectively (Table 6.1, lines 2–3), values of 10, 20 and 21 min in rats administered the agent i.v., i.p. and s.c., respectively (Table 6.1, lines 34–36), and a value of 8.75 min in dogs following i.v. administration (Table 6.1, line 45). Lieder and Borch (1985) reported a value of 7.0 min in the dog (Table 6.1, line 44). Qazi *et al.* (1988) have published values of 13.4 ± 0.7 and 13.1 ± 0.5 min in humans infused with doses of 75 and 150 mg/kg DSH, respectively (Table 6.1, lines 66 and 67). In contrast, Jensen (1984) reported half-lives of 19.1, 26.6 and 138 min for DSH in three dogs to whom it was administered i.v. in dimethylsulfoxide (average 61 min; Table 6.1, line 42).

Cobby *et al.* (1978) reported an apparent volume of distribution in dogs for DSH of 0.16 l/kg (Table 6.3; line 2) and a total body clearance of 0.0331 l/min/kg. A relatively similar value for the volume of distribution (0.20 l/kg; Table 6.3, line 1) is obtained from the rat data of Strömme (1965b). Qazi *et al.* (1988) have published values of 0.290 ± 0.007 and 0.275 ± 0.006 in humans infused with 75 and 150 mg/kg doses of DSH (Table 6.3, lines 7 and 8). The value reported by Jensen (1984) for dogs was higher (0.44 l/kg; Table 6.3, line 5).

In addition to plasma levels of free DSH, Strömme (1965b) estimated the levels of protein-bound ^{35}S of which 45–83% could be released by GSH and 32–74% could be identified as DSH. The rate of disappearance of the protein-bound ^{35}S from plasma was relatively slow, the apparent half-life for the process being 134 min (Table 6.1, line 15).

6.6.3 Plasma levels of diethyldithiocarbamic acid methyl ester

Cobby *et al.* (1978), in a set of elegant experiments, infused dogs with DSH and DSMe and reported that 27% of administered DSH is methylated to yield DSMe (Table 6.2, line 40). Using less direct methods, Jensen (1984) found 47% of administered DSH to be metabolized to DSMe (Table 6.2, line 42). The plasma half-life of DSMe appears to be substantially longer than that of DSH. Cobby *et al.* (1978) reported the plasma half-life of DSMe in dogs to be 49 min (Table 6.1, line 40). Under parallel circumstances, Jensen (1984) reported a value for the plasma half-life of DSMe of 57 min in dogs (Table 6.1, line 43). Cobby *et al.* (1978) also undertook retrospective kinetic evaluations of the plasma

DSH data which Prickett and Johnston (1953) had obtained by a rather non-specific method, and of the plasma ^{35}S data obtained by Strömme following i.p. administration of ^{35}S-DSH. Both sets of data evidenced biexponential decay, and this Cobby *et al.* (1978) interpreted as representing combined DSH and DSMe values. On this basis, they computed values of 1.3 and 20 min (Table 6.1, lines 10 and 11) for DSH and DSMe half-lives, respectively, from the data of Prickett and Johnston (1953). Likewise, from the data of Strömme (1965b) they computed half-life values for DSH and DSMe of 8 and 76 min, respectively (Table 6.1, lines 19 and 20).

DSMe is a more lipid-soluble compound than DSH. In keeping with this, Cobby *et al.* (1978) found the volume of distribution for DSMe in dogs (2.5 l/kg; Table 6.3, line 3) to be 15-fold higher than the volume of distribution for DSH in this species. Surprisingly, Jensen (1984) reported the volume of distribution for DSMe (0.61 l/kg; Table 6.3, line 6) to be only 1.4-fold higher than that for DSH. Cobby *et al.* (1978) also reported total body clearance for DSMe to be 0.0319 l/min/kg.

6.6.4 Excretion of sulfate and the *S*-glucuronide of diethyldithiocarbamic acid

The two major urinary metabolites of ^{35}S-DSH in rats are DSGa and sulfate. From the urinary excretion data of Strömme (1965b), the apparent half-life for DSGa excretion in urine, following i.p. administration of DSH to rats, is 45 min (Table 6.1, line 13) and 34% of the administered DSH is excreted in this manner (Table 6.2, line 7). Similar results were obtained by Gessner, T. and Jakubowski (1972), who reported 30% of the administered DSH to be excreted as DSGa (Table 6.2, line 12). They also reported 16% of the dose to be excreted as sulfate (Table 6.2, line 13). Overall, they found 57% of the ^{35}S label administered as ^{35}S-DSH to undergo urinary elimination in the first 48 h post administration (Table 6.2, line 14).

Following i.p. administration of ^{35}S-DSMe to rats, on the other hand, a higher fraction appears to be excreted as sulfate. Thus, Gessner, T. and Jakubowski (1972), using two doses (27 and 55 mg/kg), reported 62–79% of the DSMe to be excreted as sulfate (Table 6.2, lines 15 and 16). The apparent half-life for the process was 2.7 h (Table 6.1, line 23). Overall, 70 to 87% of the label administered as ^{35}S-DSMe was found by Gessner, T. and Jakubowski (1972) to undergo urinary excretion (Table 6.2, lines 17 and 18), a finding since confirmed by Faiman *et al.* (1983), who additionally reported 15% of the ^{35}S dose to be excreted in feces (Table 6.2, lines 30 and 31).

6.6.5 Tissue distribution

The tissue distribution of radioactivity at 5, 10, 20 and 45 min following administration of ^{35}S-DSH (200 mg/kg as Imuthiol by retroorbital i.v. injection) to mice has been investigated by Guillaumin *et al.* (1986). Because of the short half-life of DSH in the mouse (10 min, Table 6.1) only the activity at the 5 minute time point can be considered to be primarily due to DSH. Given the immunomodulating properties of DSH, it is striking that of the 11 tissues examined, the two with the highest activity were the spleen and the thymus. The activity in these two tissues was, respectively, 1.8- and 1.3-fold higher than that in the liver and 6.7- and 4.8-fold higher than in plasma. Over the subsequent 45 min the radioactivity of the plasma declined exponentially with a half-life of *ca* 7.4 min; the activities of the spleen and kidney did so in parallel. The activity in the thymus, the liver, the lymph nodes and the neocortex, on the other hand, remained constant or increased slightly. Guillaumin *et al.* (1986) extracted the neocortex with pentane and reported the presence therein of DSMe. No information is available, however, regarding what portion of the neocortical radioactivity could be accounted for in this manner, or whether DSMe represented a significant portion of the radioactivity in the thymus, lymph nodes, or liver.

7

Heavy metals: effects of diethyldithiocarbamate and disulfiram administration

7.1	INTRODUCTION	65
7.2	THALLIUM	69
	7.2.1 Use in single-photon emission computed tomography	70
	7.2.2 Treatment of thallotoxicosis	70
7.3	ZINC	71
7.4	CADMIUM	73
7.5	LEAD	79
7.6	NICKEL	81
	7.6.1 Treatment of nickel dermatitis	83
	7.6.2 Prevention of nickel subsulfide tumors	84
	7.6.3 Treatment of nickel carbonyl intoxication	84
7.7	COPPER	85
7.8	MERCURY	88
	7.8.1 Methyl mercury	90
7.9	PLATINUM	90
7.10	POLONIUM	93

7.1 INTRODUCTION

Diethyldithiocarbamate (DSH) is an avid ligand of heavy metals with which it forms complexes that have a much higher lipid solubility than have the heavy metal ions themselves (Chapter 2). The lipid solubility characteristic of the metals are thereby changed and this results in their patterns of distribution being altered following DSH or disulfiram (DSSD) administration. One consistent finding is that the levels of the metal found in brain are increased. Urinary excretion and kidney levels, on the other hand, are usually decreased, an advantage, since many heavy metals are nephrotoxic. Concurrently, an increase in the fecal elimination of the heavy metal is usually observed (Fig. 7.1).

The physico-chemical aspects of heavy metal transfer through membranes and the chelation chemistry of these metals is beyond the scope of this book; the interested reader is referred to the work of Williams (1981) for the coverage of the former and to the discussion of Andersen (1984) relative to cadmium for coverage of the latter.

Whether chelation with DSSD or DSH will result in an increase or a decrease in the body burden of a heavy metal, or for that matter its toxicity, depends on many factors. The effect the agents will have on the excretion rate of the metal is only one of these; another is the effect of these agents on the absorption of the metal from food. There is some evidence that systemically administered DSSD or DSH can increase the efficiency of the latter process. Moreover, the manner in

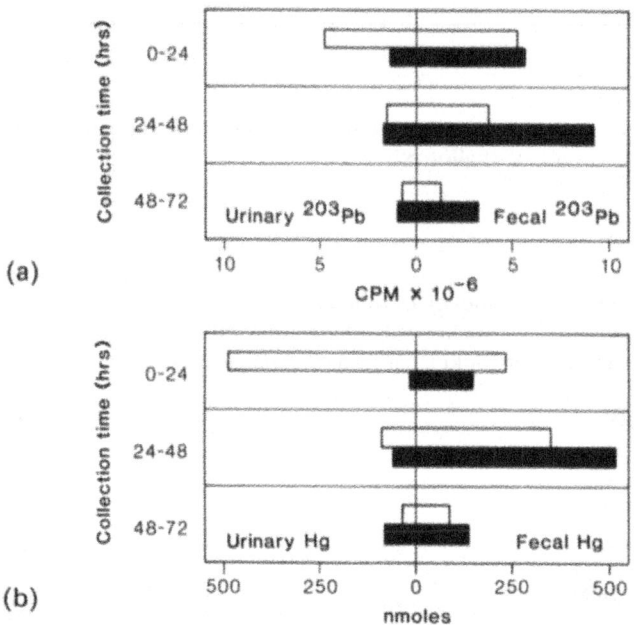

Figure 7.1   Effect of diethyldithiocarbamate (DSH) on urinary and fecal excretion of heavy metals in rats. Abscissa, amount of heavy metal excreted. Ordinate, collection period following heavy metal administration. (a) Excretion of ^{203}Pb in controls (open bars) and DSH-treated (closed bars) rats. Animals were treated with 28.6 nmol ^{203}Pb/kg as acetate and 10 min later were administered DSH (298 mg/kg, i.p.). Modified from Oskarssonn (1983). (b) Excretion of ^{203}Hg in controls (open bars) and DSH-treated (closed bars) rats. Animals were administered DSH (75 mg/kg i.v.) both 2 h prior and immediately following treatment with ^{203}HgCl$_2$ (5 µmol/kg i.v.). Modified from Aaseth *et al.* (1981).

which chelation affects absorption and excretion need not parallel each other as the dose of DSSD or DSH is increased. For instance, Sunderman (1964) reported, on the basis of metabolic balance studies, that a patient with Wilson's disease, originally in a positive balance for both copper and nickel, remained so following administration of low doses of DSH. A negative balance was achieved, however, when the DSH dose was raised. Such metabolic balance studies are very seldom undertaken be it in clinical or experimental animal studies. Yet, conclusions regarding the effect of DSSD or DSH administration on the body burdens of a heavy metal cannot be made solely on the basis of the reported effect of such administration on the metal's levels in tissues and excreta.

Whether the effects of the redistribution will result in an increase or decrease of the heavy metal level in a particular compartment, or tissue, will depend on the existent concentration gradients. Thus, for instance, following administration of copper or zinc, dosing with DSH results in increased brain levels of these elements; yet administered by itself, DSH can reduce the endogenous brain levels of these metals.

The formation of binary heavy metal–DSH complexes speeds the passage of the metals through lipoid barriers. The manner in which this affects toxicity can depend on the stability and inertness of the chelate. For instance, $Pt(DS)_2$ is rather stable and inert, while $Tl(DS)$ appears to have low stability and its rapid formation *in situ* can lead to increased toxicity. Although such complexes have high two-phase extraction constants (section 2.3), yet, even in a system such as chloroform–water, the metal is easily and quantitatively displaced by another with a higher extraction constant. Estimation of the concentrations of DS complexes in a biological matrix has seldom been attempted: Johansson and Stankiewicz (1985) have estimated the levels of $Cu(DS)_2$ in plasma following addition of DSSD to plasma or blood (sections 3.2 and 4.3.2). Given DS complexes have a tendency to become adsorbed on surfaces such as teflon and glass even after siliconization (Häring and Ballschmiter, 1980; de Bruïne *et al.*, 1985), the task will likely prove arduous and complicated. DSH may also participate in the formation of ternary DS–metal–protein complexes (Morpurgo *et al.*, 1983); formation of such complexes would tend to retard the movements of metals.

Although increases in the brain levels of a heavy metal generally elicit concern, paradoxically, as in the case of cadmium (section 7.4), such increases can be correlated with decreased toxicity. For cadmium this is presumably due to the fact that, based on LD_{50} measurements, the toxicity of $Cd(DS)_2$ is 76-fold lower than that of cadmium itself. Accordingly, such concern should be informed by knowledge of the relative toxicities of the metal itself and that of its complex with DSH.

The *in vivo* formation of DSH complexes of heavy metals may be useful even in instances, as with thallium, where the complex and the metal have indistinguishable toxicities, if the DSH helps to mobilize the metal from the tissues and speed its elimination. In such instances, however, the rate of DSH administration may need to be modulated to prevent the sudden elevation of the metal complex concentration to toxic levels. For instance, case reports of treatment of thallotoxicosis (Bass, 1963) and Wilson disease (Sunderman, 1964) with i.v. DSH indicate that, if rapidly administered to such patients, DSH can cause acute toxic effects. These are ascribable, presumably, to the pharmacological action of high concentrations of the complex formed.

DSSD is known to be metabolized to DSH *in vivo*. Also, both DSSD and DSH are considered to form the same complex with some metals (viz. copper; Sauter *et al.*, 1976). Accordingly, investigators of heavy metal toxicity and distribution have often assumed them to be equivalent. Where they have been compared, however, the results obtained have not always been similar. For instance, DSH increases fecal excretion of lead while DSSD administration has the opposite effect (Oskarsson, 1987b). A complicating factor is that heavy metal chelation can also occur following exposure to carbon disulfide, a metabolite of both DSSD and DSH. Comparative evaluation of the effects of DSSD and DSH presents problems. Firstly, it is not possible to use the same vehicle for both and secondly, use of the same route is problematical. DSSD is most often administered p.o., but administration of DSH in this manner renders it subject to acid hydrolysis in the stomach with the formation of carbon disulfide and diethylamine. Conversely, i.p. administration of DSSD as an aqueous suspension can lead to incomplete absorption, while if oil is used as the vehicle it can act as a depot and retard the absorption.

Finally, it should be kept in mind that it has been found that in some instances delay in administration of DSH following exposure to the heavy metal may be beneficial. Possibly, the delay might allow the metal to react and be trapped by relatively expendable tissue components, while early DSH administration might speed passage of the metal to regions where more vital systems can be affected.

The ensuing sections on the interactions of DSH and DSSD are arranged in the order of increasing affinity of DSH for the metal, as defined by the extraction constants given in Table 2.1.

7.2 THALLIUM

DSH can decrease thallium (Tl) toxicity. Administered to mice in a 365 mg/kg i.p. dose 24 h after a 10-day LD_{90} dose of Tl, DSH reduces mortality to 30% (Stavinoha *et al.*, 1959). This protection is probably due to increased Tl elimination. Daily administration of DSH (17.6 mg/kg/day for 6 days, in feed) increases from 79 to 90%, for instance, the cumulative amount of Tl eliminated by rats in the 7 days following its i.p. injection (Schwetz *et al.*, 1967). Also, in humans i.v. infusion of DSH (20–22 mg/kg) markedly increases the rate of urinary Tl excretion (Rieders and Cordova, 1965; Nogue *et al.*, 1983).

DSH administration, whether concurrent or subsequent to that of Tl, causes its brain levels to increase substantially. For instance, whether administered to rats 24 or 72 h after Tl, DSH (22.5 mg/kg i.v.) causes a 2-fold increase in brain Tl levels (Rauws *et al.*, 1969; Kamerbeek *et al.*, 1971); co-administration results in levels which are 5- to 10-fold higher than those seen in controls (Rauws *et al.*, 1969).

In rabbits administered ^{201}Tl and DSH concurrently, the brain ^{201}Tl level reaches 90% of its maximum within 90 s of administration and changes very slowly thereafter (de Bruïne *et al.*, 1985): the half-life of brain ^{201}Tl in rabbits can be calculated (from Table 1, p. 83, de Bruïne, 1988) to be 20 h. In humans, administered i.v. [201]Tl (1 μg) together with DSH (10 mg), 4.28% of the radionuclide is taken up by the brain. The process is exceedingly rapid, virtually no further uptake occurring after the first brain passage and a stable count being reached in 90 seconds (van Royen *et al.*, 1987; de Bruïne, 1988): a half-life of 250 h can be calculated from the ^{201}Tl levels at various times thereafter. The ready uptake of Tl(DS) into the brain is explained by its brain-blood partition coefficient which is 18/1 (Lear and Navarro, 1987). It should be noted, however, that in rabbits administered ^{201}Tl and DSH concurrently, the fraction of the injected radionuclide which is taken up by the brain (1.46–2.47%) is a function of the DSH dose (de Bruïne, 1988). Moreover, the very long biological half-life of radionuclide *in situ* thereafter, and the ability of DSH, administered long after Tl, to cause significant redistribution of it to the brain, suggests that Tl(DS) dissociates readily and that its *in vivo* existence is evanescent. Support for this hypothesis comes from the observation of Kamerbeek *et al,* (1971) that within 90 s of addition of Tl(DS) to liver homogenate, 55% of it was no longer extractable with methyl isobutyl ketone. Such evanescence might explain the finding that, in the rat, the 3-week LD_{50} for $TlNO_3$ and Tl(DS) are comparable, being 16 and 17 μg/kg, respectively (Rauws *et al.*, 1969).

7.2.1 Use in single-photon emission computed tomography

^{201}Tl is a gamma-emitting radionuclide with a half-life of 2 days which can be used for cerebral blood flow imaging with single-photon emission computed tomography (SPECT). The ready uptake of ^{201}Tl(DS) by cerebral tissue and the stable count thereafter suggested that it might be suitable as a radiopharmaceutical for local cerebral blood flow (LCBF), or regional cerebral blood flow, imaging (van Royen, 1987). Such imaging can provide clinically valuable information for the management of cerebral infarctions, brain tumors, epilepsy and dementia. To determine how accurately brain localization of ^{201}Tl(DS) might reflect LCBF, Lear and Navarro (1987) and Lear (1988) using rats, co-injected ^{201}Tl(DS), with other LCBF tracers ([^{123}I]isopropyliodoamphetamine, [^{14}C]iodoantipyrine and d,1[^{99m}Tc]-hexamethylpropyleneamine oxime complex), sacrificed the animals 2 h later and, taking advantage of the different decay rates of ^{201}Tl, ^{123}I, ^{14}C and ^{99m}Tc obtained autoradiographs for the distribution of each tracer in the same brains. On the basis of quantitative digitalized analysis of these autoradiographs they concluded that ^{201}Tl(DS) distribution accurately reflects brain perfusion (i.e. LCBF). A study of SPECT imaging with ^{201}Tl in acute ischemic stroke indicates the advantages of this imaging agent lie in its high sensitivity and high stability: this allows postponement in acute situations, once the radiopharmaceutical has been administered, of the imaging procedure since redistribution within the brain takes many hours (de Bruïne *et al.*, 1990).

7.2.2 Treatment of thallotoxicosis

A number of case reports have been published describing DSH therapy of thallotoxicosis. Some have achieved a significant degree of clinical improvement; in the hands of others, DSH treatment has led to serious problems. Since no other effective therapy of thallotoxicosis is available, these case reports will be examined in some detail. Bass (1963) administered 25 mg/kg of DSH in 500 ml 5% glucose as a slow (4 h) i.v. infusion to a man with very severe Tl poisoning. The procedure was repeated four times over a 5-day period. On each occasion the patient experienced intense joint pains during the infusion and, on two occasions, developed a toxic psychosis. However, the patient, who was moribund at the beginning of DSH therapy, improved over the course of it. Sunderman, Jr. (1967) administered p.o. gelatine capsules containing 375 mg of DSH (7.5 mg/kg) mixed with 0.6 g sodium bicarbonate (to serve as a gastrointestinal buffer) with 200 ml water every 4 h for 3 days to a patient who had ingested rat poison containing 375 mg Tl sulfate, this course of treatment being repeated twice. The patient showed definite clinical improvement during the DSH therapy, becoming more lucid, alert and cooperative. Urinary excretion of Tl increased 3-fold during the first course of treatment and 2.5-fold during the second. The patient did not experience any side effects during the DSH therapy. Kamerbeek *et al.* (1971) reported that a patient suffering from Tl intoxication lost consciousness during the infusion of DSH (dose and rate of infusion not stated) and evidenced progressive deterioration of the electroencephalogram. Although consciousness was regained a few hours later, electrographic disturbances persisted for several weeks, leading Kamerbeek *et al.* (1971) to state that the use of DSH as an antidote to thallotoxicosis is contraindicated. Nogué *et al.* (1983) administered DSH to a male schizophrenic who had ingested rat poison containing 750 mg Tl sulfate. Initially 22 mg/kg of DSH was infused i.v. in 500 ml of 5% dextrose over a 4-h period daily for 3 days. No adverse effects were observed; urinary Tl levels increased during the perfusion 4-, 5- and 20-fold on the 3 days of therapy, respectively. Later, DSH was administered p.o. as a solution of 7.5 mg/kg DSH in 50 ml of water every 6 h for 3 days. The patient experienced nausea and vomiting but no increased Tl excretion was observed. Since DSH is decomposed readily by acids to diethylamine and carbon disulfide (section 2.2), the administration of DSH solutions per os would not be expected to be effective unless steps are taken to protect it from stomach acids. The lack of effect of p.o. administration observed by Nogué *et al.* (1983) and the success of the therapy when administered by Sunderman, Jr. (1967) can be understood in this context. Oral administration of DSSD, which is stable under acid conditions, has not been evaluated for this condition. Administration of DSH by the i.v. route can also be very effective; whether serious side-effects are seen may depend on the rate at which Tl is mobilized. Since oral administration of potassium chloride also increases urinary Tl excretion, Papp *et al.* (1969) have suggested treatment of thallotoxicosis with a combination of DSH and potassium chloride.

7.3 ZINC

DSH administration leads to a redistribution of administered radiolabeled zinc (Zn). Thus in mice, administered DSH (113 mg/kg i.v.) 5 min after injection of $^{65}ZnCl_2$ (10 μmol/kg i.v.), blood and brain ^{65}Zn levels at 24 h are 2- and 3.5-fold higher, respectively, than those of controls administered $^{65}ZnCl_2$ only (Aaseth *et al.*, 1979). In the same species, administration of DSH (300 mg/kg i.p.) or DSSD (300 mg/kg p.o.) 15 min after p.o. dosing with $^{65}ZnCl_2$ (30 μmol/kg) raises the ^{65}Zn body burden at 24 h, presumably by increasing Zn absorption, but has little effect on the rate of its disposition in the ensuing 13 days (Sorensen and Andersen, 1989). Incorporation of DSSD in the diet of rats, as 0.1% in feed, for 1 week slightly increases (by 18%) the level of Zn in the spleen and slightly decreases (by 12%) that in the kidney; serum levels remain unchanged (Aaseth *et al.*, 1981). In alcoholics, DSSD therapy (800 mg twice a week for 4 weeks) does not change Zn serum levels which remain the same as those of controls (Grandjean *et al.*, 1990). No changes in Zn serum or renal levels are observed upon daily administration of DSH (113 mg/kg/day for 6 days, i.p.) to rats, although hepatic Zn levels, measured on days 1, 3 and 6, are raised about 70% (Tandon *et al.*, 1983). *In vitro*, DSH dramatically increases the uptake of Zn by erythrocytes (Aaseth *et al.*, 1979).

DSH is found to interact with the Zn of the hippocampal mossy fiber boutons (Danscher *et al.*, 1975). The Zn therein can be visualized histologically by sulfide silver staining and is considered to be involved in synaptic transmission. Its localization, both in the hippocampus and other areas of the brain, is intravesicular (Pérez-Clausell and Danscher, 1985). Administration of DSH to rats (50–1000 mg/kg i.p.) prevents sulfide silver staining of the hippocampal mossy fiber boutons (Danscher *et al.*, 1973). The effect is an immediate one: 5 min following administration of a 1000 mg/kg dose there is a loss of staining reactivity in most parts of the telencephalic neuropil. The maximal effect following this dose is seen at 45–60 min. DSH administration induces a similar inhibition of sulfide silver staining in the neuropil of the head of the dorsal horn of the spinal gray matter (Schroder *et al.*, 1978), the effect being evident within 30 min of DSH administration but no longer discernible at 2 h.

Little is known regarding the functional role of Zn in the hippocampal mossy fiber boutons. Frederickson *et al.* (1990) have proposed that chelation of Zn in these structures by DSH results in impairment of spatial working memory. Using rats which had been allowed to locate a submerged platform in a water maze, they found that infusion of DSH, via indwelling bilateral dorsal hippocampal cannulae, increases the time taken by the animal to locate the platform again. This effect is observed if the DSH is infused 15 min prior to the water maze test, but not if it is infused 4 h previously. The time course of the effect correlates with that on the silver sulfide staining of histological sections of the dorsal hippocampus of these animals. No Zn is evident in sections taken from animals killed 30 min after the DSH infusion. By 4 h, however, the staining pattern returns to normal. Additional evidence linking Zn chelation to the impairment of spatial memory is that the same effect can be induced by infusion of sodium sulfide which precipitates the Zn, but not by infusion of calcium edtate, which does not penetrate plasma membranes (Frederickson *et al.*, 1990). Chelation of the mossy fiber bouton Zn has also been advanced as the mechanism responsible for the augmentation of kainic acid toxicity (faster seizure onset and increased severity and higher mortality) by i.p. administration of DSH (Mitchell *et al.*, 1990). Although dithiazone, another agent that chelates Zn has similar effects, these workers admit it is an open question as to whether Zn chelation is the mechanism responsible for the observed effect.

The changes in staining reactivity of the hippocampal mossy fiber boutons are correlated with changes in hippocampal Zn content only at very high DSH doses. Thus, in rats, no changes could be detected in Zn levels in the hippocampal or other brain regions 30 min, 4 h or 24 h following a 250 mg/kg dose of DSH (Lakomaa *et al.*, 1982). A 23% decrease in hippocampal and a 13% decrease in cortical Zn levels is observed, however, in this species 1 h following 1000 mg/kg i.p. dose of DSH, though no other area of the brain region is significantly affected (Szerdahelyi and Kasa, 1987a). The hippocampal Zn levels remain significantly depressed for 24 h following this dose of DSH, although the sulfide silver staining in neurophils, which is blocked at 1 h, returns to normal after 6 h. In contrast, in mice no change in hippocampal Zn levels could be detected 4 h following a 900 mg/kg dose of DSH (Haycock *et al.*, 1977).

7.4 CADMIUM

DSH can protect against intoxication with otherwise lethal doses of cadmium (Cd). The timing of the DSH administration relative to that of Cd is, however, critical. Thus, DSH given to mice immediately or less than 1 h following systemic administration of Cd, is far less effective than when it is given 1–5 h after it (Table 7.1). Also, treatment with DSH within 15 min of oral dosing with Cd enhances the toxicity of the latter, whereas administered one or more hours later it does not have such an effect. The much lower oral toxicity of Cd (Table 7.1) is due to its low oral availability (1.5%). Administration of DSH at a time proximal to that of Cd results in more Cd being

Table 7.1 Effect of diethyldithiocarbamate (DSH) on mortality in the mouse following dosing with cadmium

Cadmium		DSH			Mortality			Reference
Dose[a] (mg/kg)	Route	Dose[b] (mg/kg)	Route	h post cadmium	N	Days post cadmium	%	
4	i.v.	—			10	14	60	Cantilena and Klaassen (1981)
		350	i.p.	0	10		30	
6	i.v.	—			10	14	100	
		350	i.p.	0	10		60	
8	i.v.	—			10	14	100	
		350	i.p.	0	10		10	
4.9	i.p.	—			24	30	100	Gale et al. (1981)
		500	i.p.	−0.17	16	30	25	
		500	i.p.	0.02	8	30	75	
		500	i.p.	0.17	8	30	38	
		500	i.p.	0.5	16	30	6	
		500	i.p.	1	16	30	0	
		500	i.p.	1.5	8	30	0	
		25	i.p.	2	6	30	33	
		50	i.p.	2	6	30	17	
		75	i.p.	2	6	30	0	
		100	i.p.	2	12	30	0	

		200	i.p.	2	6	30	0
		500	i.p.	2	24	30	0
		500	i.p.	3	8	30	0
		500	i.p.	5	8	30	0
		500	i.p.	8	8	30	50
9.8	i.p.	500	i.p.	2		30	100
7.9	p.o.	–	i.p.	0.25	15	10	0
		63			10	10	10
49	p.o.	–	i.p.	0.25	15	10	0
		248			10	10	50
97	p.o.	–	i.p.	0.25	15	10	20
		496			10	10	100
145	p.o.	–	i.p.	0.25	27	10	85
		628			10	10	100
145	p.o.	–	i.p.	0.25	5	10	40
		628	i.p.	1	5	10	100
		628	i.p.	2	5	10	40
		628	i.p.	3	5	10	40
					5	10	40

Andersen et al. (1988)

[a] Expressed in terms of the weight of the metal cation.
[b] Expressed in terms of the weight of the trihydrate.

absorbed (Andersen *et al.*, 1988), likely because of the formation of the Cd chelate, $Cd(DS)_2$, in the gastrointestinal tract.

Upon incubation of isolated rat hepatocytes with $Cd(DS)_2$, the rate of Cd uptake is initially (first 4 h) 4 times higher than that observed upon incubation with $CdCl_2$. Also, a greater proportion of the Cd is found to be associated with the particulate fraction of the cells (Hellström-Lindahl and Oskarsson, 1989b). An important observation made by these workers is that $Cd(DS)_2$ is not pharmacologically inert. Thus upon incubation with hepatocytes, or their cytosol, $Cd(DS)_2$ causes inhibition of glutathione reductase and succinic dehydrogenase similar in magnitude to that seen following incubation with $CdCl_2$. Yet, these two solutes differ in the extent to which they inhibit alcohol dehydrogenase. This suggests that the properties of $Cd(DS)_2$ are different from those of the Cd cation.

As much as 50% of administered Cd is sequestered in the liver and kidney. The accumulation ratio, R_a, defined as

$$R_a = \frac{\text{per cent of administered Cd present in organ}}{\text{(organ weight/body weight)} \times 100}$$

has values for these two organs of around 10 and 8, respectively (Gale *et al.*, 1982b). The R_a for spleen is around 1.2, but 0.5 or less for other organs. DSH is particularly effective in lowering Cd levels in the kidneys and the spleen and, to a lesser extent, those in the liver. In mice and rats previously administered Cd, treatment with DSH lowers Cd kidney levels by as much as 85% (Cantilena and Klaassen, 1981; Gale *et al.*, 1983a,b,c, 1985a, 1986b; Cikrt *et al.*, 1986b; Andersen *et al.*, 1988, 1989; Andersen and Nielsen, 1989). Among 18 other non-dithiocarbamate chelating agents tested, only 2,3-dimercaptopropanol (BAL) is also able to decrease renal Cd levels (Shinobu *et al.*, 1983a).

In organs with $R_a > 1$, Cd is sequestered by metallothionein, a cysteine-rich low molecular weight protein that avidly binds Cd. Such binding leads to the half-life of Cd in rodents being 50–250 days. Administration of either Cd or chelating agents stimulates metallothionein synthesis (Goering *et al.*, 1985), a process that reaches a maximum 6–12 h after Cd administration (the stimulation by chelating agents occurs because of the resulting increased uptake of dietary zinc, another metal bound by metallothionein). DSH removes Cd bound to metallothionein: incubation of partially purified mouse Cd metallothionein with 1 mM DSH *in vitro* results in removal of 56% of the Cd in 2 h (Gale *et al.*, 1985b).

Although DSH treatment lowers renal Cd levels, it does not increase urinary Cd excretion (Cantilena and Klaassen, 1981; Gale *et al.*,

1982b). Nonetheless, except when administered immediately following oral dosing with Cd, it lowers Cd body burdens (Gale *et al.*, 1983a,b,c, 1986b). This is effected by marked increases in fecal Cd excretion rates. Thus 6-fold (Gale *et al.*, 1982b, 1983a,b,c) and 10-fold (Klaassen *et al.*, 1984) higher fecal excretion rates are reported in mice pretreated with Cd 48 h to 6 weeks previously, though in mice administered DSH immediately following Cd, fecal excretion is not increased (Cantilena and Klaassen, 1981). Using rats pretreated with Cd during the preceding 39 days, Cikrt *et al.* (1986b) found that DSH does not increase biliary excretion of Cd, and suggested that the increased fecal elimination of Cd is mediated by transmucosal excretion across the intestinal wall.

The effect of treatment with DSSD on Cd body burdens has been little studied. Gale *et al.* (1989a) found that oral administration of DSSD in doses of 11.3, 106 and 441 mg/kg/day for 4 days to mice injected with Cd 3 days earlier in each case lowers hepatic Cd levels (by 16–25%) without altering either renal or brain levels. Administered in a 500 mg/kg/day i.p. dose in peanut oil, DSSD, as before, lowers hepatic Cd levels by 15%, but also reduces body burdens by 10% and increases brain levels 2.5-fold. Under comparable conditions, a 500 mg/kg i.p. dose of DSH decreases body burdens by 20%, lowers liver and kidney levels by 29% and 54%, respectively, but increases brain levels 21-fold.

The ability of DSH to induce organ redistribution of administered Cd is quite striking. The lowering of the renal Cd burden is usually accompanied by the depression of Cd levels also in the spleen and liver. In animals with very high Cd body burdens, however, liver Cd levels may actually be increased by DSH treatment (Shinobu *et al.*, 1983b). On the other hand, DSH administration results in increases in Cd levels in the heart, lung, testes and brain (Cantilena and Klaassen, 1981; Gale *et al.*, 1982b, 1985a, 1986b); the latter are increased as much as 20-fold (Cantilena and Klaassen, 1981).

The mechanism whereby DSH induces marked increases in brain Cd uptake has been investigated by Cantilena *et al.* (1982). Using rats, they showed that, (a) the first pass cerebral extraction of Cd was increased 10-fold, (b) there was no general alteration in the blood–brain barrier permeability nor an increase in cerebral blood flow. The addition of DSH to a solution of $CdCl_2$, they found, increased the apparent octanol:water partition coefficient for Cd from 0.03 to 11.34, a 375-fold increase. A similar value (11.5) for the octanol:water partition coefficient of $Cd(DS)_2$ was observed by Gale *et al.* (1983c) who also reported its octanol:0.1 M Tris buffer pH 7.4, chloroform:water, and chloroform:0.1 M Tris buffer pH 7.4 partition coefficients to be 490, 1.4 and 1413, respectively. These increases in lipophilicity due to complexation, are substantial and explain the higher uptake of Cd into the brain. Even so, these are well short of the $10^{5.5}$ value of the chloroform:water extraction constant for the $Cd(DS)_2$ complex which can be calculated from the data in Table 2.1.

Exposure of the brain to heavy metals is known to lead to neurotoxicity. Also, the testes are a target organ for Cd toxicity. Accordingly, the increases in the Cd burden of these two tissues which is brought about by DSH treatment of Cd exposed animals, has led some to conclude that DSH is contraindicated in Cd intoxication (Cantilena and Klaassen, 1981). However, using newborn rats, O'Callaghan and Miller (1986) found that, while DSH increases redistribution of Cd to the brain, it also prevents Cd-induced neurotoxicity as judged by three criteria: (a) brain weight, (b) brain histology and (c) striatal levels of synapsin I, a neuron–specific phosphoprotein. Specifically, they reported that DSH (100 mg/kg), when co-administered with 3 mg/kg $CdCl_2$ on postnatal day 5, increases the total brain levels of Cd at 24 h by 55–65%. Yet, this dose of DSH blocks the 24% decrease in brain weight and the necrosis of the neostriatum and corpus callosum otherwise seen in these animals by postnatal day 22. Likewise it blocks the 39% decrease in striatal levels of synapsin I caused by a 2.75 mg/kg dose of $CdCl_2$, a dose that does not cause any obvious cytopathology. Also, DSH given 30 min to 5 h after administration of a toxic dose of $CdCl_2$, is effective in decreasing degenerative changes in mouse testes (Walker *et al.*, 1984, 1986). The reason that DSH lowers the toxicity of Cd while raising its organ levels is likely to be that the toxicity of $Cd(DS)_2$ is lower than that of $CdCl_2$. Thus, while an i.p. dose of 5 mg/kg Cd, administered as $CdCl_2$, is consistently lethal in mice (Table 7.1), the i.p. LD_{50} for $Cd(DS)_2$ in this species is 650 mg/kg (Gale *et al.*, 1981). This suggests a low degree of dissociation of the complex *in vivo*.

The brain accumulation of Cd following $Cd(DS)_2$ treatment renders it unacceptable as a therapeutic agent. Accordingly, efforts are being made to discover alternative dithiocarbamates that capitalize on the high affinity of this structure for Cd. The goal is to lower Cd body burdens without causing redistribution of Cd to the brain and, given the renal toxicity of Cd, without increasing its urinary excretion. The field is a rather active one, involving the synthesis and *in vivo* testing of many novel dithiocarbamates (Cikrt *et al.*, 1984, 1986a; Gale *et al.*, 1984a,c, 1987, 1988; Jones, S.G. and Jones, 1984; Eybl *et al.*, 1988; Kiyozumi *et al.*, 1990; Shimada *et al.*, 1990). No mathematical and pharmacokinetic model has been developed to date for the absorption, distribution and fate of Cd *in vivo* and it is therefore not possible to discuss the effects of DSH and other dithiocarbamates on the rates of the various processes involved. Structure activity considerations are, moreover, rendered difficult because of the use of an 'immensely broad range' (Bláha *et al.*, 1985) of experimental conditions employed in published reports. These include variations in the Cd and dithiocarbamate dose, route, and duration of treatment, as well as in the intervals between Cd and dithiocarbamate treatment, and between the latter and sacrifice. One strategy that has been tried is to use mixtures of dithiocarbamates (Gale *et al.*, 1983d; Bláha *et al.*, 1988). Another is to design dithiocarbamates with more hydrophilic substituents so that their complexes with Cd will be less lipid-soluble and thus less able to cross the blood–brain barrier. Yet another strategy has been to design dithiocarbamates that will have molecular weight in excess of 350 so as to increase the Cd chelate's biliary secretion. One of the more recent compounds with these properties to be tested, *N*-(4-methoxybenzyl)-*N*-dithiocarboxy-D-glucamine, has the following structure,

$$CH_2OH \cdot (CHOH)_6 \cdot CH_2$$

$$4\text{-}CH_3O \cdot C_6H_4 \cdot CH_2 \qquad N-C \begin{matrix} S \\ \\ SH \end{matrix}$$

Given in a 1 mmol dose on two consecutive days to mice administered Cd (1.15 mg/kg) 14 days earlier, it lowers whole body, kidney and liver Cd levels by 56, 40 and 77%, respectively, without altering brain Cd levels (Singh *et al.*, 1990). It is interesting that upon testing the *in vivo* ability of this compound and two of its homologues to mobilize hepatic Cd deposits in mice, it is found that their efficacy varies in the same order as their ability to remove Cd from purified murine Cd metallothionein *in vitro* (Gale *et al.*, 1989b; Jones, M.M. *et al.*, 1989).

7.5 LEAD

Administration of DSH and DSSD in close temporal proximity, or subsequently to that of lead (Pb), appears to render Pb more lipid-soluble, presumably via the formation of the $Pb(DS)_2$ complex, and brings about a redistribution of Pb organ burdens and a shift in the Pb elimination pattern, increasing fecal and decreasing urinary excretion (Fig. 7.1). Overall, this results in a modest increase (10%) in Pb elimination during the first 72 h post DSH administration (Oskarsson, 1983, 1987b). More chronic treatment with DSH (678 mg/kg i.p. 5 times in an 11 day period) can bring about a greater (*ca* 30%) increase in Pb elimination, but doubling the DSH dose has no additional effect (Gale *et al.*, 1986a). Also, administration of the same dose p.o. decreases the effect by one-third.

DSH and DSSD administration results in a rapid lowering of the Pb burden of some of the tissues where these would otherwise be highest, thus the kidneys, bone and erythrocytes (Oskarsson, 1983, 1984, 1987b; Danielsson *et al.*, 1984). The levels in liver, another tissue where Pb accumulation usually occurs, are increased 1.5- to 2-fold (Oskarsson, 1983, 1984, 1987b; Danielsson *et al.*, 1984). In relative terms, a very much more dramatic increase is seen in the Pb levels in the brain, a tissue normally safeguarded from Pb accumulation. In animals given tracer doses of radiolabeled Pb, at 4, 24 or 72 h following administration of DSH and DSSD the brain levels of the radionuclide are consistently much higher (2- to 16-fold) than those in controls (Oskarsson, 1983, 1984, 1987b; Danielsson *et al.*, 1984; Oskarsson and Lind, 1985). Elevation of Pb brain levels, *vis-à-vis* controls, is also observed following more chronic oral treatment with DSH (Oskarsson and Lind, 1985; Gale *et al.*, 1986a; Weiss *et al.*, 1990), though not following its chronic i.p. administration (Gale *et al.*, 1986a).

Although there are many similarities between the effects of DSH and DSSD on the levels of Pb in tissues and the manner in which these change with time, there are also some major differences. Thus, 4 and 24 h following administration of DSSD (1 mmol/kg p.o), erythrocyte Pb levels are, respectively, 7- and 14-fold lower than after the same dose of DSH. Also, while following DSSD, Pb levels in bone decrease between 4 and 24 h, and conversely those in brain increase, the opposite is true for DSH (Danielsson *et al.*, 1984).

In a very interesting study, Oskarsson and Hellström-Lindahl (1988) have compared the effectiveness of Pb acetate and Pb(DS)$_2$ with respect to their inhibition of δ-aminolevulinic acid dehydratase (ALAD) in primary hepatocyte cultures. They found that while the uptake of Pb(DS)$_2$ into hepatocytes is 40 times faster than that of the Pb acetate, the degree of inhibition of ALAD is a function of the cellular Pb concentration and that the purified enzyme is inhibited equally by Pb(DS)$_2$ and Pb acetate. This indicates that the Pb in Pb(DS)$_2$ is fully pharmacologically active, at least with respect to ALAD.

The inhibition of ALAD causes *in vivo* a block in heme biosynthesis, which leads to reduction of the hematocrit and urinary excretion of δ-aminolevulinic acid (ALA), a heme precursor. Administration to rats of DSH (100 mg/kg, 2 times per week) for 12 weeks, concurrently with 50 or 500 ppm Pb in the drinking water, results in a significant increase in urinary ALA excretion (Weiss *et al.*, 1990). Also, exposure of rats pre- and postnatally (from conception to weaning) to both Pb and DSSD significantly enhances the Pb-induced lowering of their hematocrit and Pb-induced elevation of urinary ALA excretion (Oskarsson, 1989). In contrast, Tandon *et al.* (1985), using a radically different dosing schedule, namely pretreatment of rats for 4 weeks with Pb acetate (10 mg/kg, 6 times per week) followed by administration of two doses of DSH (68 mg/kg i.p. 8 h apart), observed that the DSH treatment significantly increases blood ALAD activity 2 days later and decreases urinary ALA excretion.

Concurrent exposure of rats to Pb and DSSD during pregnancy and lactation produces, in the offspring, neurophysiological, neurochemical and behavioral effects (increased home cage exploration and behavioral reactivity) not seen in animals exposed to either Pb or DSSD alone. The changes occasioned by the concurrent exposure to Pb and DSSD include increased levels of dopamine and serotonin metabolites in the caudate nucleus, greatly increased levels of arginine and methionine in the brain (Oskarsson *et al.*, 1986a), and reduced firing rates of Purkinje neuron (Oskarsson *et al.*, 1986b). On the other hand, the number of intranuclear inclusion bodies in the renal proximal tubule cells of these rat dams (characteristic reaction of kidneys to Pb intoxication) was markedly reduced (Oskarsson and Johansson, 1987). Additionally, co-administration of DSSD and Pb to the rat dams, for 5 days starting on the day of parturition, decreases the Pb levels in the milk of the dams, and the Pb body burdens of the suckling pups; this treatment also decreases Pb levels in maternal erythrocytes, but increases the Pb levels in maternal brain, liver and kidneys (Oskarsson, 1987a).

7.6 NICKEL

Both DSH and DSSD have been shown to possess an ability to antagonize the toxic effects of nickel (Ni) compounds. DSH has been shown to protect rats against lethal i.p. doses of $NiCl_2$ though less effectively than do D-penicillamine, diglycyl L-histidine-*N*-methylamide, or triethylenetetramine (Horak *et al.*, 1976). Then again, these results were obtained upon pretreating the animals with DSH 1 min prior to administration of $NiCl_2$, a dosing schedule which, by analogy with DSH's antidotal actions relative to Cd intoxication, may not have been optimal.

The extractability of Ni from pH 7.4 phosphate buffer into chloroform is increased by $10^{6.7}$ in the presence of a molar excess of DSH, the Ni partition coefficient for the system chloroform:pH 7.4 phosphate buffer being increased from 0.0007 to 3566 by the DSH (Jasim and Tjälve, 1986). As might be expected from the tremendous increase in the lipophilicity of Ni occasioned by formation of $Ni(DS)_2$, DSH causes marked changes in Ni distribution. At the cellular level, Nieboer *et al.* (1984) found that $10^{-6}M$ DSH increases the uptake of Ni into rabbit alveolar macrophages 3.5-fold. Menon and Nieboer (1986) found that DSH promotes cytosolic accumulation of Ni by peripheral mononucleated leukocytes. At the organ level, DSH administration to animals dosed with Ni causes brain levels of Ni to be consistently elevated many-fold. Thus, 57-, 85- and 89-fold increases have been reported in mice by Oskarsson and Tjälve (1980), Jasim and Tjälve (1986) and Jasim and Tjälve (1984), respectively and a 22-fold increase was reported by Belliveau *et al.* (1985) in rats. DSSD administration to Ni-dosed rats brings about an even greater elevation of Ni brain levels, a 300-fold increase being reported (Jasim and Tjälve, 1984).

The effect of DSH administration on the overall rate of elimination of Ni is a function of dose. In mice administered both $NiCl_2$ and DSH (113 mg/kg i.v.), the 24 h Ni levels in all tissues examined are higher than in controls administered only $NiCl_2$, thus indicating a decrease in Ni elimination (Jasim and Tjälve, 1986). When the DSH dose is larger (924 mg/kg), however, the Ni levels in the kidneys are decreased by as much as 3.7-fold at 4 h (Oskarsson and Tjälve, 1980). Ni balance studies undertaken in rats exposed to nickel carbonyl showed that DSH (100 mg/kg) increases significantly excretion of Ni, the fecal excretion being augmented more than urinary and the overall increase in excretion being about 20% (West and Sunderman, 1958).

Urinary and plasma levels of Ni are increased in all patients treated with DSSD for Ni dermatitis (Menné *et al.*, 1980). Hopfer *et al.* (1987) have reported that this is also true of alcoholics administered DSSD in a dose of 250 mg/day. In the latter patients, increases in serum and urine Ni levels were observed to progress from 4- and 8-fold after the first 24 h of therapy to 17- and 39-fold after 4–36 months of therapy. The possibility that the increased levels may have been due to more efficient absorption of dietary Ni led Hopfer *et al.* (1987) to suggest caution in the administration of DSSD to individuals with occupational exposures to Ni. While such a concern is appropriate, it remains to be determined whether the administration of DSSD, in the dose employed, leads to a positive Ni balance. Ni balance studies were performed by Sunderman (1964) while treating with DSH a woman suffering from severe Wilson's disease. He found the woman to be in a positive Ni balance when given DSH in a dose of 10 mg/kg. A negative balance was achieved when she was given DSH doses of 20 and 30 mg/kg, at which time she excreted, respectively, 38 and 196 µg Ni daily in excess of her intake.

7.6.1 Treatment of nickel dermatitis

DSSD is an effective treatment of nickel dermatitis, a condition affecting predominantly females and the most common permanent dermatological disability (Menné and Hjorth, 1982). Skin application of a DSH-containing ointment has been reported to show a capacity to inactivate patch-test reactions to Ni in Ni-sensitive patients (Samitz and Pomerantz, 1958). Parenterally administered DSSD is also effective in the treatment of this condition (Kaaber *et al.*, 1979, 1987; Menné *et al.*, 1980; Christensen and Kristensen, 1982). In one series of 11 patients, all of whom responded to an oral Ni challenge with a flare-up of an existing dermatitis, DSSD (100 mg, 3 times per day) therapy resulted, over the course of 4–5 weeks in considerable improvement in 82% and a complete cure in 64% (Kaaber *et al.*, 1979). In a second series, 10 of 11 patients showed considerable improvement and 2 were cured; all relapsed within 16 weeks of cessation of the treatment (Christensen and Kristensen, 1982). In a third series of 61 patients reacting positively to Ni patch testing and administered 50–400 mg DSSD per day, 70% were significantly improved and 46% were cured. Recurrence of the dermatitis occurred in 50% within a month and in 90% within 6 months of cessation of the therapy (Kaaber *et al.*, 1987). A flare-up of the eczema is often observed at the beginning of the DSSD therapy and a gradual escalation of the dose is therefore indicated.

An unusually high proportion of the patients treated with DSSD for nickel contact dermatitis develop hepatic toxicity (Christensen and Kristensen, 1982; Kaaber *et al.*, 1987; Kristensen, 1981). Thus, hepatitis developed in 5 (8%) and required hospitalization in 4 of the 61 patients treated by Kaaber *et al.* (1987), although in none of the cases were there any sequelae. Also, 6 additional patients had increased serum transaminase levels during DSSD therapy. The occurrence of the hepatitis had no relationship to the dose or duration of DSSD treatment, nor to Ni blood levels. Neither DSSD nor its metabolites, DSH and carbon disulfide (CS_2) will induce hepatic necrosis in otherwise untreated animals. The latter two compounds will do so, however, if the animals have been pretreated with phenobarbital (section 8.2.5). This may be so because phenobarbital induces hepatic cytochrome P-450 and so increases the rate of CS_2 metabolism. The latter involves the formation of carbonyl sulfide (COS) and atomic sulfur which attacks the nearest cysteine sulfhydryl on the P-450 cytochrome and causes its degradation, initially to cytochrome P-420 (section 8.2.7). Thus the occurrence of liver necrosis may be associated with an increased rate of destruction of cytochrome P-450.

Individuals suffering from nickel contact dermatitis are likely to have had significant exposure to the metal. The therapeutic effectiveness of DSSD in this condition suggests chelation of Ni is taking place. The formation of the highly lipophilic $Ni(DS)_2$ complex likely speeds the passage of both Ni and DSH to the location of the P-450, thereby leading to higher CS_2 levels and higher rates of desulfuration. This, in turn, would lead to higher rate of cytochrome P-420 formation and cytochrome destruction, thus setting the stage for overt hepatotoxicity. The enzyme primarily responsible for the degradation of the cytochrome is heme oxygenase. Its levels are increased by administration of both DSH (Miller *et al.*, 1983) and Ni (Sunderman, Jr. *et al.*, 1983a). Moreover, DSH and Ni exhibit a marked synergism in this regard (Sunderman, Jr. *et al.*, 1983b). These high levels of heme oxygenase may thus signal high rates of cytochrome P-450 destruction.

7.6.2 Prevention of nickel subsulfide tumors

DSH administration reduces the incidence of malignant tumors induced in rats by i.m. implantation of nickel subsulfide (Ni_3S_2), a compound identified as a potent carcinogen present in metallurgical dust obtained from refinery flue stacks. Over a period of 6–8 months, 72% of control female rats (N = 25) implanted with 10 mg of Ni_3S_2 developed tumors, but that incidence was reduced to 12% by weekly i.p administration of 20 mg DSH for the first 6 weeks following implantation. An analogous, but less dramatic difference in tumor incidence (84 and 52%, respectively; P = 0.03) was seen in male rats similarly treated (Sunderman, Sr. *et al.*, 1984).

7.6.3 Treatment of nickel carbonyl intoxication

In mice and rats, DSH provides complete protection against acute exposure to nickel carbonyl [$Ni(CO)_4$] administered in concentrations many times the LD_{50} value; DSH is more effective in this regard than D-penicillamine and other chelating agents (West and Sunderman, 1958; Baselt *et al.*, 1977; Mitchell *et al.*, 1978). In mice, 60 min after exposure to $Ni(CO)_4$, be it by inhalation or i.p. injection, the lungs become the tissue with the highest Ni burden. Administration of DSH (766 mg/kg i.p.) 30 min following the exposure to Ni(CO)$_4$ by these two routes, lowers the lung levels 93 and 79%, respectively. Forebrain levels, on the other hand are lowered (by 49%) in the mice administered Ni(CO)$_4$ by inhalation, but raised (5.6-fold) in those administered it i.p. (Tjälve *et al.*, 1984).

DSH has been used therapeutically in the treatment of individuals exposed accidentally to Ni(CO)$_4$ in the atomic energy industry and other occupational settings. Indeed, DSH has been identified as the drug of choice for treatment of such intoxication by the Committee on Medical and Biological Effects of Environmental Pollution (1975) of the U.S. National Research Council. The clinical employment of DSH for this condition has been reviewed by Sunderman, Sr. (1971, 1981, 1990). Based on the treatment, during the course of three decades, of more than 375 such cases under his supervision, he reports that no deaths have occurred in those who received DSH therapy within 4 days of Ni(CO)$_4$ exposure. Briefly, treatment is initiated if the concentration of Ni in urine of exposed individuals rises significantly above normal levels (these are 2.0 ± 1.1 µg/dl), i.e. if the levels are > 5.3 µg/dl. The intoxication is considered mild, moderately severe, and severe if the Ni levels in an 8 h urine are < 10, 10–50 and > 50 µg/dl, respectively. In mild cases, a total of five capsules, each containing 200 mg DSH plus 200 mg sodium bicarbonate, are administered every 2 min, the staggered administration reducing nausea. Moderately severe intoxication is treated with the same initial 5×200 mg dose, followed by 4×200 mg at 4 h, 3×200 mg at 8 h, 2×200 mg at 16 h (a total of 2.8 g during the first day), and 0.4 g/day thereafter until urinary Ni levels return to normal. If the condition is severe or critical, parenteral administration of 29 mg/kg DSH in sodium dihydrogen phosphate buffer is considered. Treatment may last for 14 days.

Although DSSD also decreases Ni(CO)$_4$ induced mortality in mice, it is less effective than DSH as a Ni(CO)$_4$ antidote (West and Sunderman, 1958).

7.7 COPPER

Of the metal anions for which DSH and DSSD have a high affinity (Table 2.1), copper (Cu) is the physiologically most available. As a consequence, formation of Cu complexes dominates much of the biochemistry and pharmacology of these two compounds and reference is made to the subject repeatedly in this monograph. Added to blood, DSSD is reduced and converted stoichiometrically to the Cu complex, Cu(DS)$_2$

(section 3.2), which is taken up by the red blood cells (section 3.4). Thus, the complex is a major metabolite of both DSSD and DSH (section 5.4). The inhibition by DSH of many enzymes is mediated by its complexation of the Cu at their active center (section 8.1). In particular, such complexation is responsible for the inhibition of dopamine β-hydroxylase (section 8.4) and thereby contributes to the phenomenology of the disulfiram-ethanol reaction (section 10.8).

Co-administration of DSH (100 mg/kg i.p.) with s.c. $CuCl_2$ significantly increases the toxicity of the Cu in mice, lowering the 10-day LD_{50} from 19.4 to 5.3 mg Cu/kg (Koutenský *et al.*, 1971). The *in vitro* toxicity of Cu to red blood cells is also much higher in the presence of DSH. Thus, though in the absence of DSH, no lysis is observed with 100 µM Cu, in the presence of 50 µM DSH (by itself also not lytic to red blood cells) 25 µM Cu causes 50% of the cells to lyse (Meshnick *et al.*, 1990).

Clinically, DSSD does not appear to affect Cu's metabolic balance. Thus, Ho *et al.* (1985) found plasma Cu levels of alcoholics receiving either a 250 or a 500 mg maintenance dose of DSSD (n = 14 and 12, respectively) for six weeks to be unaltered by the therapy. Similarly, Grandjean *et al.* (1990) found that the serum Cu levels of 12 alcoholic patients receiving DSSD therapy (800 mg twice a week) for 4 weeks did not change from pretreatment levels and did not differ from those of a group of non-alcoholic controls. Also, a group of 18 alcoholics treated repeatedly over a long period of time (up to 10 years) with the same DSSD regimen had serum levels no different from those of a control group.

In rats, administration of DSSD (50 mg/kg/day p.o. in 2% methyl cellulose for 3 to 6 weeks) results in a significant increase in Cu levels of all seven brain areas examined (average increase 45% and 126% at 3 and 6 weeks, respectively). This treatment also leads to a 29% ad 18% increases at 3 and 6 weeks, respectively, in liver Cu levels and in a 19% and 22% increases at 3 and 6 weeks, respectively, in erythrocyte Cu levels (Ho *et al.*, 1985)

The effect of DSH on Cu's metabolic balance is determined by its dose. This was documented by Sunderman (1964) while treating a woman suffering from severe Wilson's disease, a condition which leads to excessive accumulation of Cu in brain and liver. The woman remained in positive Cu balance when given doses of 10 and 20 mg/kg DSH. A negative balance was achieved, that is her Cu excretion exceeded its intake, upon administration of 30 mg/kg DSH per day.

In dogs, administered DSH in daily oral doses of 30, 100 and 300 mg/kg, Cu serum levels were elevated at 90 days by 25–50%, as a function of dose (Sunderman *et al.*, 1967). In rats, a single i.p.

250 mg/kg dose of DSSD has no effect on the Cu levels of different brain regions 24 h later (Lakomaa *et al.*, 1982), though injection with this dose 5 times per week for 4 weeks does result in increases of 33–55% in the Cu levels of the cortex, hippocampus and brain stem.

Working with rats, Szerdahelyi and Kasa (1987b) found that administration of DSH (1000 mg/kg i.p) 20 min prior to that of Cu acetate (5 mg/kg i.p.) results in increased hippocampal Cu levels. When examined 60 and 300 min later, these are, on average, 37% higher than in animals administered Cu acetate only, and 70% higher than those of untreated controls. Cu levels in the hypothalamus, parietal cortex and cerebellum, which are not increased in animals administered Cu acetate alone, are increased 20–35% if DSH is administered prior to Cu. Using a modified sulfide silver method, Szerdahelyi and Kasa (1987b) studied the histochemical location of Cu in the hippocampal region of both naive and Cu acetate-treated animals. They reported that in naive animals, glial cells are intensely stained while pyramidal and granule cells are negative. Following administration of Cu acetate, Cu accumulates also in the neurons. No information is available, however, on the effects of DSH on the cellular distribution of Cu.

The distribution of administered radiolabeled Cu is altered by DSH. Brain levels of ^{64}Cu in mice dosed with ^{64}Cu salts are increased by DSH administration, primarily as a function of DSH dose, thus from about 2-fold by a 25 mg/kg dose to as much as 38-fold by 766 mg/kg (Koutenský *et al.*, 1971; Aaseth *et al.*, 1979; Jasim *et al.*, 1985). The latter dose also increases two or more fold the ^{64}Cu levels in the heart, lungs, pancreas, testes and adrenals of such animals, although it decreases by half those in the liver and, if administered within 4 h of the ^{64}Cu, those in the kidney also (Jasim *et al.*, 1985). Brain Cu levels in rats exposed to 10 mM DSH in their drinking water for 35 days, but not dosed with Cu, are 75% higher than those of controls (Allain and Krari, 1991). Because of the likely hydrolysis of the DSH by gastric acid to carbon disulfide and diethylamine (Chapter 2), this effect may not be due to DSH itself.

In the treatment of a subject with Wilson's disease, Sunderman (1964) noted an immediate clinical improvement during i.v. therapy with 20 mg/kg DSH. He reported that, within 5 min of the start of the infusion, redness of the conjunctiva developed in the proximity of the Kayser–Fleisher rings (Cu deposits encircling the cornea in Wilson's disease). The conjunctival irritation was associated with a local burning sensation and mild lacrimation which persisted for 15 minutes following the end of the injection. After 2 years of DSH treatment, the rings practically disappeared.

7.8 MERCURY

DSH lowers the renal mercury (Hg) levels observed following i.v. $HgCl_2$ administration, a finding of considerable interest given the well-known renal toxicity of Hg. Thus in rats administered DSH (75 mg/kg i.v.) immediately following $HgCl_2$ (5 µmol/kg i.v.) the kidney Hg levels at 24 h are 33% lower than in controls (Aaseth *et al.*, 1981). Likewise in mice, administration of DSH (225 mg/kg p.o.) at 2 h prior and concurrently with $HgCl_2$ (750 nmol/kg i.v.) lowers the kidney Hg levels at 4 h by 54% (Danielsson, 1984). For the rats, this decrease in renal Hg levels coincides with an almost total prevention (>99%) of urinary Hg excretion (Fig. 7.1). Neither of these effects is seen in rats if the DSH (60 mg/kg i.m.) and $HgCl_2$ administrations are staggered by 90 min (Kachru and Tandon, 1986), a not too surprising result, given the short half-life of DSH. Urinary Hg excretion in rats co-administered $HgCl_2$ and DSH is found to rise in the 24–48 h post administration period and to exceed by 2.5-fold that observed in control animals in the 48- to 72-h period. The finding that at 72 h renal Hg levels are 2.9 times higher than those in DSH-free controls (Aaseth *et al.*, 1981) suggests the phenomena are related. Overall, DSH co-administration causes fecal excretion to account for a greater proportion of the total Hg excreted in the first 72 h, although DSH decreased somewhat the amount excreted in this manner in the first 24 h. All these results are consistent with DSH increasing, through the formation of the $Hg(DS)_2$ chelate, the lipophilicity of Hg. Also in keeping with this is the observation that, in both $HgCl_2$-dosed rats and mice, co-administration of DSH results in a marked elevation of brain Hg levels measured 4 h to 4 days post administration (Aaseth *et al.*, 1981; Danielsson, 1984).

Uptake of Hg by cultures of isolated hepatocytes incubated with $Hg(DS)_2$ in serum-free medium is 3-fold higher than when these are incubated with mercuric acetate (HgAc). In the presence of serum, because the tendency for binding to serum proteins is greater for HgAc than $Hg(DS)_2$, the differential is greater yet (Hellström-Lindahl and Oskarsson, 1989a). The uptake of $Hg(DS)_2$ is even greater than that of methyl mercury (MeHg). Exposure of the hepatocytes to $Hg(DS)_2$ results in the inhibition of glutathione reductase and alcohol dehydrogenase. When the degree of inhibition is expressed in terms of the intracellular Hg concentration it is evident that glutathione reductase is less susceptible to inhibition by Hg if it is derived from the uptake of $Hg(DS)_2$ rather than that of HgAc (Fig. 7.2). This suggests that $Hg(DS)_2$ does not immediately dissociate and that the enzyme is less sensitive to Hg in the chelated form. (Glutathione reductase is even less susceptible to inhibition by the Hg of MeHg.) No difference exists, however,

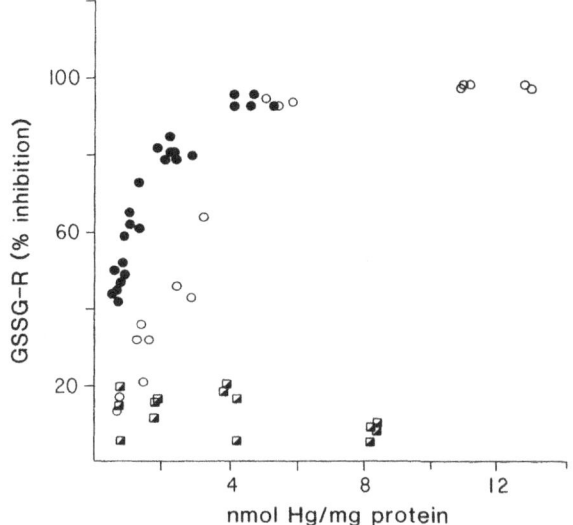

Figure 7.2 Relationship between cellular mercury (Hg) uptake and glutathione reductase (GSSG-R) inhibition in primary cultures of rat hepatocytes exposed to mercuric acetate (HgAc; closed circles), mercuric diethyldithiocarbamate (Hg(DS)$_2$; open circles), and methyl mercury (MeHg; squares). Modified with permission from Hellström and Oskarsson (1989a).

between the susceptibility of alcohol dehydrogenase to inhibition by Hg derived from Hg(DS)$_2$ and HgAc (Hellström-Lindahl and Oskarsson, 1989a).

In mice, DSH co-administration decreases markedly the overall amount of Hg transferred to the fetus at both 4 and 24 h post administration (Danielsson, 1984). Concurrently, at 4 h it changes the distribution ratio for Hg between maternal erythrocytes and plasma from 1.6 to 4.8. This suggests that the decreased fetal Hg level results from the Hg in blood of DSH-treated animals being much less free to diffuse across the placenta.

Changes in Hg distribution, occasioned by the co-administration of DSSD (1 mmol/kg) to mice with HgCl$_2$, parallel, in most respects, those seen following DSH co-administration. Such differences as are observed suggest that DSSD may possess some advantages over DSH. Thus, the increase in brain Hg levels observed at 4 and 24 h is much lower following DSSD co-administration (1.3- and 1.9-fold, respectively; $P > 0.05$) than that following DSH (7.1 and 7.2, respectively; $P < 0.05$), while the renal Hg levels and those in the fetus were similar to those observed in animals co-administered DSH (Danielsson, 1984).

7.8.1 Methyl mercury

MeHg is considered not to undergo significant degradation *in vivo* to inorganic mercury and the effect of DSH on its disposition therefore needs to be considered separately. Administration of DSH (25 mg/rat, ~125 mg/kg s.c.) to rats, first concurrently with MeHg chloride (1 mg/kg i.v.) and then twice daily for 8 days, results in a 59% decrease in urinary and a 24% decrease in fecal excretion of Hg over the 8-day period, relative to that in controls (Norseth, 1974). In DSH-treated animals, as compared with controls, the kidney Hg levels are significantly lower at both 24 h and 8 days post MeHg administration (by 61 and 29%, respectively), while those in the brain were increased (6.4- and 2.0-fold, respectively), as are those in the liver (1.5- and 1.7-fold, respectively). The levels in the erythrocytes, on the other hand, are not significantly different at either time point. In rats pretreated with MeHg, i.p. DSH administration causes a rapid decrease in biliary Hg excretion which is evident within 10 min or less and lasts from 15 min to 2 h depending on dose (Norseth, 1974). DSSD has a similar effect (Gale *et al.*, 1984b). When administered to mice 3, 4 and 5 days following MeHg pretreatment, DSH (225 mg/kg i.p.) is without effect on the elimination of MeHg.

7.9 PLATINUM

Much of the current interest in the interaction of DSH with platinum (Pt) results from the ability of DSH to prevent the development of the late nephrotoxicity induced by the administration of cisplatin [*cis*-dichlorodiammineplatinum(II)], a clinically important cancer chemotherapeutic drug of the following structure:

$$\begin{array}{ccc} \text{Cl} & & \text{NH}_3 \\ & \diagdown \diagup \\ & \text{Pt} \\ & \diagup \diagdown \\ \text{Cl} & & \text{NH}_3 \end{array}$$

Nephrotoxicity is a limiting factor in the therapeutic utilization of cisplatin (Walker and Gale, 1981) and DSH's ability to counter it has therapeutic importance (Chapter 15). Since DSH is effective in preventing cisplatin nephrotoxicity when it is administered 1–3 h after it, it is referred to as a cisplatin rescue agent. In a parallel manner, exposure of cultures of LLC-PK$_1$, a porcine kidney cell line, to DSH (1 mM) for 1 h immediately following a 1-h incubation with cisplatin (0.2 mM) prevents the development of the 72-h toxicity otherwise induced by the cisplatin (Montine and Borch, 1988). Although exposure to DSH does not change the Pt content of these cells, following such exposure about 40% of the Pt present in the cells is in the form of $Pt(DS)_2$. This stable adduct of Pt with DSH, first described by Fackler *et al.* (1968), absorbs strongly in the UV with wavelength maxima at 254 and 347 nm (Bannister, S.J. *et al.*, 1979). Though freely soluble in chloroform, it is nearly insoluble in water. Its toxicity is low: BDF_1 mice administered i.p. a suspension of $Pt(DS)_2$ in carboxymethylcellulose in doses of 10, 25, 50, and 100 mg/kg all survive 30 days (Borch, private communication). By way of comparison, the 15-day LD_{50} for cisplatin administered i.p. to mice is 8.5 mg/kg (section 15.2.1). Also, unlike cisplatin, $Pt(DS)_2$ is not nephrotoxic: mice administered the adduct have normal day 5 blood–urea–nitrogen levels, the elevation of which is a measure of nephrotoxicity. Additionally, no renal damage is observed when the kidneys of these animals are examined histologically on day 5 (Borch, private communication).

The information regarding the *in vivo* effect of DSH on the excretion and tissue levels of Pt in cisplatin pretreated animals is fragmentary. Administered to rats soon (1 h) after cisplatin (7.5 mg/kg), DSH (2.9 mmol/kg) reduces the renal Pt burden at 75 days by 27% relative to DSH-naive controls (Jones, M.M. *et al.*, 1986). Administered to rats 24 h after cisplatin (8 mg/kg), DSH (1 mmol/kg) increases the 5 h renal Pt burden 43% relatively to DSH-naive controls, though it does not alter hepatic Pt burdens and increases the biliary Pt excretion rate so that at 2–3 h it is 70-fold greater than in controls (Basinger *et al.*, 1989). The apparent ability of DSH to mobilize tissue Pt notwithstanding, repeated DSH administration (at 1 min, 1 h and 3 h post cisplatin) does not result in transfer of any Pt to the brain; 48 hrs after dosing with cisplatin the Pt levels in this organ remain undetectable.

The Pt of cisplatin displaces the Hg of $Hg(DS)_2$, albeit very slowly (Borch, private communication), indicating that the extraction constant for the reaction of Pt with DSH to form the $Pt(DS)_2$ complex is larger than the parallel one for the formation of $Hg(DS)_2$. Since the latter extraction constant is the second highest among all the metals investigated, being exceeded only by that for palladium (Table 2.1), it is clear that the affinity of DSH for Pt is very high indeed. DSH displaces glutathione from the polymeric Pt–glutathione complex $[Pt(GS)_2 \cdot 3H_2O]$ by a reaction with a second-order rate similar to that for its displacement of Pt from cisplatin (Dedon and Borch, 1987). An analogous removal by DSH of Pt from it complexes with intracellular target molecules is considered to be the mechanism whereby DSH reverses cisplatin nephrotoxicity. Bodenner *et al.* (1986b) used γ-glutamyl-transpeptidase (GGTP), a renal enzyme which contains a sulfhydryl group essential for enzymatic activity, as a model of such a target. They reported that cisplatin inhibits, over the period of several hours, both the purified enzyme and its activity in rat kidney brush border preparations in a time-dependent fashion and that 1 and 10 mM DSH reversed the inhibition, the higher DSH concentration doing so more rapidly. Another model substance which has been used to explore the interactions between Pt, DSH and proteins has been a purified α_2-macroglobulin, a plasma protein which consists of four identical subunits. Each subunit can be joined to one other by sulfur bonds so that a single band, corresponding to the half molecule, is observed with denaturing polyacrylamide gel electrophoresis under non-reducing conditions. Cisplatin readily cross-links the non-covalently associated subunits, so that a single band, corresponding to the whole molecule, is observed upon electrophoresis. DSH, even in a 10 μM concentration, substantially reverses the cisplatin effect. Nearly all the Pt cross-links are eliminated by 1 mM DSH, although 3.6 mM DSH has no detectable effect on the S—S intersubunit bonds themselves (Gonias *et al.*, 1984). In parallel with these structural effects, $\geqslant 90\%$ of α_2-macroglobulin's trypsin binding activity is lost upon incubation with 1 mM cisplatin for 6 h. Subsequent incubation for 6 h with 1 mM DSH restores the activity fully.

GGTP is one of several renal proximal tubule enzymes which have one or more sulfhydryl groups essential for activity. Since at 4 and 24 h following administration of a 7.5 mg/kg dose of cisplatin, there is no *in vivo* inhibition of this enzyme, it is considered not to be the *in vivo* target of cisplatin nephrotoxicity. This is also true of the ATPases of the renal proximal tubule membrane, that is, the Na^+/K^+- and Mg^{2+}-adenosine-5'-triphosphatases. Although 24 h after the 7.5 mg/kg dose of cisplatin, both alkaline phosphatase and leucine aminopeptidase, two other enzymes in this tissue, are significantly inhibited (by 39 and 10%, respectively), *in vivo* DSH treatment does not prevent their inhibition (Dedon and Borch, 1987).

DSH does not reverse or inhibit the tumoricidal action of cisplatin (section 15.2.5). This latter action is considered to be mediated by cisplatin's formation of bifunctional adducts with DNA. Incubation of Pt–DNA adducts, such that the Pt:DNA ratio is <0.05, with 10 mM DSH for 10 h results in removal of less than 1% of the Pt (Bodenner *et al.*, 1986a). To explore the role of DSH further, these workers studied the reaction of DSH with Pt–DNA complexes. They found that while the cisplatin–guanosine monoadduct, $Pt(NH_3)_2(guanosine)(OH_2)^{2+}$, and two isomeric cisplatin–adenosine bisadducts, $Pt(NH_3)_2$ (adenosine)$_2^{2+}$, react quite rapidly with DSH, the cisplatin–guanosine bisadduct, $Pt(NH_3)_2$(guanosine)$_2^{+2}$, is quite unreactive towards DSH. The primary cytotoxic action of cisplatin is known to be the cross-linking of guanine bases of the same or opposite strands of DNA. DSH, if present, can prevent this from occurring, but once the bisguanine bridges are formed, DSH addition does not reverse the process.

Using the LLC-PK$_1$ porcine kidney-derived cell line, Montine and Borch (1988) found that incubation for 60 min with cisplatin results in dose-dependent inhibition of DNA, RNA and protein synthesis as well as a subsequent (72 h) loss of viability. Incubation with DSH for 60 min fails to reverse the inhibition of RNA synthesis but both the inhibition of protein synthesis and the effect on viability are reversed, a DSH concentration of $\geqslant 300\,\mu M$ being necessary to achieve either. Moreover the dose modification factor (DMF) of 1.6 was observed for both actions of DSH. On the basis of these results, it is concluded that inhibition of protein synthesis is the critical nephrotoxic event induced by cisplatin and reversed by DSH (Montine and Borch, 1988).

7.10 POLONIUM

Administration of DSH (200 mg/kg i.v.) to rats daily for 10 days following dosing with 0.075 mCi/kg polonium (Po) reduces Po body burdens at 11 days by 32% relative to DSH-naive controls. The DSH treatment increases the day 11 brain Po levels 5-fold, but decreases the Po levels in liver, spleen and lymph nodes (chief locations of Po accumulation in control animals) 4- to 5-fold. It also increases the mean survival time of the animals from 15 to 32 days (Krivchenkova and Safronov, 1964).

8

Disulfiram and diethyldithiocarbamate as enzyme inhibitors

8.1	INTRODUCTION	96
	8.1.1 General aspects of enzyme inhibition by disulfiram	97
	8.1.2 General aspects of enzyme inhibition by diethyldithiocarbamate	99
	8.1.3 Copper enzymes inhibited by diethyldithiocarbamate *in vitro* .	101
8.2	INHIBITION OF DRUG METABOLIZING ENZYMES	102
	8.2.1 Introduction	102
	8.2.2 *In vivo* inhibition in humans	104
	8.2.3 *In vivo* inhibition of hepatic monooxygenases by disulfiram in experimental animals	108
	8.2.4 *In vivo* inhibition of hepatic monooxygenases by diethyldithiocarbamate and carbon disulfide	109
	8.2.5 *In vivo* effects on P-450 cytochromes	111
	8.2.6 *In vitro* inhibition by disulfiram	115
	8.2.7 *In vitro* inhibition by diethyldithiocarbamate and carbon disulfide	116
	8.2.8 Inhibition by diethyldithiocarbamic acid methyl ester	118
	8.2.9 *In vivo* effects on enzymes of the glucuronic acid pathway	118
	8.2.10 Effects on extrahepatic drug metabolizing enzymes	119
	8.2.11 Summary	119
8.3	INHIBITION OF DOPAMINE β-HYDROXYLASE	120
	8.3.1 *In vivo* inhibition: animal studies	121
	8.3.2 *In vivo* inhibition: clinical studies	125
	8.3.3 *In vitro* inhibition	125
	8.3.4 *In vivo* effect on tyrosine	126
8.4	INHIBITION OF SUPEROXIDE DISMUTASE	126
	8.4.1 Introduction	126
	8.4.2 *In vivo* effects	127
	8.4.3 Mechanism	129
	8.4.4 Effects in cell culture	131
	8.4.5 Summary	133
8.5	INACTIVATION OF GLUTATHIONE PEROXIDASE	133
8.6	EFFECT ON CATALASE	135

8.1 INTRODUCTION

Much of the early biochemical work on the effects of dithiocarbamates and thiuram disulfides followed the introduction of agents of this class as agricultural pesticides and fungicides in the 1930s and 1940s (Thorn and Ludwig, 1962). The discovery in 1948 of the clinical interaction between disulfiram (DSSD) and ethanol further stimulated interest in these agents. The early studies explored these compounds as inhibitors of growth, respiration and carbohydrate metabolism, and as biocidal agents. Investigation of their effects on isolated enzymes soon revealed that their inhibitory activity was due to their ability to complex the metals of metalloenzymes, or, alternatively, to react with enzyme sulfhydryl groups. Also, it was noted that sulfhydryl-containing endogenous compounds, such as glutathione (GSH) and cysteine, could often partially reverse the inhibition (Thorn and Ludwig, 1962).

Early work on the inhibition of enzymes by DSSD or diethyldithiocarbamate (DSH) has been reviewed (James, 1953; Hunter and Lowry, 1956; Ludwig and Thorn, 1960; Thorn and Ludwig, 1962). In addition to aldehyde dehydrogenase, the mammalian enzymes considered in these reviews included alcohol dehydrogenase, aldehyde oxidase, alkaline phosphatase, amine oxidase, amylase, choline dehydrogenase, glutamic dehydrogenase, D-glyceraldehyde-3-phosphate dehydrogenase, monoamine oxidase, succinic dehydrogenase, tryptophan pyrrolase, and xanthine oxidase.

It should be borne in mind that DSSD and DSH differ in their properties and mode of action. DSSD inhibits chiefly by reacting with thiol groups of proteins, thereby producing mixed disulfides and releasing DSH as a byproduct of the reaction; the inactivated enzyme may, but need not have the DS moiety bound to it covalently, as the reactions given by equations (8.1) and (8.2) illustrate.

$$\text{Enzyme–SH} + \text{DS–SD} \rightarrow \text{Enzyme–S–SD} + \text{DSH} \qquad (8.1)$$

$$\text{Enzyme} \begin{matrix} \diagup \text{S–SD} \\ \diagdown \text{SH} \end{matrix} \rightarrow \text{Enzyme} \begin{matrix} \diagup \text{S} \\ \quad | \\ \diagdown \text{S} \end{matrix} + \text{DSH} \qquad (8.2)$$

The latter reaction (8.2) may occur if a second, suitably positioned vicinal thiol group is present on the enzyme. Such a sequence of reactions occurs with E_1, the cytosolic aldehyde dehydrogenase (section 9.3.1).

DSH acts chiefly as a metal ion chelator and a thiol, which can inhibit enzyme action by complexing metals in the active center, or by scavenging free radicals that may be necessary for a reaction. It is a particularly potent metal chelating agent for copper (section 2.3). If present in molar excess, it is capable of extracting copper from enzymes and other proteins (ceruloplasmin: Morell and Scheinberg, 1958; galactose oxidase: Amaral *et al.*, 1966; superoxide dismutase: Cocco *et al.*, 1981a; Cu-substituted carbonic anhydrase: Morpurgo *et al.* 1983). Typically the resulting apoenzymes are inactive. On the other hand, its ability to remove zinc from proteins is much more circumscribed, probably because of its lower affinity for the metal (section 2.3). Thus, no matter how large the excess of DSH, it will not remove the zinc associated with the Cu–Zn superoxide dismutase (Cocco *et al.*, 1981b) or with carbonic anhydrase (Morpurgo *et al.*, 1983). The latter case is of interest since DSH does inhibit the enzyme and zinc is the only metal associated with it (section 8.1.2). DSH binds reversibly to the catalytic zinc of horse liver alcohol dehydrogenase (Syvertsen and McKinley-McKee, 1984) and, when present in large excess, causes a selective loss of zinc from the enzyme (Drum *et al.*, 1969a, b; Drum and Vallee, 1970).

DSSD and DSH inhibit *in vitro* many enzymes in addition to those mentioned above (sections 8.1.1–8.1.3). Administration of these agents also causes the inhibition of a number of enzymes or enzyme systems *in vivo*. The inhibition of aldehyde dehydrogenase forms the basis for the clinical use of DSSD; it has been the object of much investigation, discussed in Chapter 9. Other instances in which *in vivo* inhibition contributes significantly to the pharmacological actions of these agents are covered in separate sections of this chapter. One of these is the inhibition of the cytochrome P-450 associated monooxygenases and other xenobiotic metabolizing enzymes of the endoplasmic reticulum (section 8.2); it is viewed as the potential basis for drug interactions. Another is the inhibition of dopamine β-hydroxylase (section 8.3) which plays a role in the disulfiram–ethanol reaction. Superoxide dismutase inhibition (section 8.4) is of considerable interest as this enzyme constitutes the organism's first line of defense against the toxic superoxide anion radical to which all aerobes are exposed. Finally, glutathione peroxidase (section 8.5) and catalase (section 8.6) are two other enzymes involved in defense against reactive oxygen species whose inhibition by DSH has been investigated.

8.1.1 General aspects of enzyme inhibition by disulfiram

The reaction of DSSD with protein sulfhydryl groups to form mixed disulfides and DSH (equation 8.1) was first proposed by Strömme (1963a) with respect to the *in vitro* inhibition of bovine brain and yeast hexokinases (K_i 20 and 80 µM, respectively). Enzymes which have been thus inactivated can be regenerated by the use of a reducing thiol. Strömme used cysteamine. Others have used cysteine, glutathione, dithiothreitol and 2-mercaptoethanol.

The disulfide exchange reaction between DSSD and a protein thiol takes place because the leaving group, DSH, is a stronger acid than the protein thiol (for review see Kitson, 1988).

How many sulfhydryl groups in a protein will react with DSSD can depend on structural constraints. Thus, porcine kidney D-amino acid oxidase (EC 1.4.3.3) has 12 sulfhydryl groups per mole, 6 to 8 of which react readily with sulfhydryl reagents. It is inhibited *in vitro* by DSSD with which it reacts to give the expected DSH product (Neims *et al.*, 1966b). The inhibition observed is a linear function of the amount of DSSD added, complete inhibition being seen when 6–8 mole equivalents of DSSD are added. Exposure to ^{35}S-labelled DSSD results, as predicted, in the liberation of 6–8 mole equivalents of ^{35}S-DSH. For all 12 sulfhydryl groups to react with DSSD, however, it is necessary to use a denaturing agent, following which the remaining protein sulfhydryls become accessible to interaction with DSSD.

An elegant demonstration of the formation of mixed disulfides in the *in vivo* inactivation of enzymes is the ability of 10 mM dithiothreitol to regenerate, when incubated with microsomes from DSSD-treated rats, the 7 α-hydroxylase inactivated by *in vivo* DSSD treatment (Andersson and Bostrøm, 1984). This enzyme is a specific cytochrome P-450-dependent hydroxylase (section 8.3.4) which *in vitro* is *ca* 50% inhibited by 1 µM DSSD (Andersson and Bostrøm, 1984; their Fig. 1). Considering that following its *in vivo* administration DSSD is present in undetectable or submicromolar concentrations in blood (Johansson, 1988), it would appear that enzyme inactivation by formation of the mixed disulfide either requires local resynthesis of DSSD from DSH, or the possible formation of a mixed disulfide from the co-oxidation of DSH with an endogenous thiol.

Among the enzymes most sensitive to *in vitro* inhibition by DSSD is E_1, the cytosolic, or Class 1, aldehyde dehydrogenase which can be instantaneously inhibited in a stoichiometric reaction with 1–4 µM DSSD. Because of the importance of aldehyde dehydrogenases to the pharmacological activity of DSSD *in vivo*, the inhibition of these enzymes by DSSD and its metabolites are discussed at length is Chapter 9. By contrast, the *in vivo* effects of DSSD on alcohol dehydrogenase (ADH) are considered to be negligible, although DSSD pretreatment does lead to an inhibition of *in vivo* ethanol elimination. This effect, however, is occasioned by an accumulation of acetaldehyde and the effect it has on ethanol metabolism (section 10.7). *In vitro* the ADH can be inhibited by DSSD. Thus, the K_i values for mouse and rat liver ADH are 43 and 150 μM, respectively (Sharkawi, 1980). Such concentrations of DSSD are not achievable, however, *in vivo*. In the case of horse liver ADH, Carper *et al.* (1987) observed a slowly developing inhibition in the presence of 0.6–4.6 μM DSSD, so that after 48 h of incubation a plateau of about 50% inhibition was reached. However, the inhibition was totally prevented by addition of a thiol, such as dithiothreitol. Considering the slowness of the reaction and its easy reversibility by thiols, a significant inhibition of ADH *in vivo* is unlikely.

Several other enzymes have been reported to be inhibited by DSSD. Thus, Nousiainen and Törrönen (1984) found that in rats DSSD inhibits a microsomal carboxyesterase both *in vivo* and *in vitro* (*ca* 50% by 100 μM). Glucose-6-phosphate dehydrogenase has been reported by Marselos *et al.* (1976) to be inhibited following chronic administration of either DSSD or DSH to rats. Cha *et al.* (1982) could not confirm this effect of DSSD when administered in feed to mice, but found that daily injections of DSSD (100 mg/kg in corn oil for 7 days) did reduce the activity of this enzyme significantly. Choo and Riendeau (1987) found DSSD to be an *in vitro* inhibitor of 5-lipoxygenase with an IC_{50}, determined in the soluble fraction of rat polymorphonuclear leukocyte sonicate, of 0.53 ± 0.11 μM (the corresponding figure for DSH was 2–4 μM). Finally, Leo et al. (1989) have reported a rat cytosolic retinal dehydrogenase (EC 1.2.1.36) to be inhibited *in vitro* by 20–50 μM DSSD, concentrations not achievable *in vivo*.

It must be borne in mind that *in vivo* DSSD administration can cause not only DSSD-mediated enzyme inhibition, but also effects mediated by metabolites of this drug.

8.1.2 General aspects of enzyme inhibition by diethyldithiocarbamate

Although DSH chelates copper (Cu) avidly, often only a fraction of the enzyme-associated Cu can be removed. Thus, even 10 mM DSH removes only one of the two Cu atoms associated with bovine serum amine oxidase, though following exposure to this DSH concentration, the residual Cu is in a DSH-bound form (Morpurgo *et al.*, 1987a). Also, DSH removes 2 of 8 Cu ions of green zucchini ascorbate oxidase with significant inhibition (Morpurgo *et al.*, 1987b, 1988), but less than 10% of the 4 Cu ions of the Japanese lacquer tree *Rhus vernicifera* laccase (Morpurgo *et al.*, 1987b).

DSH also chelates zinc (Zn), but much less avidly. Accordingly, while enzymes having Zn at their active site are inhibited by DSH, as a rule the Zn is not extracted from the enzyme even if a large excess of DSH is used. A good example of these relationships is the behavior of the native, Zn-containing carbonic anhydrase (EC 4.2.1.1) and its cobalt (Co) and Cu analogues (Morpurgo *et al.*,1983). The native bovine carbonic anhydrase contains one Zn(II) per molecule. Although the enzyme is inhibited by DSH (K_i 1.7 mM), no Zn is lost even when the enzyme is dialyzed against 10 mM DSH for 24 h. It can be reactivated by simply dialyzing it against DSH-free medium. The Co enzyme, formed by exposure of the apoenzyme to subequivalents of $CoCl_2$, is also active. It is inhibited by DSH, with loss of Co, at DSH concentrations one order of magnitude lower than the Zn enzyme. Finally, the Cu enzyme, formed by exposure of the apoenzyme to $CuCl_2$ (it is inactive), loses its Cu quite readily when exposed to DSH.

A second example is that of the CuZn superoxide dismutase, in which Cu has a catalytic role and Zn a structural one. Exposure of the enzyme to DSH results in inhibition and loss of the Cu, but no Zn can be extracted. If, using other chelators, the Zn is removed and substituted by Co, a modified but nonetheless active CuCo superoxide dismutase is obtained. Upon exposure of this enzyme to DSH, both Cu and Co are removed (Cocco *et al.*, 1981b).

Horse liver alcohol dehydrogenase constitutes an exception to the above rule, in that millimolar concentrations of DSH do cause a selective loss of Zn (Drum *et al.*, 1969a, b; Drum and Vallee, 1970). Interestingly, however, if exposed to the inhibitor prior to the addition of substrate, it is more readily inhibited by DSSD than DSH, apparently by the reaction of DSSD with one of the enzyme's thiol groups, the extent of inhibition being dependent on the length of exposure (Carper *et al.*, 1987).

In millimolar concentrations, DSH can inhibit many metalloenzymes. Such concentrations of DSH occur in animals when high doses of DSH are administered. For instance, Fisher rats injected with 100 mg/kg of DSH by i.v. bolus had peak DSH plasma levels greater than 530 µg/ml (that is >3 mM; Borch, private communication, re: Dissertation by P. Dedon). Similarly, Bodenner *et al.* (1986b) reported peak plasma DSH levels of 1.17 mM in rats administered 250 mg/kg DSH i.v., and peak levels of 0.58 mM following s.c. administration of the same dose. High doses of DSH (75–150 mg/kg) have been administered by i.v. infusion to humans receiving cisplatin or carboplatin for cancer therapy (Qazi *et al.*, 1988; Rothenberg *et al.*, 1988) and peak plasma levels of 0.4–1.0 mM DSH were noted. High doses of DSH are also used during treatment of heavy metal poisoning in humans. Under such circumstances DSH plasma levels in the millimolar range can be expected.

Accordingly, effects on many enzymes susceptible to such concentrations of DSH should be expected.

By contrast, only micromolar concentrations of DSH arise during DSSD therapy of alcoholism. Thus treatment with a 250 mg p.o. dose of DSSD gives rise to peak DSH plasma levels of 0.77–1.14 μM (Faiman *et al.*, 1984). Johansson (1989a) recorded *ca* 0.3 μM DSH in the plasma of patients receiving a 400 mg p.o. dose of DSSD. Such concentrations of DSH may cause significant inhibition of only the most sensitive enzymes, with K_i values in the micromolar range.

8.1.3 Copper enzymes inhibited by diethyldithiocarbamate *in vitro*

In addition to the copper-containing enzymes whose inhibition by DSH was discussed in section 8.1.2, another group of enzymes which are inhibited by DSH *in vitro* are the copper-containing tyrosinases (EC 1.14.18.1), also called phenol oxidases (for review see Schmidt, 1988). Many of these enzymes possess both a tyrosinase and a dopa oxidase function; DSH inhibits these functions differentially. An example of this is the inhibition of the murine and hamster melanoma enzyme. The DSH K_i for the dopa oxidase function is 80–100 μM (Lerner *et al.*, 1950; Pomerantz, 1963); DSH is less effective in inhibiting the tyrosine hydroxylase function of this enzyme (Pomerantz, 1966; Laskin and Piccini, 1986). Other tyrosinases which have been reported to be inhibited by DSH are listed below; the functions inhibited and their K_i values are given where available: (a) a rat intestinal tyrosinase enzyme (Schmidt, 1979); (b) a bovine uveal dopa oxidase, K_i 18.8 μM (Nakazawa *et al.*, 1985); (c) a detergent-activated tyrosinase from *Xenopus laevis* (dopa oxidase, K_i 30 μM; tyrosine hydroxylase, K_i 50 μM: Wittenberg and Triplett, 1985); (d) tyrosinases from streptomyces and mushrooms (dopa oxidase, K_i 0.34 and 3.0 μM; tyrosine hydroxylase, K_i 6.2 and 4.1 μM, respectively: Yoshimoto *et al.*, 1985); and (e) a potato phenol oxidase (Van Driessche *et al.*, 1984).

Diamine oxidases (EC 1.4.3.6) constitute yet another group of copper-containing enzymes inhibited by DSH *in vitro*. These include the diamine oxidases of: (a) the human placenta (100% inhibited by 50 μM; Bardsley *et al.*, 1974); (b) porcine kidney (100% inhibited by dialysis against 50 μM; Mondovi *et al.*, 1967); and (c) lentil seedlings (Rinaldi *et al.*, 1984). Also reported to be inhibited by DSH *in vitro* are (a) a monoamine oxidase (EC 1.4.3.4) from the human placenta (40% inhibition by 50 μM; Bardsley *et al.*, 1974); (b) the calmodulin-dependent phosphatase of rat brain (Ruiz de Elvira *et al.*, 1987); and (c) the copper-containing peptidylglycine alpha amidating monooxygenase of pituitary cells, which is involved in the terminal amidation of pituitary peptide hormones (Mains *et al.*, 1986).

Finally, early reports had suggested that cytochrome oxidase, an important copper-containing enzyme, is partially inhibited at high DSH concentrations. The findings of Griffiths and Wharton (1961) that the purified enzyme is 20% inhibited by 1 mM DSH, are problematical since the assay used by these authors involved cytochrome *c*, which is known to be readily reduced by DSH (Strömme, 1963a). More recently, Gallagher and Reeve (1976) have reported that an 18 h dialysis against 5–10 mM DSH results in a 50–55% inhibition of the enzyme. However, exposure of a biological system (Chinese hamster cells) to 3 mM DSH for 90 min does not result in any inhibition of the enzyme (Marklund and Westman, 1980).

8.2 INHIBITION OF DRUG METABOLIZING ENZYMES

8.2.1 Introduction

Many drugs and other xenobiotics are metabolized oxidatively by a family of membrane-bound iron-containing hemoproteins located in the endoplasmic reticulum of cells, most prominently those of liver (for review see Black and Coon, 1989). Since in the reduced state these hemoproteins bind carbon monoxide to give a unique 450 nm peak in the Soret region of the spectrum, they are referred to generically as cytochromes P-450 (P-450). The reactions catalyzed by these enzymes involve the insertion of an atom of oxygen into the substrate, typically to give more polar metabolites,

$$RH + O_2 + NADPH + H^+ \rightarrow ROH + H_2O + NADP^+ \tag{8.3}$$

They are, therefore, called monooxygenases. Some substrates (viz. ethers such as *p*-nitroanisole, substituted amines such as ethylmorphine) yield unstable intermediates and the process becomes one of dealkylation. In the case of demethylations, an unstable oxygenated metabolite is formed which, after biotransformation, yields formaldehyde as the byproduct, i.e. the leaving group is oxygenated. The requirement of the P-450 enzymes for both oxidative and reducing equivalents gave rise to their earlier appellation of mixed function oxidases. These enzymes monooxygenate endogenous lipids, including steroid hormones and various cholesterol derivatives, with a high degree of specificity (for review see Waxman, 1988). In the metabolism of xenobiotic compounds they have overlapping site specificities.

Both DSSD and DSH are potent and clinically important *in vivo* inhibitors of the metabolism of many xenobiotics (section 8.2.2). In instances where the xenobiotic is a carcinogen, this can result in the modulation of its action (for review see Fiala, 1981, Bertram, 1988). Pretreatment of experimental animals, primarily rats, with DSSD results in impairment of hepatic metabolism of a wide range of substrates of the P-450 monooxygenases (all those tested to date) and a decrease in hepatic P-450 content (section 8.2.3). Analogous phenomena are observed following systemic pretreatment with DSH, the primary DSSD metabolite. These phenomena are also seen following oral DSH administration, but under these conditions their course is much more rapid, resembling that seen following administration of carbon disulfide (CS_2), itself a DSH metabolite (section 8.2.4). This raises the possibility that one or two common entities may mediate the impairment of the P-450 monooxygenases by these three agents. In this context, one needs to be mindful of the potential reversibility of the reduction of DSSD to DSH. One should also recognize that dithiocarbamates can be formed *in vivo* by the reaction of CS_2 with endogenous amines and amino acids.

Pretreatment of animals with DSSD and DSH results in some degradation of cytochrome P-450. Although the impairment of the various monooxygenase activities by DSSD, DSH and CS_2 is usually accompanied by a decrease in P-450 levels, typically the latter is not commensurate with the former. In part this dichotomy is due to the method used to measure P-450 levels, in part it could be due to these agents acting on the various P-450 cytochromes selectively (section 8.2.5). Assays performed on homogenized endoplasmic reticulum (microsomes) indicate DSSD is also a very effective *in vitro* inhibitor of the monooxygenase system (section 8.2.6). DSH is a much less potent *in vitro* inhibitor of the monooxygenase system than DSSD and their actions differ in a number of respects. In the presence of NADPH, however, DSH behaves very similarly to CS_2 with the formation of cytochrome P-420 and the binding of one of its sulfur atoms to the microsomal protein, probably at Cys_{436} at the active center of the cytochrome (section 8.2.7).

DSSD and DSH appear to have enhancing effects on some conjugations, notably the enzymes of the glucuronic acid and glutathione pathways, but these effects remain less well explored (sections 8.2.9 and 8.5). The effect of chronic DSSD treatment on intestinal monooxygenase activity, although also much less studied than its effects on the hepatic activity, are of interest in that the effect is biphasic, an initial reduction in activity being replaced by its stimulation (section 8.2.9).

8.2.2 *In vivo* inhibition in humans

Clinically administration of therapeutic doses of DSSD has been found to inhibit the hepatic endoplasmic reticulum enzyme-mediated metabolism of other therapeutically employed drugs virtually every time it has been investigated (Table 8.1). Additionally, administration of DSSD has been found to inhibit endogenous metabolism mediated by this system. Thus, DSSD therapy leads to increased serum cholesterol levels (Major and Goyer, 1978), an effect attributable, in some part, to its inhibition of cholesterol 7α-hydroxylase, a specific P-450 enzyme (Andersson and Boström, 1984; Waxman, 1986). Also, administration of DSSD causes a decrease in the urinary excretion of D-glucaric acid (Freundt, 1978). The excretion of this end-product of the D-glucuronic acid pathway is considered an indirect measure, in humans and guinea pigs, of endoplasmic reticulum enzyme function and is quantitatively correlated with hepatic P-450 content (Hunter *et al.*, 1974). Although the ability of DSH to inhibit drug metabolism in humans has not been investigated, its administration also leads to a significant reduction in D-glucaric acid excretion (Larseille *et al.*, 1982).

In humans, the inhibition of drug metabolism caused by DSSD develops rapidly, and is observed within 4 hours of its administration (Olesen, 1966). It persists, or intensifies, upon repeated administration (Table 8.1) without any evidence of subsequent induction of the P-450 system. Moreover, it is prolonged. A single dose, for instance, causes a 6-day-long depression of D-glucaric acid elimination (Freundt, 1978). Likewise, 10 days after a course of DSSD, antipyrine (aminophenazone) metabolism continues to be significantly depressed in the majority of subjects (Vesell *et al.*, 1971). On the other hand, the degree to which monooxygenation is inhibited by a given dose of DSSD shows extensive interindividual variation (Vesell *et al.*, 1971, 1975; Beyeler *et al.*, 1985, 1987). Functionally, this is also true of the inhibition of aldehyde dehydrogenase (ALDH) by DSSD (Beyeler *et al.*, 1985, 1987; Brewer, 1984). A high correlation ($r = 0.88$; $P < 0.01$) is observed between the inhibition of these two enzyme activities in individual subjects. The correlation has been ascribed by Beyeler *et al.* (1985) to the effect of DSSD on each enzyme activity being related to the functional capacity of the liver.

In patients stabilized on a drug, DSSD-mediated inhibition of the drug's metabolism can lead to its accumulation and result in unexpected yet typical overdose reactions. Phenytoin is one drug for which such a sequence of events has been observed. Epileptic patients previously stabilized on it develop dizziness, ataxia and nystagmus after 1–5 weeks on DSSD (Kiørboe, 1966; Dry and Pradalier, 1973; Loiseau *et al.*, 1975). Phenytoin levels are elevated in such patients (Table 8.1). Even after discontinuation of DSSD therapy, these levels may continue to rise further for a day or two; eventually, as the phenytoin levels fall, the clinical condition resolves (Olesen, 1966; Loiseau *et al.*, 1975). Warfarin is another drug, the levels of which rise during DSSD therapy in previously stabilized patients. The rise is accompanied by an enhancement of the drug's anticoagulation action (prolongation of one-stage prothrombin time) and an increase in toxic effects such as hematuria and gross bleeding (Rothstein, 1968, 1972b; O'Reilly, 1971, 1973). By reducing the warfarin dose, however, it is possible to successfully stabilize patients on a warfarin–DSSD combination with no ill effects (Rothstein, 1968, 1972b).

DSSD therapy leads to inhibition of caffeine metabolism (Beach *et al.*, 1986) as well as the metabolism of both chlordiazepoxide and diazepam, two frequently prescribed antianxiety drugs (MacLeod *et al.*, 1978; Sellers *et al.* 1980). Both these agents have active metabolites and their metabolism may also be inhibited. Recovering alcoholics have a particularly high coffee and hence caffeine consumption (Doucette and Willoughby, 1980; Mozdzierz *et al.*, 1981). The DSSD-engendered inhibition of the elimination of the latter renders such individuals at risk for caffeine-induced symptoms of increased irritability, anxiety and insomnia. Chlordiazepoxide and diazepam are frequently used concurrently with DSSD in the treatment of recovering alcoholics (Baekeland *et al.*, 1975; Baekeland and Lundwann, 1977). The appearance of symptoms of anxiety and irritability would make the prescription of these antianxiety agents all the more likely. On occasion the combination of disulfiram therapy with chlordiazepoxide has been specifically advocated on the basis that the latter would act as both a reinforcer and blocking drug (Liebson and Faillace, 1971). Elevation of chlordiazepoxide or diazepam body burdens (and of those of their active metabolites) will result, however, in symptoms of central nervous system depression (lethargy, dizziness, etc.). Such symptoms are associated with DSSD therapy in patients receiving chlordiazepoxide; they ameliorate upon DSSD dose reduction or discontinuation (Whittington and Grey, 1969). However, the occurrence of such symptoms is not intrinsic to DSSD therapy. For patients requiring concurrent antianxiety medication, oxazepam, lorazepam, or alprazolam are better choices. Oxazepam and lorazepam are primarily metabolized by glucuronidation and their elimination is not impaired by DSSD treatment (Table 8.1). Rather, DSSD was found to enhance the elimination of lorazepam in the majority of the, admittedly small, sample of patients studied (Sellers *et al.*, 1980). With regard to

Table 8.1 Impairment of metabolism of drugs and endogenous substrates by disulfiram (DSSD) and diethyldithiocarbamate (DSH) in humans

Drug	Subjects Nature	Number	DSSD dose	Effect Parameter	Change %	P	Study
Phenytoin[a], p.o. maintenance	Epileptic patients	4	400 mg × 9 days	Phenytoin blood level	+254 ± 69		Olesen (1966)
Phenytoin[a], p.o. maintenance	Epileptic patients	2	400 mg × 9 days	Phenytoin[b] blood level	+45 ± 11		Olesen (1967)
Primidone[a], p.o. maintenance	Epileptic patients	3	400 mg × 9 days	Phenobarbital blood level	+5 ± 1		Olesen (1966)
Antipyrine, p.o.	Normal males	7	7 mg/kg × 4 days	Half-life	+68	<0.001	Vesell et al. (1971)
Antipyrine, p.o.	Normal males	10	7 mg/kg × 10 days	Half-life	+68	<0.001	Vesell et al. (1971)
Antipyrine, p.o.	Normal males	6	3.5 mg/kg × 10 days	Half-life	+53	<0.05[c]	Vesell et al. (1975)
Antipyrine, i.v.	Normal males	6	3.5 mg/kg × 10 days	Half-life	+95	<0.05[c]	Vesell et al. (1975)
Antipyrine, p.o.	Normal subjects	9	400 mg/kg × 2 days	clearance	−16	<0.05	Loft et al. (1986)
[14]C-Aminopyrine, p.o.	Normal subjects	7	250 mg × 4 days	Metabolic clearance	−48	<0.01	Hepner and Vesell (1974)
[14]C-Aminopyrine, i.v.	Abstinent[d] alcoholics	8	400 mg × 3–6 days	Breath ^{14}C-CO$_2$	−22		Beyeler et al. (1985)
Warfarin, p.o.	Normal males	8	500 mg × 1 day	Warfarin plasma level	+27	<0.02	O'Reilly (1973)
Warfarin, p.o.	Normal males	7	500 mg × 3 weeks	Warfarin plasma level	+23	<0.001[e]	O'Reilly (1973)
Chlordiazepoxide, i.v.	Normal males	6	500 mg × 14 days	Half-life	+84	<0.01	MacLeod et al. (1978)
Diazepam, p.o.	Normals + alcoholics	8	500 mg × 12 days	Half-life	+37	<0.05	MacLeod et al. (1978)
Oxazepam, p.o.	Normals + alcoholics	7	500 mg × 14 days	Half-life	+17	>0.05	MacLeod et al. (1978)
Lorazepam, p.o.	Volunteers	4	500 mg × 12 days	Half-life	−14		Sellers et al. (1980)

		n	Dose	Parameter	Change	P	Reference
Alprazolam p.o.	Abstinent[f] alcoholics	11	500 mg × 14 days	Half-life	−8	>0.05	Diquet et al. (1990)
Imipraine, i.v.	Normal males	2	500 mg × 14 days	Half-life[g]	+16		Ciarulo et al. (1985)
Desipramine, i.v.	Normal male	1	500 mg × 4 weeks	Half-life[h]	+20		Ciarulo et al. (1985)
Caffeine, p.o.	Normal males	5	250 mg × 4 days	Half-life[i]	+39	<0.01	Beach et al. (1986)
Caffeine, p.o.	Normal males	5	500 mg × 4 days	Half-life[j]	+34	<0.005	Beach et al. (1986)
Caffeine, p.o.	Abstinent[k] alcoholics	5	500 mg × 4 days	Half-life[l]	+29	<0.002	Beach et al. (1986)
Theophylline, i.v.	Abstinent[m] alcoholics	8	250 mg × 8 days	Half-life[n]	+13	<0.02	Loi et al. (1989)
Theophylline, i.v.	Abstinent[m] alcoholics	8	500 mg × 8 days	Half-life[o]	+51	<0.02	Loi et al. (1989)
ENDOGENOUS SUBSTRATES							
D-glucaric acid	Normal males	7	10 mg/kg × 1 day	24 h excretion	−38	<0.05	Freundt (1978)
D-glucaric acid	Normal males	4	DSH 300 mg bid × 1 week	8 h excretion	−30	<0.05	Larseille et al. (1982)
Cholesterol	Abstinent alcoholics	6	500 mg × 3 weeks	Serum cholesterol	+18	<0.02	Major and Goyer (1978)

[a] Concurrently with maintenance on other agents.
[b] Also: urinary excretion of phenytoin metabolite, 5-(p-hydroxyphenyl)-5-phenylhydantoin, decreased by 40 ± 2%.
[c] $P<0.05$ for combined i.v. and p.o. data.
[d] With entry aminopyrine breath test values in normal range.
[e] $P<0.001$ for each of 5 of the 7 patients studied.
[f] Also: total body clearance of alprazolam increased by 18% ($P>0.05$).
[g] Also: total body clearance of imipramine decreased by 24%.
[h] Also: total body clearance of desimipramine decreased by 24%.
[i] Also: total body clearance of caffeine decreased by 30% ($P<0.005$).
[j] Also: total body clearance of caffeine decreased by 29% ($P<0.005$).
[k] From alcohol but 9/11 smoked cigarettes.
[l] Also: total body clearance of caffeine decreased by 24% ($P<0.001$).
[m] From alcohol and tobacco smoking.
[n] Also: total plasma clearance of theophylline and formation clearance of its metabolites decreased by 21% ($P<0.001$) and 20% ($P<0.001$), respectively.
[o] Also: total plasma clearance of theophylline and formation clearance of its metabolites decreased by 31% ($P<0.001$) and 22% ($P<0.02$), respectively.

alprazolam, its half-life and clearance have been reported to be unaffected by DSSD therapy (Diquet *et al.*, 1990), a somewhat surprising finding given that it is metabolized via hydroxylation and that another inhibitor of drug metabolism, cimetidine, does prolong its elimination (Greenblatt *et al.*, 1983).

When DSSD administration is combined with that of cimetidine, another agent which inhibits drug metabolism *in vivo*, the resulting inhibition of drug metabolism is additive (Loft *et al.*, 1986).

8.2.3 *In vivo* inhibition of hepatic monooxygenases by disulfiram in experimental animals

The experimental animal used most frequently in investigation of the effect of DSSD on hepatic drug metabolism has been the rat. No systematic *in vivo* study has been performed of the inhibition of hepatic monooxygenase activity as a function of the dose of DSSD. Moreover, in determining monooxygenase activity a variety of substrates are used as probes and while the resulting estimates are frequently similar, they reflect the activities of different clusters of P-450 isozymes, are thereby distinct, and can be significantly different.

The dose used most commonly in rat studies of the impairment of drug metabolism by DSSD is 1 g/kg, p.o. Doubling the dose fails to enhance the effect further. Thus 24 h after 1 and 2 g/kg p.o. doses of DSSD no differences are observed (Stripp *et al.*, 1969) in the degree of inhibition of ethylmorphine *N*-deethylation (39 and 37%, respectively) or the extent by which P-450 levels are depressed (24 and 26%, respectively). On the other hand, 400 mg/kg of DSSD is the lowest oral dose reported to cause a significant impairment of P-450 activity after a single administration; it causes a 33% decrease in aniline hydroxylase activity (Zemaitis and Green, 1976b). However, chronic administration of as little as 100 mg/kg/day will result in a 25% impairment of aniline hydroxylase after 2 days and a 46% impairment after 5 days (Zemaitis and Green, 1976b). The route of administration and vehicle are also important. A single 100 mg/kg dose of DSSD causes a one-third decrease in monooxygenase activity (benzo[*a*]pyrene hydroxylase) at 24 h, if it is administered i.p. in oil (Grafström and Green, 1980). Yet a 200 mg/kg dose administered by the same route, but either in aqueous suspension or in dimethylsulfoxide, is without effect on aminopyrine demethylation 24 and 48 h later (Willson *et al.*, 1979).

Parenthetically it should be added that p.o. administration of 200 mg/kg of DSSD to rats result in the inhibition 24 h later of the microsomal carboxylesterase in liver, plasma carboxylesterase and plasma cholinesterase by 29%, 21% and 27%, respectively, and that raising the dose to 1000 mg/kg increases the inhibition to 38%, 45% and 53%, respectively (Zeimatis and Green, 1976a).

The onset of the DSSD effects in rats is slow. No impairment is detected in the first 8 h post administration of 1 g/kg, whether administered orally (Honjo and Netter, 1969), i.p. in an aqueous suspension (Stripp *et al.*, 1969), or i.p. in oil (Hunter and Neal, 1975). Impairment is significant at 12 h (ethylmorphine *N*-deethylation; Stripp *et al.*, 1969), 15 h (aminopyrine *N*-demethylation; Honjo and Netter, 1969; Netter *et al.*, 1970), and 18 h (hexobarbital metabolism: Nilsson and Wahlstrøm, 1989). It reaches its maximum at 24 h and remains significant for 72 h (Stripp *et al.*, 1969).

The impairment of monooxygenase activities by DSSD administration in the rat is not uniform. Some activities are more resistant than others. Thus, while aniline hydroxylase activity is 32% impaired ($P < 0.05$) 24 h following the administration of DSSD in a 400 mg/kg/day dose, no impairment of ethylmorphine *N*-deethylation activity is observed at that point in time. Though after 2 days of treatment, the ethylmorphine *N*-deethylation activity is decreased by 50% ($P < 0.05$), by then the aniline hydroxylase activity is decreased by 61% ($P < 0.05$). As the daily DSSD administration is continued for 12 days, the impairment of the monooxygenase activity remains unabated (Zemaitis and Green, 1976b).

The DSSD-induced impairment of monooxygenase activity in rats is usually accompanied by a depression of P-450 levels, although the latter is virtually always more modest than the former (Stripp *et al.*, 1969; Hunter and Neal, 1975; Lang *et al.*, 1976, Zemaitis and Green, 1976b; Grafström and Green, 1980; Cha *et al.*, 1983). There is, moreover, a degree of correspondence in the time course of these phenomena (Stripp *et al.*, 1969).

In mice administered DSSD, the effects on monooxygenase activity are observed sooner than in rats. Four hours following a 500 mg/kg p.o. dose of DSSD, monooxygenase activity (benzo[*a*]pyrene hydroxylase, 2-acetylaminofluorene *N*-hydroxylase and aldrin monooxygenase) is impaired in both C57BL/6 and DBA/2 mice, on average, by 66% (Roberfroid *et al.*, 1983). Also, the *in vivo* half-life of antipyrine is lengthened by 60–70%.

8.2.4 *In vivo* inhibition of hepatic monooxygenases by diethyldithiocarbamate and carbon disulfide

Because DSH is unstable in acidic media, such as gastric juice, decomposing therein to CS_2 and diethylamine, consideration of the effects of

DSH on monooxygenase function following its oral administration are best deferred until after discussion of the effects observed following its systemic administration.

The most widely employed systemic dose of DSH in studies of its effects on the hepatic drug metabolizing system of rats is 750 mg/kg i.p., though administration of a dose as small as 200 mg/kg results, for instance, in a significant (27%) reduction 24 h later in hepatic ethylmorphine *N*-deethylation activity (Stripp *et al.*, 1969). Neither the 200 nor a 250 mg/kg dose have any effect, however, on hepatic P-450 levels 24 h post administration, though higher doses do (Fig. 8.1a).

The time course of the effects of systemically administered DSH on the hepatic monooxygenase system is somewhat more rapid than that

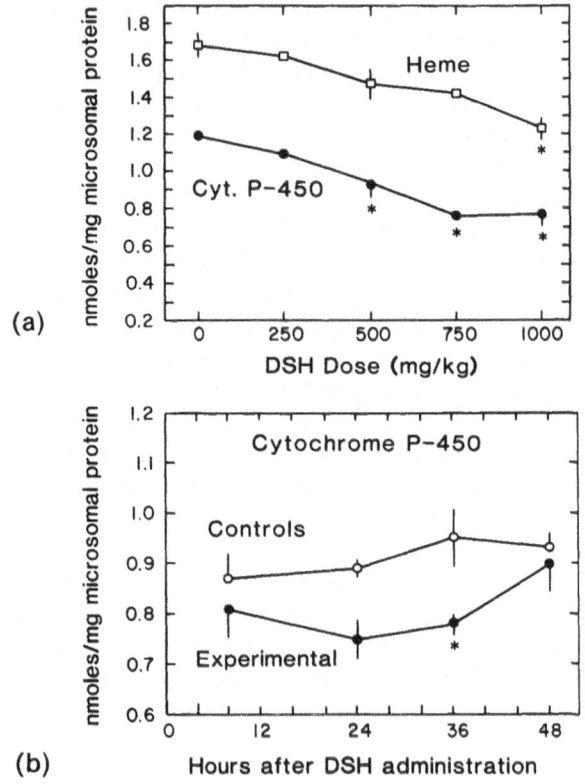

Figure 8.1 Effects of intraperitoneal administration of diethyldithiocarbamate (DSH) on hepatic microsomal cytochrome P-450 in the rat. (a) Dose–response relationships for the effects of diethyldithiocarbamate on microsomal cytochrome P-450 and microsomal heme at 24 h. (b) Time course of the effects of 750 mg/kg DSH. *Significantly different from control, $P < 0.05$. Redrawn with permission from Miller *et al.* (1983).

seen following DSSD administration. Thus, by 6 h after a 1 g/kg i.p. dose of DSH, both the benzamphetamine *N*-demethylase activity and the P-450 levels are depressed significantly (Hunter and Neal, 1975). The P-450 levels reach their nadir at 24 h (Fig. 8.1b) and are still significantly depressed at 36 h. By 48 h, however, they are indistinguishable from controls (Miller *et al.*, 1983; Hunter and Neal, 1975).

Contrary to what might be expected, following oral administration of DSH the onset of the P-450 lowering effect is faster and its duration is shorter than following i.p. administration (Fig. 8.2) In particular, the rapidity of onset, which exceeds that seen following i.p. administration several-fold, is very similar to that seen following CS_2 administration, regardless by which route (Fig. 8.3). So too are the time course and relative extent of the inhibition of both aniline hydroxylase and aminopyrine *N*-demethylase activities occasioned by the oral administration of 200 mg/kg DSH and 30 mg/kg CS_2, respectively (Figs 8.2 and 8.3). This similarity could be explained by a gastric hydrolysis of part of the administered DSH to CS_2. Finally, it should be noted that the dose-dependence relationship for CS_2 spans a wider range (from 3 to 500 mg/kg) than is true for the other agents considered.

8.2.5 *In vivo* effects on P-450 cytochromes

The impairment of the various monooxygenase activities by DSSD pretreatment is usually accompanied by a decrease in P-450 levels, however the magnitude of the latter is typically smaller than that of the former. That is to say, DSSD administration results in a greater functional impairment of P-450 than is apparent from the reduction in P-450 levels, as determined spectrophotometrically following reaction of the cytochrome with carbon monoxide.

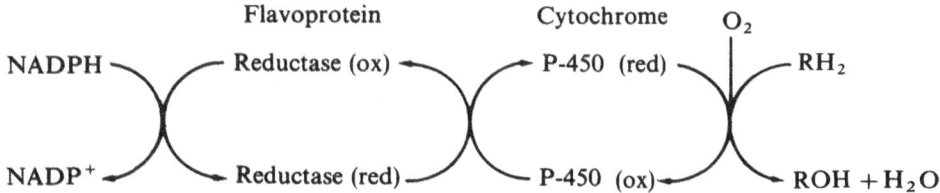

The P-450 monooxygenase complex has two primary functional components: a flavoprotein enzyme and a cytochrome. The reduced cytochrome reacts with the substrate and oxygen becoming oxidized in the process. The flavoprotein acts as a reductase of the oxidized cytochrome. To determine their respective levels it is usual to measure

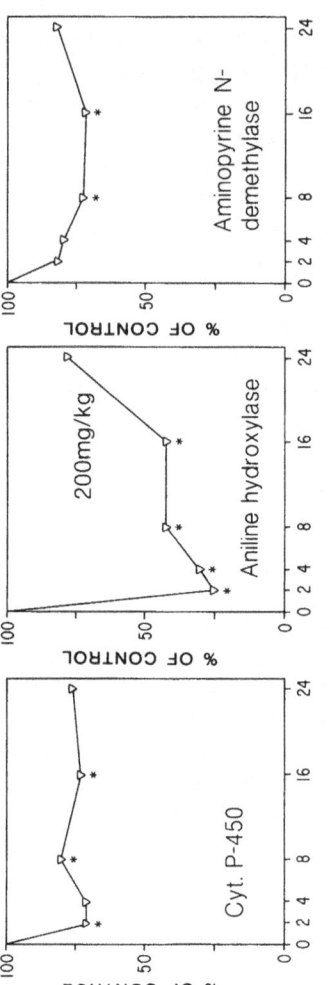

Figure 8.2 Time course of the effect of oral administration of a 200 mg/kg dose of diethyldithiocarbamate (DSH) on hepatic microsomal cytochrome P-450 and some drug-metabolizing enzymes in the rat. *Significantly different from control, $P < 0.05$. Redrawn from Siegers *et al.* (1982).

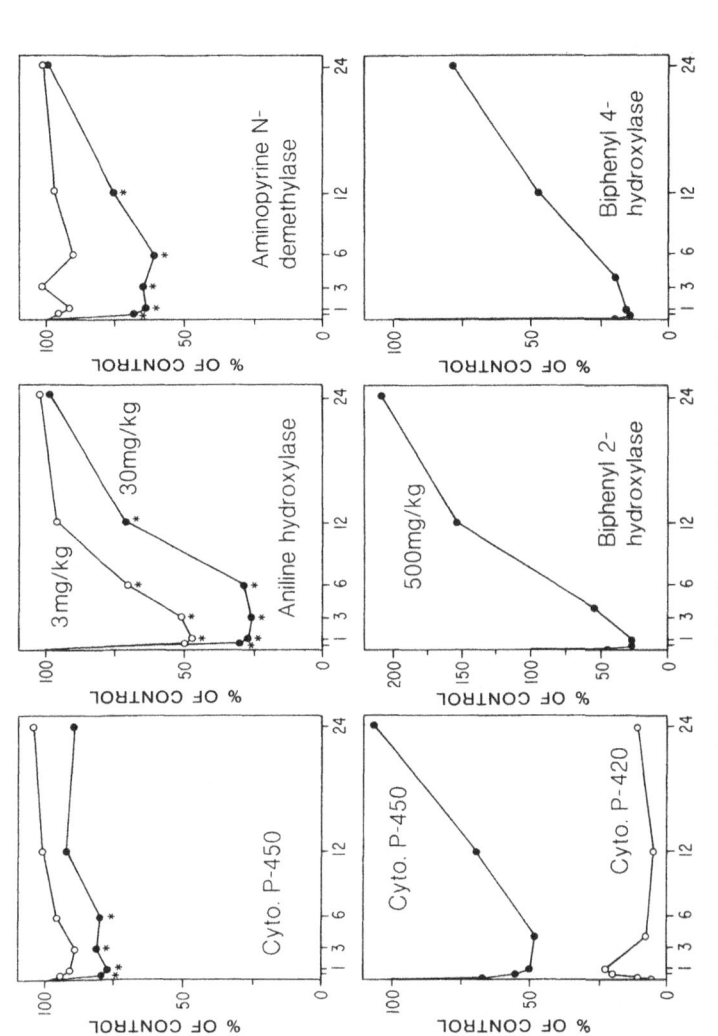

HOURS AFTER CARBON DISULFIDE ADMINISTRATION

Figure 8.3 Time course of the effects of carbon disulfide on hepatic microsomal cytochrome P-450 and some drug-metabolizing enzymes in the rat. (Top) following oral administration of 3 and 30 mg/kg (open and closed circles, respectively). *Significantly different from control, $P < 0.05$. Redrawn from Masuda *et al.* (1986). (Bottom) Following intraperitoneal administration of 500 mg/kg. Both P-450 and P-420 values are expressed in percentage of control P-450 levels. Drawn from data of Obrebska *et al.* (1980).

the Soret spectrum of the carbon monoxide adduct of the cytochrome and to measure the activity of the reductase in an assay which employs exogenous cytochrome *c* as an electron acceptor. When measured in this manner, the activity is referred to as NADPH cytochrome *c* reductase. DSSD pretreatment (200 mg/kg i.p., 24 h prior) was observed by Stripp *et al.* (1969) to decrease this activity only slightly (by 17%). The activity of the reductase can also be measured using the membrane-bound P-450 cytochrome (i.e. the microsomal fraction: Gigon *et al.*, 1968). If measured in this manner, the activity is referred to as NADPH cytochrome P-450 reductase. Following the same DSSD pretreatment (200 mg/kg i.p., 24 h prior) this latter activity is markedly diminished (66%). Since the enzyme used in both assays is the same flavoprotein, the lower activity recorded when cytochrome P-450 is employed indicates that the ability of the cytochrome to act as an electron acceptor has been impaired by the DSSD pretreatment. This provides a functional explanation for the observed parallel lowering of the monooxygenase function (by 55%), as measured with ethyl morphine as substrate. Moreover, the extent of the impairment of cytochrome P-450 to act as an electron acceptor is greater than the 49% decrease in the binding of P-450 with carbon monoxide to give the Soret spectrum used to measure P-450 levels (Stripp *et al.*, 1969), suggesting that the functional impairment does not prevent the cytochrome from forming an adduct with carbon monoxide to give a Soret spectrum. The same phenomenon has been observed by Stripp *et al.* (1969) at 48 h after an i.p. 200 mg/kg dose of DSSD and by Zemaitis and Green (1976b) 24 h after p.o. administration of 400 mg/kg/day DSSD for 2 days.

The depression of P-450 levels by these agents suggests destruction of the cytochrome. Although normally hepatic P-450 heme turnover is quite rapid, administration of DSH (750 mg/kg) accelerates it, reducing the half-life of the fast phase of heme loss from 6 to 3 h (Miller *et al.*, 1983). Within 2 h of the administration of this dose of DSH, the levels of hepatic heme oxygenase, the enzyme responsible for the rate-limiting step in P-450 catabolism, are increased 3-fold. By 8 h, the levels are 7-fold higher than those of controls, though they return to control values 24 h after DSH administration. The levels of hepatic δ-aminolevulinic acid synthetase, the enzyme responsible for the rate-limiting step in P-450 synthesis, also rise, but less rapidly and for longer. Thus, by 8 h after administration they are elevated by 55% and they remain elevated at 24 h (Miller *et al.*, 1983).

The hepatic monooxygenase system comprises multiple P-450 isoforms of overlapping site specificities. Biotransformations catalyzed by specific isoforms can result in the formation of different metabolites. Some of the isoforms can be preferentially induced by pretreatment with xenobiotics (for review see Ioannides and Parke, 1987). In the rat, P-450b and P-450e are induced by pretreatment with phenobarbital (PB), and P-450c by pretreatment with 3-methylcholanthrene (MC).

Hunter and Neal (1975) compared the ability of DSSD, DSH and CS_2 to depress monooxygenase activity (benzamphetamine N-demethylation) and P-450 levels at 6 and 48 h post administration in normal and PB or MC pretreated rats. Although there were some variations in the degree to which DSSD, DSH and CS_2 reduced monooxygenase activity and P-450 levels in the three groups, no clear meaningful pattern emerged, suggesting that these agents impair multiple P-450 isoforms.

In PB pretreated animals, though not otherwise, CS_2 induces hepatic necrosis (for review see Beauchamp *et al.*, 1983), as does DSH, but not DSSD (Hunter and Neal, 1975). The latter dichotomy could be due to the formation of hepatotoxic concentrations of the same or similar metabolites from CS_2 and DSH, but not DSSD. It might be noted, parenthetically, that ethanol pretreatment also sensitizes rats to CS_2 induced hepatotoxicity (Snyderwine *et al.*, 1988).

8.2.6 *In vitro* inhibition by disulfiram

When added to rat hepatic microsomes, isolated from either normal or PB-induced animals, DSSD is a potent inhibitor of P-450 reactions. Thus, it gives K_i values of $0.2–1.2 \times 10^{-5}$M for the competitive inhibition of the dealkylation of p-nitroanisole (Honjo and Netter, 1969), ethylmorphine (Zemaitis and Green, 1976b, 1979) and p-nitrophenetol (Jørgensen and Johansen, 1983). Also, as an inhibitor of benzo[a]pyrene hydroxylase, another monooxygenase activity, it ranks among the top five of 34 known and potential inhibitors of P-450 metabolism (Stohs and Wu, 1982). Further, it binds to P-450, producing a type I spectrum (Zemaitis and Green, 1976b; Masuda and Nakamura, 1989), a property common to a large group of substrates metabolized by P-450. This suggests that it inhibits the metabolism of the other substrates by competing for binding sites on P-450. Incubation of DSSD in the admittedly high concentration of 1.0×10^{-4}M, impairs the subsequent activity of several microsomal enzymes (aniline hydroxylase, p-nitroanisole O-demethylase and glucose-6-phosphatase) regardless of whether or not NADPH is present during the incubation (Masuda, 1988). This again suggests that DSSD does not have to undergo a P-450-mediated activation to act as an inhibitor at this concentration.

One isoform of the cytochrome, P-450$_{Ch7\alpha}$, the enzyme that catalyzes the 7α-hydroxylation of cholesterol, is exquisitely sensitive to inhibition by DSSD. Exposure of either rat microsomes (Waxman, 1986) or of the enzyme purified to homogeneity (Ogishima *et al.*, 1987) to 4×10^{-6}M DSSD causes extensive inactivation. Subsequent exposure of the microsomes to 10 mM 2-mercaptoethylamine for 4 min fully reactivates the enzyme (Waxman, 1986). *In vivo*, chronic daily dosing of rats with DSSD leads to a partial inactivation of the cytochrome. However, *in vitro* the inactivation of the thus inhibited enzyme is substantially reversed (85%) by 10 mM dithiothreitol (Andersson and Boström, 1984). These observations suggest that DSSD blocks a highly reactive thiol group near the active center of the enzyme, presumably by the formation, at least initially, of a mixed disulfide. Nor is this manner of inhibition unique to P-450$_{Ch7\alpha}$, since the activity of other microsomal steroid hydroxylases, partially blocked by 10 μM DSSD, is also reactivated by treatment with 2-mercaptoethylamine (Waxman, 1986). It is noteworthy that when DSSD is added to fresh microsomal membranes, it is reduced to DSH and that when DSSD is formed by such membranes in the presence of NADPH, a large portion of it becomes bound to the membranes, from which it can be displaced by GSH (Masuda, 1988). On the other hand, unlike CS$_2$, DSSD is not immediately effective in perfused liver preparations in impairing monooxygenase activity (*p*-nitroanisole *O*-demethylation: Masuda *et al.*, 1988).

8.2.7 *In vitro* inhibition by diethyldithiocarbamate and carbon disulfide

In many particulars the actions of DSH on P-450 differ from those of DSSD. Firstly, DSH inhibits competitively the metabolism of some of the same P-450 substrates as DSSD, but is considerably less potent, its K_i value ranging from 1.3 to 1.8×10^{-4}M (Honjo and Netter, 1969; Zemaitis and Green, 1976b). Secondly, it forms no binding spectrum with P-450 (Honjo and Netter, 1969; Zemaitis and Green, 1976b; Masuda and Nakamura, 1989). Thirdly, though incubation with 10^{-3}M DSH for 15–30 min depresses P-450 levels and impairs microsomal enzyme activity, it does so only if NADPH is present during the incubation (Hunter and Neal, 1975; Zemaitis and Green, 1979; Miller *et al.*, 1983; Masuda, 1988). Although these are incubation conditions that result in the formation of DSSD from DSH (Masuda, 1988; Masuda and Nakamura, 1989; see Chapter 6), the effects of DSH on the P-450 system bear many more similarities to those of CS$_2$ than those of DSSD.

Like DSH, CS$_2$ brings about a decrease in P-450 (De Matteis and Seawright, 1973) and an impairment of monooxygenase activity

(Obrebska *et al.*, 1980) when incubated with liver microsomes in the presence of NADPH, but not in its absence. Also, upon incubation with microsomes in the presence of NADPH, both DSH (Miller *et al.*, 1983) and CS_2 (De Matteis and Seawright, 1973) bring about marked increases in the levels of cytochrome P-420 (P-420), a degradation product of P-450. The appearance of P-420 is also a consequence of *in vivo* CS_2 administration (Fig. 8.3). The significance of this stems from the fact that the unusual 450 nm Soret region spectrum band characteristic of P-450 is due to a thiolate sulfur atom ligated to the heme iron in the fifth or proximate coordination site. A specific cysteine residue of the cytochrome (Cys_{436} in the sequence numbering convention of rabbit P-450 isozyme 2) is considered to provide this thiolate ligand (for review see Black and Coon, 1989). The appearance of a 420 band indicates that this sulfhydryl is no longer ligated to the heme iron. The transient nature of this increase (Fig. 8.3) suggests that the formation of P-420 following CS_2 exposure is an intermediate step in the CS_2-induced degradation of P-450. Incubation of microsomes with NADPH and CS_2 leads to formation of carbonyl sulfide (COS). If CS_2 labeled with ^{35}S or ^{14}C is used, 50% of the ^{35}S label, but none of the ^{14}C label, becomes bound to P-450 (De Matteis and Seawright, 1973; De Matteis, 1974; Dalvi *et al.*, 1974). Upon incubation of these labelled microsomes with cyanide, ^{35}S is released in the form of thiocyanate (SCN^-). This indicates that the ^{35}S is attached to the P-450 as the terminal sulfur of a hydrosulfide (R-S-S-H) (Catignani and Neal, 1975). This would be formed by the reaction of atomic sulfur with a protein cysteine residue. The mechanism involved appears to be a P-450 catalyzed desulfuration reaction that leads to the release of atomic sulfur in singlet form. This is highly electrophilic and attacks the nearest cysteine sulfhydryl, namely that at Cys_{436}. The ^{35}S label also becomes bound to the microsomes upon their incubation with ^{35}S-labeled DSH in the presence of NADPH (Miller *et al.*, 1983). This indicates that DSH, CS_2 or some other metabolite derived from DSH undergoes oxidative desulfuration. GSH inhibits the binding of the ^{35}S label of DSH to microsomes; it also inhibits the DSH-induced conversion of P-450 to P-420 (Miller *et al.*, 1983). Interpretation of these actions of GSH is difficult. On one hand, by providing alternate binding sites, GSH could act to protect the microsomal membrane. On the other hand, GSH would reduce any DSSD formed from DSH back to it.

Differences exist between the effects of DSH and CS_2. Thus the latter does not bring about any changes in heme oxygenase, UDP-glucuronyl transferase activity, or glucose-6-phosphatase activity (Masuda *et al.*, 1986); nor does it affect microsomal carboxyesterase (Nakayama and Masuda, 1985).

8.2.8 Inhibition by diethyldithiocarbamic acid methyl ester

Available information indicates that the DSH metabolite, diethyl-dithiocarbamic acid methyl ester (DSMe), is a more potent inhibitor of drug metabolism than DSH. Traiger *et al.* (1984, 1985) have investigated the effects of these two agents on the metabolism of aminopyrine and α-naphthylisothiocyanate. The hyperbilirubinemia and cholestasis produced by the latter agent in rats and mice is considered to be due to the formation of toxic metabolites via the hepatic monooxygenase system. Specifically, α-naphthylisothiocyanate is thought to be desulfurated by the hepatic monooxygenase system to α-naphthylisocyanate with the formation of atomic sulfur, which is extremely reactive. Pretreatment of rats with DSSD, DSH or DSMe inhibits, in each case, the development of the hyperbilirubinemia which otherwise follows α-naphthylisothiocyanate administration (Traiger *et al.*, 1984). The dose–response relationships for this effect of DSH and DSMe indicate the latter to be 3 times more potent than DSH. Both DSMe and DSH inhibit the NADPH-dependent metabolism of α-naphthylisothiocyanate and aminopyrine by rat hepatic microsomes *in vitro*, but DSMe is much more potent than DSH (Traiger *et al.*, 1985). The inhibition of the NADPH-dependent metabolism of α-naphthylisothiocyanate by DSMe is a competitive one (K_i:0.18 mM). DSMe also decreases, *in vivo*, the excretion of ^{35}S-labeled inorganic sulfate following administration of ^{35}S-α-naphthylisothiocyanate (Traiger *et al.*, 1984). The competitive nature of this effect is suggested by the fact that DSMe itself is metabolized to inorganic sulfate (section 5.8) and gives rise to a desulfurated metabolite, diethyl-monothiocarbamate (DmSMe), *in vivo* (section 5.9).

8.2.9 *In vivo* effects on enzymes of the glucuronic acid pathway

Chronic administration of DSSD or DSH increase the activity of UDP glucuronosyltransferases (EC 2.4.1.17) and have been reported to produce significant effects on several of the other enzymes of the glucuronic acid pathway. In rats, oral administration of 300 mg/kg/day DSSD or DSH for 4 days increases (by 2.5- and 1.6-fold, respectively) the activity of hepatic UDP-glucuronosyltransferases when this is assayed 24 h after the last dose using *p*-nitrophenol as a substrate (Marselos *et al.*, 1976). In mice, incorporation of DSSD as a 0.6% w/w additive in the diet for 14 days is found to increase UDP-glucuronosyltransferase activity. This is so whether the activity is assayed with *p*-nitrophenol, 4-methylumbelliferone, or 4-hydroxybiphenyl (Ford and Benson, 1988). Finally, it should be recalled (section 8.2.2) that the elimination of lorazepam, a drug metabolized primarily by glucuronidation, is increased by DSSD pretreatment in the majority of patients studied (Sellers *et al.*, 1980).

Marselos *et al.* (1976) reported other enzymes of the glucuronic acid pathway also to be significantly affected by the chronic treatment with DSSD or DSH. Thus, these workers observed stimulation of UDP-glucose dehydrogenase (2.3- and 1.7-fold, respectively), UDP-glucuronic acid pyrophosphatase (1.7- and 1.6-fold, respectively), and L-gluconate dehydrogenase (1.4-fold for DSSD only). On the other hand, they found decreases in the activities of glucose-6-phosphate dehydrogenase, β-glucuronidase (by 84 and 62%, respectively), and D-glucuronolactone dehydrogenase (by 84% for DSH only).

8.2.10 Effects on extrahepatic drug metabolizing enzymes

The microsomal benzo[*a*]pyrene hydroxylase of the small intestine is inhibited by DSSD *in vitro*, but with only one-tenth of the potency seen in liver microsomes (Grafström and Green, 1980; Grafström and Holmberg, 1980; Stohs and Wu, 1982). The activity is also inhibited by DSH, but with a 50-fold lower potency than that of DSSD (Grafström and Green, 1980; Grafström and Holmberg, 1980). The inhibitory effect of 0.1 mM DSSD, on the other hand, is much enhanced if it is preincubated with the homogenate. If, additionally, the incubation occurs in the presence of NADPH, the hydroxylase activity is completely abolished (Grafström and Green, 1980).

In contrast to what is observed with respect to the liver, *in vivo* pretreatment with DSSD has biphasic effects on the intestinal benzo-[*a*]pyrene hydroxylase activity. Acute administration of 100 mg/kg p.o. in oil results in a 75% inhibition of the activity 24 h later, without any concomitant change in intestinal P-450 levels. Moreover, whereas chronic daily administration of 100 or 200 mg/kg DSSD in this manner for 5 days leads to a marked fall in hepatic hydroxylase activity, that of the small intestine is increased by 31 and 65%, respectively. At the same time, intestinal P-450 levels are also much increased and the Soret spectrum of the cytochrome has an absorption maximum at 450 nm, rather than one at 448 nm as observed following MC induction (Grafström and Green, 1980). This stimulation persists upon continuation of the 100 mg/kg/day DSSD treatment for 30 days (Grafström and Holmberg, 1980).

8.2.11 Summary

Several possibilities emerge as potential mechanisms for the inhibition and impairment of hepatic endoplasmic reticulum enzymes by DSSD and DSH, but they need not be mutually exclusive. CS_2 is a metabolite of both agents. Accordingly, its oxidative desulfuration, with the formation of singlet atomic sulfur and attack by the latter on the cysteine residue normally ligating the heme iron, could mediate both the DSSD- and DSH-engendered enzyme inactivation. The identification of COS, the product of such a desulfuration, in the blood of alcoholics dosed with DSSD (Johansson, 1989b) is consistent with this hypothesis. On the other hand, P-450 can oxidize DSH to DSSD and thus the inhibition could be mediated through the actions of the latter. Theoretically, these compounds could also undergo oxidative desulfuration, but formation of the expected products of such reactions has not been observed. However, the DSH metabolite, diethylmonothiocarbamic acid methyl ester (DmSMe), has been identified as an *in vivo* metabolite of DSSD (Johansson, 1989a). It would be the product of the oxidative desulfuration of diethyldithiocarbamic acid methyl ester (DSMe), a known metabolite of DSSD (Gessner, T. and Jakubowski, 1972). Accordingly, this raises the possibility that DSMe might mediate, in part at least, the DSSD- and DSH-induced inactivation of P-450. Then again, DSSD could also inhibit P-450 by formation of a mixed disulfide with a critically located cysteine residue. The latter appears to be the mechanism whereby DSSD inhibits P-450$_{Ch7\alpha}$, a P-450 isoform, since the enzyme can be regenerated by the use of a disulfide reducing agent.

8.3 INHIBITION OF DOPAMINE β-HYDROXYLASE

The biosynthesis of norepinephrine (NE) from tyrosine is a three-step process (Fig. 8.4) of which the last step is catalyzed by dopamine β-hydroxylase (DBH) [3,4-dihydroxyphenylethylamine, ascorbate: oxygen oxidoreductase (β-hydroxylating), EC 1.14.2.1]. This enzyme is present in catecholamine-containing vesicles of the sympathetic nervous system, brain, and adrenal medulla and is released therefrom together with the catecholamines. It is a copper-containing mixed-function oxidase in that it employs atmospheric oxygen, the reaction it catalyzes being

$$\text{dopamine} + O_2 + \text{ascorbate} \rightarrow \text{L-norepinephrine} +$$
$$\text{dehydroascorbate} + H_2O \qquad (8.4)$$

Although the rate-limiting step in the biosynthesis of NE is the hydroxylation of tyrosine (Udenfriend *et al.*, 1966), the β-hydroxylation of dopamine (DA) becomes the rate-limiting step if DBH is sufficiently inhibited.

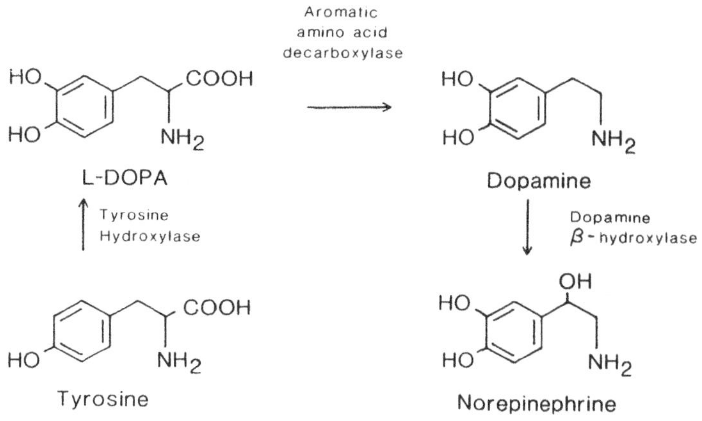

Figure 8.4   Biosynthetic pathway for dopamine and norepinephrine from tyrosine.

8.3.1 *In vivo* inhibition: animal studies

In 1964 Goldstein, M. *et al.* reported that when rats are administered DSSD (400 mg/kg i.p.) in a divided dose at 2 and 0 h prior to an injection of ^{3}H-DA, their heart levels of ^{3}H-NE 2 h later are 6-fold lower and their heart levels of ^{3}H-DA are 5-fold higher than those of DSSD naive controls. These results and analogous ones from the spleen, suggest that DSSD inhibits the hydroxylation of the injected DA. Musacchio *et al.* (1964) and Thoenen *et al.* (1965, 1967) further characterized the effects of DSSD pretreatment on tissue catecholamines. Using rats, Musacchio *et al.* observed that DSSD pretreatment (400 mg/kg i.p. at 18 and 1 h prior to sacrifice) reduces the endogenous NE content of the 100 000 *g* particulate fraction of heart homogenates, that is the fraction containing the catecholamine nerve-ending vesicles, by 50%, but that it does not reduce the *in vivo* uptake of ^{3}H-NE into these vesicles. Using cats, Thoenen *et al.* found that following DSSD pretreatment (2–4 × 400 mg/kg p.o. in the 48 h prior) there is a marked decrease in the NE output of the spleen when it is sympathetically stimulated. Moreover, in DSSD-pretreated animals, the ratio of NE to DA in the venous effluent of the spleen following such stimulation is the same as that found in the tissue. Thus the inhibition by DSSD of the β-hydroxylation of DA results in much of the excess DA being retained in the nerve-ending vesicle from which, like NE, it is released by nerve stimulation.

In addition to DA, DBH β-hydroxylates tyramine, *m*-tyramine, octopamine, *m*-octopamine and the α-methyl analogs of DA and tyramine.

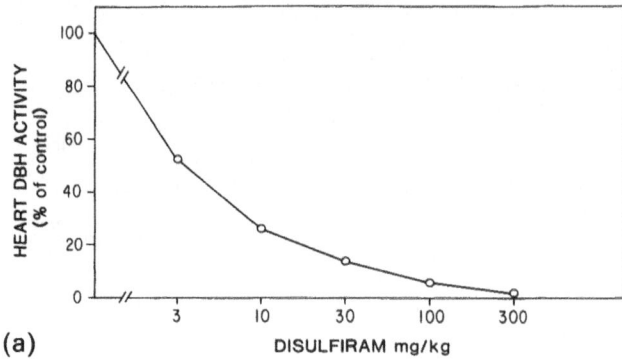

(a)

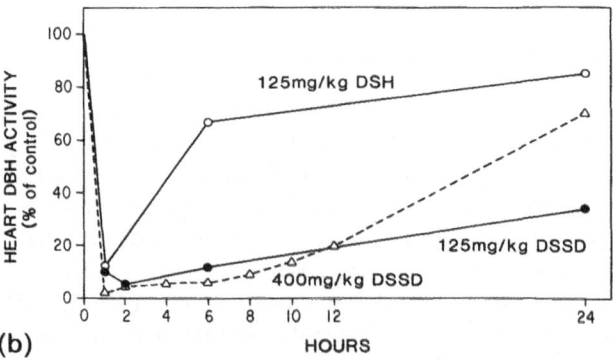

(b)

Figure 8.5 Effect of disulfiram (DSSD) on the activity of dopamine β-hydroxylase (DBH) and tissue norepinephirne (NE) and dopamine (DA) levels. (a) Inhibition of heart DBH activity by DSSD in the rat. DSSD was administered i.p. (in saline containing 0.5% Tween 80 and 1% carboxymethylcellulose) 1 h prior to dosing with ^{3}H-tyramine. The hearts were removed 60 min later and the content of the β-hydroxylated derivative, ^{3}H-octopamine determined. Redrawn from Musacchio *et al.* (1966a). (b) Composite for the time course of inhibition of the rat heart DBH activity by DSSD and diethyldithiocarbamate (DSH) administered i.p. (The 400 mg/kg DSSD data set was redrawn from Musacchio *et al.* (1966a) except for the 1 h point obtained by extrapolation from (a). The 125 mg/kg DSSD data are from Symchowicz *et al.* (1966). The 125 mg/kg DSH data set was redrawn from Lippman and Lloyd (1969). (c) Composite for the time course of the effect of DSSD and DSH on the levels of catecholamines in rat heart and brain. DSSD and DSH were administered in 400 mg/kg i.p. and 500 mg/kg s.c. doses, respectively. (The heart and brain NE post-DSSD data are from Musacchio *et al.* (1966a). The brain NE post-DSH data are from Carlsson *et al.* (1966). The brain DA data are from Goldstein, M. and Nakajima (1967).)

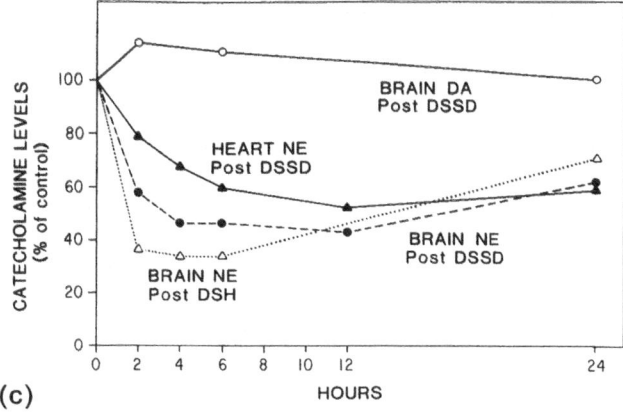

(c)

Figure 8.5 *cont.*

All of these substrates have been used in the *in vivo* study of DBH inhibition by DSSD. Pretreatment of rats with DSSD (400 mg/kg i.p.) 1 hr prior to the administration of any of these substrates in a labeled form results in the heart levels of their respective β-hydroxylated metabolites at 60 min being very markedly depressed relative to the levels observed in DSSD-naive controls. The degree of DBH inhibition which can be calculated from these experiments ranges from 79% for α-methyldopamine to 98% for *m*-tyramine (Musacchio *et al.*, 1964, 1966a). The degree of DSSD-induced inhibition is dose-dependent (Fig. 8.5a) and it reaches a maximum at 1–2 h post administration (Fig. 8.5b). Following administration of DSH, the onset of the inhibition is similarly rapid (Fig. 8.5b) though it wanes more quickly. The time course of the DSSD-induced lowering of endogenous NE levels in the rat heart follows a course similar to that of the DBH inhibition (Fig. 8.5c). DSH administration has also been shown to lower NE levels in the ileum of rats and rabbits (Collins, 1965; Carlsson *et al.*, 1966). A 200 mg/kg s.c. dose results in a significant effect in the first 6 h. A 500 mg/kg s.c. dose produces a maximal effect: it lowers ileum NE to about 40% of control and raises DA levels about 2-fold.

Additional information as to whether the effects of DSSD on endogenous *in vivo* NE levels are solely due to DBH inhibition, derives from studies of the effects of DSSD pretreatment on the actions of tyramine. This sympathomimetic agent liberates NE from its storage sites and thereby causes a pressor effect. Neither is affected by DSSD pretreatment (Musacchio *et al.*, 1966b; Bhagat *et al.*, 1966). The NE storage sites take up circulating NE and in animals in whom reserpine treatment has depleted these stores to the point that tyramine is ineffective, infusion of NE restores the response to tyramine. DSSD pretreatment does not prevent NE uptake from the circulation or restoration by this means of the tyramine response in reserpinized animals. The tyramine response can also be restored in normal animals by infusion of DA which is taken up into the NE storage sites and hydroxylated there into NE. This process requires the participation of DBH and is blocked by DSSD pretreatment.

In rats, brain levels of NE also fall following administration of DSSD or DSH (Fig. 8.5c). Oral DSSD (1 g/kg at 18 and 3 h prior) also brings about a reduction (45%) in rat brain NE levels (Jonsson *et al.*, 1967). Similarly, in mice DSSD (200 mg/kg i.p.: Moore, 1969) and DSH (200 mg/kg i.p.: Moore, 1969; 400 mg/kg i.p.: Johnson *et al.*, 1970; 250 mg/kg i.p.: Maj and Vetulani, 1969, 1970) cause significant falls in brain NE levels. To determine whether such CNS effects can be ascribed to DBH inhibition, Goldstein, M. and Nakajima (1966, 1967) used DOPA which, unlike the above-mentioned substrates of DBH, can cross the blood–brain barrier. Administration of DOPA to rats whose brain NE levels had been depleted with reserpine leads, in controls, to a restoration of these levels in a two-step process (Fig. 8.4). In rats pretreated with DSSD (400 mg/kg i.p.), however, DOPA administration fails to restore the brain NE levels, indicating that DSSD causes inhibition of DBH in the CNS. Although the rise in brain DA levels following acute administration of DSSD or DSH is small (Fig. 8.5c) and not increased significantly by monoamineoxidase inhibition (Carlsson *et al.*, 1967), it can be significant (Johnson *et al.*, 1970; Maj and Vetulani, 1970) be it in rats or mice. Moreover, following chronic DSH administration (300 mg/kg/day i.p. for a week) the rise in brain DA levels can be quite marked (79%) when measured 24 h after the last dose of DSH (Mazumder *et al.*, 1985). Spinal cord DA levels appear to be more sensitive to DSH administration. Thus at 2 h following an acute 250 mg/kg i.p. dose of DSH spinal cord DA levels are 2.5-fold higher than in controls (Storm *et al.*, 1984). Similarly, mediobasal hypothalamus DA levels are also more sensitive, being elevated by 79% at 3 h post administration of a 550 mg/kg dose of DSH (Blaustein *et al.*, 1986).

The effect of DSSD treatment on *in vivo* DBH has been studied by Major *et al.* (1982), who found that chronic treatment does result in lowered DBH levels in monkeys. An alternative way of assessing DBH function *in vivo* is to administer DA ^{3}H- (or T-) labelled in the β-position and to measure the titrated water (THO) formed (section 8.3.2). Using this approach Hoeldtke and Stetson (1980) found a significant decrease in THO formation following pretreatment with 20 mg/kg of DSSD i.p.

8.3.2 *In vivo* inhibition: clinical studies

Inhibition of DBH would be expected, *a priori*, to result in lower NE levels in body fluids. Indeed, DSSD therapy (500 mg/day) has been reported to lower NE levels in urine (Rogers *et al.*, 1979) and cerebrospinal fluid (Major *et al.*, 1979a). Blood NE levels, on the other hand, are found to rise significantly following treatment with this dose of DSSD (Lake *et al.*, 1977, 1980), the rise being correlated with increases in standing and supine blood pressure, though no increases in blood pressure are observed following treatment with the lower, 250 mg/day dose (Lake *et al.*, 1977; Major *et al.*, 1977a). In humans, efforts to show DSSD treatment-induced changes in DBH levels, be it in plasma (Lake *et al.*, 1980) or cerebrospinal fluid (Lake *et al.*, 1977), have not been successful. This could be due to the fact that the inhibition of DBH by DSH is reversible (section 8.3.2) and that the *ex vivo* DBH assay involves significant dilution.

An alternative method for the estimation of *in vivo* inhibition of DBH is the administration of DA ^{3}H-labelled in the $β$-position. Upon hydroxylation of this position by DBH, water containing an atom of ^{3}H (THO) is released (Hoeldtke and Kaufman, 1978). Applying this methodology to humans, Hoeldtke and Stetson (1980) also determined the concurrent excretion of the individual ^{3}H-catecholamines and their ^{3}H-metabolites. They found that administration of DSSD for 4 days in a dose of 5.5 mg/kg/day (equivalent to 385 mg/70 kg/day) reduces the rate of THO formation by 35% and the ratio of total ^{3}H-NE/^{3}H-DA metabolites by 45%. Some of the catecholamine metabolites are formed by the action of ALDH. Hoeldtke and Stetson (1980) found that the levels of these metabolites are lower following DSSD therapy, an indication that in this dose DSSD causes an inhibition of ALDH at the sites where catecholamines are metabolized (section 9.6.1).

8.3.3 *In vitro* inhibition

DSH is a non-competitive DBH inhibitor for both substrate and ascorbate; it has a K_i of 0.5–1 μM (Green, 1964; Goldstein, M. *et al.*, 1965; Johnson *et al.*, 1969; Hidaka *et al.*, 1973). In the presence of ascorbate, DSSD is immediately reduced to DSH and prompt DBH inhibition results (Goldstein, M. *et al.*, 1964, 1965). DBH is a Cu enzyme containing 2 μmoles of Cu per μmole of enzyme and the mechanism of the inhibition is that DSH, a potent chelator of Cu (section 7.7), chelates the enzyme's Cu and thereby blocks it. The inhibition can be overcome by addition of Cu^{2+} ions (Friedman, S. and Kaufman, 1965) or by prolonged dialysis (Goldstein, M. *et al.*, 1965).

8.3.4 *In vivo* effect on tyrosine

Acutely, DSH administration leads, in rats, to an elevation in brain tyrosine levels (Goodchild, 1969; Magos and Jarvis, 1970; Bloom *et al.*, 1977; Flood *et al.*, 1986); though DSH does not inhibit tyrosine hydroxylase (Nagatsu *et al.*, 1964), the accumulation of NE precursors may do so. Chronic administration of DSH (400 mg/kg/day i.p. for 3 days) to rats results in a delayed and presumably compensatory activation of tyrosine hydroxylase (Heubusch and DiStefano, 1978).

8.4 INHIBITION OF SUPEROXIDE DISMUTASE

8.4.1 Introduction

Superoxide dismutases (SOD) are a ubiquitous and important group of enzymes that catalyze the first step in the reduction of the harmful superoxide anion radical, O_2^- (Fridovich, 1983, 1989; Byczkowski and Gessner, 1988). This reactive oxygen species (ROS) forms during normal reduction of oxygen in respiring cells, or in the course of various one-electron oxidations triggered by irritants or invading organisms. Four different SOD metalloenzymes have been identified to date. Two of these are copper–zinc-containing enzymes, namely: (1) a cytosolic copper–zinc-containing superoxide dismutase (CuZn-SOD) which is found in the cytosol and the mitochondrial inter-membrane space of eukaryotic cells and (2) an extracellular copper–zinc-containing superoxide dismutase (EC-SOD) which is an immunologically distinct mammalian CuZn metalloenzyme found in plasma and, more generally, in extracellular fluid (Bannister *et al.*, 1987). A third enzyme, whose location in mammals is exclusively in the matrix of the mitochondria, is a manganese-containing superoxide dismutase (Mn-SOD); it is also present in plants. Finally, aerobic prokaryotes and some plants possess an iron superoxide dismutase (Fe-SOD).

As knowledge regarding the various SOD enzymes has increased, so analytical methods have progressed to allow determination of their individual activities (Ohman and Marklund, 1986; Bannister and Calabrese, 1987). Earlier, cyanide was used to distinguish between the CuZn metalloenzymes, which it inhibits, and Mn-SOD, which it does not. Using cyanide it has been found that in most human tissues the levels of the CuZn metalloenzymes exceed those of Mn-SOD, ranging from 1.25-fold higher levels in liver to 10-fold higher levels in lung (Marklund, 1980). As detailed below, both of the CuZn metalloenzymes are inhibited by DSH. Mn-SOD, on the other hand, is unaffected by 3 mM DSH. This is true of the pure bovine heart enzyme, and of the Mn-SOD activity in cell culture and in human liver homogenates (Marklund and Westman, 1980; Westman and Marklund, 1980).

8.4.2 *In vivo* effects

Administration to experimental animals of an appropriate amount of DSH results in inhibition of SOD activity in all tissues examined, thus blood (mouse: Heikkila *et al.*, 1976; rat: Miura *et al.*, 1978), brain (mouse: Heikkila *et al.*, 1976, rat: Puglia and Loeb, 1984), liver (mouse: Heikkila *et al.*, 1976), lung (rat: Frank *et al.*, 1978; Deneke *et al.*, 1979; Forman *et al.*, 1980) and heart (rat: Guarnieri *et al.*, 1981). The inhibition reaches a maximum after 1–2 h (Fig. 8.6; also Puglia and

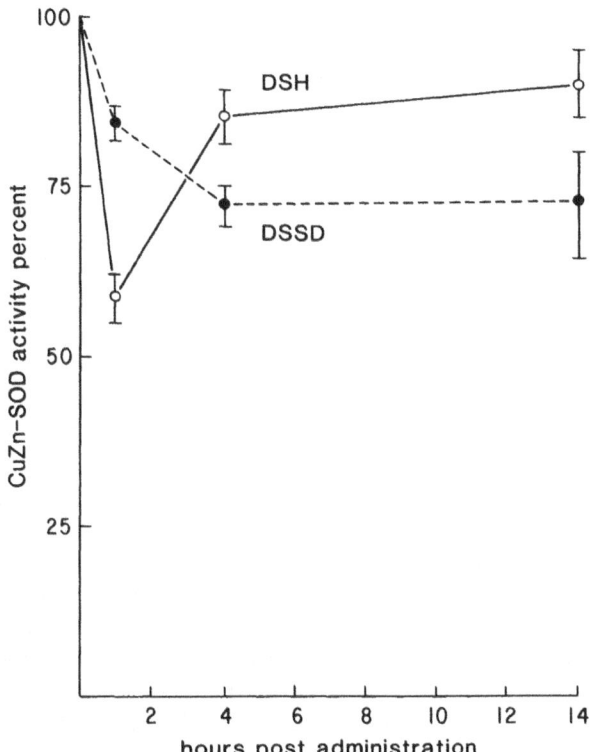

Figure 8.6 Effect of diethyldithiocarbamate (DSH) and disulfiram (DSSD) administration on pulmonary copper-zinc superoxide dismutase (CuZn-SOD) activity in rats. Redrawn from Heikkila *et al.* (1976).

Loeb, 1985) and wanes thereafter (Heikkila *et al.*, 1976; Forman *et al.*, 1980) at a rate of 1–2%/h. The degree of inhibition of SOD activity is dose-dependent (Heikkila *et al.*, 1976; Puglia and Loeb, 1985). A 200 mg/kg dose of DSH results in a 40% inhibition ($P<0.001$) of lung CuZn-containing SOD activity at 1 h (Puglia and Loeb, 1985) and an 18% inhibition ($P<0.05$) of total lung SOD activity at 4 h (Deneke *et al.*, 1979). Following a 1200 mg/kg dose of DSH, cardiac CuZn-SOD activity is 81% inhibited at 2 h (Guarnieri *et al.*, 1981). Finally, 3 h following a 1500 mg/kg DSH dose, total SOD activity is 48, 71 and 86% inhibited in brain, liver, and blood, respectively (Heikkila *et al.*, 1976).

DSSD administration also leads to inhibition of CuZn-containing SODs. Thus, 4 h following a 200 mg/kg i.p. dose of DSSD in an aqueous suspension, a 31% inhibition ($P<0.01$) of lung CuZn-containing SOD activity is seen in rats (Forman *et al.*, 1980). The inhibition develops more slowly than following a 200 mg/kg dose of DSH (Fig. 8.6). The slow onset may be in part due to the very low water solubility of DSSD nd its impaired absorption following i.p. administration (Moore, 1969). Slow and incomplete absorption may also be the reason for the low degree of inhibition (8%; $P<0.05$) of total liver SOD activity observed by Heikkila *et al.* (1976) following i.p. administration of two doses of 600 mg/kg DSSD in aqueous suspension to mice. Ohman and Marklund (1986) investigated whether DSSD therapy (250 mg/day) of alcoholics had any effect on the levels of EC-SOD activity in plasma. Though patients on DSSD had, on average, levels of EC-SOD activity 17% lower than control patients, the finding was not a statistically significant one ($P=0.22$).

Age increases the susceptibility of animals to DSH-induced inactivation of hepatic CuZn-SOD (Radojičić *et al.*, 1987). Thus at 3 h following administration, a 1000 mg/kg dose of DSH produces 51% inhibition in 3-month-old rats, but a 76% inhibition in 30-month-old animals; the difference is significant ($P<0.05$). In the young, but not the old rats, this DSH dose increases significantly ($P<0.05$) protein synthesis, as evidenced by the incorporation of labeled amino acids into liver cytosolic proteins. Pretreatment with cycloheximide, a protein synthesis inhibitor which has no effect on CuZn-SOD activity in otherwise untreated animals, increases the DSH-induced inactivation of CuZn-SOD in young rats to 80%, but does not alter the extent of its inactivation in old rats (75%). This suggests that the recovery of CuZn-SOD activity is brought about by synthesis of fresh enzyme and that aged animals have a much lower capacity in this regard than do young ones.

8.4.3 Mechanism

Studies of the *in vitro* interaction of DSH with CuZn-SOD (Heikkila *et al.*, 1976; Misra, 1979; Cocco *et al.*, 1981a,b) indicate that DSH reacts with the two protein-bound Cu atoms to form a Cu-diethyldithiocarbamate chelate which then interacts with the protein part of the enzyme and is tightly held. The process involves a two-step increase in absorbance at 450 nm. Both steps follow first-order kinetics. The faster of the steps accounts for about 85% of total absorbance and parallels the loss of enzymic activity (Cocco *et al.*, 1981a). The Cu-diethyl-dithiocarbamate complex cannot be extracted by organic solvents (Heikkila *et al.*, 1976; Misra, 1979, Cocco *et al.*, 1981a) or separated from the enzyme by gel filtration (Misra, 1979; Cocco *et al.*, 1981a). It can be displaced, however, by high speed centrifugation (39 000 *g* for 20 min; Cocco *et al.*, 1981a). This latter property is similar to that of ceruloplasmin from which Morell and Scheinberg (1958) were also able to displace the Cu complex of DSH by centrifugation. The enzyme can be fully reactivated by exposure to a stoichiometric quantity of Cu (Cocco *et al.*, 1981b). Also, following exposure to Cu, the Cu-diethyl-dithiocarbamate complex becomes extractable with organic solvents (Heikkila *et al.*, 1976). No Zn is lost from the enzyme, even after incubation with a 100:1 excess of DSH. This is not due to lack of accessibility, since the unnatural CuCo-SOD enzyme, formed by replacement of the Zn in the native enzyme with Co, loses its Co upon exposure to a 10:1 excess of DSH (Cocco *et al.*, 1981b). Exposure of DSH-inactivated CuZn-SOD to 10 µM cysteine, 2-mercaptopropionyl-glycine, or reduced glutathione results in partial reactivation of the enzyme (Hoshino *et al.*, 1985). The potency of these agents decreases in the order in which they are listed.

An analysis of the time course of the reaction of DSH with the bovine erythrocyte CuZn-SOD at pH 7.4 and 25°C, led Cocco *et al.* (1981a) to conclude that the rate of enzyme inhibition is first order with respect to the molarity of the DSH raised to the power of 1.5, as well as with respect to time (*t*), that is:

$$E_t = E_o e^{-k[\text{DSH}]^{1.5} t} \tag{8.5}$$

where E_t and E_o stand for enzyme activity at zero time and after a period *t* of incubation with DSH. The value of *k* reported by Cocco *et al.* (1981a) was $220 \pm 30 \, \text{min}^{-1} \text{M}^{-1.5}$. The resulting relationship between the DSH concentration and the time required for 50% inactivation ($T_{50\%}$) of bovine CuZn-SOD can be calculated and is shown in Fig. 8.7. Bartkowiak *et al.* (1983), who also used bovine erythrocyte

CuZn-SOD at a pH of 7.4, reported a value for k of $251 \pm 37\,\text{min}^{-1}\text{M}^{-1.5}$ (the value for aged erythrocyte CuZn-SOD was 25% higher). On the other hand, Marklund (1984), working with human erythrocyte CuZn-SOD exposed to 0.5 mM DSH at pH 7.4 and 37°C, reported a $T_{50\%}$ of 40 min, which indicates a value of k of $1550\,\text{min}^{-1}\text{M}^{-1.5}$. This suggests that the human CuZn-SOD is more sensitive to DSH inactivation than is the bovine one. Moreover, Marklund (1984) found all three human EC-SOD isozymes (A, B and C) to be even more sensitive. Exposed to 0.1 mM DSH under analogous conditions, the

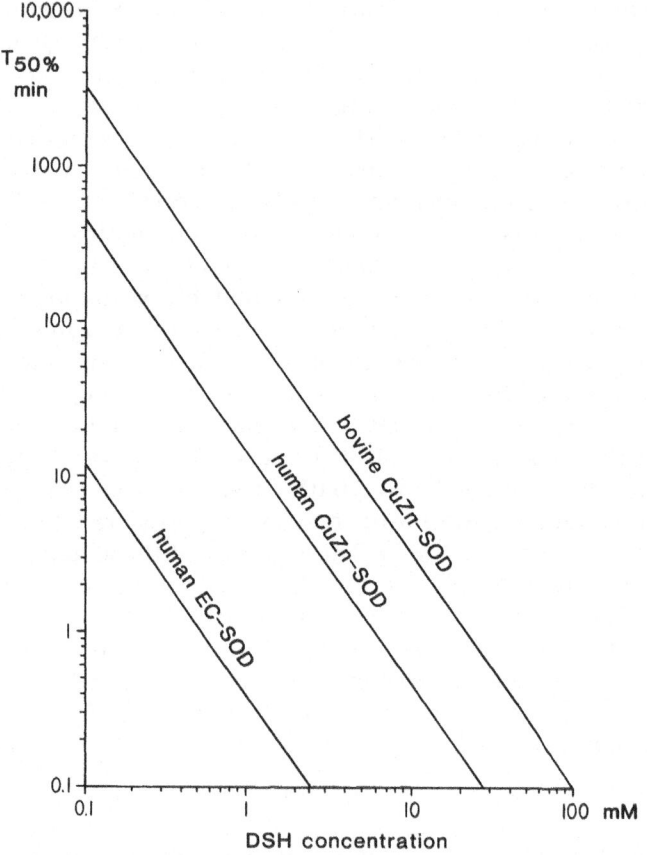

Figure 8.7 Projected times required for 50% inactivation of copper–zinc superoxide dismutases (CuZn-SODs) as a function of the molar concentration of diethyldithiocarbamate (DSH). The projection is based on the premise that the kinetics established by Cocco Hempel *et al.* (1989) since they had no counterpart in the opposing structure as a result of the non-aligned N-and C-termini or due to gaps introduced in optimizing the alignment.

latter enzymes yielded $T_{50\%}$ values of around 12 min. Should the same reaction order apply, this would correspond to a value of k of 57 750 min^{-1}M$^{-1.5}$. The resulting differences in projected $T_{50\%}$ values are illustrated in Fig. 8.7.

8.4.4 Effects in cell culture

In cell culture, inhibition of CuZn-SOD is observed following exposure of the cells to 1–10 mM concentrations of DSH, though the degree of inhibition and attendant toxicity reported by different workers shows significant variation (Table 8.2).

This variation may reflect, in part, differences in sensitivity of the CuZn-SOD to DSH in different organisms. Another factor that may be partly responsible for the differences in observed toxicity is the chelation by DSH of the Cu in the cell culture medium with the formation of the lipophilic Cu(DS)$_2$ and the resultant redistribution of the Cu from the medium to the cells. Evidence for the latter is supplied by Trombetta *et al.* (private communication) who noted a 5-fold increase in the Cu content of rat cerebral cortical astrocytes 4 h following a 60 min exposure to 235 µM DSH. Once inhibited by DSH, the CuZn-SOD activity of cells is regenerated slowly, 50% of the activity being regained in about 7 h (Westman and Marklund, 1980).

An unusual and interesting CuZn-SOD-mediated effect of DSH is that on *Plasmodia*. Scheibel *et al.* (1979) reported that DSSD and DSH inhibit the *in vitro* growth of the human malarial parasite *Plasmodia falciparum* in concentrations as low as 1 µg/ml. Fairfield *et al.* (1983) later demonstrated, by infecting mice and rats with *Plasmodia burghei*, a murine malaria parasite, that the parasite lacks any native SOD, incorporating instead substantial amounts of host CuZn-SOD. Although *P. falciparum* contains some native Mn-SOD, it also mainly depends on human CuZn-SOD it incorporates (Ranz and Meshnick, 1989). When DSH-inactivated CuZn-SOD is added to *P. falciparum* cultures in human blood cells, the cultures are cleared of parasites. Since DSH-treated bovine serum albumin is without effect, the antimalarial activity is attributable to the inactivated enzyme. This suggests that the parasite, while able to recognize and incorporate host CuZn-SOD, cannot distinguish the active enzyme from the DSH-inactivated form. The antimalarial activity cannot be reversed by excess Cu or Zn (Meshnick *et al.*, 1986). Subsequently, Meshnick *et al.* (1990) have reported that the toxicity of DSH to *P. falciparum* cultures *in vitro* is markedly potentiated by Cu.

Table 8.2 Diethyldithiocarbamate (DSH) inactivation of superoxide dismutase (SOD) in cultured cells

Tissue	DSH conc. (μM)	Exposure duration (min)	SOD inactivation (%)	Mortality (%)	Reference
Chinese hamster cells	3 000	90	96	32	Westman and Markland (1980)
Chinese hamster cells	1 000	120	65	<5	Evans et al. (1983b)
Chinese hamster cells	220	60	55	~85	Lin et al. (1979)
	110	30	9	~20	
Rat premeiotic male germ cells	2 500	60	54	<20	Coogan et al. (1986)
Rat cerebral cotrical astrocytes	156	60	none		Trombetta et al. (1988)
Human HL-60 cells	10 000	120	67	>95	Kelner et al. (1989)
	1 000	120	<10	75	
	100	120	none	50	
Human mononuclear cells	1 000	240	79		Conkling et al. (1985)
	100	240	none		

8.4.5 Summary

For any significant inhibition to accrue *in vivo*, the peak molarity of administered DSH has to be sufficiently high so that the $T_{50\%}$ value for the inhibition of the enzyme does not exceed the *in vivo* half-life of the DSH. The values for the latter tend to be, however, quite short (Table 6.1).

The high sensitivity of the human EC-SOD to DSH inactivation focuses particular attention on its C isozyme (EC-SOD C). It has a high affinity for endothelial cell-surface-sulfated glycosaminoglycans (Karlsson and Marklund, 1988b) and becomes bound to them without, for the major part, losing enzymic activity (Adachi and Marklund, 1989). *In vitro*, endothelial cells bind EC-SOD C avidly so that, at maximum binding, a considerable portion of the endothelial cell surface is covered with EC-SOD C molecules. The resulting cell-surface SOD activity exceeds the intracellular activity several-fold (Karlsson and Marklund, 1989). *In vivo*, 90% of i.v. administered EC-SOD C rapidly binds to the surface of vascular endothelial cells and disappears from the circulation within 5–10 min. It can be fully released back into plasma by heparin, the half-life of the heparin-releasable enzyme being about 10 h (Karlsson and Marklund, 1987, 1988a). Most of the EC-SOD in the body is extravascular and almost all of it is bound; the lungs and the heart are the two tissues showing the most sustained uptake of administered EC-SOD C (Karlsson and Marklund, 1989).

8.5 INACTIVATION OF GLUTATHIONE PEROXIDASE

Both administration of DSH and exposure to it under aerobic conditions *in vitro* can lead to inhibition of glutathione peroxidase (GSHPx) (EC 1.11.1.9). The selenium-containing GSHPx (Se-GSHPx) which, in conjunction with GSH, acts as a biological antioxidant, is pivotal in preventing hepatic peroxidation (for review see Flohe, 1982). This is so because the enzyme is a cytosolic one that has a very low K_m for H_2O_2 (in the μM range) and a very high velocity, whereas catalase has a K_m in the mM range and is sequestered in peroxisomes (Simmons and Jamall, 1988). Further, Se-GSHPx plays an important role in safeguarding tissues against ROS damage by protecting CuZn-SOD from H_2O_2 which inactivates it (Blum and Fridovich, 1985).

Besides Se-GSHPx, liver and other tissues also contain Se-independent GSHPx activity. The latter derives from some of the numerous glutathione-*S*-transferase (GST) isozymes (Mannervik, 1985; Arthur *et al.*, 1987), which are active, as is Se-GSHPx, towards organic hydroperoxides, but unlike Se-GSHPx, are not active towards H_2O_2 (Prohaska and Ganther,

1977). Accordingly, when the assay is based solely on activity towards cumene hydroperoxide, it is appropriate to refer to 'total GSHPx'.

Administration of a large DSH dose (1.2 g/kg) results in progressive inactivation of mouse lung and liver GSHPx during the first 6.5 h, at which time the activity is reduced to 30 and 70% of control levels, respectively. The activity returns to control levels after 24 h (Goldstein *et al.*, 1979). Although moderate doses of DSH (250 and 500 mg/kg) have no significant effect on Se-GSHPx activity, a 1000 mg/kg dose does cause a 24% inhibition of activity in the rat brain 2 h post administration (Puglia and Loeb, 1984). *In vitro*, an analogous inactivation is observed under a variety of circumstances. Thus, incubation of rat liver homogenate with 1×10^{-2}M DSH for 6.5 h causes a 68% inactivation of total GSHPx (Goldstein *et al.*, 1979); 30 min exposure of human fibroblast cultures to concentrations higher than 1×10^{-3}M results in a dose-dependent inactivation of GSHPx (Michiels and Remacle, 1988); and a 1-h exposure of rat cerebral cortical astrocytes to 2.35×10^{-4}M DSH results at 4 and 24 h in a 38 and 27% inactivation of Se-GSHPx, respectively (Trombetta *et al.*, private communication).

Three lines of evidence indicate that the observed inactivation of GSHPx by DSH is not a direct effect. Firstly, purified GSHPx (from bovine erythrocytes) is not discernibly affected by incubation at 25°C and pH 7.8 with 1×10^{-2}M DSH, a concentration which brings about complete inactivation of the cytosolic CuZn-SOD (Blum and Fridovich, 1985). Secondly, in biological systems the inactivation has a requirement for oxygen. Thus, in liver homogenates no inactivation is observed under anaerobic conditions (Goldstein *et al.*, 1979). Also, exposure of nematodes to 5×10^{-3}M DSH results in loss of 50% of the GSHPx activity, but only if the organisms are subsequently exposed to 3 atm oxygen (Blum and Fridovich, 1983). Thirdly, even under aerobic conditions no inactivation of GSHPx is observed in liver homogenates incubated with DSH if SOD is added (Goldstein *et al.*, 1979). Conversely, addition to such homogenates of dihydrofumaric acid, a O_2^- generator, enhances the inactivation. The DSH/O_2-induced inactivation is therefore considered to be mediated by the DSH inhibition of CuZn-SOD and the resultant increase in O_2^-. GSHPx reacts with H_2O_2 to yield an inactive form of the enzyme. Although this inactive form can be reactivated by GSH, its reaction with O_2^- leads to an irreversible inactivation (Blum and Fridovich, 1985). In the presence of tissue homogenates, DSH itself can simulate GSHPx, being oxidized by hydrogen peroxide to DSSD. The latter, in turn, oxidizes GSH to GSSG with regeneration of DSH. Hydrogen peroxide reduction thereby becomes coupled to the hexose monophosphate pathway of glucose metabolism (Kumar *et al.*, 1986).

In vitro, the glutathione-*S*-transferase activity of some of the GST isozymes is non-competitively inhibited by 0.01 mM DSH (Dierickx, 1984). No information is available, however, regarding the effect of DSH on the GSHPx activity of these isozymes.

In vivo in mice, on the other hand, the hepatic glutathione-*S*-transferase activity is increased 4- to 6-fold by inclusion of DSSD in their diet (1% of feed for 14 days) if measured using 1-chloro-2,4-dinitrobenzene, 1,2-dichloro-4-nitrobenzene, or *p*-nitrobenzylchloride, but not at all when using 1,2-epoxy-3-(*p*-nitrophenoxy)propane as the substrate (Cha *et al.*, 1983). This suggests DSSD administration results in increased levels of the μ- and π-, but not the α-class GSTs. Administration to mice of either DSSD or DSH in feed (0.5% for 14 days) also increases the glutathione-*S*-transferase activity, as assayed with 1-chloro-2,4-dinitrobenzene and 1,2-dichloro-4-nitrobenzene as substrates, in the intestine (4-fold), in the forestomach (2-fold) and to a lesser extent ($\leqslant$ 1.5-fold) in the lung, liver and kidneys (Benson and Barretto, 1985). In rats, administration of DSSD in feed (2 g/kg for 4 weeks) increases 2-fold hepatic microsomal glutathione-*S*-transferase activity, as assayed with 1-chloro-2,4-dinitrobenzene (Bertram *et al.*, 1985). In rats, administration of DSSD in feed (2 g/kg for 4 weeks) increases 2-fold hepatic microsomal glutathione-*S*-transferase activity, as assayed with 1-chloro-2,4-dinitrobenzene (Bertram *et al.*, 1985).

8.6 EFFECT ON CATALASE

Catalase is an important enzyme in the organism's armory against ROS. The effects of DSH on this enzyme are quite marginal. Administered to mice in a 1.2 g/kg i.p. dose, DSH has no significant or consistent effect on lung and liver catalase (Goldstein *et al.*, 1979) and though in rats, a significant ($P < 0.05$) decrease in blood catalase activity is seen 2 h following a 1.5 g/kg i.p. dose (Miura *et al.*, 1978), the inhibition is quite small (17%). Chronic administration of 1 mmol/kg/day for 5 days leads to a modest (20%) but significant ($P < 0.01$) decrease in hepatic mitochondrial fraction catalase (Khandelwal *et al.*, 1987). *In vitro*, exposure of catalase in blood lysates to 3 mM DSH leads to a 50% inhibition which develops slowly over a 90 min period (Miura *et al.*, 1978). At very high DSH concentrations (*ca* 150 mM) more extensive inhibition of the enzyme has been reported (Michiels and Remacle, 1988). Since O_2^- inhibits catalase (Kono and Fridovich, 1982), the observed inhibition may be secondary, as in the case of GSHPx, to the increase in O_2^- levels brought about by the DSH-induced inactivation of SOD.

9

Inhibition of aldehyde dehydrogenase

9.1 INTRODUCTION 137
    9.1.1 Multiplicity and terminology of aldehyde dehydrogenase isozymes   138
    9.1.2 Genetic polymorphism of E_2 144
9.2 PHENOMENOLOGY OF THE INHIBITION BY DISULFIRAM 145
    9.2.1 *In vivo* inhibition 145
    9.2.2 *In vitro* inhibition 150
9.3 MECHANISM OF THE INHIBITION 150
    9.3.1 Class 1 aldehyde dehydrogenases 150
    9.3.2 Class 2 aldehyde dehydrogenases 152
    9.3.3 Action of the mixed disulfides of diethyldithiocarbamate 153
9.4 ROLE OF DISULFIRAM METABOLITES 154
    9.4.1 Diethyldithiocarbamic acid, carbon disulfide and diethylamine . 154
    9.4.2 Diethyldithiocarbamic acid methyl ester 155
    9.4.3 Diethylmonothiocarbamic acid methyl ester 157
9.5 INHIBITION OF ALDEHYDE DEHYDROGENASES IN BLOOD 158
    9.5.1 Human erythrocyte aldehyde dehydrogenase 158
    9.5.2 Human leukocyte aldehyde dehydrogenase 160
9.6 INHIBITION OF METABOLISM OF ENDOGENOUS ALDEHYDES . . . 162
    9.6.1 Biogenic monamine-derived aldehydes 162
    9.6.2 Substrates of specific aldehyde dehydrogenases 164
9.7 ALDEHYDE AND XANTHINE OXIDASES 166

9.1 INTRODUCTION

The first two steps in the metabolism of ethanol to acetate *via* acetaldehyde are predominantly catalyzed by alcohol dehydrogenase and aldehyde dehydrogenase (ALDH), respectively. The efficiency of the enzymes involved in acetaldehyde disposition in humans is such that, during ethanol metabolism, blood acetaldehyde levels normally remain in the $1-2 \mu M$ range (section 10.4). Higher blood acetaldehyde levels are observed, however, during the disulfiram–ethanol reaction

(DER), a condition induced by the ingestion of ethanol in individuals pretreated with disulfiram (DSSD). This led early to the surmise that the administration of DSSD results in an inhibition of acetaldehyde metabolism, and that the resulting raised acetaldehyde levels are responsible for the phenomenology of the DER (section 10.5). Moreover, because the DER is so intensely unpleasant, DSSD has been adopted as an aversely protective agent in the treatment of alcoholism (Chapter 11). This, in turn, has focused intense research interest on the enzymes involved in acetaldehyde metabolism and the mechanism of their inhibition.

Both the investigation and discussion of the mechanism of DSSD-induced inhibition have been complicated by the multiplicity of mammalian enzymes that, at least *in vitro*, are able to oxidize acetaldehyde. Principally these are the NAD^+-dependent aldehyde dehydrogenases, although some other enzymes, for instance, aldehyde oxidase, also possess this property.

9.1.1 Multiplicity and terminology of aldehyde dehydrogenase isozymes

The techniques of gel electrophoresis and isoelectric focusing reveal the presence of at least four ALDH activity bands in human liver extracts (Harada *et al.*, 1980) and greater numbers still in those of other tissues (Aarnio and Koivula, 1986; Ryzlak and Pietruszko, 1989). Since, to assure visualization of the ALDH activity, it is usual to expose the gel to relatively high concentrations of an aldehyde (most often acetaldehyde) in the development of the gel, the affinity towards the aldehyde of some of the enzymes thus detected can be quite low (millimolar K_m values). Thus, for instance, of the four human hepatic ALDH isozymes initially reported, two have micromolar K_m values for acetaldehyde (30–48 and 1–3 µM at pH 7.0 for E_1 and E_2, respectively; Pietruszko, 1983), while the K_m values for the other two are in the millimolar range (3.3 and 5.0 mM at pH 7.0 for E_3 and E_4, respectively; Pietruszko, 1983; MacKerell *et al.*, 1986; Forte-McRobbie and Pietruszko, 1986). Since the LD_{50} for acetaldehyde is in the 300–500 mg/kg range and thus millimolar acetaldehyde concentrations are lethal, the above-mentioned E_3 and E_4 isozymes cannot have any role in acetaldehyde metabolism *in vivo*.

With time and improved techniques more activity bands of human hepatic ALDH have been discerned and ALDH enzymes purified. One such isozyme, whose two components have K_m values of 40–50 µM at pH 7.0 and which is distinct from the E_3 isozyme mentioned above, has also been given, somewhat confusingly, the appellation E_3 (Kurys *et al.*,

1989). It is relatively insensitive to DSSD, undergoing a 10% loss of activity with respect to propionaldehyde in the presence of saturating (40 μM) concentrations of DSSD. The E_3 appellation has been used yet again with respect to ALDH isozymes found in the human stomach (Yin *et al.*, 1988). No information is available regarding the effects of DSSD on this latter isozyme.

In general terms, all enzymes that oxidize aldehyde with NAD^+ or $NADP^+$ as a co-factor are, formally, aldehyde dehydrogenases. However, many of these enzymes possess a much greater activity towards a specific endogenous aldehyde than they do towards the aldehydic substrates used experimentally. When such an endogenous substrate is identified, the enzyme is then seen as a specific aldehyde dehydrogenase. For example, E_4 has been identified as glutamic γ-semialdehyde dehydrogenase, or more precisely, 1-pyrroline-5-carboxylate dehydrogenase (EC 1.5.1.12) by Forte-McRobbie and Pietruszko (1986). It is said to be totally insensitive to DSSD (Pietruszko *et al.*, 1987).

E_1 and E_2 have been sequenced (Hempel *et al.*, 1984, 1985; Hsu *et al.*, 1985) and, accordingly, there is no ambiguity regarding their identity, even though the non-specific aldehyde dehydrogenase (EC 1.2.1.3) designation continues to be applied to them. In the literature these isozymes have been referred to in the past by a number of different terms (Table 9.1). For ALDH isozymes which have neither been sequenced nor given a specific aldehyde dehydrogenase designation, such numerative non-specific aldehyde dehydrogenase appellations remain, but are ultimately trivial and transient.

E_2 is a mitochondrial enzyme while E_1 is a cytosolic one (it is often referred to as cytoplasmic). E_1 has been isolated from human erythrocytes (Inoue *et al.*, 1979; Agarwal *et al.*, 1989) and brain (Ryzlak and Pietruszko, 1987, 1989) as well as the liver. The brain mitochondrial enzyme has many similarities to the hepatic E_2 enzyme and might be

Table 9.1 Terminology of Class 1 and 2 human aldehyde dehydrogenases[a]. Correspondences between the several coexisting systems of nomenclature used in the literature.

Class 1	Class 2	Reference
E_1	E_2	Greenfield and Pietruszko (1977)
ALDH II	ALDH I	Harada *et al.* (1980)
$ALDH_1$	$ALDH_2$	Impraim *et al.* (1982)

[a] Mammalian Aldehyde Dehydrogenase Nomenclature (1988).

Table 9.2 Purified hepatic aldehyde dehydrogenases and their inhibition by disulfiram

Species	Isozyme	Location[a]	$K_m^{b,c}$ (μM)	Disulfiram inhibition			Reference
				Extent	%	μM^d	
Human	E_2	M	1–3	None	0	40	Greenfield and Pietruszko (1977)
	E_1	C	30–48	Complete	Stoichiometric		Kurys et al. (1989)
	E_3	C?	40–50	Marginal	10	40	
Equine	F2	M	0.2	Marginal	40	50	Eckfeldt et al. (1976)
	F1	C	70	Complete	Stoichiometric		
Ovine	Mitochondrial	M	210[e]	Marginal	25	50	Kitson (1975, 1983)
	Cytoplasmic	C	174[e]	Incomplete	Stoichiometric		Dickinson and Berrieman (1979) Dickinson et al. (1981)
Bovine	Mitochondrial	M	0.05–0.4	Marginal	20	50	Sugimoto et al. (1976)
	Cytoplasmic	C	440	Complete	100	1	Takahashi et al. (1979)
	Microsomal	P	1500	None	0	50	Guan et al. (1988)
Porcine	Mitochondrial	M	0.6	None	0	50	Guan et al. (1988)
	Cytosolic	C	44	Incomplete	Stoichiometric		Ramsey et al. (1989)
Canine	ALDH IA	C	2600	Marginal	15	50	Sanny (1985)
	ALDH IB	C	3400	Complete	97	1	
	ALDH IIA	M	40	Partial	80	5–50	
	ALDH IIB	M	1.4	Marginal	50	50	

Rat	Enzyme I	M	1.5	Partial	6	67	Siew et al. (1976)
	Enzyme II	M	1500	Partial	6	53	
Rat	Mitochondrial I	M	150[f]	Marginal	25	50	Lindahl and Evces (1984a)
	Mitochondrial II	M	150[f]	None	0	50	
	Microsomal I	P	2400	None	6	50	
	Microsomal II	P	1700[f]	None	3	50	
Rat	pI 6.2	C	500	Marked	50	0.1	Cao et al. (1989)
	pI 5.8	C	170	Sizeable	50	20	
	pI 5.3, 5.4 and 5.6	C	170	Marked	50	5	
Rat-inducible	Phenobarb-inducible	C	1400[f]	Complete	96	50	Lindahl and Evces (1984b)
	TCDD-inducible	C	4100[f]	Marginal	28	50	
	Promotion-associated	C	1300[f]	Complete	100	50	
	Tumour-specific	C	2200[f]	Marginal	45	50	
Rat-inducible	Phenanthrene-inducible	C	0.28	Complete	97	1	Torronen (1985)
	Benzo[a]pyrene-inducible	C	38	Marginal	40	100	

[a] C cytosolic; M, mitochondrial; P, microsomal.
[b] Determined with NAD$^+$ as cofactor.
[c] Determined for acetaldehyde unless otherwise stated.
[d] Disulfiram concentration at which inhibition was determined.
[e] Determined for D, L-glyceraldehyde (Crow et al, 1974).
[f] Determined for propylaldehyde rather than acetaldehyde.

identical to it (Ryzlak and Pietruszko, 1987, 1989). Although it has been separated into isozymes E2(a) and E2(b), the separate identity of these remains to be confirmed.

NAD$^+$-dependent ALDH enzymes analogous to E_1 and E_2 have been isolated from the livers of such other large mammals as the horse, ox, sheep and dog (Table 9.2) and a mitochondrial enzyme analogous to E_2 has been isolated from rat liver (Farrés *et al.*, 1989). The complete primary structures of the horse mitochondrial and cytosolic enzymes (referred to as F2 and F1, respectively) have been determined (von Bahr-Lindström *et al.*, 1984; Johansson, J. *et al.*, 1988). Like the human E_1 and E_2 enzymes, F1 and F2 are each 500 amino acid residues long. Although in both humans and horses the mitochondrial and cytosolic enzymes are clearly homologous (i.e. similar in structure and ancestral origin), both homotopic pairs (that is those having the same subcellular localization) are much more highly conserved. Thus, the E_2 and F2 enzymes share 96.5% identity and E_1 and F1 have 96.5% identity, while the two human enzymes, E_1 and E_2, share 83.2% identity and the two horse enzymes share 82.6% identity (Fig. 9.1). The rat mitochondrial ALDH is also 500 amino acid residues long and has a 96% identity with human E_2 (Farrés *et al.*, 1989).

On the basis of these structural interrelationships, a new nomenclature of the mammalian aldehyde dehydrogenases has been adopted (Nomenclature of Mammalian Aldehyde Dehydrogenases, 1988), whereby constitutive cytosolic ALDHs such as the human E_1 and the horse F1 enzyme fall into Class 1 ALDHs, while constitutive mitochondrial ALDHs such as the human E_2, the horse F2 and the mitochondrial rat enzyme are considered Class 2 ALDHs. The finding that the primary structure of a rat hepatoma cell ALDH (Jones, D.E. *et al.*, 1988) and that a rat liver cytosolic ALDH induced by 2,3,7,8-tetrachlorodibenzo-*p*-dioxin (TCDD) are identical (Hempel *et al.*, 1989), but only distantly related (27–30% identity) to Class 1 and 2 ALDHs, has led to the agreement to consider such inducible enzymes as Class 3 ALDHs.

ALDH activities in animal tissues are frequently identified by reference to their subcellular localization (cytosolic and mitochondrial) and their affinity for acetaldehyde (low- and high-K_m). The latter classification can be confusing, due to the existence of several conventions regarding what is considered the dividing line between low- and high-K_m. One convention accords the low-K_m designation to the seemingly ubiquitous Class 2 mitochondrial enzymes with a K_m in the single digit μM range (e.g. E_2), and relegates ALDHs with higher K_m (viz. E_1) to the high-K_m category (cf. Harada *et al.*, 1982). Another convention considers K_m values in the μM range to be low and those in the mM

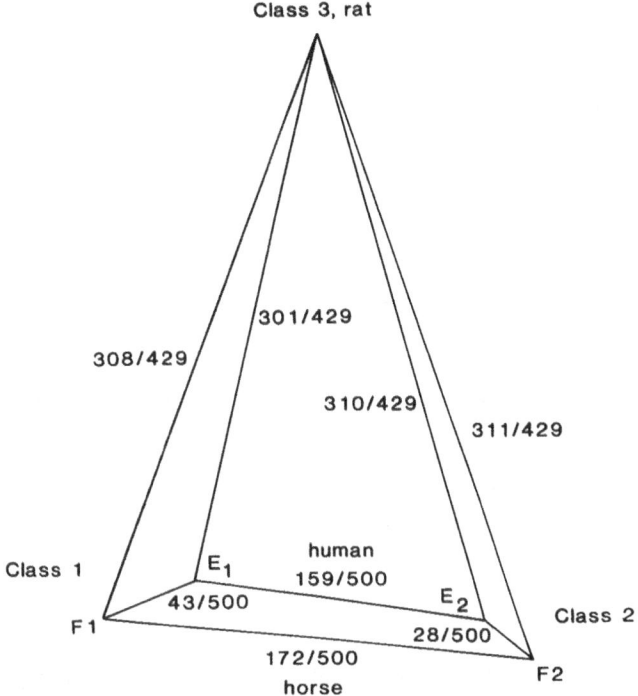

Figure 9.1 Relationship between the hepatic human and equine Class 1 and 2 aldehyde dehydrogenases (ALDHs) and the inducible rat Class 3 ALDH. Each of the five apices represents a different ALDH enzyme as indicated. The length of the line connecting any two apices is roughly proportional to the percentage of amino acid residues by which the two enzymes differ. More precisely, the number of such differences per number of aligned residues is written as a fraction along the connecting line. (Modified from Hempel *et al.*, 1989).

range to be high (cf. Pietruszko, 1983). Yet another convention derives from the work of Tottmar *et al.* (1973), who found that, in rat liver homogenates exposed to saturating NAD^+ concentrations, 5 mM acetaldehyde was required for maximum ALDH activity, but that 30–50% of the ALDH activity persisted as the acetaldehyde concentration was lowered to 10 µM. They also noted that the subcellular distribution of these dual forms of ALDH activity was not uniform. It has therefore become usual to determine ALDH activity, be it in homogenates or subcellular fractions, at two acetaldehyde concentrations and to report that observed in the presence of 15–70 µM acetaldehyde as the low-K_m activity (for review see Forte-McRobbie and Pietruszko, 1985). The difference between the latter values and those obtained in the presence of 5 mM acetaldehyde are reported as the high-K_m activity. To obviate confusion, the terms low- and high-K_m ALDH activities are used in this monograph only as defined by this last convention.

Tissue distribution studies of ALDH with K_m in the μM range show that the highest concentrations of these enzymes occur in the liver (Deitrich, 1966). In human liver, in particular, the ALDH content comprises more than 1% of total protein (Pietruszko, 1983), but is extremely variable (Forte-McRobbie and Pietruszko, 1985).

9.1.2 Genetic polymorphism of E_2

A substantial body of research performed in animals indicates that the mitochondria are the primary site of acetaldehyde metabolism (Parrilla *et al.*, 1974; Weiner, 1987). On the basis of this localization, it follows that the enzymes involved are the Class 2 ALDHs. Confirmation that this is also true of humans comes from investigation of the genetic polymorphism of the E_2 enzyme.

In 1979 Goedde *et al.* reported E_2 to be missing in 50% of the Japanese liver specimens they examined. Similar findings were made with respect to Chinese liver specimens by Teng (1981). The presence of both E_1 and E_2 in hair root follicles (Harada *et al.*, 1982) has rendered possible the investigation of the genetic polymorphism of ALDH in humans. It has been found that one-third to a half of Orientals of Mongoloid origin (Japanese, Chinese, Vietnamese, etc.) and South American Indians are deficient in the normal E_2, though none of the Caucasians or Africans examined show such a deficiency (for review see Bosron and Li, 1986; Goedde *et al.*, 1986; Agarwal and Goedde, 1989; Goedde and Agarwal, 1990). Moreover, the atypical or 'Oriental' E_2 has very little (Ferencz-Biro and Pietruszko, 1984) or no acetaldehyde dehydrogenase activity (Yoshida *et al.*, 1984, 1985; Yoshida and Davé, 1985). Individuals who are deficient in the normal E_2 exhibit high acetaldehyde levels in blood following ingestion of ethanol (range up to 125 μM following a 0.4 g/kg ethanol load) and experience an ethanol sensitivity, the symptomatology of which parallels, in many respects, that of the DER (Mizoi *et al.*, 1983, 1988). Not surprisingly, such individuals tend to show a natural aversion to alcoholic beverages and are seldom found among the ranks of the alcoholic.

The correlation between the E_2 deficiency and high blood acetaldehyde levels following ethanol ingestion lends strong support to the conclusion that *in vivo* acetaldehyde is metabolized primarily by E_2. At the same time, in 20% of E_2-deficient subjects, the blood acetaldehyde level peaks, following ingestion of 0.4 g/kg ethanol, at less than 20 μM, suggesting the involvement of other ALDH isozymes in the *in vivo* removal of the acetaldehyde (Mizoi *et al.*, 1988).

9.2 PHENOMENOLOGY OF THE INHIBITION BY DISULFIRAM

9.2.1 *In vivo* inhibition

Much of the information regarding the *in vivo* inhibition of ALDH comes from work in rats. The subcellular distribution of ALDH activity in rodent (rabbit, rat, mouse) liver differs from that in larger mammals. In rodent liver, the activity is primarily located in the mitochondria and microsomes, almost exclusively so in the rat (Lindahl and Evces, 1984c), whilst in the livers of all non-rodent species investigated it is primarily found in the mitochondria and cytosol (Fig. 9.2). Administration of DSSD to rats causes considerable inhibition of the mitochondrial low-K_m ALDH activity of their liver, but has relatively little effect on the microsomal high-K_m ALDH activity therein (Fig. 9.2a). There is much less of a difference in the subcellular distribution of low-K_m and high-K_m ALDH activity in the liver of the dog. Also, the inhibition of ALDH activity that results from pretreatment of the animals with DSSD is much more evenly distributed (Fig. 9.2c). The subcellular distribution of low-K_m and high-K_m ALDH activity in human liver is not unlike that seen in dog liver (Fig. 9.2b), though the effect of DSSD administration on these activities has yet to be investigated.

The differences in the responses of the low-K_m and high-K_m ALDH activity to DSSD administration in the rat are underscored by both dose–effect and time-course studies. Thus, whereas 24 h after administration the mitochondrial low-K_m ALDH activity is increasingly inhibited as the DSSD dose is increased from 150 to 600 mg/kg, the high-K_m ALDH activity, be it in the mitochondria, the microsomes, or the whole homogenate, remains unaffected (Marchner and Tottmar, 1978). Likewise, though the low-K_m ALDH activity in whole homogenate and mitochondria is maximally inhibited at 24–48 h following administration of DSSD (Fig 9.3a and b, respectively), the high-K_m ALDH remains unaffected at all times (Marchner and Tottmar, 1978; Brien *et al.*, 1985).

At first glance these findings appear to contradict the earlier ones of Deitrich and Erwin (1971) who reported that, following DSSD adminstration (300 mg/kg DSSD, p.o.) to rats, the ALDH activity of both the mitochondrial fraction of liver homogenate and that of its microsome- and cytosol-containing 10 000 $g \times$ 10 min supernatant were inhibited. However, they determined ALDH activity using 0.33 mM indole-3-acetaldehyde (IAL) as the substrate and it has since been suggested that different forms of ALDH are involved in the metabolism of acetaldehyde and IAL (Tottmar and Hellström, 1983). Accordingly, it is

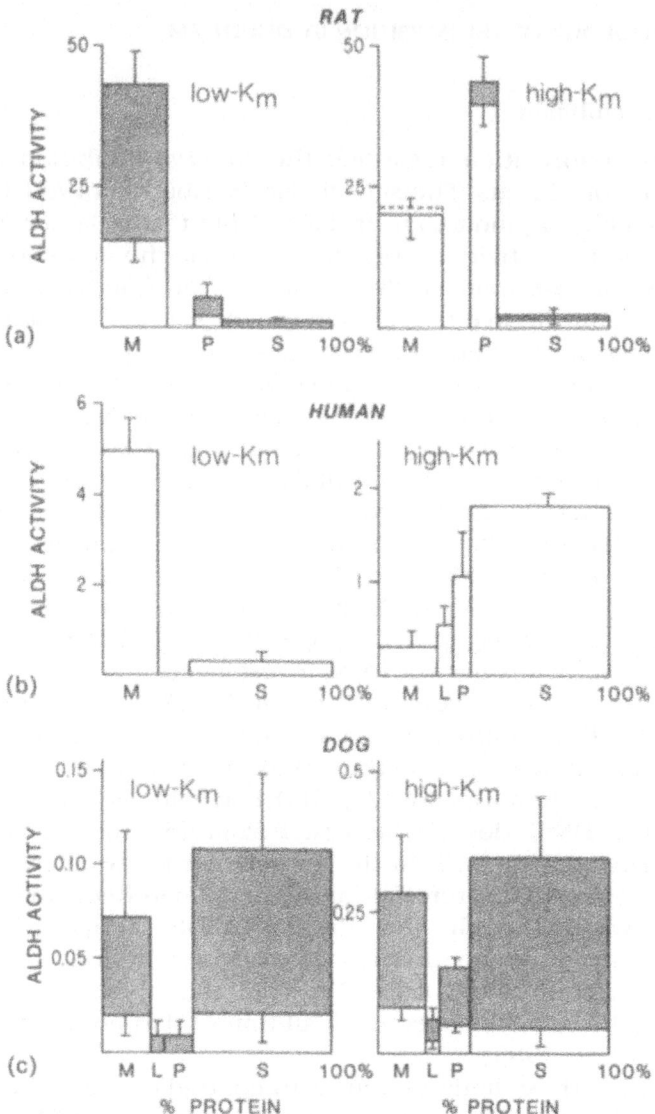

Figure 9.2 Schematic comparison of the subcellular distribution of low-K_m and high-K_m aldehyde dehydrogenase (ALDH) activity in three species and the effects thereon of *in vivo* pretreatment with disulfiram (DSSD). Horizontal scale: cellular fractions obtained by differential centrifugation of homogenate; the width of each fraction is proportional to protein content of the fraction. M, mitochondrial; L, light-mitochondrial; P, microsomal; S, cytosolic. ALDH activity in cell fractions from control subjects: sum of shaded plus open bars. ALDH in cell fractions from subjects administered DSSD: open bars (in instance where activity greater than in

possible that the supernatant ALDH isozyme whose activity towards IAL was inhibited by DSSD administration is one that shows no activity when acetaldehyde is the substrate. Also at variance with the findings described in the preceding paragraph are those of Johansson *et al.* (1989), who reported that the high-K_m, but not the low-K_m, ALDH activity of liver homogenate was significantly ($P<0.01$) decreased by pretreatment of animals with DSSD and ethanol.

Mouse hepatic low-K_m ALDH activity is 27% inhibited 24 h after the i.p. administration of 300 mg/kg DSSD. It returns to control values within 4 days. In contrast, the blood ALDH activity of these animals, assayed with IAL, is 81% inhibited at 24 h and does not return to control values for 21 days (Tottmar and Hellström, 1983)

The *in vivo* inhibition of ALDH that is occasioned by administration of DSSD appears to be irreversible. In rats, for instance, the observed slow spontaneous recovery appears to involve *de novo* enzyme synthesis, since it is completely blocked by the protein synthesis inhibitor, cycloheximide (Deitrich and Erwin, 1971). Although dithiothreitol and 2-mercaptoethanol can reverse *in vitro* DSSD-induced inhibition of ALDH, the inhibition of hepatic ALDH induced by *in vivo* DSSD administration cannot be reversed *ex vivo* by dithiothreitol (Deitrich hand Erwin, 1971), nor can similarly induced *in vivo* inhibition of human erythrocyte ALDH be reversed *ex vivo* with 2-mercaptoethanol (Hellström and Tottmar, 1983; Towell *et al.*, 1983a). On the other hand, Weiner and Ardelt (1984) noted a significant *ex vivo* effect of 0.01 M mercaptoethanol if added, before homogenization, to the brains of rats dosed with 100 mg/kg DSSD 16 h earlier. Whereas in the absence of any mercaptoethanol, the ALDH activity of mitochondria was significantly

---

controls: dashed outline). Low-K_m ALDH activity was determined in the presence of 15—50 μM acetaldehyde; high-K_m ALDH activity was determined as the difference between the low-K_m ALDH activity and the total ALDH activity determined in the presence of 5 mM acetaldehyde. (a) Subcellular distribution of ALDH activity in the rat. DSSD (300 mg/kg p.o.) was administered 24 h prior. [ALDH activity data from Tottmar and Marchner (1976); subcellular protein distribution data from Tottmar *et al.* (1973); ALDH activity expressed in nmol of NADH formed/min/mg protein.] (b) Subcellular distribution of ALDH activity in humans. [Redrawn from Henehan *et al.* (1985); ALDH activity is expressed in terms of relative specific activity.] (c) Subcellular distribution of ALDH activity in the dog. DSSD was administered 100 mg/kg for 2 days followed by 40 mg/kg for 3 days. [ALDH activity data from Sanny *et al.* (1988); subcellular protein distribution shown (Sunny, private communication) is that observed in control animals; it changed following DSSD treatment; ALDH activity expressed in μmol of NADH formed/min/g liver.]

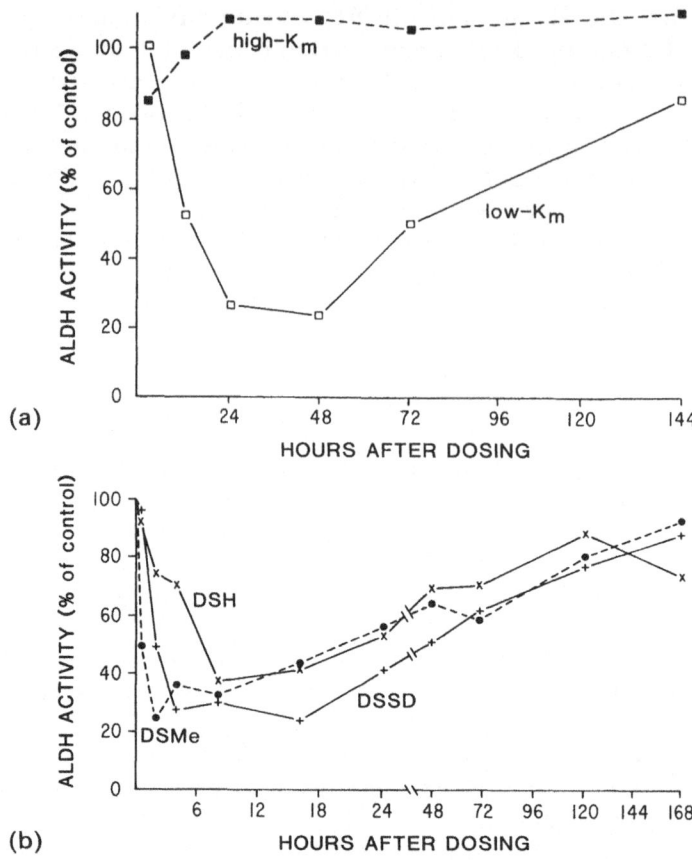

Figure 9.3 Time course of the effect of *in vivo* administration of disulfiram (DSSD) and some of its metabolites on hepatic aldehyde dehydrogenase (ALDH) activity in rats. (a) Effect of DSSD (300 mg/kg p.o.) on the low-K_m ALDH activity (determined in the presence of 25 µM acetaldehyde) and the high-K_m ALDH activity (difference between the former and that determined in the presence of 5 mM acetaldehyde) of whole homogenate. Redrawn from Marchner and Tottmar (1978). (b) Effect of DSSD (75 mg/kg i.p.), diethyldithiocarbamate (DSH: 114 mg/kg i.p.) and the methyl ester of diethyldithiocarbamic acid (DSMe: 41.2 mg/kg i.p.) on the lowK_m mitochondrial ALDH activity (determined in the presence of 50 µM acetaldehyde). Redrawn from Yourick and Faiman (1989).

inhibited, and that of the cytoplasm was not, when mercapto-ethanol was used the reverse result was obtained: the cytoplasmic ALDH activity was significantly inhibited, while the mitochondrial activity was not.

Table 9.3 Purified human aldehyde dehydrogenases and their inhibition by disulfiram (DSSD)

ALDH	Enzyme	Tissue	Isozyme	K_m^a Acetaldehyde (µM)	Physiological substrate (µM)	DSSD[b] inhibition	2-Mercapto-ethanol	Reactivation glutathione	Reactivation cysteine	Reference
Non-specific	Aldehyde dehydrogenase	Liver	E_1	30–48	0.4–2.4[c]	Complete[d]	Yes[e]	5%[f]	–	1,2,3,4
		Erythrocyte	E_1	17		Complete	Yes[g]	–	–	5
		Liver	E_2	1–3	0.8–1.0[c]	None	–	–	–	1,2
Non-specific	Aldehyde dehydrogenase	Brain	E_1	92		Complete[d,h]	Yes[i]	None[j]	None[j]	6,7,8
			$E_2(a)$	1	1.0[c]	Complete[h]	Yes[i]	None[j]	None[j]	6,8
			$E_2(b)$	1	0.5[c]	None	–	–	–	6,8
Specific	Glyceraldehyde 3-phosphate dehydrogenase	Brain	E6.6	575	42	Complete[h]	Yes[i]	None[j]	None[j]	6,8
			E6.8	2 000	172	Complete[h]	Yes[i]	None[j]	None[j]	6,8
			E8.5	300	35	Complete[d,h]	Yes[i]	Yes[j]	Yes[j]	6,8
			E9.0	350	32	Complete[h]	Yes[i]	Yes[j]	Yes[j]	6,8
Specific	Succinic semialdehyde dehydrogenase			875	0.7–2.0	Complete[h]	Yes[i]	None[j]	None[j]	6,8,9
Specific	1-pyrroline-5-carboxylate dehydrogenase	Placenta		22 000	170	Complete[k]	–	–	–	10

[a] Where K_m determined at several pH values, values obtained at pH nearest to 7.4 reported.
[b] In some instances inhibition stoichiometric, in others only complete in presence of saturating concentrations of DSSD; see text or original publications for details.
[c] Stoichiometric.
[d] 3,4-Dihydroxyphenylacetaldehyde and 5-hydroxyindoleacetaldehyde; see Refs 2 and 4.
[e] 18 mM 2-mercaptoethanol.
[f] 9 mM reduced glutathione for 18 h.
[g] 200 mM 2-mercaptoethanol.
[h] 3.3 µM disulfiram.
[i] 43 mM 2-mercaptoethanol.
[j] 33 µM reduced glutathione or cysteine.
[k] 40 µM disulfiram.

1. Greenfield and Pietruszko (1977). 2. Mackerell et al. (1986). 3. Vallari and Pietruszko (1982). 4. Vallari and Pietruszko (1983). 5. Inoue et al. (1978). 6. Ryzlak and Pietruszko (1989). 7. Ryzlak and Pietruszko (1988). 8. Ryzlak (1986). 9. Ryzlak and Pietruszko (1988). 10. Farrés et al. (1988).

9.2.2 *In vitro* inhibition

Paradoxically, Class 2 ALDHs, the enzymes considered to be primarily responsible for the metabolism of acetaldehyde formed from ethanol *in vivo* (section 9.2.2), are quite resistant to *in vitro* DSSD inhibition, being only partially inhibited by saturated (40–50 µM) aqueous solutions of DSSD. By contrast, Class 1 ALDHs are very sensitive to *in vitro* inhibition by 3 µM DSSD or less (Table 9.2).

When first purified, human liver ALDH was found to be rather insensitive to DSSD inhibition *in vitro*. Thus, Kraemer and Deitrich (1968) reported only a 50% inhibition by 100 µM DSSD (in propylene glycol) and Blair and Bodley (1969) a 35% inhibition at 40 µM. Subsequently, the characterization of separate hepatic mitochondrial and cytoplasmic ALDH isozymes revealed that the sheep (Kitson, 1975; Dickinson and Berrieman, 1979; Kitson, 1982), horse (Eckfeldt *et al.*, 1976) and ox (Sugimoto *et al.*, 1976) cytoplasmic isozymes are exquisitely sensitive to DSSD, being inhibited by stoichiometric quantities of DSSD (Table 9.2). The mitochondrial isozyme from each of these species, on the other hand, is rather insensitive, showing an inhibition of 25–50% at saturating DSSD concentrations (40–50 µM). The same is also true of the human E_1 and E_2 isozymes purified to apparent homogeneity (Greenfield and Pietruszko, 1977). Such observations have led to the surmise that the *in vivo* inhibition of Class 2 ALDHs must be due to some metabolite of DSSD. Efforts to identify such a metabolite continue.

Human brain non-specific ALDH isozyme inhibition by DSSD presents a more complex situation. The E1 human brain enzyme is, like the hepatic E_1, readily inhibited by DSSD. However, two brain enzymes, E2(a) and E2(b), have been purified (Ryzlak and Pietruszko, 1987, 1989). In many particulars they are very similar to the hepatic E_2 enzyme (Table 9.3), but one, the E2(a) enzyme, is readily inactivated by DSSD, while the other is insensitive to it.

9.3 MECHANISM OF THE INHIBITION

9.3.1 Class 1 aldehyde dehydrogenases

Kitson (1978) reported that most of the activity of the Class 1 ALDH from sheep liver was abolished by two or less molecules of DSSD per ALDH tetramer, this inhibition being reversed by 2-mercaptoethanol (Kitson, 1975). A similar stoichiometry was observed by Vallari and Pietruszko (1982, 1983) for E_1, the Class 1 human liver ALDH. Specifically they found that, following a 20-h incubation with two equivalents of DSSD, the enzyme was completely inactivated, though in the course of 4–6 min in the presence of NAD and substrate (propionaldehyde) a slight reversal of the inhibition occurred. They also found upon incubation of the enzyme with 2 mole equivalents of symmetrically labelled ^{14}C-DSSD, that no incorporation of the label occurred and the radioactivity was recovered in the form of DSH. Yet the dialyzed, label-free enzyme remained fully inhibited and was found to have sustained a loss of four -SH groups per enzyme tetramer. Moreover, the inhibition was reversed by 2-mercaptoethanol. They concluded that DSSD inhibits the enzyme by oxidizing vicinal -SH groups to disulfides. They proposed this to occur by a two-step process. The first step involves the production of a mixed disulfide by a disulfide exchange reaction between DSSD and a protein sulfhydryl, this resulting in the attachment of a DS residue to the protein (equation 8.1). The second step is another disulfide exchange reaction. It involves a vicinal sulfhydryl group and results in the formation of an internal disulfide and the release of DSH (equation 8.2). Using the sheep Class 1 ALDH and ^{14}C-DSSD, Kitson (1983) found it possible to separate the two steps. The first step was rapid and accounted for the observed inhibition. The second step occurred slowly and resulted in enzyme that was still inactive, but no longer labelled with the DS moiety. Even if the sheep Class 1 ALDH is rigorously purified so that it contains less than 0.5% of the Class 2 ALDH, it cannot be inhibited by more than 98%; it retains 2% of the original activity even in the presence of a large excess of DSSD (Dickinson *et al.*, 1981), a finding that remains unexplained.

In addition to functioning as dehydrogenases, ALDHs can also function as esterases, hydrolyzing, for instance, *p*-nitrophenol acetate (Feldman and Weiner, 1972). Both activities of the sheep Class 1 ALDH are equally inhibited by DSSD. Yet, whereas substrate for the dehydrogenase activity does not protect the enzyme against DSSD inactivation, that for the esterase does (Kitson, 1982). Kitson (1987) has reported a high degree of correlation between the DSSD-induced decrease in the pre-steady-state burst in NADH formation and the degree of inhibition brought about by DSSD in both the dehydrogenase and esterase activities of this enzyme. This high degree of correlation indicates that, with respect to this enzyme, DSSD is an active-site-directed reagent. With the elucidation of the enzyme's primary structure, the identification of the site of action of DSSD becomes a possibility. The finding that iodoacetamide, another sulfhydryl modifying reagent, alkylates the Cys-302 residue of the human Class 1 ALDH (Hempel *et al.*, 1982, 1984, 1985), and that this alkylation not only causes inactivation of the enzyme, but is prevented by both the substrate (Hempel and Pietruszko, 1981) and DSSD (Hempel *et al.*, 1982), implicates Cys-302 as the DSSD-reactive cysteine residue (Hempel *et al.*, 1985; von Bahr-Lindström *et al.*, 1985; Hempel and Jørnvall, 1986). It is of interest, therefore, that Cys-302 is very highly conserved, being the only cysteine residue retained in all ALDHs whose structure has been elucidated to date (Hempel *et al.*, 1989).

9.3.2 Class 2 aldehyde dehydrogenases

Class 2 ALDHs are resistant to *in vitro* inhibition by DSSD (Table 9.2) and high DSSD concentrations (100 μM) are required for greater than 80% inactivation (Sanny and Weiner, 1987). At the same time, the number of active sites on the enzyme, as determined by the magnitude of the pre-steady-state burst in NADH formation, does not decrease upon exposure to DSSD until about 75% of the enzyme's activity is lost, indicating that unlike its action with respect to Class 1 ALDHs (Kitson, 1987), the action of DSSD on Class 2 ALDHs is not that of an active-site-directed reagent (Sanny and Weiner, 1987).

Though resistant to inhibition by DSSD, Class 2 ALDHs are highly susceptible to inhibition by mixed disulfides formed from DSSD by disulfide exchange reactions with other thiols. This was first observed for the mixed disulfide of DSH and 2-mercaptoethanol, which, in a 10 μM concentration, caused a 65% inhibition of the sheep Class 2 ALDH (Kitson, 1975). Later, E_2, the human Class 2 ALDH, was found to be exquisitely sensitive to stoichiometric amounts of *N,N*-diethylthiocarbamyl-*S*-methyl disulfide (DSSMe; Fig. 5.1), the mixed disulfide of methanethiol (MeSH) and DSH (MacKerell *et al.*, 1985). The inhibition is totally reversible by 2-mercaptoethanol. Also, as with E_1 and DSSD, the inhibition is reversed to a small extent by continued exposure to substrate (Pietruszko and MacKerell, 1986). The second-order rate constant for the inhibition of E_2 by mixed disulfides of DSH and increasing chainlength homologues of MeSH suggests that steric hinderance is responsible for the resistance of this enzyme to inhibition by DSSD *in vitro* (MacKerell *et al.*, 1985). Formation of DSSMe from DSSD and MeSH *in vivo*, although not demonstrated to date, could explain the *in vivo* inhibition of Class 2 ALDHs by DSSD. Such a synthesis could take place, either via a disulfide exchange reaction or oxidatively by reaction of MeSH with DSH. MeSH is a known product of endogenous catabolism, the blood levels of this entity becoming elevated following liver injury. Indeed, in cirrhotics, micromolar concentrations of MeSH are observed following a protein load (Kromhout *et al.*, 1980).

9.3.3 Action of the mixed disulfides of diethyldithiocarbamate

DSSMe and the other mixed disulfides of DSH that have been found to be E_2 inhibitors (section 9.3.2) are also effective inhibitors of the human Class 1 ALDH (MacKerell *et al.*, 1985). Also, DSSMe is just as effective an inhibitor of the sheep Class 1 ALDH as is DSSD itself (Kitson and Loomes, 1985). Kitson (1988) argues that, because DSH is a stronger acid than MeSH, the disulfide would label the protein with the -SMe group and that because MeSH is such a weak acid, that formation of the internal protein disulfide would not occur (Kitson and Loomes, 1984).

Additional information regarding the mechanism of Class 1 ALDH inhibition by DSSD and the mixed disulfides of DSH comes from the observations of Kitson (1979) that 2,2'-dithiodipyridine (PSSP), a protein thiol modifying agent, rapidly activates ALDH and protects it against DSSD (Kitson, 1979). As the reaction with PSSP proceeds, 2-thiopyridone (PSH) is liberated, the amount of PSH release soon exceeding, however, that predicted by equation (8.1), indicating that in this instance also the reaction represented by equation (8.2) follows (Kitson and Loomes, 1985). The release of PSH from the PSSP-activated enzyme ($t_{1/2}$ of 3 h at 25 °C: Kitson and Loomes, 1984) is accompanied by a loss of all its activity (Kitson, 1982). However, this secondary release of PSH does not occur if the enzyme has been pretreated with

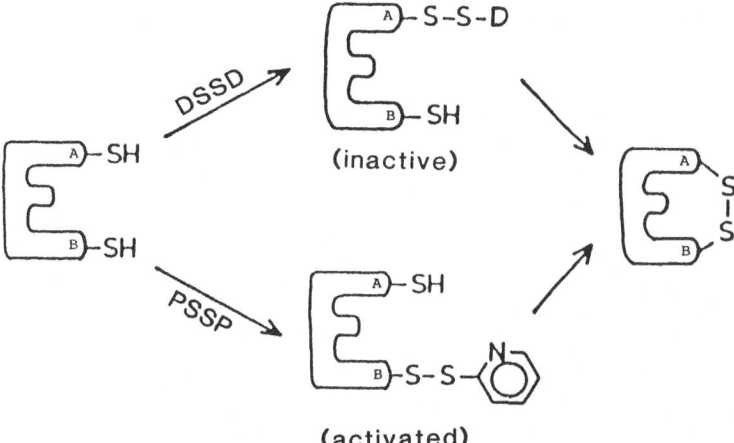

(activated)

Figure 9.4 Scheme showing how disulfiram (DSSD) and 2,2'-dithiodipyridine (PSSP) could oxidize different cysteine thiols at different sites (sites A and B) and yet result in the formation of the same internal disulfide. Modified from Kitson and Loomes (1984).

DSSD. The most parsimonious explanation for these phenomena postulates (Kitson and Loomes, 1984; Kitson, 1988) that the cysteine residue with which PSSP first reacts to activate the enzyme (site B) is different from that with which DSSD first reacts (site A), but that the internal disulfide that is eventually formed involves both of these residues (Fig. 9.4). The protection that activation by PSSP affords the enzyme against DSSD, but not against DSSMe (Kitson, 1988), is seen as being an indication that the presence of a SP residue at site B provides steric protection of site A from the bulkier DSSD. Reaction of the enzyme with the mixed 2-thiopyridyl methyl disulfide (PSSMe), which is accompanied by release of PSH and is viewed as resulting in the labelling of the site B with an -SMe residue, induces some activation of the enzyme, but, being less bulky, does not protect it from inhibition by either DSSD or DSSMe (Kitson and Loomes, 1985).

9.4 ROLE OF DISULFIRAM METABOLITES

9.4.1 Diethyldithiocarbamic acid, carbon disulfide and diethylamine

The metabolite first formed from DSSD is DSH (section 5.1). Its administration to rats results in an inhibition of the low-K_m ALDH activity of hepatic mitochondria (Deitrich and Erwin, 1971; Yourick and Faiman, 1989; Hart *et al.*, 1990). The peak inhibition is observed 8 h after the administration of DSH (114 mg/kg i.p.). Because each molecule of DSSD can form two of DSH, it is usual when comparing the potency of these agents to allow for this equivalence. In this context, it is found that the ALDH inhibition induced by DSH administration develops more slowly than that observed after administration of a thus equivalent amount of DSSD. At 2 h post administration, the ALDH activity is 48% less inhibited in rats treated with DSH than those receiving DSSD (Fig. 9.3). Likewise, the blood acetaldehyde levels caused in these animals by administration of ethanol (1 g/kg i.p.) 2 h after the DSH pretreatment are only 50% as high as those observed when ethanol is administered 2 h following DSSD pretreatment (Yourick and Faiman, 1989). By 8 h post administration, however, both the ALDH inhibition and the acetaldehyde blood levels seen following ethanol administration are the same regardless of which agent is used.

Whether such an equivalence extends to all doses of the two agents is another matter. Deitrich and Erwin (1971), who determined the ALDH activity at 40 h post administration using 330 μM 3-indoleacetaldehyde, reported that the dose–response curves for the inhibition of the ALDH activity by DSH and DSSD were superimposable. On the other hand, Hart *et al.* (1990), who determined the ALDH activity at 8 h post administration using 50 μM acetaldehyde, reported the dose–response curve for DSH to be considerably less steep than that for DSSD, so that, even if one allows for the above-mentioned equivalence factor, low doses of DSH would appear to have greater activity than equivalent ones of DSSD. However, in another publication from the same laboratory (Yourick and Faiman, 1989), it is stated that a 5–10 mg/kg i.p. dose of DSSD induces a 10% inhibition of the low K_m ALDH activity. If this is so, then even at such low doses the activity of the two agents would be comparable.

In vitro, DSH has not proved to be an effective inhibitor of ALDH. Because DSH is a potent chelator (Chapter 7), early reports that ALDH was a Zn-containing enzyme (Schwarcz and Stoppani, 1960) lead to the inference that it inhibited ALDH by chelation of its Zn (Stoppani *et al.*, 1966; Li and Vallee, 1969). Subsequently, atomic absorption analysis of the E_2 enzyme failed to demonstrate the presence of Zn and, as a consequence, the correlation reported earlier by Stoppani *et al.* (1966), between the potency of various Zn chelators (including DSH) and their inhibition of ALDH, is viewed as spurious (Sidhu and Blair, 1975). In any event, the DSH-induced inhibition of ALDH reported by Stoppani *et al.* (1966) was marginal at best (12% at 0.33 mM DSH). More specifically, 0.5 mM DSH does not inhibit the sheep Class 2 ALDH (Kitson, 1975) nor does 1 mM DSH inhibit the human one (Harada *et al.*, 1982). Exposure of the sheep Class 1 ALDH to 0.1 mM DSH, on the other hand, has been reported to cause a significant inhibition, which increases on standing. The observed inhibition is probably due, however, to the oxidation of a trace amount of DSH to DSSD and can be largely prevented by 10 μM dithiothreitol, an antioxidant (Kitson, 1982).

Carbon disulfide (CS_2) and diethylamine (Et_2NH) are two *in vivo* metabolites of DSH (section 5.6). E_1 and E_2 are not inhibited by up to 10 mM CS_2. E_1 is also not inhibited by 10 mM Et_2NH and while this agent does inhibit E_2, the K_i for the inhibition is 0.1 mM (Blair and Bodley, 1969; Harada *et al.*, 1982).

9.4.2 Diethyldithiocarbamic acid methyl ester

The methyl ester of diethyldithiocarbamic acid (DSMe) is a metabolite of DSSD (Gessner, T. and Jakubowski, 1972; Cobby *et al.*, 1977a; Faiman *et al.*, 1977; Johansson *et al.*, 1989). Its administration induces in rats a marked (up to 90%) and dose-related inhibition of low-K_m ALDH activity (measured using a 50 μM concentration of acetaldehyde) which is as long lasting as that observed following administration of DSSD (Yourick and Faiman, 1987). Moreover, following administration of DSMe, the onset of the ALDH inhibition is significantly faster than that seen following administration of either DSSD or DSH (Yourick and Faiman, 1989). Already half an hour following administration of DSMe (41.2 mg/kg i.p.) the low-K_m mitochondrial ALDH activity is 50% inhibited and peak inhibition is observed at 2 h. Administration of ethanol (1 g/kg) at that time results in blood acetaldehyde levels which are twice as high as those seen when animals pretreated with an equimolar dose of DSSD are used (Yourick and Faiman, 1989).

There is some indication that DSMe may play a role in clinically relevant ALDH inhibition. Thus, in an experiment with groups of human volunteers treated for a 2-week period with various doses of DSSD and challenged with ethanol (0.15 g/kg) DER reactions occurred only in those groups that had mean plasma DSMe levels greater than 80 nM 2 h after DSSD administration (Johansson and Stankiewicz, 1989).

In a second study, Johansson *et al.* (1991) determined, at 2-week intervals, the blood DSMe level and the reaction to an ethanol challenge of 52 non-alcoholic individuals given DSSD daily on a schedule whereby it was incrementally increased by 100 mg every 14 days (section 11.6.2). The results of this study also indicate some relationship between blood DSMe levels and the occurrence of a DER. Thus, after 2 weeks on a 100 mg DSSD dose, the median blood DSMe level of the group ($n=21$) that experienced a DER when challenged with ethanol following this treatment was 68 µM. On the other hand, the median blood DSMe level of a second group ($n=27$) which, when challenged with ethanol following treatment with 100 mg of DSSD, did not experience a DER was 15 µM. Upon raising the DSSD dose to 200 mg for two weeks, the median blood DSMe increased to 92 µM and all the subjects experienced a DER when challenged with ethanol. In a third group that required 2 weeks of treatment with 300 mg before developing a DER ($n=4$), the blood DSMe levels were undetectable after 2 weeks at 100 mg, and the median value after 2 weeks at 200 mg DSSD was 40 µM. After 2 weeks at 300 mg DSSD, however, the median DSMe level rose to 108 µM. The median blood acetaldehyde levels observed in these subjects following the ethanol challenges exhibited a similar pattern.

In 1987, Yourick and Faiman suggested that DSMe is 'the active chemical species' responsible for the alcohol-sensitizing properties of DSSD. Since 1 mM DSMe had been previously found not to have any effect *in vitro* on either Class 1 or Class 2 ALDHs (Kitson, 1976), its identification as 'active chemical species' has proved controversial (Kitson, 1989). Since Yourick and Faiman (1987) confirm the earlier finding that DSMe is 'a poor *in vitro* inhibitor of low Km ALDH even at concentrations of 1 mM', the problem may be a semantic one. DSMe inhibits the low-K_m ALDH when incubated with liver homogenates in an air atmosphere, but fails to do so if incubated in a nitrogen atmosphere (Johansson *et al.*, 1989), suggesting that it is metabolized to the entity responsible for inhibition of the ALDH. The failure to detect any ^{35}S-CS_2 in the expired air following administration of ^{35}S-DSMe to either rats (Faiman *et al.*, 1983) or dogs (Jensen, 1984) indicates that DSMe does not give rise to DSH, since CS_2 is a well-established and readily detectable metabolite of these compounds (section 5.6). This strongly suggests that DSMe is a more proximal precursor of the entity responsible for ALDH inhibition than either DSSD or DSH.

9.4.3 Diethylmonothiocarbamic acid methyl ester

DSMe is further metabolized to diethylmonothiocarbamic acid methyl ester (DmSMe), the monothio analogue of DSMe (Johansson, 1989a; Johansson *et al.*, 1989). Administration of DmSMe to rats (18.6 mg/kg i.p.) results in a very rapid onset of inhibition of the hepatic mitochondrial low-K_m ALDH activity, peak (70%) inhibition being observed half an hour after administration (Hart *et al.*, 1990). The peak level of inhibition is similar to that achieved with a dose of DSMe twice as large and the dose–response relationship for *in vivo* inhibition of the low-K_m ALDH activity suggests that DmSMe is a more potent inhibitor than DSMe (Hart *et al.*, 1990). On the other hand, in groups of human volunteers treated for a 2-week period with various doses of DSSD and challenged with ethanol (0.15 g/kg) no correlation was observed between the occurrence of DER reactions and the group mean plasma DmSMe levels 2 hours after DSSD administration (Johansson and Stankiewicz, 1989).

In vitro DmSMe causes a slow, progressive, but marginal inhibition of a partially purified preparation of bovine Class 2 ALDH. After a 24-h period of exposure to 2.76 mM DmSMe, only 26% of the ALDH activity is blocked (Johansson, 1989c). No inhibition is observed of the hepatic mitochondrial low-K_m ALDH activity following a 60-min incubation of mitochondria with 0.1 mM DmSMe, although following a 60 min incubation with 1 mM DmSMe, significant inhibition (*ca* 25%) is observed (Hart *et al.*, 1990). On the other hand, incubation of 28 µM DmSMe with rat liver homogenates for 60 min potently inhibits the low-K_m

ALDH (Johansson *et al.*, 1989). Based on this evidence it appears that DmSMe is also a precursor of the entity responsible for ALDH inhibition.

*See page 42 for Note added in press.

9.5 INHIBITION OF ALDEHYDE DEHYDROGENASES IN BLOOD

9.5.1 Human erythrocyte aldehyde dehydrogenase

ALDH activity is found in human blood cells; Pietruszko and Vallari (1978) reported the presence of four isozymes in the cellular fraction of human blood, two of these having the same mobility as hepatic E_1 and E_2. The two major isozymes did not correspond, however, to any previously described.

The erythrocyte ALDH activity is readily inhibited by DSSD (62% by 1 μM and 99% by 5 μM) and has an apparent acetaldehyde K_m of 0.43 mM in intact cells and 0.69 mM in their lysate (Inoue *et al.*, 1978). Purified to homogeneity, it has an acetaldehyde K_m of 17 μM at pH 7.4, is rapidly and non-competitively inhibited by DSSD, and is regenerated by 2-mercaptoethanol (Inoue *et al.*, 1979). In all these particulars it is similar to E_1, and, like E_1, its binding to NADH is increased by magnesium (Rawles *et al.*, 1987). Based on analysis of peptides obtained by a tryptic digest of the enzyme purified to homogeneity, the enzyme appears to be identical to E_1 (Agarwal *et al.*, 1989).

In patients receiving DSSD (250 mg/day), total loss of erythrocyte ALDH activity occurs in the first 36–120 h of therapy; the decline in activity seems to follow a zero-order rate characteristic for each patient (Towell *et al.*, 1983a). The enzyme is very sensitive to *in vivo* inhibition by DSSD. For instance, following daily administration of just 1 mg of DSSD for 14 days it is significantly ($P < 0.001$) though only slightly (8%) inhibited (Johansson *et al.*, 1991). Yet, even total inhibition of erythrocyte ALDH does not assure therapeutic effectiveness. Towell *et al.* (1983a), for instance, could not detect any ALDH activity in two patients who claimed that, though they were taking 250 mg DSSD per day, they could drink without adverse effects. Johansson and Stankiewicz (1989) suggest that erythrocyte ALDH is completely inhibited within 3–5 days of initiation of therapy, if the dosage is sufficient to result in measurable levels of DmSMe, a metabolite of DSSD, but that otherwise it may not be totally inhibited for 120 days. However, in a later study, in which individuals maintained on 100 to 300 mg of DSSD were challenged with ethanol, the median values for the inhibition of erythrocyte ALDH (range 95–98%) in groups that responded with a DER and those that did not were found to be all very similar (Johansson *et al.*, 1991).

A characteristic of the depression of erythrocyte ALDH by DSSD therapy is that it lasts in excess of 2 months after its termination (Towell *et al.*, 1983b) and long after dissipation of the pharmacological effects that can result in a DER (section 11.6.1). The prolonged inhibition of erythrocyte ALDH has been confirmed by Tottmar and Hellström (1983) and by Helander *et al.* (1988) who found that, in patients who had been administered 200 mg/day for a month or 400 mg every other day for 2 weeks and in whom the erythrocyte ALDH was 90% inhibited at the end of this period, it took 60–70 days following discontinuation of therapy for the ALDH level to return to normal. Erythrocytes, being enucleated cells, lack the machinery needed to resynthesize the irreversibly inhibited ALDH. Hence the effect of DSSD can be expected to be long lasting, i.e. until the cells are substantially replaced.

The erythrocyte ALDH inhibition that follows *in vivo* DSSD therapy cannot be reversed *ex vivo* with 2-mercaptoethanol (Tottmar and Hellström, 1983; Towell *et al.*, 1983a). That this agent is able to reverse, either totally or in large part, the *in vitro* DSSD-induced loss of activity of a number of cytoplasmic ALDHs is well documented (Eckfeldt *et al.*, 1976; Kitson, 1978; Inoue *et al.*, 1979; Vallari and Pietruszko, 1982, 1983; Tottmar and Hellström, 1983; Towell *et al.* 1983a; Rawles *et al.*, 1987). These observations have led to the suggestion that the *in vivo* and *in vitro* mechanisms of inhibition differ and have been viewed as raising doubts as to whether the *in vitro* studies are pertinent to the effects observed *in vivo* (Tottmar and Hellström, 1983; Towell *et al.*, 1983a; Johansson *et al.*, 1989; Johansson and Stankiewicz, 1989). The first question that arises in this respect is whether reversibility is time-limited. Vallari and Pietruszko, who reactivated the enzyme with 2-mercaptoethanol 12 min after inhibiting it with DSSD [Kitson (1978) did so after 4 min], state that the ALDH activity is not recovered with 2-mercaptoethanol (or with 1,4-dithiothreitol) after prolonged dialysis (details not given) of the modified enzyme in the absence of the reducing agent (Vallari and Pietruszko, 1982, 1983). On the other hand, Towell *et al.* (1983a) reported being able to reverse with 2-mercaptoethanol the inhibition of ALDH activity of both erythrocytes and their lysates even after these had been incubated with DSSD at 37 °C for 24 h. A second question, and one that has not been raised, is whether the inactivated ALDH is retained by the erythrocytes. In the hepatocyte, DSSD-induced inactivation of cytochrome P-450 is followed by a fall in the cytochrome content of the cell (section 8.3.5). Thus, before ascribing the inability of reducing agents to reactivate the ALDH to a different mechanism of inhibition, it would be well to determine if there is any enzyme there to be reactivated.

Although Class 1 ALDH, the ALDH type present in erythrocytes, is readily inhibited by DSSD, it is not inhibited by DSH (Kitson, 1982). In keeping with this, when 100 μM DSH is incubated with either whole blood or erythrocyte hemolyzate, no inhibition of the erythrocyte ALDH is observed (Johansson, 1990a). If, however, this same concentration of DSH is incubated for 5 min with washed erythrocytes in the presence of EDTA, a 78% inhibition of the erythrocyte ALDH results (Helander and Johansson, 1989). This suggests that under the latter conditions DSH is metabolized to an active inhibitor of the enzyme. This could be DSSD, since in this system a 10 μM concentration of DSSD causes an 84% inhibition of the enzyme. In erythrocytes, oxy-hemoglobin and methemoglobin can oxidize DSH to DSSD, though no accumulation of DSSD occurs in DSH-exposed erythrocytes under normal conditions since these cells have an efficient, glucose-dependent, GSH generating system and GSH readily reduces DSSD to DSH (section 5.3). In washed erythrocytes, however, the GSH generating system would be expected to fail for lack of glucose, and DSSD accumulation could occur. Moreover, the observed inhibition of erythrocyte ALDH under these circumstances is unlikely to be due to the formation of DmSMe, since the latter is without effect when added to the washed erythrocytes so as to give a 100 μM concentration (Helander and Johansson, 1989).

9.5.2 Human leukocyte aldehyde dehydrogenase

In addition to erythrocytes, ALDH activity is also found in leukocytes and platelets (Helander and Tottmar, 1986, 1987a,b; Helander *et al.*, 1988). Because erythrocytes outnumber leukocytes in the blood by a large factor, in excess of 99% of blood ALDH activity derives from erythrocytes. Nonetheless, the leukocytes ALDH activity is 17 times higher, per cell.

Exposure of leukocytes to the mitogen, phytohemagglutinin, increases their ALDH activity 3-fold. Unlike the erythrocyte and platelet ALDH activities, which are 85% inhibited by 1 μM DSSD, the leukocyte activity is rather resistant to inhibition by even 50 μM DSSD (Helander and Tottmar, 1988). In this respect the leukocyte activity is similar to that of the hepatic mitochondrial enzyme E_2. It should be noted that incubation of washed leukocytes with 100 μM DSH also fails to result in inhibition of the leukocyte ALDH activity (Helander and Johansson, 1989), although parallel incubation of washed erythrocytes does result in the inhibition of the erythrocyte ALDH (section 9.5.1). The difference may be due to the inhibition of the erythrocyte enzyme, under these circumstances, being caused by the oxidation of DSH to DSSD. Leukocytes may be less able to carry out this reaction; in any event the leukocyte ALDH is insensitive to the product of the reaction, DSSD.

By contrast with the extensive and long-lasting inactivation of erythrocyte ALDH by DSSD therapy, leukocyte ALDH appears to be inhibited less and for a shorter period of time by such treatment. Thus, in patients receiving 200–400 mg daily, the leukocyte ALDH activity is 40–60% inhibited within 2–3 days and remains unaltered at this level of inhibition during continued treatment and for a couple of days after termination of therapy, after which it reverts to control values after about a week (Helander *et al.*, 1988; Helander and Carlsson, 1990). In these same patients, erythrocyte ALDH is inhibited to a much greater extent (95%), and continues to remain depressed after termination of the therapy, so that a week later it is still 90% inhibited. Accordingly, the inhibition of the leukocyte ALDH provides a much better indication of recent dosing history with DSSD and might, therefore, be useful in checking compliance with DSSD therapy.

In interpreting the findings of the group responsible for much of the work of blood ALDH inhibition (Helander, Hellström and Tottmar), cognizance must be taken of their use of IAL, 3,4-dihydroxyphenylacetaldehyde (DOPAL) and 5-hydroxyindoleacetaldehyde (5-HIAL), as substrates in the assay of ALDH activity, rather than the usually employed acetaldehyde or propionaldehyde. The many-fold greater affinity of blood ALDH for these substrates than for acetaldehyde (Helander and Tottmar, 1986) increases markedly the sensitivity of the assay. It complicates, however, the interpretation of the results, since the observed ALDH-inhibitory effects of DSSD are, in part, a function of the substrate employed. For instance, a 5-min incubation of partially purified human blood ALDH with 5 µM DSSD results in an almost complete inhibition of acetaldehyde ALDH, but only in a 70–85% inhibition of IAL and DOPAL ALDH activities (Helander and Tottmar, 1986). Conversely, whole blood ALDH activity, following either *in vivo* administration of DSSD or *in vitro* exposure to 5 µM DSSD for 1–5 min, is significantly less inhibited when assayed using acetaldehyde than when IAL is employed as a substrate (Tottmar and Hellström, 1983). Such differences have led Tottmar and Hellström (1983) to conclude that different forms of ALDH are involved in the acetaldehyde and IAL assays. Interestingly, this contrasts with the observation that administration of DSSD to rats results in a similar degree of inhibition of the brain low-K_m ALDH activity whether acetaldehyde or DOPAL are used to assay it, leading to the conclusion that the same enzyme is involved in the oxidation of both substrates (Pettersson and Tottmar, 1982).

9.6 INHIBITION OF METABOLISM OF ENDOGENOUS ALDEHYDES

9.6.1 Biogenic monamine-derived aldehydes

The action of monoamineoxidase on three important endogenous neurotransmitter monoamines, dopamine (DA), norepinephrine (NE) and 5-hydroxytryptamine (5-HT), results in the formation of the corresponding aldehydes. DSSD administration-induced changes in the metabolite pattern of these monoamines indicates that the oxidation of the aldehydes derived from them, an ALDH catalyzed reaction, is inhibited. Such an inhibition was demonstrated in the caudate nucleus of the conscious rat by Berger and Weiner (1977) and Weiner *et al.* (1978) using push–pull perfusion with ^{14}C-DA. DSSD pretreatment, these workers found, increases the ratio of neutral to acidic DA metabolites, i.e. the ratio of DOPAL plus 3,4-dihydroxyphenylethanol (DOPET) to 3,4-dihydroxyphenylacetic acid (DOPAC) plus HVA. Perfusion of another subcortical nucleus, the nucleus accumbens, yields similar results, though DSSD pretreatment had little effect on the ratio of these metabolites in other brain areas (Weiner *et al.*, 1978). DSSD administration, it should be noted, has no effect on the activity of aldehyde reductase (Hellström and Tottmar, 1982b).

DSSD-induced changes in the pattern of catecholamine metabolites are complicated by the inhibition of dopamine β-hydroxylase (DBH) which hydroxylates DA to NE (Fig. 9.5 and section 8.2). For instance, Hoeldtke and Stetson (1980) observed that in individuals pretreated with DSSD (5.5 mg/kg/day for 4 days) and administered ^{3}H-DA, the excretion of ^{3}H-NE is reduced by 26%, but the excretion of ^{3}H-methoxy-4-hydroxymandelic acid (VMA), the acidic end-metabolite of 3,4-dihydroxymandelicaldehyde (DHMAL), is reduced by 75%, or 3-fold more. This disparity is not surprising, given that the pathway for the formation of VMA involves both of the enzymes inhibited by DSSD whereas only DBH participates in the synthesis of NE. Because of the inhibition of ALDH, more of the ^{3}H-DHMAL that is formed is reduced to ^{3}H-methoxy-4-hydroxyphenylglycol (MHPG), and, as a result, the net excretion of this metabolite is increased by 20%.

Because of the DSSD-induced inhibition of DBH, the fraction of the administered ^{3}H-DA that is metabolized to DOPAL via monoamineoxidase (MAO) is increased and accordingly, in spite of the inhibition of ALDH, the excretion of VMA, the acidic end-metabolite of DOPAL, is not significantly altered. At the same time, however, a 12-fold increase in the excretion of ^{3}H-DOPET indicates how much larger a proportion of the DOPAL is metabolized via the reductive pathway in

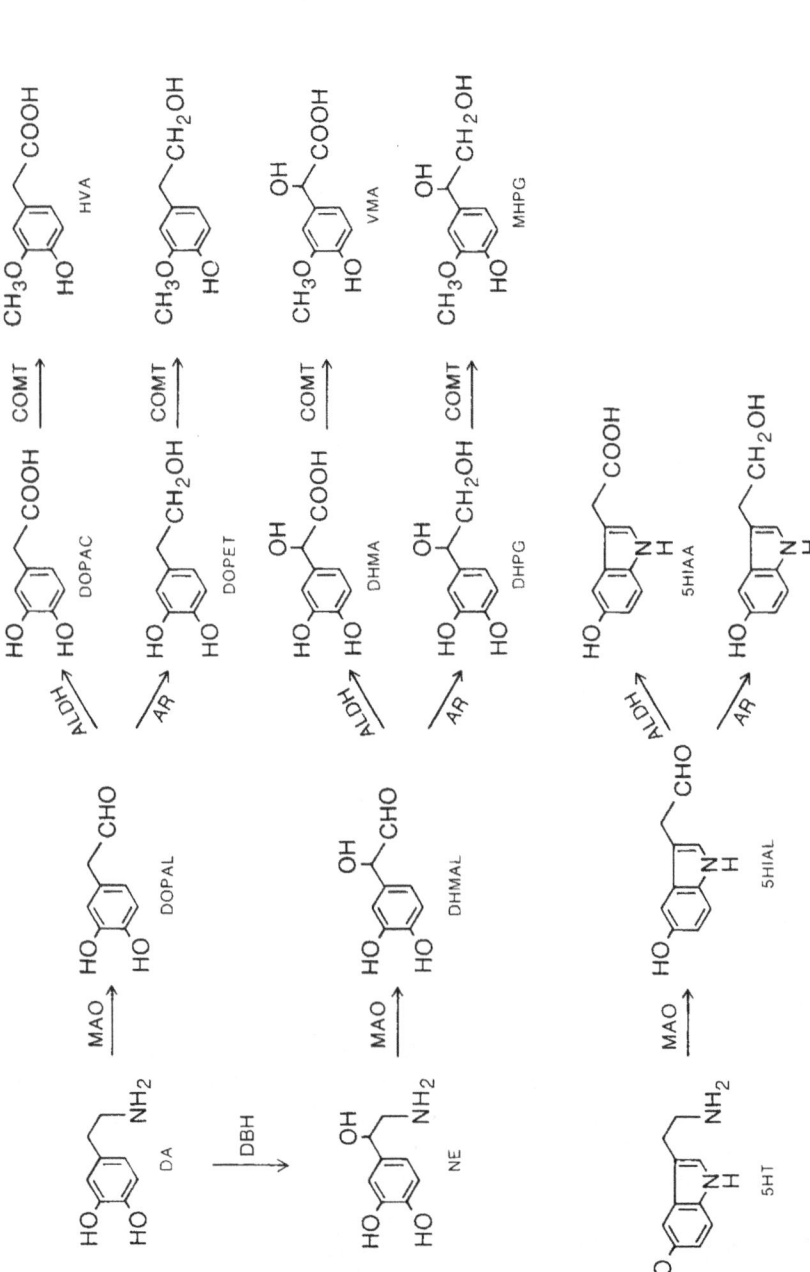

Figure 9.5 Pathways of catecholamine metabolism, i.e. dopamine (DA) and norepinephrine (NE), at top. Pathways of 5-hydroxytryptamine (5HT) metabolism, at bottom. Other entities are represented as follows: dihydroxyphenylacetaldehyde (DOPAL); dihydroxyphenylacetic acid (DOPAC); 3-methoxy-4-hydroxyphenylacetic acid (HVA); dihydroxyphenylethanol (DOPET); dihydroxymandelaldehyde (DHMAL); dihydroxymandelic acid (DHMA); 3-methoxy-4-hydroxymandelic acid (VMA); dihydroxyphenylglycol (DHPG); methoxyhydroxyphenylglycol (MHPG); 5-hydroxyindolealdehyde (5HIAL); 5-hydroxyindoleacetic acid (5HIAA); 5-hydroxytryptophol (5HTOL). The enzymes are represented as: dopamine β-hydroxylase (DBH); monoamineoxidase (MAO); aldehyde dehydrogenase (ALDH); aldehyde reductase (AR); catechol O-methyltransferase (COMT).

the DSSD-pretreated individual. These results dovetail with those obtained at an earlier date by Major *et al.* (1977b), who found that DSSD therapy actually reduced the levels of HVA in cerebrospinal fluid.

Inhibition of ALDH would be expected to also decrease the formation of 5-hydroxyindoleacetic acid (5-HIAA) from 5-HIAL, itself the product of the oxidation of 5-HT by the action of MAO (Fig. 9.5). The matter is complicated, however, by the fact that the serotonergic system exhibits a reciprocity to the norepinephrinergic one so that depletion of NE levels leads to the elevation of 5-HT ones and *vice versa*. Because of the decrease in NE levels brought about by DSSD, this could lead to increases in 5-HIAA levels. Indeed, under some dosing circumstances, DSSD administration to experimental animals leads to significant increases in 5-HIAA levels (Johnson *et al.*, 1972; Minegishi *et al.*, 1979), as well as those of 5-HT itself (Fukumori *et al.*, 1979; Marchand *et al.*, 1990). Clinically, however, DSSD therapy has not been found to lead to an elevation of 5-HIAA cerebrospinal fluid levels (Major *et al.*, 1977b).

There exists an alternate pathway for the metabolism of 5-HIAL, namely its reduction to 5-hydroxytryptophol (5-HTOL). Both the increased formation of 5-HT and the inhibition of the oxidation of 5-HIAL would be expected to increase the levels of 5-HIAL and 5-HTOL. Beck *et al.* (1986) have in fact found that in rats receiving a diet containing 2 g DSSD per kg of diet for 7 days, 5-HTOL levels (free and conjugated) are significantly elevated (1.6- and 2.1-fold, respectively) in the two brain regions examined (diencephalon and pons medulla). Minigishi *et al.* (1979) have suggested that an increase in 5-HIAL is responsible for the depressive properties of DSSD and its ability to prolong the duration of hexobarbital-induced anesthesia. The latter postulate has been challenged, however, on the basis that DSSD pretreatment does not increase the sensitivity of rat brain to hexobarbital (Nilsson *et al.*, 1987, Nilsson and Whalström, 1989).

9.6.2 Substrates of specific aldehyde dehydrogenases

DSSD, besides inhibiting *in vitro* Class 1 ALDHs, has been found to inhibit a number of purified so-called specific ALDHs which, though possessing low affinity for acetaldehyde, have high affinities for specific products of intermediary metabolism. Among these are the glyceraldehyde-3-phosphate (G3P) dehydrogenase isozymes and the succinic semialdehyde (SSA) dehydrogenase of human brain (Table 9.3). Although DSSD is a potent inhibitor of rat brain SSA dehydrogenase *in vitro*, the enzyme is not inhibited *in vivo* 2 and 24 h after administration of a 150 mg/kg dose of DSSD (Hellström and Tottmar, 1982b). Another specific ALDH that is inhibited by DSSD is glutamic γ-semialdehyde dehydrogenase, or more exactly, 1-pyrroline-5-carboxylate (P5C) dehydrogenase which has been purified from human placenta (Farrés *et al.*, 1988). It has properties which are practically identical to those of the P5C dehydrogenase (the 'E$_4$ ALDH') purified from human liver (Forte-McRobbie and Pietruszko, 1986).

Given the low affinity of these dehydrogenases for acetaldehyde, their inhibition would be without consequence on the *in vivo* metabolism of acetaldehyde. However, their *in vivo* inhibition could have consequence on the relevant pathway of intermediary metabolism.

The inhibition of the G3P and SSA dehydrogenases is reversed by 2-mercaptoethanol. For the E8.5 and E9.0 isozymes of G3P dehydrogenase, the inhibition is also reversed by 33 μM cysteine and GSH (Table 9.3). Considering that intracellular GSH concentrations can be in the millimolar range (0.5–10 mM, see Meister and Anderson, 1983) the inhibition of these latter two isozymes might also be reversible *in vivo*.

Aldehydes formed in the oxidative deamination of monoaminergic neurotransmitters constitute an important category of neural tissue aldehyde substrates. A substantial body of data has accumulated which documents the inhibitory effects of DSSD administration on the metabolism of these aldehydes *in vivo* (for review see Weiner and Ardelt, 1984). Purification of the various ALDHs has permitted *in vitro* investigation of their affinity for these substrates. Both DOPAL and 5-HIAL, the aldehydes derived from dopamine (or norepinephrine) and serotonin, respectively, have affinities as high or higher than for acetaldehyde for hepatic E$_1$ and E$_2$ (MacKerell *et al.*, 1986) and brain E2(a) and E2(b) enzymes (Ryzlak and Pietruszko, 1989). On the other hand, both G3P dehydrogenase and SSA dehydrogenase are inactive towards DOPAL (Ryzlak and Pietruszko, 1989). Also, when mixtures of acetaldehyde and DOPAL or 5-HIAL are incubated with E$_2$, and to a lesser extent with E$_1$, the rate of oxidation of the monoamine-derived aldehydes is much inhibited (MacKerell *et al.*, 1986). These findings have led Ryzlak and Pietruszko (1989) to suggest that the aldehydes derived from biogenic amines may be the physiological substrates for the non-specific ALDHs.

Acetaldehyde itself can also be considered an endogenous substrate in that microbial fermentation in the gastrointestinal tract does result in the formation of some ethanol which is absorbed and metabolized in the liver. However, even after 7 days of DSSD feeding, rat blood levels of acetaldehyde remain below the detection limit, if the assay method used involves first precipitation and removal of the blood proteins. If instead the blood is simply hemolyzed prior to head space chromatography, feeding DSSD does result in a significant elevation in some protein-bound form of acetaldehyde that is liberated by the heating that the assay involves (Eriksson, 1985).

9.7 ALDEHYDE AND XANTHINE OXIDASES

Aldehyde oxidase (EC 1.2.3.2) a molybdenum-containing cytosolic metalloflavoprotein (for review see Beedham, 1987), is strikingly similar to xanthine oxidase. It catalyzes the hydroxylation of many xenobiotics, the oxygen atom incorporated in the substrate being derived from water, rather than from molecular oxygen as is the case with the P-450 monooxygenases. As its name implies, *in vitro* it also oxidizes aliphatic aldehydes, including acetaldehyde (Jones, D.G., 1967). Its affinity for acetaldehyde is, however, quite low as evidenced by a K_m for this substrate of 100 mM (Palmer, 1962). Xanthine oxidase, which also can oxidize acetaldehyde *in vitro*, has a similar K_m for it. An early report that aldehyde oxidase is inhibited *in vitro* by DSSD (Kjeldgaard, 1949) involved a misappellation (Graham, 1951). In any event, because of their low affinity for acetaldehyde, these enzymes would be expected to have no role in its *in vivo* disposition.

10

The disulfiram–ethanol reaction

10.1 INTRODUCTION 167
10.2 DISCOVERY AND THERAPEUTIC APPLICATION 168
10.3 PHARMACOLOGICAL CHARACTERISTICS 171
    10.3.1 General phenomenology 171
    10.3.2 Respiratory effects 172
    10.3.3 Effects on cardiovascular function 172
    10.3.4 Electrocardiographic changes during the reaction 174
    10.3.5 High dose adverse effects: cardiovascular collapse 175
10.4 BLOOD ACETALDEHYDE DETERMINATION 177
10.5 THE ACETALDEHYDE HYPOTHESIS 178
    10.5.1 Critical evaluation of the acetaldehyde hypothesis 178
    10.5.2 Summary 184
10.6 QUEST FOR ANIMAL MODELS OF THE REACTION 184
    10.6.1 The hypothermic effect of the combination in the rat 188
    10.6.2 Effects of disulfiram on the cardiovascular actions of ethanol
           in the rat 189
10.7 EFFECT OF DISULFIRAM ON ETHANOL METABOLISM 191
10.8 THE DOPAMINE β-HYDROXYLASE HYPOTHESIS 193
    10.8.1 Effects of disulfiram on the cardiovascular actions of
           acetaldehyde 194
    10.8.2 Restatement of the dopamine β-hydroxylase hypothesis . . . 197
    10.8.3 Clinical relevance of the dopamine β-hydroxylase hypothesis 198
    10.8.4 Summary 199
10.9 EFFECT OF ETHANOL IN ANIMALS PRETREATED WITH
    DISULFIRAM METABOLITES 199
10.10 TREATMENT OF THE REACTION 201

10.1 INTRODUCTION

The disulfiram–ethanol reaction (DER) is the name given to a syndrome experienced by individuals who, following treatment with disulfiram (DSSD), ingest ethanol. The DER is decidedly unpleasant. Accordingly, ever since the discovery of this syndrome, efforts have been made to utilize DSSD in aversive therapies of alcoholism, though the early therapeutic strategies employed differed markedly from the current ones (section 10.2). Partly as a result of this, a great deal has been learned regarding the pharmacological phenomena and toxicities characteristic of the human DER (section 10.3).

From the earliest times, it has been evident that acetaldehyde accumulation plays some role in the phenomenology of the syndrome. The inadequacy of the original assay methods for acetaldehyde (section 10.4) impeded, until recently, evaluation of the 'acetaldehyde hypothesis' that the DER is primarily due to an impairment of aldehyde metabolism (section 10.5) secondary to an inhibition of aldehyde dehydrogenase (Chapter 9).

Obtaining information relevant to the human DER from animal studies is problematic because ethanol administration following DSSD pretreatment does not cause, in the species most often employed, a syndrome fully parallel to the DER and the dose that is required to elicit pharmacological effects is rather large (section 10.6). In recognition of this, the term DER is used in this monograph (though not in the literature) solely with reference to the syndrome observed in humans. One complicating factor in studies of the DER is that pretreatment with DSSD lowers the rate of disposition of subsequently administered ethanol, a phenomenon which is mediated by the increased acetaldehyde levels (section 10.7)

The acetaldehyde hypothesis cannot, by itself, account for the fall in systolic blood pressure seen during the DER. It can account for that fall, however, if it is coupled to the dopamine β-hydroxylase hypothesis (section 10.8). The latter was developed when it was found that DSSD administration can result in inhibition of dopamine β-hydroxylase (section 8.2). Studies of the cardiovascular actions of acetaldehyde in animals and of the effect of DSSD pretreatment on sympathetic function and catecholamine metabolism support the latter hypothesis (section 10.8).

Finally, because the DER is a potentially serious medical condition, methods that can be used for controlling or counteracting it are discussed (section 10.9).

10.2 DISCOVERY AND THERAPEUTIC APPLICATION

The occurrence of a toxic interaction between a tetraalkylthiuram disulfide and ethanol was first reported by Williams (1937). He noted that consumption of as little as 6 oz of beer caused, among workers exposed to tetramethylthiuram di- and monosulfide, flushing of the face and hands, a rapid pulse, palpitations, and a fall in blood pressure. The consequent total abstinence practiced by these workers led Williams to suggest that the substance might be effective in the treatment of alcoholism.

In 1945 in Copenhagen, Jacobsen and Hald, while investigating the potential of DSSD (tetraethylthiuram disulfide) as a vermicidal agent, each ingested several tablets of the agent and, neither a teetotaler, soon discovered to their surprise, the DER (Jacobsen, 1987; Appendix A). Following further exploration, the Danish investigators published their findings, namely that, in individuals treated with this agent, ingestion of ethanol caused a 'formidable' reaction (Hald and Jacobsen, 1948a; Hald *et al.*, 1948). Moreover, the reaction, though evidently unpleasant, seemed innocuous. Mindful of the potential usefulness of such an agent in the treatment of alcoholism, these workers undertook a series of studies that characterized the reaction. They concluded, initially on the basis of Hald's olfactory perception upon entering a room where Jacobsen was experiencing a DER (Jacobsen, 1987; Appendix A), that the reaction was caused by an *in vivo* accumulation of acetaldehyde formed during ethanol metabolism and that this was mediated by an inhibition of its enzymatic oxidation (Hald and Jacobsen, 1948a, b; Hald *et al.*, 1948, 1949a,b; Asmussen *et al.*, 1948a; Larsen, 1948; Jacobsen, E. and Martensen-Larsen, 1949; Jacobsen, E. and Larsen, 1949; Hald and Larsen, 1949).

The treatment paradigm introduced by the Danish group was based on the concept of aversion conditioning. The physician was to instruct the patient to drink alcohol while on DSSD; the resulting DER experience was expected to induce in the patient an aversion to alcoholic beverages. The occurrence of violent DER episodes thus occasioned was viewed as therapeutically beneficial (Martensen-Larsen, 1948). Soon, reports of the severity of DER reactions in some individuals led to the recommendation that patients with myocardial disease, cirrhosis of the liver, nephritis, epilepsy and assorted other conditions be excluded from DSSD therapy (Glud, 1949). Later, the treatment paradigm itself was amended: the DER was to be induced only during 'conditioning' or 'experience sessions', with a physician and nurse in attendance and equipment for emergency treatment and putative antidotes available. Also, the patient was to be kept under close observation for the subsequent 24 h (Brown and Knoblock, 1951; Shaw, 1951). Nonetheless, instances continued to be reported of DERs even more 'formidable' than the original authors had observed (Ferguson, 1949). Severe impairment of cardiovascular function lasting several hours, episodes of apnea (Bell and Smith, 1949), syncope and coma

(Hine *et al.*, 1950; Child *et al.*, 1951), convulsions (Shaw, 1951) and instances of a fatal outcome (Jones, R.O., 1949; Steckler and Harris, 1951; Shaw, 1951) were reported.

By 1952, the accumulation of reports of severe or fatal DERs led to a revision of the 1948 view that the reaction was 'unpleasant but innocuous' (Jacobsen, E., 1952). As a result, therapeutic emphasis shifted from use of DSSD to induce aversive conditioning to its use primarily as a 'sobering crutch.' Based on the premise that 'the effectiveness of disulfiram as deterrent to drinking lies in creating fear of a reaction, not in the development of actual aversion to alcoholic beverages', the dose was to be adjusted to 'the smallest amount which will cause a slight flushing, slight increase of pulse rate', and 'a mild dyspnea of 15–20 minutes duration following ingestion of a single trial dose of alcohol' (Council on Pharmacy and Chemistry, 1952).

A chance discovery (Jacobsen 1987; Appendix A) led to production of microcrystalline disulfiram (Hald *et al.*, 1953) which proved to be much more effective; a 250 mg maintenance dose proved fully adequate (Martensen-Larsen, 1950). An effervescent formulation of DSSD (Dumex dispargettes®) which includes a wetting agent was introduced in Denmark in 1959 (E. Petersen, private communication) but remain unavailable in Australia, the United Kingdom and the United States (section 1.1). The bioavailability of the effervescent formulation has been found to be almost 3-fold greater than that of the non-effervescent tablets available in the United Kingdom (Andersen, 1991). *Prima faciae* this is likely to be also true of the non-effervescent tablets marketed in the U.S. and Australia.

In the United States, doses have been reduced to 0.25–0.5 g daily (Armstrong, 1957). A survey of the literature in 1972 by Rothstein failed to uncover any reports of subsequent deaths occasioned by the DER. Moreover, Rothstein (1972a) related that Ayerst, the then U.S. manufacturer of DSSD (currently Wyeth-Ayerst), also did not know of any deaths attributable to this reaction. The American Medical Association treatment paradigm described above (Council on Pharmacy and Chemistry, 1952) has endured to the present. The test elicitation of the DER has been very largely, though not entirely (Sauter *et al.*, 1977), abandoned except in the research setting (Brewer, 1984; Beyeler *et al.*, 1985, 1987; Christensen *et al.*, 1991; Johansson *et al.*, 1991). A challenge with ethanol doses small enough to occasion only a mild DER has been advanced by Brewer (1984) as a method of ensuring that the DSSD dose prescribed is a pharmacologically effective one.

10.3 PHARMACOLOGICAL CHARACTERISTICS

10.3.1 General phenomenology

The clinical phenomenology of the DER has been the subject of only a handful of studies since the reports of the Danish group in 1948–49 (Hald and Jacobsen, 1948a,b; Jacobsen, E. and Martensen-Larsen, 1949). The initial reports focused, to a large degree, on subjective and cutaneous phenomena. The earliest manifestations of the DER to be noted were a facial flush accompanied by a sensation of heat, a rise in skin temperature, conjunctival injection, and a scarlet visage (Hald *et al.*, 1948). Administration of as little as 16 g of ethanol 36 h following

Table 10.1 Onset time and incidence of signs and symptoms of the disulfiram–ethanol reaction

	Hine et al. (1952)		Raby (1953a)		Marconi et al. (1961) Incidence (%)	
	Onset (min)	Incidence (%)	Onset (min)	Incidence (%)	DSSD	Placebo
Sensation of heat	5 ± 2	90			52	30
Acetaldehyde odor	12 ± 7	60	5 ± 5	100		
Face flushing	7 ± 4	94	8 ± 5	100		
Conjunctival injection	10 ± 4	89			61	17
Palpitations	13 ± 6	55			65	13
Throbbing	14 ± 7	31				
Cough			21 ± 20	21		
Dyspnea	12 ± 6	53	24 ± 28	26	65	22
Universal flush			27 ± 13	39	96	43
Headache			35 ± 34	34	48	30
Sleepiness	32 ± 17	56	41 ± 21	21	26	13
Abdominal pain			42 ± 29	10		
Hyperaesthesia			42 ± 25	39		
Pallor			68 ± 28	74		
Profuse perspiration			70 ± 40	15		
Malaise	32 ± 17	33	76 ± 60	49		
Nausea			76 ± 64	51		
Paraesthesia			92 ± 108	15	4	9
Twitches			108 ± 72	15		
Sleep			125 ± 79	46		
Vomiting			121 ± 73	44		
Vomit and blood			283 ± 144	10		

Dosing information: the number of subjects (*n*), the dose of disulfiram (DSSD) and the challenge dose of ethanol (EtOH) were as follows. Hine *et al.* (1952): *n*, 44; DSSD, 1 g on days 1 and 2, 0.75 g on days 3 and 4, 0.5 g on day 5; EtOH, 0.5 g/kg. Raby (1953): *n*, 37; DSSD, 0.5–7 g over 3 days (mean 2.55 g); EtOH, variable, but generally 50 ml. Marconi *et al.* (1961): *n*, 23; DSSD, 0.5 g/day; EtOH, 0.25–0.5 g/kg.

pretreatment with 1.5 g of DSSD was found to elevate facial skin temperature by 4–5°C for 90 min or more (Hald and Jacobsen, 1948a,b; Hald
et al., 1948). A smell of acetaldehyde on the breath, palpitations, and a
throbbing sensation in the neck and head area (the latter frequently
developing into a headache) were the other early manifestations noted.
Other symptoms, including hyperesthesia, paresthesia, nausea and
vomiting sometimes followed. An ordering of these phenomena was
first attempted by Bowman *et al.* (1951) and Child *et al.* (1951), but
the most detailed tabulation is to be found in the studies of Hine *et al.*
(1952) and Raby (1953a). The percentage incidence and mean onset
times calculated from the latter tabulations are presented in Table 10.1.
Expectancy can play a substantial role in eliciting some of these
symptoms, since knowledge of the DER has become common among
the lay population. The magnitude of the expectancy effect was
explored by Marconi *et al.* (1961) who, having led all their subjects to
believe they had been pretreated with DSSD (half had in fact received
placebo), noted the relative frequency with which effects previously
associated with the DER followed the consumption of ethanol by
DSSD-pretreated and DSSD-naive subjects (Table 10.1).

10.3.2 Respiratory effects

A particularly dramatic symptom of the DER, and one singularly
distressing to patients, is dyspnea (Hald and Jacobsen, 1948b). It is
frequently preceded by a dry, loud, barking cough (Raby, 1953a). As
observed by Asmussen *et al.* (1948a), however, ventilation is in fact
increased. These workers found that, 30 min after administration of
ethanol to DSSD-pretreated individuals, the minute volume increased
by 41%, the arteriovenous oxygen difference decreased 23%, and the
alveolar pCO_2 fell by 18%. Both Raby (1954b) and Sauter *et al.* (1977)
confirmed that a rise in ventilation is characteristic of the DER (Table
10.2) and that it is accompanied by a significant fall in blood pCO_2 (23%
at 30 min: Sauter *et al.*, 1977), a rise in blood pO_2 (23% at 20 min:
Sauter *et al.*, 1977), and a fall in blood pH (arterial to 7.51 ± 0.04: Raby,
1954c; central venous to 7.46 at 20 min: Sauter *et al.*, 1977).

10.3.3 Effects on cardiovascular function

Initially, little importance was attached to the cardiovascular changes
associated with the DER. In the early publications by the Copenhagen
group, 'moderate amounts' of ethanol (30–60 ml of gin) were described
as eliciting either no, or only a slight and non-significant change in

Table 10.2 Effects of the disulfiram–ethanol reaction on cardiovascular function and ventilation

Study	Heart rate increase Maximum effect		Ventilation increase Maximum effect		Fall in diastolic b.p. Maximum effect		Fall in systolic b.p. Maximum effect	
	Time (min)	Magnitude (beats/min)	Time (min)	Magnitude (%)	Time (min)	Magnitude (mmHg)	Time (min)	Magnitude (mmHg)
Hine et al. (1952)	20	26			30	23	30	20
Raby (1953a, 1954b)	25 ± 13	37 ± 20	33 ± 18	55 ± 25	39 ± 22	61 ± 29	64 ± 29	43 ± 31
Sauter et al. (1977)	20	41	20	169	30	34	65	21
Beyeler et al. (1987)	25	42			30	41 ± 18	45	46 ± 32

For dosing information see Tables 10.1 and 10.4.

blood pressure (Hald *et al.*, 1948; Hald and Jacobsen, 1948b). It was noted, however, that 30–60 min after larger quantities of ethanol (40–50 g or more) a 'considerable fall in blood pressure can be seen, e.g., to 65 mm Hg systolic, while the diastolic pressure may fall to zero' (Hald *et al.*, 1948). With the surfacing of the impairment of cardiovascular function as a major contributory factor of severe, life-threatening and fatal DER episodes, the cardiovascular effects of the DER became the subject of both clinical and laboratory studies. Earlier, Asmussen *et al.* (1948a) had suggested that the DER-induced cutaneous vasodilation is a manifestation of a more general vasodilation. They speculated that it, in turn, could be the cause of the 48% increase in cardiac output they observed in subjects experiencing the DER. However, having failed to note any effects on blood pressure, they concluded the increase in cardiac output could be easily explained by the concomitant hyperventilation. Subsequent clinical investigations have documented marked decreases in both systolic and diastolic pressure during the DER. The magnitude and peak times of these changes, as obtained from tables or graphs of published data, are presented in Table 10.2; their course has been reported by Beyeler *et al.* (1985, 1987). In a fraction of the patients experiencing the DER, the blood pressure changes are dramatic; thus, Hine *et al.* (1952) reported pressures of 80/40 mm Hg or less in 6 of 31 patients. Raby (1953a) noted a lowering of systolic pressure by 70 mm Hg or more in 7 of 37 patients and Beyeler *et al.* (1987) observed systolic pressure to fall to 70 mm Hg or less in 4 of 16 patients. From the analysis by Beyeler *et al.* (1987) it appears that the blood pressure fall is due, proximally, to a severe reduction in peripheral vascular resistance (to a median of 46% of control) which is only partially compensated by an increase in cardiac output (average increase 1.6-fold; range 1.0- to 2.4-fold; $n = 11$).

10.3.4 Electrocardiographic changes during the reaction

A flattening of the T wave is one of the manifestations of the DER. Child *et al.* (1951) reported it to occur in 78% of 80 DSSD-pretreated patients administered just 8 ml of ethanol (a tachycardia was observed in 80% of this group). Raby (1953b) observed a flattening of the T wave in 95% of 37 subjects experiencing a DER; in 50% of them a depression of the S–T segment was also seen. On average, these changes became maximal 45 min after ethanol administration and their median duration was 113 min. Raby (1952) also observed a fall in arterial blood potassium (mean 3.0 mg%, $n = 10$). He noted that the electrocardiographic changes and the fall in blood potassium appeared to be correlated to each other and to the intensity of the DER. Levy *et al.* (1967) also noted an association between abnormal electrocardiograms and hypotensive episodes during the DER, while Sauter *et al.* (1977) found that a fall in plasma potassium is one of the longer lasting events associated with the DER. Low potassium levels are known to depress the T wave, to decrease cardiac conduction and, thereby, also contractility.

10.3.5 High dose adverse effects: cardiovascular collapse

The possibility that the DER might occasion cardiovascular collapse elicits considerable concern, particularly so because in the early days of DSSD therapy a number of fatalities were associated with it. From the case reports of Jones, R.O. (1949), Shaw (1951), Steckler and Harris (1951), and Becker and Sugarman (1952) it is evident that deaths subsequent to the cardiovascular collapse occurred in individuals receiving doses of DSSD in excess of 1 g/day and that they occurred with some delay (Table 10.3). Typically death was characterized by apnea which occurred while the patient was asleep. Additionally, the cardiovascular collapse was often preceded by vomiting or clinically significant nausea. Lowering of the dose of DSSD, first to 0.5 and later to 0.25 g/day, appear to have led to a reduction in the incidence of DERs complicated by cardiovascular collapse; there have been no further reports of fatal outcome associated with this complication (Rothstein, 1972a). Nonetheless, because of the concern raised by the possibility of the occurrence of such phenomena, their insidious course, and the continued absence of an animal model, these four prototypical case reports are summarized below.

Table 10.3 Fatal cardiovascular collapse consequent upon the disulfiram–ethanol reaction

| | Dose | | |
| | Disulfiram | Ethanol[a] | Time of |
Report	(g)	(g)	death
Jones (1949)	5.25 in 5 days	12	155 min
Shaw (1951)	5.25 in 4 days	12	260 min
Steckler and Harris (1951)	4.5 in 3 days	6	36 h
Becker and Sugarman (1952)	5.0 in 3 days	12	270 min

[a] Approximate, see text.

Jones, R.O. (1949) reported on a 29-year-old male administered 5.25 g of DSSD over 5 days who was then challenged with 1 oz of rum. He had an intense reaction. About 70–80 min following ingestion of the rum, he vomited. After this he felt better, and by 135 min had fallen asleep. Ten minutes later the patient had stopped breathing, was pulseless, cyanotic and could not be revived.

Shaw (1951) reported on a 48-year-old male administered 5.25 g of DSSD over 4 days and challenged with 1 oz of whiskey. Twenty minutes later his blood pressure dropped to 60/40 and his pulse, which had risen to 140, fell to 60. Emergency measures restored his blood pressure to normal and there was no evidence of his being in danger. Two hours later he went into shock, however, and could not be revived.

Steckler and Harris (1951) reported on a 49-year-old female dosed with 1.5 g of DSSD per day for 3 days and then given 45 ml of wine. Shortly thereafter, the patient felt nauseous and her blood pressure fell to 40/0. The patient recovered and slept. Next morning she felt nauseous, was given atropine, and felt better. While asleep the following night she was found to be apneic and pulseless.

Becker and Sugarman (1952) reported on a 49-year-old male patient given 5 g of DSSD over 3 days and challenged with 1 oz of whiskey. Fifteen minutes later the patient felt nauseous. This was followed 5 min later by pallor and then by a drop in blood pressure to 86/50. Following emergency measures, the patient's blood pressure recovered and the patient fell asleep. Four and a half hours after the initiation of the DER the patient turned on his back, became pale and dyspneic and ceased breathing.

The effect of DER on blood pressure in patients who received 4 g of DSSD over a 5-day period (1 g on days 1 and 2, 0.75 g on days 3 and 4, 0.5 g on day 5) was investigated by Hine *et al.* (1952). They reported that blood pressure dropped to shock levels (80/40) in 6 of 31 patients challenged with the equivalent of 16 g ethanol/70 kg, but in none of the 20 patients challenged with half that dose. They also noted that five of the patients receiving the higher dose, but none of those receiving the lower dose, vomited. No information is available, however, as to whether there was any correlation between vomiting, or nausea, and the fall of blood pressure to shock level. However, Peachey *et al.* (1981a), while investigating the analogous calcium carbimide–ethanol reaction, noted a correspondence between the occurrence of cardiovascular collapse and preceding vomiting or nausea. They have suggested that the precipitating factor in the development of the collapse is an enhanced vagal tone induced by a vomiting- or nausea-precipitated reflex. Their reversal of the collapse in one individual by intravenous administration of atropine, confirms previous statements regarding the effect of atropine in reversing severe hypotensive episodes during the DER, and lends support to the proposed mechanism.

If nausea or vomiting occur in individuals given high doses of DSSD, they tend to do so early in the course of the DER. When associated with such gastrointestinal symptomatology, precipitous falls in blood pressure appear to predispose the patient to later potentially fatal events even if, in the interim, blood pressure is restored to normal values. (See sections 10.5.1 and 10.9 for a discussion of the antidotal use of 4-methylpyrazole in the treatment of the DER.)

10.4 BLOOD ACETALDEHYDE DETERMINATION

The acetaldehyde assay methods available to the early investigators of the DER were rather non-specific. Although this was apparent to some of the investigators concerned (Hald and Jacobsen, 1948a), it nonetheless led to the perception that acetaldehyde was a normal and not insignificant component of human blood.

Application of a head-space gas-chromatographic (GLC) method (Duritz and Truitt, 1964) to the assay resolved the problem of non-specificity, but led to the unmasking of another and more intractable problem: the non-enzymatic formation of acetaldehyde from ethanol by blood *in vitro* (Truitt, 1970; Eriksson *et al.*, 1977). As methodologies for the measurement of acetaldehyde have improved, however, the acetaldehyde levels reported as present in blood following ethanol ingestion by non-Orientals have continued to decline (Eriksson *et al.*, 1982; Eriksson, 1983; Suokas *et al.*, 1985; Adachi *et al.*, 1990). Investigators using the GLC method (Peachey *et al.*, 1983; Beyeler *et al.*, 1985, 1987), while confirming that ethanol ingestion leads to the appearance of significant blood acetaldehyde levels in individuals pretreated with DSSD, found that in controls ethanol ingestion fails to raise blood acetaldehyde above the limit of detection of the method (*ca* 1 µM). Similar results are obtained in rats (Eriksson, 1985). Using a new high-pressure liquid-chromatographic (HPLC) method for acetaldehyde (Peterson and Polizzi, 1987) sensitive in the picamole range, Peterson *et al.* (1988) have reported that, following ingestion by human volunteers of a 0.3 g/kg dose of ethanol, the mean peak plasma acetaldehyde level is 31 nmol/g protein (*ca* 2.7 µM). It remains to be seen whether this is confirmed by others, but even this level is smaller by one to two orders of magnitude than those reported (section 10.5.1) for control subjects by the early investigators of the DER reaction who used non-chromatographic methods (Hald and Jacobsen, 1948a; Hine *et al.*, 1952; Raby, 1954a; Sauter *et al.* 1977).

10.5 THE ACETALDEHYDE HYPOTHESIS

The hypothesis that the DER is a manifestation of acetaldehyde toxicity resulting from its accumulation as a consequence of the DSSD-induced inhibition of its oxidation, originated with the Copenhagen Group (Hald and Jacobsen, 1948a, b; Hald *et al.*, 1949b). The hypothesis was based on their observations (a) that the excretion of acetaldehyde in breath during the DER could be demonstrated by trapping it in a sodium bisulfite solution and isolation of its 2,4-dinitrophenylhydrazone, (b) that the occurrence of the DER was temporally correlated with high blood acetaldehyde, (c) that intravenous infusion of acetaldehyde to human volunteers replicates many of the symptoms of the DER, namely: tachycardia, increased respiratory minute volume, lowered alveolar $p\,CO_2$ and facial vasodilation (Asmussen *et al.*, 1948b), and (d) that DSSD pretreatment inhibited acetaldehyde metabolism (Hald *et al.*, 1949b; Kjeldgaard, 1949). Basically, this hypothesis has stood the test of time, although in the interim it was buffeted by apparent inconsistencies.

At the time the acetaldehyde hypothesis was formulated, the nature and significance of the effects of the DER on cardiovascular function and blood pressure were not appreciated. Accordingly when Asmussen *et al.* (1948b) studied the effects of acetaldehyde infusion in humans, relatively little attention was paid to its cardiovascular effects, other than to note the marked vasodilation of the face and the increase in pulse rate induced by the infusion. The severe muscular pains of the arm and shoulder that accompany acetaldehyde infusion (Asmussen *et al.*, 1948b) prevented later investigators from extending these clinical studies (Raby, 1955 cited by Perman, 1962a). Subsequently, when the clinical nature and importance of the cardiovascular concomitants of the DER became evident, investigation of whether these effects could be encompassed by the acetaldehyde hypothesis was hindered by the absence of an animal model in which the DER would elicit the cardiovascular changes seen clinically. Accordingly, the question of whether the acetaldehyde hypothesis can explain the cardiovascular concomitants of the DER has mostly lain dormant. As will be described in this chapter, it is now evident that, to a large extent, it can.

10.5.1 Critical evaluation of the acetaldehyde hypothesis

The strength of correlation between the elevation in blood acetaldehyde levels and the intensity of the DER constitutes the first criterion by which the correctness of the acetaldehyde hypothesis can be judged. The marked variation in the blood acetaldehyde values originally reported as observed during the DER (Table 10.4) rendered the hypothesis difficult to accept. In addition, a number of clinical investigators struggled with the paradox that blood acetaldehyde levels comparable to that seen during the DER could be induced (or so it seemed), without eliciting any DER-like symptoms, by giving sizable doses of ethanol to DSSD-naive individuals (Hine *et al.*, 1952; Raby, 1954a, 1956; Sauter *et al.* 1977). Hine *et al.* (1952), noting the close temporal correspondence between increases in blood acetaldehyde levels during the DER and its acute clinical manifestations, came to support the acetaldehyde hypothesis nonetheless. Others, however, could not reconcile the hypothesis to these paradoxical observations without invoking additional factors. Thus Raby (1956) suggested the presence of acetaldehyde in a 'non-active state,' while Sauter *et al.* (1977) suggested that DSSD, or its metabolites, induced a predisposition to acetaldehyde in the organism.

Based on the current consensus that blood acetaldehyde levels during normal ethanol metabolism are at or below the limit of detection of the earlier analytical methods (section 10.4), the working assumption can be made that in the earlier studies (Hald and Jacobsen, 1948a; Hine *et al.*, 1952; Raby, 1954a; Sauter *et al.*, 1977) the blood acetaldehyde levels reported as observed following administration of ethanol to DSSD-free controls, represent assay blanks. Accordingly, these have been subtracted in Table 10.4 from the levels observed in the DSSD-pretreated subjects. The resulting 'corrected' mean acetaldehyde blood levels associated with the DER fall consistently into a relatively narrow range (2.0–5.1 µg/ml). It is of interest to observe, in this context, that Raby's (1953a) olfactory sense served him better than his assay method, for he noted that, though the administration of a sufficient quantity of ethanol could elevate the 'acetaldehyde' concentration (as per assay) in DSSD-naive subjects to levels comparable to those registered in subjects experiencing the DER, only on the breath of the latter was the odor of acetaldehyde detectable. Finally, a statistically significant correlation between the peak plasma acetaldehyde levels and the maximal drop in diastolic blood pressure ($r = 0.83$) was observed by Beyeler *et al.* (1985). They found the correlation to be particularly high for individuals over 40 years of age ($r = 0.94$).

A second criterion, by which the correctness of the acetaldehyde hypothesis can be judged, is the strength of the temporal correlations between the elevation in blood acetaldehyde levels and the occurrence of DER symptoms and signs. Sauter *et al.* (1977) reported significant correlations between mean blood acetaldehyde levels at nine different

Table 10.4 Blood acetaldehyde levels observed following ethanol administration to individuals pretreated with disulfiram

Study	n^a	Disulfiram Mean dose g	days	Ethanol Dose g	Control µg/ml (µM) mean	Experimental µg/ml (µM) mean	maximum	Corrected µg/ml (µM) mean	maximum	Time of maximum min
Hald and Jacobsen (1948a)	s	1.5	1	32	1.1 (25)	5.3 (120)		4.2 (95)		55
Hine et al. (1952)	31	0.8[b]	5	16[f]	1.9 (43)	4.5 (102)	13.1 (297)	2.6 (59)	11.2 (254)	20
Raby (1954a)	31	0.92[c]	5	40	10.6 (241)	13.6 (309)	25.1[h] (570)	3.0 (68)	14.5[h] (329)	50
Sauter et al. (1977)	16	0.8	3	10.3	2.5 (57)	7.2 (164)	19.9 (452)	4.7 (107)	17.4 (395)	20
Peachey et al. (1983)	6	0.24[d]	2	10.6[g]	—	2.0 (45)		2.0 (45)		30
Beyeler et al. (1985, 1987)	16	0.4[e]	5.3	13.2	—	5.1[i] (116)	8.8 (200)	5.1[i] (116)	8.8 (200)	15–30

[a] n = number of subjects; s = several.
[b] 1 g on days 1 and 2, 0.75 g on days 3 and 4, 0.5 g on day 5.
[c] Range 0.75–7.0 g in 3 days.
[d] 0.35 mg/kg/day; mean weight 68.9 kg.
[e] 0.4 g/day for 3–6 days.
[f] 0.5 ml/kg of 90 proof ethanol, weight unstated, assumed 70 kg.
[g] 0.15 mg/kg; mean weight 68.9 kg.
[h] Patient received 4.5 g disulfiram in 3 days and 60 g ethanol.
[i] Median.

time points and diastolic blood pressure ($r=0.948$), systolic blood pressure ($r=0.618$), pH ($r=0.711$), $p\text{CO}_2$ ($r=0.780$), and plasma potassium ($r=0.744$). Peachey *et al.* (1983), using lower DSSD doses, also reported significant temporal correlations between blood acetaldehyde levels and skin temperature (r range 0.56–0.82), as well as heart rate (r range 0.67–0.94), for each of their six subjects. Four of the subjects also evidenced a significant correlation between blood acetaldehyde and pulse pressure (r range 0.68–0.91). Though Hine *et al.* (1952) did not perform any statistical analysis, they too reported that 'most of the subjective and objective signs and symptoms reach a peak at the same time as the acetaldehyde levels'. Finally, although Beyeler *et al.* (1985, 1987) also did not calculate temporal correlations, their data, as shown in Fig. 10.1a, strongly suggest these are significant.

A third criterion is the degree to which the phenomenology of the DER can be mimicked in DSSD-naive individuals by generating sizable blood acetaldehyde levels. As mentioned before, acetaldehyde infusion has been found not to be a practical way in which this can be investigated. About one quarter to one half of the Oriental populations, however, have a deficiency in E_2, the low-K_m aldehyde dehydrogenase (ALDH) (section 9.1.2). Following ethanol ingestion, such individuals develop significant blood acetaldehyde levels (Mizoi *et al.*, 1979, 1988). This is accompanied by facial flushing, palpitations, dizziness, headache, nausea and vomiting, sleep, tachycardia, and a drop in diastolic blood pressure (Mizoi *et al.*, 1983, 1988). The intensity of the tachycardia is significantly correlated ($r=0.86$) to the acetaldehyde blood levels (Inoue *et al.*, 1985). Reference to Tables 10.1 and 10.2 reveals all of these are phenomena a'so associated with the DER. Mizoi *et al.* (1983, 1988) observed, however, no drop in systolic blood pressure in their subjects, although the DER is associated with a significant drop in systolic blood pressure (Table 10.2, Fig. 10.1). Therefore, the correspondence, though high, is not complete.

A fourth criterion is the degree to which lowering blood acetaldehyde levels during the course of the DER terminates it. Infusion of an inhibitor of alcohol dehydrogenase, 4-methylpyrazole, does lower blood acetaldehyde under these circumstances. To date, no systematic study of the effect of 4-methylpyrazole on the DER has been performed, but a case report has been published of its use in an emergency situation (Lindros *et al.*, 1981). A man was admitted with facial flushing, tachycardia, nausea, vomiting and chest pain. He had been given DSSD surreptitiously by his wife the night before, had since drank two bottles of red wine, and his blood acetaldehyde was 70 µM. Administration of 4-methylpyrazole resulted in an immediate marked

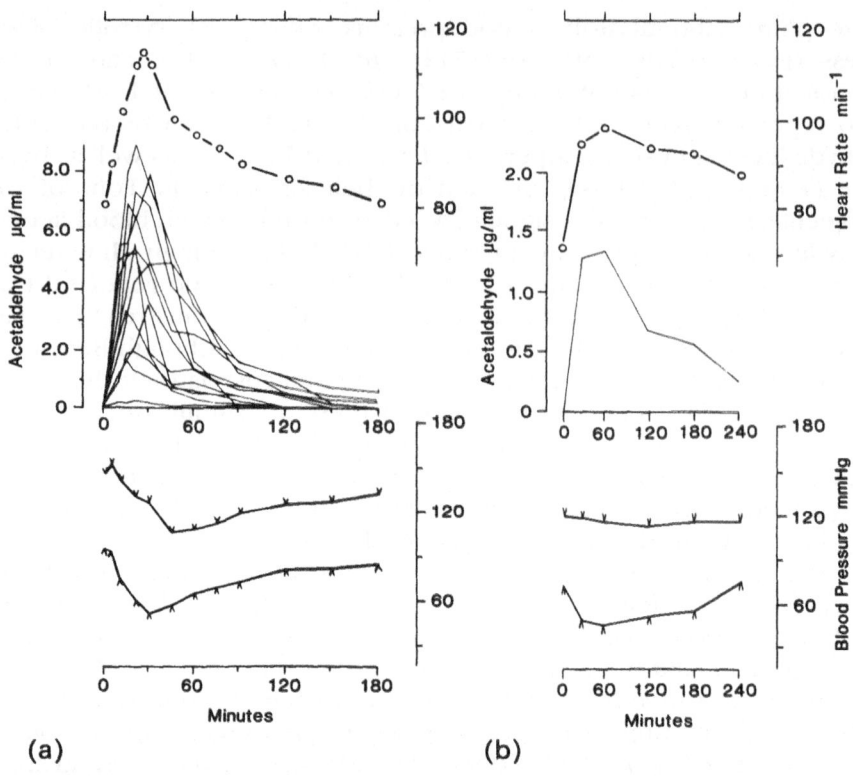

Figure 10.1 (a) Time course relationship of cardiovascular changes and blood acetaldehyde levels during the course of the disulfiram–ethanol reaction. Patients were administered 0.4 g of disulfiram daily for 3–6 days and were challenged with a 13.2 g dose of ethanol at zero time. Composite from Beyeler *et al.* (1985, 1987; with permission). (b) Time course relationship of cardiovascular changes and blood acetaldehyde levels following ingestion of 0.4 g/kg ethanol at zero time by males deficient in E_2, the low-K_m aldehyde dehydrogenase. Composite from Mizoi *et al.* (1988).

reduction in blood acetaldehyde, and in the gradual disappearance of flushing, tachycardia, and electrocardiographic abnormalities (Fig. 10.2).

Moreover, the effects of 4-methylpyrazole administration have been investigated systematically in two studies of the calcium carbimide–ethanol reaction (CCER) as well as in a study of the nitrefazol–ethanol reaction (NER). These reactions are rather analogous to the DER, but differ from it in that the marked fall in systolic blood pressure which is a consistent component of the DER (Fig. 10.1a, Table 10.2), is not usually seen in either the CCER or the NER. In any event, in one of the

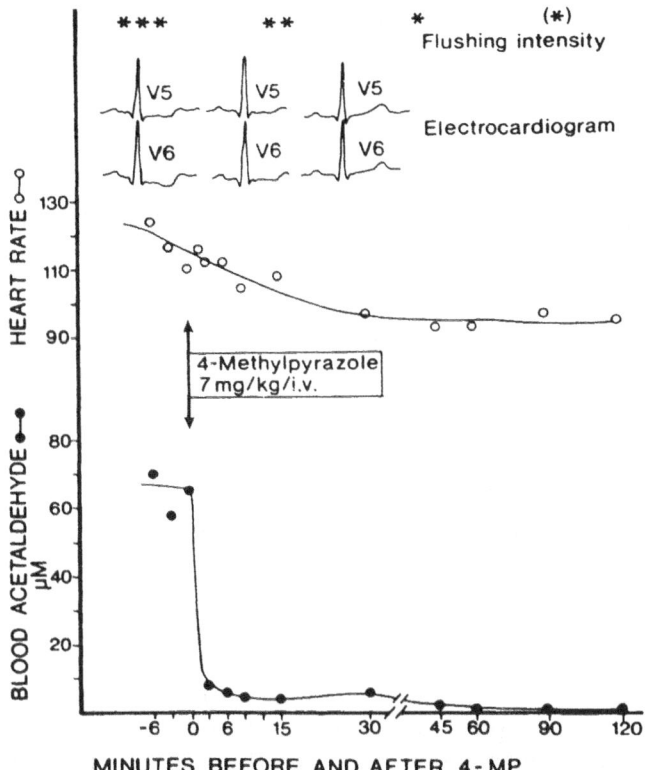

Figure 10.2 Effect of the administration of 4-methylpyrazole (4-MP) to an alcoholic experiencing a disulfiram–ethanol reaction. Flushing intensity was evaluated independently by two individuals on a 4-point scale ranging from strong [••••] to hardly noticeable [(•)]. The EKG tracings shown were made 10 min prior, and, respectively, 4 and 10 min following administration of 4-MP. From Lindros *et al.* (1981) with permission.

CCER studies the i.v. infusion of 4-methylpyrazole resulted in a 90% reduction in blood acetaldehyde levels, a disappearance of flushing and a decrease in heart rate (Lindros *et al.*, 1981). In the other, administration of ethanol led to a rise in blood acetaldehyde, tachycardia, increased cardiac output as well as decreased diastolic pressure and total peripheral resistance; all these effects were reversed by i.v. administration of 4-methylpyrazole 25 minutes into the CCER (Kupari *et al.*, 1983). In the NER study, ethanol raised blood acetaldehyde levels, skin temperature and cardiac output, while lowering diastolic blood pressure and total peripheral resistance. Again, i.v. administration of 4-methylpyrazole 30 min into the NER lowered blood acetaldehyde and reversed all of the above-mentioned changes (Suokas *et al.*, 1985).

The ability of 4-methylpyrazole to reverse all the symptoms and signs of the CCER and NER is a powerful argument that these reactions are mediated solely by acetaldehyde.

10.5.2 Summary

On the basis of four different criteria, the evidence at hand suggests that most of the signs and symptoms of the DER are mediated by the accumulation of acetaldehyde in the bloodstream. The acetaldehyde hypothesis fails to explain, however, the drop in systolic blood pressure uniformly observed during the DER. As discussed in section 10.8, this too is an effect of acetaldehyde, but one which becomes evident only following the DSSD-induced inhibition of a second enzyme.

10.6 QUEST FOR ANIMAL MODELS OF THE REACTION

Preliminary to any discussion of experimental animal studies of the DER, one has to consider how well various species fulfil the role of models for the reaction observed in humans. Already in 1948, Larsen reported difficulties in finding an animal model of the DER. He found that he was unable to elicit any effect on blood pressure, heart rate, or cutaneous vasomotor control by administering ethanol to DSSD-pretreated mice, guinea pigs or rabbits, although in mice and possibly guinea pigs, the pretreatment enhanced the narcotic effect of ethanol.

In considering the selection criteria for animal models of the DER, one should be mindful that, in humans, the salient characteristic of the DER is its toxicity. In its early therapeutic use, DSSD was prescribed in doses which, while higher than those used currently, were themselves not toxic. Yet, during that period there occurred a significant number of fatalities; these were ascribed to the DERs elicited by the ingestion of relatively small doses of ethanol. Given what is known about the individual toxicities of these two agents, it follows that in humans their combination is significantly more toxic than would be expected on the basis of simple additivity (Gessner, 1988). In choosing an animal model, therefore, it would be desirable to use as a selection criterion that the species selected exhibit a similar sensitivity to the joint toxicity of these two agents. None of the animal models used to date, however, have been shown to meet this criterion.

The combined lethality of DSSD and ethanol, administered in appropriately staggered sequence, has been explicitly investigated in mice (Moldowan and Acholonu, 1982) and in rats (Child *et al.*, 1952). In DSSD-pretreated mice, the mortality following ethanol administration was slightly but not significantly greater than in DSSD-naive controls. Isobolographic analysis of the rat data (Fig. 10.3) reveals that the observed toxicity of the combination was less than would have been expected on the basis of simple additivity of the concurrently observed individual toxic actions of the two agents (Gessner, 1973, 1974, 1988).

In all animals tested (rabbits, rats, mice, dogs and cats) DSSD pretreatment results in an elevation of blood acetaldehyde levels following ethanol administration (for review see Truitt and Walsh, 1971). Since the elevation of acetaldehyde levels has been advanced as the cause of the human DER, to be able to test this hypothesis in an animal model requires that it also share some other characteristics with

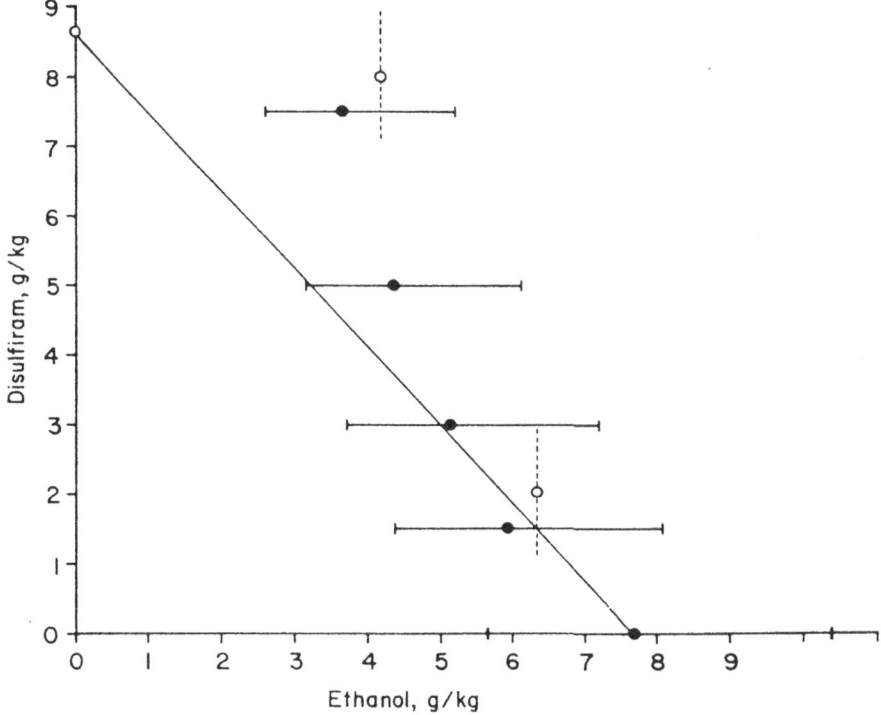

Figure 10.3 Isobalogram for the interaction of ethanol and disulfiram with respect to their lethal effects in rats. Constructed from the data of Child *et al.* (1952). Where Child *et al.* reported raw mortality data, the LD_{50} values (●) and their 95% confidence limits were calculated by the use of the ISOBOL program (Gessner, 1988); in other instances the LD50 values (○) are given as reported by Child *et al.* (1952) and are without confidence limits. The dashed lines represent the manner in which mixture composition was varied in the latter cases. Reprinted from Gessner (1973).

the human DER. By itself, therefore, an elevation of blood acetaldehyde under such conditions is not a sufficient criterion for selection.

An alternative selection criterion for an animal model of the DER would be the severity of the hypotension elicited by the administration of ethanol to DSSD-pretreated animals, since a precipitous and extreme drop in blood pressure is the chief toxic effect of the DER in humans. The administration of ethanol results in a hypotensive response in DSSD-pretreated rabbits, dogs and rats (Table 10.5). Of these, rabbits appear to be most sensitive. Infusion of a 0.2 g/kg dose of ethanol over a 5- to 10-min period to either conscious animals or ones under urethane anesthesia results in a much greater fall in blood pressure in DSSD-pretreated animals than in controls (Perman, 1962a,b). The hypotension induced in the DSSD-pretreated animals is a terminal one. This is not seen in DSSD-naive rabbits and it suggests that, in this species, DSSD and ethanol may exhibit more than additive synergism. Also, infusion of acetaldehyde to DSSD-pretreated rabbits causes a fall in blood pressure (Perman, 1962a).

In dogs, i.v. administration of ethanol, either as a bolus (0.24 g/kg) or an infusion (40 mg/kg/min for 60 min) results in a marked fall in blood pressure in DSSD-pretreated animals while in the DSSD-naive controls either no effect or an initial increase in systemic pressure and heart rate is observed (Nakano *et al.*, 1969, 1974).

Finally, in the DSSD-pretreated rat, ethanol does cause a significant fall in blood pressure. This is the principal basis for its use as a model of the DER. The dose of ethanol that is used to elicit this effect is quite large: 1 g/kg (Hellström and Tottmar, 1982a; Jensen and Faiman, 1984, 1986; Yourick and Faiman, 1989; Johansson *et al.*, 1989; Petersen, 1989). As a consequence, blood ethanol levels present at the time of the hypotensive response are quite high (Table 10.5). Since ethanol itself possesses hypotensive properties, and since infusion of acetaldehyde to DSSD-pretreated rats does not cause a fall in blood pressure, questions have arisen regarding whether the observed fall in blood pressure may be partially mediated by ethanol (section 10.6.2).

Another criterion for the selection of an animal model of the DER that has been advanced is a lowering of the core body temperature (Jensen and Faiman, 1984). The rationale for this suggestion is that one of the early characteristics of the human DER is the elevation of facial skin temperature that accompanies the facial flush (section 10.3.1). It should be noted however that no fall in body temperature has been reported to occur even in fatal DER episodes in humans (section 10.3.5). Subsequent investigation of this phenomenon, moreover, has cast doubt regarding its usefulness as a selection criterion (section 10.6.1).

Table 10.5 Effects of ethanol on blood pressure and heart rate in normal and disulfiram-pretreated subjects

Study	Species	Disulfiram Dose	Ethanol Dose	Blood level (mM)	Acetaldehyde blood level (µM)	Blood pressure Change mmHg	Blood pressure P	Heart rate Change min⁻¹	Heart rate P
Perman (1962)	Rabbit	—	0.2 g/kg i.v.			−10			
		0.35 g/kg × 2 days	0.2 g/kg i.v.			−38	<0.001		
Nakano et al. (1969)	Dog	—	0.24 g/kg i.v.			−7		−7	
		0.5 g/kg × 5 days	0.24 g/kg i.v.			−27	<0.01	−18	<0.01
Nakano et al. (1974)	Dog	—	40 mg/kg/min[a]			+14		+7	
		0.15 g/kg × 5 days	40 mg/kg/min[a]			0	<0.05	−6	<0.05
Nakano et al (1974)	Dog	—	40 mg/kg/min[b]			0		−6	
		0.15 g/kg × 5 days	40 mg/kg/min[b]			−33	<0.01	−17	<0.01
Hellström and Tottmar (1982)	Rat	—	1.0 g/kg i.p.	16	15	−1%		+6%	
		0.1 g/kg i.p.	1.0 g/kg i.p.	17	173	−13%	<0.01	+7%	>0.05
Yourick and Faiman (1989)	Rat	—	1.0 g/kg i.p.	16		−5		+38%	
		0.041 g/kg i.p.	1.0 g/kg i.p.	19	199	−20	<0.05	+32%	>0.05

						Systolic Change mmHg	Systolic P	Diastolic	Diastolic P	Heart rate Change min⁻¹	Heart rate P
Johansson et al. (1989)	Rat	—	1.0 g/kg i.p.			−7.5%	<0.01	−5%	<0.05	+2%	
		0.13 g/kg[c] i.p.	1.0 g/kg i.p.			−34.5%	<0.05	−15%		+8%	<0.05
Petersen (1989)	Rat	—	1.0 g/kg i.p.	10	2	−9		−6			
		0.01 g/kg i.p.	1.0 g/kg i.p.	10	31	−13	<0.01	−10			>0.05
		0.03 g/kg i.p.	1.0 g/kg i.p.			−22	<0.01	−10			>0.05
		0.1 g/kg i.p.	1.0 g/kg i.p.			−26	<0.001	−16	<0.001		>0.05
Mizoi et al. (1988)	Human	—	0.4 g/kg p.o.	7	116	−2		−2		+7	
	Human[d]	ALDH deficient	0.4 g/kg p.o.			−28		−4		+27	
Beyeler et al. (1985, 1987)	Human	0.4 g/kg × 3–6 days	0.19 g/kg p.o.			−41		−43		+95	

[a] Infused i.v. for 20 min.
[b] Infused i.v. for 60 min.
[c] 100 mg/kg 19 h prior + 30 mg/kg 3 h prior.
[d] Deficient in E_2, the low K_m mitochondrial aldehyde dehydrogenase.

Although a number of other characteristics of the human DER have been described (increased minute volume and plasma pO_2, flattening of the T wave, lowered plasma pCO_2, pH and potassium: Asmussen *et al.*, 1948b; Child *et al.*, 1951; Raby, 1952, 1953b; Sauter *et al.*, 1977), none have been used as criteria in selection of an animal model. Also, as discussed in section 10.3.5, there is some evidence that, in humans, the vagal reflex induced by nausea and vomiting contributes to the cardiovascular collapse associated with the DER and the analogous CCER. In this context, the inability of rodents to vomit needs to be borne in mind.

Some of the conclusions reached by investigators using rats in the investigations of the interaction of DSSD and ethanol are as follows: 'the disulfiram–ethanol reaction in rats is caused by the combined action of ethanol and acetaldehyde on the cardiovascular system' (Hellström and Tottmar, 1982a); 'In the rat ... the severity of the DER was not related to blood acetaldehyde, but appears temporally to correlate with blood ethanol' (Jensen and Faiman, 1986); 'the symptoms, collectively referred to as the DER and their intensities, are due to the interaction of ethanol, acetaldehyde, dose of ethanol and disulfiram, and the disulfiram pretreatment time' (Yourick and Faiman, 1989). Given the need for high ethanol doses to elicit a pharmacological effect in the DSSD-pretreated rat and the apparent low sensitivity of the animal to elevated blood acetaldehyde, the degree to which these conclusions are applicable to the human DER remains, at best, an open question.

10.6.1 The hypothermic effect of the combination in the rat

A significant lowering of core body temperature is observed 90 min following the administration of a 1 g/kg dose of ethanol to rats pretreated 8 h earlier with 100 mg/kg of DSSD. The effect is proportional to both the dose of ethanol and that of DSSD. The treatment, moreover, induces a temporally closely correlated decrease in blood pressure (Jensen and Faiman, 1984). Though these workers did not detect any significant decreases in body temperature when the two agents were administered individually in these doses, it should be borne in mind that both are known to have hypothermic effects themselves. Thus, DSSD in doses greater than 30 mg/kg has been reported to induce, in the 4 h following its administration, a significant and dose-related hypothermia in rats (Sharkawi and Cianflone, 1978; Petersen, 1989). Ethanol administration also induces hypothermic effects in this species (Freund, 1973).

Subsequently, it was reported that treatment of the rats with pimozide (0.5 mg/kg), an agent considered to be a dopamine receptor blocker, either prior or following administration of the ethanol, markedly attenuated both the hypothermic and hypotensive effects of the combination, though it did not affect the elevation in blood acetaldehyde levels observed in such animals (Jensen and Faiman, 1986). Since the hypothermic effects of both ethanol (Mullin and Ferko, 1981) and DSSD (Sharkawi and Cianflone, 1978) are also blocked by pimozide, there are strong reasons to suspect that the mechanism of the hypothermia induced by the combination and the two agents individually is similar and the greater effects observed with the combination likely constitutes an instance of simple additive synergism, not a potentiation (Gessner, 1988).

10.6.2 Effects of disulfiram on the cardiovascular actions of ethanol in the rat

The fall in diastolic and, to a lesser extent, in systolic blood pressure induced by a 1 g/kg dose of ethanol in the DSSD-pretreated rat is proportional to the DSSD dose (Petersen, 1989). These effects of ethanol peak at 8–16 h and remain significant for 24 h following administration of DSSD i.p. as a fine aqueous suspension (Yourick and Faiman, 1989). The duration of the effect of 1 g/kg of ethanol in these animals is some 4 h.

Ethanol (1 g/kg i.p.) has similar effects on blood pressure in rats pretreated with diethyldithiocarbamate (DSH), diethyldithiocarbamic acid methyl ester (DSMe) and diethylmonothiocarbamic acid methyl ester (DmSMe), all metabolites of DSSD (Yourick and Faiman, 1989; Johansson *et al.*, 1989; Petersen, 1989).

Various attempts have been made to determine to what extent the observed fall in blood pressure induced by ethanol administration in the DSSD-pretreated rat may be mediated by the effects of ethanol itself. One approach has employed 4-methylpyrazole, an alcohol dehydrogenase inhibitor, by eliminating acetaldehyde production from ethanol: this agent should block any effects attributable to acetaldehyde. In DSSD-naive rats, a 3 g/kg i.p. dose of ethanol increases heart rate and lowers blood pressure (by 18%). Administration of 4-methylpyrazole to such animals increases blood ethanol levels and depresses the blood pressure further (to 30%). Administration of a 1 g/kg dose of ethanol to DSSD-naive rats results in much smaller effects. In DSSD-pretreated animals, however, this dose of ethanol results in a sharp rise in blood acetaldehyde levels, a significant blood pressure drop (13%), and pronounced tachycardia and tachypnea. All these phenomena are promptly reversed by 4-methylpyrazole (Hellström and Tottmar, 1982a). This suggests that most of the cardiovascular changes observed following administration of a 1 g/kg dose of ethanol to DSSD-pretreated rats are attributable to ethanol metabolites. Of these, acetaldehyde has marked cardiovascular actions (section 10.8) although acetate, which is also formed during ethanol metabolism, has vascular effects too. Acetate has been identified as causing the splanchnic vasodilation observed following ethanol administration (Carmichael *et al.*, 1987), an effect that involves raised adenosine plasma levels and stimulation of the A_2 adenosine receptors (Carmichael *et al.*, 1988; Orrego *et al.*, 1988).

A somewhat different conclusion is reached on the basis of experiments involving separate and concurrent exposure of rats to infused acetaldehyde and i.p. administered ethanol (Hellström and Tottmar, 1982a). Although 175–195 μM blood acetaldehyde levels can be achieved in several ways, some involving administration of 1 g/kg ethanol, others cannot (Table 10.6), only in the presence of ethanol do these acetaldehyde levels cause a significant fall in blood pressure. Hellström and Tottmar (1982a) saw this as evidence that 'the depressant effect of acetaldehyde is potentiated by ethanol, or vice versa, since the ethanol dose used produced only moderate effects in rats given ethanol alone.' Their data do indicate synergism, though it is not possible, in the absence of dose–response information for each of the agents individually, to determine whether the synergism was greater than dose-additive and therefore appropriately classed as potentiation

Table 10.6 Comparison of the effects of ethanol, acetaldehyde, and their combinations on blood pressure and acetaldehyde levels in naive and disulfiram-pretreated rats[a]. From Hellström and Tottmar (1982a).

Disulfiram[b] pretreatment (mg/kg)	Ethanol[c] i.p. (mg/kg)	Acetaldehyde[d] i.v. (mg/kg/h)	Blood[e] acetaldehyde (μM)	Blood pressure[e] change (%)	P
–	1000	–	15 ± 5	-1 ± 3	ns
–	–	4	189 ± 37	-4 ± 4	ns
–	1000	4	194 ± 38	-14 ± 5	<0.01
100	–	4	187 ± 63	0 ± 3	<0.001
100	1000	–	173 ± 40	-13 ± 3	<0.001

[a] Anesthetized with 150 mg/kg hexobarbital i.p.
[b] Administered i.p. in 5% gum acacia 24 h prior to zero time.
[c] Administered i.p. 10 min prior to zero time.
[d] Infused for 20 min starting at zero time.
[e] Determined at end of infusion or at 20 min post ethanol administration.
ns = not significant

(Gessner, 1988). Somewhat analogous phenomena to those observed by Hellström and Tottmar (1982a) have been reported by Carmichael *et al.* (1987) using cyanamide, another ALDH inhibitor. These latter workers observed a significant lowering of peripheral resistance following administration of ethanol to cyanamide-pretreated rats. The intensity of the effect appeared to be correlated to the increased blood acetaldehyde levels, and was not observed following administration of either ethanol or cyanamide alone. Surprisingly, however, the effect could not be duplicated by infusing acetaldehyde itself.

Also surprising and perplexing is the ability of pimozide (Jensen and Faiman, 1986) to divorce the increase in blood acetaldehyde levels seen following administration of ethanol to DSSD-pretreated rats and the hypotensive effects that normally accompany such administration (section 10.6.1). The more recent observations that in the first 24 h following pretreatment with DSSD, or its metabolites DSH and DSMe, there is a correlation between ethanol-administration-induced acetaldehyde blood levels and depresssion of blood pressure (Yourick and Faiman, 1989), leaves open the question regarding what effect pimozide might have on the correlation. Analogous concerns arise with regard to correlation between raised blood acetaldehyde levels and the hypotensive effects in the rat model following ethanol administration in animals pretreated with DmSM (Petersen, 1989; Hart *et al.*, 1990), particularly so because of the potent hypothermic effects shared by DSMe (Hart *et al.*, 1990) and DmSMe (Petersen, 1989). The actual hypothermic effect can be compensated for by the use of a heating pad (Petersen, 1989). However, the fact that the analogous effect of DSSD is blocked by pimozide (section 10.6.1) suggests the possibility that their hypotensive effects might likewise be pimozide-sensitive.

In conclusion, one fact the data in Hellström and Tottmar (1982a) and those of Yourick and Faiman (1989) clearly show is that, relative to humans, rats have a marked lack of sensitivity to the cardiovascular effects of acetaldehyde (section 10.8.1). Also, the dose of ethanol that is used in the rat model (1 g/kg) raises concerns because of the hypotensive actions of ethanol itself. By comparison the dose that elicits the DER in humans is 0.19 g/kg and doses of 0.2 and 0.24 g/kg have been used to decrease blood pressure in DSSD-pretreated rabbits and dogs, respectively (Table 10.5).

10.7 EFFECT OF DISULFIRAM ON ETHANOL METABOLISM

It is a common finding that the rate of elimination of ethanol is reduced from that observed in controls if the animals are pretreated with either

DSSD (Hald *et al.*, 1949a; Schlesinger *et al.*, 1966; Tottmar and Marchner, 1976; Sharkawi and Caillé, 1979) or DSH (Nishigaki *et al.*, 1985). Similar findings are also obtained *in vitro* using isolated hepatocytes (Crow *et al.*, 1977). The data of Brown *et al.* (1983) suggest that the rate of ethanol elimination may also be reduced in humans pretreated with DSSD.

Such observations have led to questions regarding whether DSSD might inhibit alcohol dehydrogenase (ADH). However, the ADH activity in DSSD-pretreated animals, when examined *ex vivo*, is found not to be affected (Lamboeuf *et al.*, 1974; Tottmar and Marchner, 1976; Sharkawi and Caillé, 1979). Rather, raised acetaldehyde levels result in reduced rates of ethanol metabolism, be it *in vivo* (Ryle *et al.*, 1985; Masuda *et al.*, 1988), in perfused liver systems (Lindros *et al.*, 1972), in the soluble fraction of liver homogenates (Dawson, 1981, 1983; Harrington *et al.*, 1988), or by purified ADH (Wratten and Cleland, 1963; Hanes *et al.*, 1972).

Two mechanisms have been advanced as mediating the effect of acetaldehyde on ethanol metabolism. First, it has been suggested that the decrease in the rate of ethanol elimination is due to the back reaction (Lindros *et al.*, 1972; Cederbaum and Dicker, 1979, 1981; Cronholm, 1985; Ryle *et al.*, 1985). The ADH-catalyzed reaction of ethanol with NAD^+ to give acetaldehyde and NADH is a reversible one and its thermodynamic equilibrium constant, K_{eq}, is far in the direction of ethanol formation, its value in the case of the human and horse enzymes being $0.97 \times 10^{-11}M$ (Pietruszko *et al.*, 1973). The efficiency of the back reaction is presumably responsible for rat blood acetaldehyde levels being virtually the same at the end of a 20-min period of acetaldehyde infusion (4 mg/kg/h) irrespective of whether the animals are pretreated with DSSD or not (Table 10.6); similar findings have been reported following DSH pretreatment (Nishigaki *et al.*, 1985). The other mechanism that has been suggested is that acetaldehyde itself acts as an inhibitor of the alcohol dehydrogenase (Dawson, 1981, 1983). It is beyond the scope of this monograph to rehearse the arguments presented in support of these alternative hypotheses; however, either one could adequately explain the decreased elimination of ethanol during the DER without invoking an inhibition of the alcohol dehydrogenase by DSSD.

In individuals pretreated with DSSD, the peak blood ethanol levels resulting from the ingestion of a given dose of ethanol would be expected, as a consequence of the accumulation of acetaldehyde and its effect on ethanol elimination, to be higher than in normal controls. Consequently, the pharmacological effects of a given dose of ethanol would be expected also to be more intense. In a double-blind experiment, Brown *et al.* (1983) have found this to be so with respect to both subjective assessment of mood and objective assessment of behavior of individuals dosed with 500 mg of DSSD and given 8 h later 0.625 g/kg of ethanol (*ca* 44 g/70 kg or three drinks) over a 2-h period.

10.8 THE DOPAMINE β-HYDROXYLASE HYPOTHESIS.

The dopamine β-hydroxylase (DBH) hypothesis, as originally formulated by Truitt and Walsh (1971), was based on the premise that the primary cardiovascular action of acetaldehyde in DSSD-naive animals is vasopressive and cardiostimulatory and these actions are mediated by norepinephrine (NE) release. It held that DSSD, by inhibiting DBH, blocks the synthesis of NE and thereby causes a partial depletion of NE stores. The acetaldehyde which accumulates in blood following ethanol ingestion was posited by the hypothesis to release such NE as remained in the stores, resulting in a transient vasoconstrictive effect and a further depletion of the NE stores. With the latter depleted, the direct vasodilating and cardiodepressive effects of acetaldehyde were unmasked, according to the hypothesis, and led to the observed hypotensive effects.

The impetus for the formulation of this companion hypothesis to the earlier acetaldehyde one, was the difficulty encountered (section 10.5) by clinical investigators in reconciling the total absence of DER-like symptoms with the appreciable blood 'acetaldehyde' levels achieved by the administration of large doses of ethanol to DSSD-naive individuals (Raby, 1956; Perman, 1962a; Sauter *et al.*, 1977). It was later discerned that the paradox was due, largely, to problems inherent in the methodology of acetaldehyde determination (Truitt and Walsh, 1971) and, in time, the view was accepted that the previously reported blood acetaldehyde levels should be taken *cum grano salis* (Kitson, 1977). By that time substantial evidence had accumulated, however, that the vasopressor and cardiostimulatory actions of acetaldehyde were mediated by NE. Thus it was shown that the vasoconstrictor effects of acetaldehyde are potentiated by cocaine (Eade, 1959) and blocked by pretreatment with adrenergic α-blocking agents (Egle *et al.*, 1973). Moreover, upon depletion of catecholamine stores with reserpine the vasoconstrictor action of acetaldehyde is blocked (Eade, 1959) and vasodepressor effects are observed (Akabane *et al.*, 1964). Also, it had been shown that acetaldehyde can release NE from its stores (Truitt and Walsh, 1971). At the same time, it had been observed that DSSD inhibits DBH (Goldstein, M. *et al.*, 1964; section 8.3). Accordingly, it appeared quite plausible that DSSD-induced inhibition of DBH could contribute significantly to the phenomenology of the DER. To appreciate the nature of this contribution it is necessary to review the various cardiovascular actions of acetaldehyde. These are discussed in the following section.

10.8.1 Effects of disulfiram on the cardiovascular actions of acetaldehyde

Basically, acetaldehyde has three actions on the cardiovascular system. It is a vasodepressor at both high and low concentrations. At intermediate concentrations it has sympathomimetic properties mediated by NE; these are blocked by DSSD pretreatment.

In high bolus doses (16–40 mg/kg i.v.), acetaldehyde causes vasodilation and bradycardia in the rat. The effect is one mediated by a vagal reflex, being blocked by atropine and by vagotomy (Egle *et al.*, 1973). Brugere *et al.* (1986) confirmed these findings and reported the effect to be dose-related. Rapid i.v. injection of 16 mg/kg acetaldehyde in 1.0 ml/kg saline elicited, for instance, a 56% fall in blood pressure which, in 8 of 10 rats, was accompanied by apnea (mean duration 5.3 s). The effect could be elicited by injection of the acetaldehyde into the right, but not the left ventricle, suggesting that the reflex is probably initiated in the pulmonary circulation.

In moderate doses, administered as an i.v. bolus, acetaldehyde evidences sympathomimetic properties: it is a vasoconstrictor and it has inotropic and chronotropic cardiac effects (Truitt and Walsh, 1971; Brien and Loomis, 1983c). These were carefully documented in dogs by Nakano *et al.* (1974), who showed that in DSSD-naive animals graded bolus doses of acetaldehyde (1–16 mg/kg i.v.) result in sharp, short-lived, proportional increases in heart rate and blood pressure (Table 10.7). These investigators also showed that in the isolated hind-limb preparations from such animals, graded acetaldehyde doses result in sharp, short-lived increases in femoral artery perfusion pressure. Following DSSD pretreatment, these same doses of acetaldehyde caused decreases in both heart rate and blood pressure in the whole animal, and a long-lasting decrease in perfusion pressure in the isolated hind limb preparation.

By contrast, in low doses acetaldehyde has little or no effect on blood pressure in DSSD-naive animals, although it does reduce peripheral resistance. Thus Bandow *et al.* (1977) found that i.v. infusion of 0.5–2.0 mg/kg/min acetaldehyde to dogs has no significant effect on blood pressure (Table 10.7), though it significantly reduces total peripheral and coronary vascular resistance and increases heart rate, cardiac output and coronary blood flow. Blockade with propranolol

Table 10.7 Effects of acetaldehyde on blood pressure and heart rate in normal and disulfiram-pretreated subjects

Study	Species	Disulfiram dose	Acetaldehyde		Change in blood pressure (mmHg)	Change in heart rate (min^{-1})
			Dose	Blood level (µM)		
Asmussen et al. (1948b)	Humans	–	1.2 mg/kg/min			+31
Perman (1962a)	Rabbit	–	1.2 mg/kg/min		None	
		0.35 g/kg × 2 days	1.2 mg/kg/min		−34	
Nakano et al. (1974)	Dog	–	4 mg/kg bolus		+32	+19
		0.15 g/kg × 5 days	4 mg/kg bolus		−8	−1
Nakano et al. (1974)	Dog	–	16 mg/kg bolus		+68	+29
		0.15 g/kg × 5 days	16 mg/kg bolus		−20	−5
Bandow et al. (1977)	Dog	–	0.5 mg/kg/min		+2	+5
		–	1.0 mg/kg/min		+4	+15
		–	2.0 mg/kg/min		+8	+36
Friedman et al. (1979)	Dog	–	0.2 mg/kg/min	43	−6	−2%
		–	0.6 mg/kg/min	129	−6	−6%
Hellström and Tottmar (1982a)	Rat	0.1 g/kg	4 mg/kg/min	189	−4	+9%
			4 mg/kg/min	187	0	+12%

abolishes all of these effects except for the increased coronary blood flow and the reduced vascular resistance. Likewise, Friedman *et al.* (1979) reported that infusion of dogs with acetaldehyde at 0.2 and 0.6 mg/kg/min for 15 min has no significant effect on either heart rate or blood pressure, though it significantly reduces total peripheral resistance and increases cardiac output (Note that blood pressure recordings in experimental animal usually reflect systolic pressure.) The mechanism whereby acetaldehyde brings about a reduction in peripheral resistance was studied by Altura *et al.* (1978) who, using rat aorta strips, found that acetaldehyde attenuates contractile responses to epinephrine (E), angiotensin, vasopressin, serotonin and potassium chloride by a non-competitive shift of the dose–response curves. They found that these actions of acetaldehyde are not inhibited by alpha adrenergic, histaminergic, cholinergic or serotonergic blocking agents and are not attributable to the release of beta adrenoceptor or prostaglandin-like substances.

Administration of ethanol to individuals deficient in the low-K_m ALDH, E_2 (section 9.1.2), provides information regarding the effects of low acetaldehyde levels on the cardiovascular system in DSSD-free humans. The rise in blood acetaldehyde thus occasioned is correlated with a fall in diastolic pressure and an increase in heart rate. However, no change in systolic pressure is observed (Fig. 10.1b). At the same time, blood NE and E levels rise 1.8- and 2.3-fold, respectively (Mizoi *et al.*, 1988). These changes are attributable to acetaldehyde, rather than ethanol, since none of them are seen following administration of the same dose of ethanol to individuals with normal ALDH (Mizoi *et al.*, 1982, 1988). The effect of DSSD pretreatment on the response to ethanol in E_2-deficient individuals has not been studied.

Inhibition of DBH and the resultant blockage of NE synthesis would be expected to impair sympathetic action. This has been observed following DSSD pretreatment of dogs. Stimulation of the left sympathetic nerve in such animals does not result in the increases in heart rate, blood pressure, and myocardial contractile force which are seen in controls (Nakano *et al.*, 1969). Likewise, while in control dogs with bilateral mid-cervical vagotomy, occlusion of both common carotid arteries brings about an increase in heart rate and blood pressure, it fails to do so in DSSD-pretreated animals (Nakano *et al.*, 1974). Also, while the cardiovascular response to usual physical activities (viz. graded bicycle exercise) is not altered by therapeutic doses of DSSD in humans, the response to extreme hypotensive stress (postural hypotension induced by 0.3-0.4 mg nitroglycerine sublingually) is significantly impaired. Specifically the systolic, but not the diastolic, pressure fall is significantly greater and the chronotropic response is smaller in the DSSD-treated subjects (Rogers *et al.*, 1979). A DSSD-induced impairment of sympathetic action would be expected to reduce the ability of the organism to compensate for a decrease in peripheral resistance through stimulation of heart rate and cardiac output and to result in a fall in systolic pressure. In keeping with this Perman (1962a), who infused 1.2 mg/kg/min acetaldehyde to rabbits, observed that, whereas in DSSD-naive rabbits acetaldehyde infusion has no effect on blood pressure, in DSSD-pretreated ones it causes a fall.

In the DSSD-pretreated rat, infusion of acetaldehyde has no effect on blood pressure (Table 10.7). It has nonetheless proved possible to evaluate whether inhibition of DBH contributes in this species to the DSSD-pretreatment-induced lowering of blood pressure by ethanol. Because the DSSD-induced inhibitions of ALDH and DBH have different time courses, manipulation of the time interval between the administrations of DSSD and ethanol renders it possible to compare the effects of similar levels of alcohol-generated acetaldehyde in the presence of different levels of DBH inhibition. To measure this inhibition Tottmar and Hellström (1979) administered ^{14}C-tyramine (^{14}C-TA), noted the amount taken up by the heart and measured the fraction transformed to ^{14}C-octopamine (^{14}C-OA). Their data indicate that blood pressure changes induced by ethanol-derived blood acetaldehyde ($\geqslant 80\ \mu$M) are significantly greater if the DBH is inhibited. To illustrate: acetaldehyde levels of $93 \pm 8\ \mu$M caused a blood pressure fall of 26 ± 6 mm Hg in animals with significant DBH inhibition (as evidenced by a ^{14}C-OA:^{14}C-TA ratio of 1.7). On the other hand, in animals with little DBH inhibition (^{14}C-OA:^{14}C-TA ratio of 10.7) the blood pressure fall associated with acetaldehyde levels of $96 \pm 32\ \mu$M was less than half as large (12 ± 5). These findings were confirmed by the use of two ALDH inhibitors devoid of DBH inhibitory activity: cyanamide and coprine (Tottmar and Hellström, 1979). In animals pretreated with these agents the accumulation of blood acetaldehyde following ethanol administration was also accompanied by a drop in blood pressure, although again the effect was less than half as large as that seen in DSSD-pretreated animals.

10.8.2 Restatement of the dopamine β-hydroxylase hypothesis

In summary, the evidence reviewed above calls for a restatement of the DBH hypothesis (section 10.5). Although acetaldehyde, if administered in bolus doses, does have direct NE-release-mediated sympathomimetic effects, such effects probably play little or no part in the phenomenology of the DER since (a) the rate of generation of acetaldehyde following administration of ethanol subsequent to DSSD pretreatment is more likely to resemble that of a slow i.v. infusion, and (b) NE release following such slow i.v. infusion is a result of compensatory sympathetic stimulation brought about by the acetaldehyde-induced lowering of peripheral resistance. During the DER, it is this latter mechanism of NE release that is most likely to be responsible for the acute depletion of the already DBH-inhibition-attenuated NE stores.

Certain parallels should be noted between the phenomena observed following high doses of acetaldehyde in experimental animals and some characteristics of the DER-related cardiovascular collapse syndrome discussed in section 10.3.5. One such characteristic of the human syndrome is that a period of apparent recovery precedes death. An analogous observation was made in rats by Sprince *et al.* (1974) while determining the LD_{50} of acetaldehyde. The acute toxic manifestations of respiratory distress, gasping, and an anesthetic-like paralysis wore off rather rapidly and many animals appeared to fully recover, only to die three or more hours later in respiratory distress and stupor. The vagal influences and the antidotal effect of atropine observed in experimental animals (Egle *et al.*, 1973; Brugere *et al.*, 1986) also find echos in the all too meager information regarding the human DER-related cardiovascular collapse syndrome. It is tempting to speculate that under the influence of very high acetaldehyde blood levels, adrenergic stores in the heart are depleted to such an extent that the ability to maintain homeostasis is lost and activation of the parasympathetic innervation of the heart, as in a vagal reflex, has catastrophic consequences. Atropine would help guard against this, as would a rebuilding of the adrenergic stores of the heart by infusion of E and NE. It is of interest to note, therefore, that infusion of one or both of these agents has frequently been mentioned as a component of the treatment of the DER (Lester *et al.*, 1952; Markham and Hoff, 1953).

10.8.3 Clinical relevance of the dopamine β-hydroxylase hypothesis

Whether the DBH hypothesis should be accepted with respect to the DER revolves around the question of whether at the doses of DSSD employed therapeutically, functionally relevant inhibition of DBH occurs in humans. Therapeutic doses of DSSD increase urinary excretion of 3-methoxy-4-hydroxyphenylacetic acid (HVA) and decrease that of 3-methoxy-4-hydroxymandelic acid (VMA), the terminal metabolites of dopamine and NE, respectively (Vesell *et al.*, 1971; Rogers *et al.*, 1979; Robins and Barron, 1983). This urinary excretion pattern indicates lower rates of NE formation from dopamine (Fig. 9.5), and is thus consistent with the DBH hypothesis, as is the finding by Rogers *et al.* (1979), that the urinary excretion of NE and its conjugates are lower in individuals on DSSD. Functional *in vivo* inhibition of DBH by DSSD (385 mg/70 kg for 4 days) has been reported by Hoeldtke and Stetson (1980). These investigators administered dopamine specifically tritium-labelled in the beta position, and found decreased release of tritiated water and a decrease in total tritiated NE metabolite excretion. As already mentioned (section 10.8.1), Rogers *et al.* (1979) found that treatment for two weeks with 500 mg/day doses of DSSD impaired the response to extreme hypotensive stress, leading to greater than control fall in systolic pressure. From this body of data it results that high-end therapeutic doses of DSSD do induce a small, but functionally significant, inhibition of DBH. It follows that this inhibition can play a role in the clinical manifestations of the DER.

10.8.4 Summary

Acetaldehyde, in the quantities formed during the DER, reduces peripheral resistance by a direct action on vascular smooth muscle; this results in a fall in diastolic pressure and a compensatory increase in cardiac output. The adrenergically mediated response to this challenge is impaired in individuals on DSSD and a drop in systolic pressure ensues. The impairment appears to be correlated to inhibition of DBH by DSSD.

10.9 EFFECT OF ETHANOL IN ANIMALS PRETREATED WITH DISULFIRAM METABOLITES

It is evident that DSSD itself is not responsible for the DER reaction. First, most investigators are unable to detect any measurable levels of it in body fluids at any time following its administration or even its addition to blood (Chapter 4). Second, the Class 2 ALDH, the low-K_m mitochondrial enzyme responsible for the *in vivo* metabolism of ethanol-derived acetaldehyde, is rather insensitive *in vitro*, though not *in vivo*, to DSSD (section 9.2). Accordingly, it is assumed that the *in vivo* effects of DSSD that render the DER possible are mediated by an active metabolite, so the search for this entity continues. In the process, it has been found that three DSSD metabolites, namely DSH, DSMe and DmSMe, if administered *in vivo*, cause an inhibition of the Class 2 ALDH (section 9.4) and, as discussed below, that subsequent challenges with ethanol result in some of the same effects as are observed following DSSD pretreatment.

The ability of DSH, the first of these compounds to induce effects similar to those of DSSD, is the least surprising since biological systems are known which can reoxidize DSH to DSSD (section 5.1). In rats pretreated with DSH (114 mg/kg i.p.) ethanol (1g/kg i.p.), administered 8 h later, causes a significant fall in mean arterial pressure (accompanied by a rise in blood acetaldehyde). The effect is, however, only half as large and lasts only half as long as that observed in rats pretreated with an equivalent i.p. dose (75 mg/kg) of DSSD (Yourick and Faiman, 1989). The DSH effect is evident from 0.5 to 24 h following its administration and is accompanied by inhibition of the low-K_m ALDH activity of hepatic mitochondria, though this inhibition develops more slowly than that seen following DSSD administration (Fig. 9.3). DSH pretreatment also sensitizes humans to the effects of ethanol. Thus, a mild 'disulfiram reaction' has been reported to have occurred in an HIV positive patient following the ingestion of 120 ml of beer 8 h after DSH (*ca* 5 mg/kg) administered i.v. as Imuthiol (Brewton *et al.*, 1989).

Much more intriguing is the ability of pretreatment with DSMe and DmSMe (the dithio- and the monothiocarbamic acids methyl ester metabolites of DSH) to cause blood acetaldehyde levels to rise and blood pressure to fall following ethanol administration. The prevalence of the available evidence suggests that *in vivo* neither ester is hydrolyzed back to DSH and cannot regenerate DSSD either (section 5.5). Rather, they behave as more proximal precursors of the active metabolite of DSSD.

Within 30 min and for 24 h following pretreatment with DSMe (42.1 mg/kg i.p. in oil), ethanol administration (1 g/kg i.p.) causes a significant fall in mean arterial blood pressure and a rise in blood acetaldehyde (Yourick and Faiman, 1987, 1989). Both diastolic and systolic pressure are significantly depressed by ethanol administered 1 h following a 60 mg/kg dose (Johansson *et al.*, 1989). Concurrently, the low-K_m aldehyde dehydrogenase activity of hepatic mitochondria is inhibited (Fig. 9.3). Quantitatively, these effects are similar to those obtained following pretreatment with twice the molar equivalent of DSSD (75 mg/kg i.p. in aqueous suspension) suggesting that DSMe is more potent than DSSD. Moreover, DSMe appears to act more rapidly. Thus, the changes in blood acetaldehyde levels and the fall in mean arterial blood pressure at 1 h after administration of ethanol are, respectively, 100 and 80% greater in the animals pretreated (2 h previously) with DSMe than in those pretreated with DSSD (Yourick and Faiman, 1989).

The effects of DmSMe pretreatment on the response to the administration of ethanol (1 g/kg i.p.) have been studied in rats by Petersen (1989) and Hart *et al.* (1990). Both report such pretreatment causes ethanol administration to have hypotensive effects. Petersen (1989) observed the diastolic blood pressure to be significantly depressed in animals pretreated with a 50 mg/kg dose of DmSMe from 30 min to 48 h prior to ethanol administration; systolic blood pressure was depressed by ethanol following a 2-h pretreatment with a 50 mg/kg dose of DmSMe as well as 1 h after a 30 mg/kg dose. Hart *et al.* (1990) reported that the enhancement of the effects of ethanol (1 g/kg) in lowering mean arterial blood pressure was analogous whether rats were pretreated 8 h earlier with 18.6 mg/kg of DmSMe or 20.6 mg/kg of DSMe.

All these agents cause *in vivo* inhibition of the low-K_m aldehyde dehydrogenase and this is reflected in the increased blood acetaldehyde levels following ethanol administration, which in turn is the presumed cause of the blood pressure fall observed in rats. However, the animal model employed in these studies make this less certain (sections 10.6.1 and 10.6.2).

DmSMe resembles DSSD in its hypothermic actions, but is more potent: significant effects are observed with 3 mg/kg doses, while the lowest dose of DSSD shown to lower body temperature is 30 mg/kg (Petersen, 1989). DSMe has also been stated to have hypothermic effects (Hart *et al.*, 1990).

* See page 42 for Note added in press.

10.10 TREATMENT OF THE REACTION

Since the DER is due to the accumulation of acetaldehyde in the circulation, the simplest antidotal strategy is to block ethanol oxidation, and thereby the formation of the acetaldehyde. This can be accomplished by administration of the alcohol dehydrogenase inhibitor, 4-methylpyrazole. To date, knowledge regarding the effectiveness of this agent in countering the DER clinically is limited to one case report (Lindros *et al.*, 1981). Over the period of 30 min, i.v. administration of 7 mg/kg 4-methylpyrazole reversed the tachycardia, facial flushing, and electrocardiographic changes of a man admitted in DER (Fig. 10.2). Experimental clinical studies of the effect of 4-methylpyrazole on the analogous reactions to ethanol in individuals pretreated with calcium carbimide (Lindros *et al.*, 1981; Kupari *et al.*, 1983) or nitrefazole (Suokas *et al.*, 1985) suggest that it has both the requisite effectiveness and safety (section 10.5.1). A 'Phase I clinical study' of 4-methylpyrazole by Jacobsen *et al.* (1988), who obtained it from Aldrich Chemical Company (Milwaukee, WI), indicates a lack of toxicity with doses of 10 and 20 mg/kg. Adverse subjective effects (moderate dizziness and mild nausea) appear at a dose of 50 mg/kg and become more apparent at 100 mg/kg.

An alternate antidotal strategy is to antagonize the effects of the high levels of acetaldehyde. The use of ascorbic acid, administered in large i.v. doses (1–1.5 g), has long been advocated to this end (Child *et al.*, 1950) and continues to be so recommended (Haley, 1979; PDR, 1991). Large doses of ascorbic acid (2 mmol/kg) have been shown in rats to significantly decrease the mortality induced by large doses of acetaldehyde (Sprince *et al.*, 1974, 1979). Accordingly, the therapy is a rational one. The clinical effectiveness of this therapy is less well documented. Thus, Lester *et al.* (1952) found no benefit to derive, in individuals undergoing the DER, from the i.v. administration of a 1.0 g dose of ascorbic acid as a buffered solution with ferrous chloride. Niblo *et al.* (1951), on the other hand, found that ascorbic acid (1.0 g i.v.) suppressed the headache, motor restlessness, palpitations, weakness and apprehension associated clinically with the DER, though they found it not to affect the fall in blood pressure, the changes in the electrocardiogram, pulse rate or flushing. Markham and Hoff (1953) administered 1.5 g ascorbic acid i.v. to human subjects undergoing the DER and noted a tendency for the electrocardiogram to return to normal more rapidly. The mechanism of this antidotal effect of ascorbic acid remains unknown. It is interesting, however, that ascorbic acid also has antidotal effects against morphine-induced mortality in mice (Dunlap and Leslie, 1985) and that nalmefene, an opiate antagonist, blocks both the tachycardia and the rise in skin temperature experienced upon ingestion of ethanol by Asians with a history of sensitivity to alcoholic beverages, without affecting the rise in acetaldehyde plasma levels that follows such ingestion (Ho *et al.*, 1988).

Other agents shown to significantly antagonize acetaldehyde mortality in rats include *N*-acetyl-L-cysteine, as well as L-cysteine, cysteic acid, thiamine, and sodium metabisulfite (Sprince *et al.*, 1974, 1975). Ezrielev (1973) suggests that sodium metabisulfite is highly effective in controlling the principal symptoms of the DER in alcoholics. The antidotal effectiveness of the other agents relative to the DER has not been explored.

A depletion of catecholamine stores by high blood acetaldehyde levels suggests that their repletion by slow i.v. infusion of either NE (levarterenol) or E could be beneficial. E acts at α and both β_1 and β_2 receptors, thus stimulating the heart, but also causing a drop in peripheral resistance, hence potentially exacerbating this aspect of the DER. NE, on the other hand, has little activity at β_2 receptors and increases peripheral resistance and blood pressure. The latter can induce a compensatory vagal discharge and result in bradycardia. In such circumstance it too could exacerbate the DER. Both untoward effects should be mitigated by the slowness of the infusion. Also, the compensatory vagal reflex could be blocked by atropine, and the administration of the latter may be a rational strategy in the treatment of the DER. The administration of ephedrine, currently recommended by the PDR (1991), presents a potential problem. This sympath-omimetic agent acts mostly by catecholamine release. Therefore, as catecholamine stores are depleted, it becomes increasingly less effec-tive. Its uptake, moreover, does not render sympathetic cat-echolaminergic neurons any more able to respond by releasing cat-echolamines when stimulated.

Postural counteracting of the drop in peripheral resistance is yet another strategy that is available to deal with the DER. As a first step, patients should be in a recumbent position. Tilting of the bed to a head-down position (Markham and Hoff, 1953) has been found to be a procedure that, applied to individuals ($n=3$) with systolic blood pressure drops >70 mm Hg, successfully counteracted the DER-gener-ated hypotensive effect (Beyeler *et al.*, 1985).

11

Disulfiram therapy of alcohol abuse

11.1 INTRODUCTION 205
11.2 GOALS OF DISULFIRAM THERAPY 209
11.3 TREATMENT COMPONENTS CORRELATED WITH REDUCTION OF
DRINKING DAYS 209
11.4 DISULFIRAM THERAPY PARADIGMS 214
    11.4.1 Disulfiram Assurance Program 214
    11.4.2 Unsupervised compliance 218
    11.4.3 Institutionally assured compliance 220
    11.4.4 Probation-linked disulfiram treatment 222
11.5 ELECTION OF AND CONTINUATION IN TREATMENT 223
11.6 CHARACTERISTICS OF DISULFIRAM'S THERAPEUTIC EFFECTS 224
    11.6.1 Time course of effect 224
    11.6.2 Dose–response relationships and therapeutic dosages 226
    11.6.3 Can disulfiram enhance ethanol-induced euphoria? 229
    11.6.4 Can disulfiram augment craving for ethanol? 229
    11.6.5 Can drinking through a reaction terminate the effect of disulfiram? 230
    11.6.6 Interaction of disulfiram with skin lotions and after-shaves . . 231
11.7 SIDE EFFECTS OF DISULFIRAM THERAPY 232
    11.7.1 Controlled-trial studies of disulfiram side-effects 233
    11.7.2 Encephalopathies 235
    11.7.3 Peripheral neuropathy 237
    11.7.4 Hepatotoxicity 238
    11.7.5 Other side-effects 241
    11.7.6 Subclinical effects 242
    11.7.7 Role of carbon disulfide 243
11.8 CHEMICAL COMPLIANCE MONITORING 244
11.9 DISULFIRAM IMPLANTS 245

11.1 INTRODUCTION

Disulfiram (DSSD) administration results in the inhibition of E_2, the
mitochondrial aldehyde dehydrogenase (ALDH) that is the enzyme

responsible for the metabolism of ethanol-generated acetaldehyde *in vivo* (Chapter 9). As a consequence, following treatment with DSSD, the consumption of even moderate quantities of ethanol results in a rapid *in vivo* accumulation of acetaldehyde. This, in turn, causes a series of quite unpleasant symptoms and signs (Chapter 10), collectively referred to as the disulfiram–ethanol reaction (DER). When DSSD is prescribed for the treatment of alcoholism, patients are informed about these phenomena and strongly advised to abstain from ethanol. Some may test the correctness of the warning by partaking, albeit cautiously, of an alcoholic beverage. Provided that the DSSD dose is adequate (section 11.6.2) and the ethanol is consumed within 48 h of the last dose of DSSD (section 11.6.1), some of the symptoms of the DER are experienced within minutes.

By all accounts, the DER, whether personally or vicariously experienced, is sufficiently aversive for alcoholics to resist the otherwise powerful craving they feel for ethanol. While some may test-drink alcoholic beverages, none persist in imbibing these while taking effective doses of DSSD (section 11.6.5). The central fact of DSSD therapy, however, is the rather obvious one that, in order to be effective, the drug has to be taken. Yet compliance, always a problem with chronic medications that do not have an obvious effect (Cramer *et al.*, 1989; Pristach and Smith, 1990), can be particularly poor in the case of DSSD therapy.

The nature of the relationship between the frequency with which DSSD is ingested and the fraction of the days on which drinking occurs, is rendered plain (Fig. 11.1) by an analysis of the data of Azrin *et al.* (1982). These workers performed a 6-month study in which patients at a rural community alcoholism-treatment clinic were randomized to three treatment conditions. Daily DSSD (250 mg) was prescribed in each treatment condition but greater efforts were made with some groups than others to achieve compliance. The subjects were asked to record their drinking behavior and DSSD usage on a monthly calendar which the experimenters reviewed, on a monthly basis, with at least one close relative or other important person in the patients' daily life (significant other) for corroboration. Further corroboration was secured from employers and local law enforcement personnel. Also, DSSD usage data were compared with prescription renewal information. In this manner, each month the mean number of drinking days and the mean number of days on which DSSD was taken were recorded for each of the 3 groups. This was repeated for each of the 6 months of the study, thus generating 18 pairs of values for these two variables. When the resultant data are

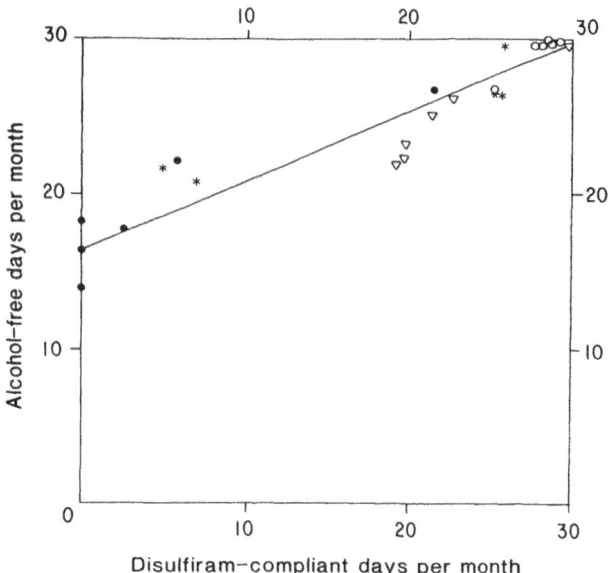

Figure 11.1 Effect of compliance with disulfiram therapy on the prevalence of abstinence in alcoholic patients during a 30-day period. Points represent treatment group data; the symbols identify the source of the data. [(●) the traditional treatment group (n = 14), (▽) the disulfiram assurance group (n = 15), (○) the disulfiram assurance plus behavioural therapy group (n = 14) in the study by Azrin *et al.*, 1982; their figures 2 and 3: (*) the reinforcement group (n = 6) in the study by Sisson and Azrin, 1986; their Figure 1.] See sections 11.1 and 11.4.1 for details of treatments.

graphed, as in Fig. 11.1, it becomes evident that adhering to DSSD therapy and the consumption of ethanol are mutually exclusive activities, seemingly governed by a reciprocal mathematical relationship. Quantitatively, there is a high correlation ($r=0.95$, $P<0.0001$) between the number of drinking days, d, and the number of DSSD-free days, f, per month. The regression equation for this relationship is

$$d = 0.52 + 0.44f \tag{11.1}$$

This equation suggests that individuals who take DSSD every day of the month remain abstinent during that whole period, while those who take it on only half of the days or stop taking it altogether drink, on average, on 7 and 14 days per month, respectively.

The robustness of the relationship is suggested by the fact that the data derived from a later and unrelated study by Sisson and Azrin (1986) appear to exhibit a similar relationship (asterisks in Fig. 11.1).

This analysis indicates that compliance with DSSD therapy is of crucial importance in reducing the number of drinking days.

Given that the appropriate goal for the DSSD therapy of alcoholism is the reduction to a minimum of the days on which drinking occurs (section 11.2), the major question to be resolved becomes how to structure treatment so as to maximize compliance. This is underscored by the fact that, though the effectiveness of different DSSD therapy paradigms in achieving a reduction in drinking days varies widely (section 11.3), maximization of treatment compliance is a consistent component of successful therapies. Various strategies are employed to this end. One which yields excellent results is based on having significant others help the alcoholics by making sure the medication is taken as prescribed (section 11.4.1). To achieve this, the therapist must structure appropriately the motivational and environmental contingencies for the patients. DSSD therapy that relies on the alcoholics taking the drug daily on their own is usually not successful (section 11.4.2). In an alternative successful treatment paradigm, the individual doses of the drug are dispensed by an institution, for instance, a treatment center (section 11.4.3). This latter paradigm has also been employed successfully by social agencies attached to the courts (section 11.4.4). Where it is not possible to assure compliance at the time of ingestion, chemical compliance testing (section 11.8) can be important. Unfortunately, disulfiram implants, which potentially might have obviated the problems of compliance, are not pharmacologically effective (section 11.9).

In a wider context, the factors that influence a patient's decision to elect DSSD therapy and persevere with it, once started, determine what fraction of alcoholics can benefit from it (section 11.5). Controlled studies indicate that, in normal therapeutic doses, DSSD is almost free of side-effects (section 11.7.1). Patients need to be aware that ethanol-containing skin lotions and aftershaves can elicit the DER (section 11.6.5). Case reports of side-reactions, particularly at higher doses, need to be carefully considered (sections 11.7.2–11.7.5), as do subclinical effects revealed by prospective studies (section 11.7.6). Some side-effects of DSSD may be mediated by carbon disulfide (CS_2), a known metabolite of DSSD (section 11.7.7).

Information regarding the time course of DSSD's effect is provided in section 11.6.1 and dose–response relationships are discused in section 11.6.2. Occasionally it is suggested that patients might be able to terminate the DER by drinking through it, but this is not so (section 11.6.6). Likewise, DSSD does not enhance ethanol-induced euphoria (section 11.6.3), or increase cravings for ethanol (section 11.6.4).

11.2 GOALS OF DISULFIRAM THERAPY

The drinking of alcoholics is characterized by being impulse-driven. Though this may be but a proximate manifestation of the alcoholics' craving for alcohol, their longing for a drink, the impulses can be obsessive. DSSD frees alcoholics from the moment to moment struggle with these impulses. In the words of Ruth Fox (1958) 'A man ... who is fighting the urge to drink may have to choose between drinking and not drinking several hundred times a day, while a man on Antabuse makes that decision just once, i.e. on taking the pill.' Moreover, it is easier for such individuals to find someone that will help them, once a day, to maintain their resolve to take DSSD, than it is to locate someone to whom they can turn on each of the many daily occasions when an obsessive impulse to drink becomes manifest and, if they are not protected by DSSD, threatens their sobriety.

One of the characteristics of alcoholism is the consumption of large quantities of ethanol by those affected. For instance, in one large study of 2339 patients entering alcoholism treatment, the mean alcohol consumption in the 30 days prior to admission was found to be 15 drinks/day (Armor *et al.*, 1976a). Consumption of such large quantities of ethanol is destructive of the patients' health and well-being. It also results in a chronic mental deficit. The latter clears slowly upon abstinence. In the interim, however, it renders it difficult for the patient to learn new ways of coping with life, ways that do not include reliance on drinking. For long-term recovery, the period of abstinence needs to last at least one and probably two years (Öjehagen *et al.*, 1988), which suggests a similar period of DSSD therapy is appropriate.

Another feature of alcoholic drinking is the large amount consumed on each drinking occasion or, more correctly, on each drinking day (consumption, once started, goes on for many hours). Typically, however, alcoholics who have to expend some effort to secure their beverage (the usual situation) are found to alternate between drinking episodes of 3–6 days and periods of relative abstinence of 2–3 days duration (Mello and Mendelson, 1972). Accordingly, average daily consumption figures can markedly underestimate the amount consumed on drinking days. Reducing the incidence of the latter to a minimum is, therefore, the immediate principal goal of DSSD therapy.

11.3 TREATMENT COMPONENTS CORRELATED WITH REDUCTION OF DRINKING DAYS

The effectiveness of different protocols of DSSD therapy is best judged by using as a criterion the percentage of days to which drinking is

Table 11.1 Comparison of the effectiveness of disulfiram-based therapies in reducing ethanol consumption

Patients	Treatments compared[a]			Method of assurance or compliance testing	Compliance %	Contingency type	Outcome		
	n	Drug	Dosage				Period	Drinking days	P
1. Liebson et al. (1973)									
Severe alcoholics receiving methadone maintenance	3	DSSD	(500 mg/d × 14d) ∫ 250 mg/d × 8–15w	Dispensed at clinic suspended in water		Forfeit of methadone maintenance	8–15w	1%	<0.001
	3	DSSD	(500 mg/d × 14d) ∫ 250 mg/d × 8–15w	None		None		17%	
2. Azirin (1976)[b]									
Alcoholics with extensive record and withdrawal at intake	9	DSSD	250 mg/d × 6m & behavioral therapy	Witnessed by wife or peer		Withdrawal of reinforcement by family or peer	6m	2%	<0.005
	9	DSSD	Advice to take DSSD and traditional AA-oriented program	None		None		55%	
3. Bigelow et al. (1976)									
Problem drinkers, 80% with history of blackouts, loss of control, craving and physical dependence	20	DSSD	(500 mg/d × 14d) ∫ 500 mg/2d × 3m	Dispensed at clinic suspended in water	92.2	Forfeit $5–10 of $100 deposit	3m	1.6–4.4%[c]	
	—			Historical comparison with prior 3y		Continuous abstinence achieved following start of treatment exceeds longest in preceding 3y by by a geometric mean of 2.5 fold (P <0.005)[d]			

4. Liebson et al. (1978)

Population	N	Drug	Dosage	Method	Value	Consequence	Time	%	P
Severe alcoholics, receiving methadone maintenance	12	DSSD	(500 mg/d × 14d) ∫ 500 mg/2d × 3m	Dispensed at clinic suspended in water		Forfeit of methadone maintenance	180d	2%	<0.002
	12	DSSD	(500 mg/d × 14d) ∫ 500 mg/2d × 3m	None		None		25%	

5. Fuller and Roth (1979); Fuller et al. (1983)

Population	N	Drug	Dosage	Method	Value	Consequence	Time	%	P
Alcoholics requesting treatment for alcoholism or admitted for alcohol related illness	43	DSSD	500 mg/d × 7d	Urine test on 19 + Scheduled visits in 1 y	55[e]	None	1y	31%	
	43	DSSD	1 mg/d × 1y	ditto	60[e]	None		32%	
	42	Vit B$_2$	50 mg/d × 1y	ditto	49[e]	None		37%	

6. Robichaud et al. (1979)

Population	N	Drug	Dosage	Method	Value	Consequence	Time	%	P
Problem drinkers referred for treatment by employer	21	DSSD	500 mg/d × 14d ∫ 500 mg/2d × 3–12m	Dispensed at clinic suspended in water	93.2	Biweekly progress report to employer	3–12m	0.1–1.2%[e]	
	—		Historical comparison with previous 2y	Job absenteeism rate fell from 9.5% during the 24-month pretreatment period to 1.7% during treatment (P<0.001)					

7. Azrin et al. (1982)

Population	N	Drug	Dosage	Method	Value	Consequence	Time	%	P
Alcoholics: drank mean 8.8 oz/d ethanol on mean of 21/30 prior days	14	DSSD	250 mg/d × 6m & behavioral therapy	Witnessed by wife or peer	94; 84[f]	Withdrawal of reinforcement by family or peer	6th m	3%	<0.01
	15	DSSD	250 mg/d × 6m	ditto	73; 66[f]	None		26%	
	14	DSSD	250 mg/d × 6m & traditional AA-oriented program	None	22; 0[f]	None		55%	

Table 11.1—*Contd.*

8. Schuckit (1983)

	n	Drug	Dosage	Monitoring		Outcome	p
Primary alcoholics DSM III criteria	172	*DSSD*	*Unspecified*	*None*	*None*	*1y* 70%	
	176	*–*	*Rejected DSSD therapy*	*ditto*	*ditto*	72%	

9. Fuller et al. (1986)[g]

	n	Drug	Dosage	Monitoring		Outcome	p
Alcoholics by NCA criteria	203	DSSD	250 mg/d × 1y	Urine test on 39 scheduled visits in 1y 23^h	None	1y 18.7%	<0.03
	204	DSSD	1 mg/d × 1y	*ditto* 17^h	None	29.9%	
	199	Vit B_2	50 mg/kg × 1y	*ditto* 18^h	None	31.9%	

[a] Convention and nomenclature employed: DSSD, disulfiram; d, day; w, week; m, month; y, year; ∫, followed by; &, together with; ( ), mandatory induction period preceding experimental period.

[b] DSSD dosage not specified; 250 mg dosage arrived at by extrapolation from Azrin *et al.* (1982).

[c] Latter number includes unvalidated days.

[d] Paired t test of the logarithmic metameters of abstinence period in Figure 1 of Bigelow *et al.* (1976).

[e] Mean percentage of all collected urines found marker-positive per subject (Fuller *et al.*, 1983): on average patients attended 12 of 19 prescheduled visits. However, they were allowed to make additional visits. Urines collected on these visits were also marker-tested and added into the totals (Fuller, private communication). Since many patients, likely the more compliant, made extra visits (raising the average number of visits per patient to 16), the recorded percentage, even if reduced by 12/19 or 0.63, likely overestimates mean compliance on the 19 prescheduled dates.

[f] Average for 6 months of treatment and for the 6th month of treatment, respectively.

[g] Drinking days data are those derived from the reports of relatives and friends.

[h] Percentage of patients whose urines were marker-positive on 15 or more of the 39 scheduled collection dates during the year.

restricted. By this criterion, the nine published controlled studies of DSSD therapy that provide such information (Table 11.1) show a wide disparity of outcomes, for they report treatment to result in the occurrence of drinking on as little as 1% and as much as 70% of the days.

When one considers these studies, two factors stand out as contributing to a significant reduction in the incidence of drinking days. The first is the use of some method of ascertaining compliance. The second is the creation of some contingency which helps to motivate the patient to remain compliant. Albeit these studies span a large range of designs and methodologies, the importance of these two factors is evident from consideration of studies 1, 2, 4 and 7 (Table 11.1). In each of these studies, patients were randomized to various experimental groups and all were either prescribed DSSD or advised to take it, but measures to ascertain and motivate compliance were applied to some of the groups only. Patients in these latter groups registered a significantly greater reduction in the incidence of drinking days. These same two factors (ascertaining compliance, motivational contingency) are components of studies 3 and 6 in which the incidence of drinking days was reduced to 1–2%, but are absent from study 8 in which patients continued to drink on 70% of the days.

In all but one of the studies in Table 11.1 some method was used to ascertain compliance. In studies 5 and 9 the method chosen was a reactive one, the *post facto* testing of the urine for a marker (riboflavin) incorporated in the dispensed medication. In the other studies the methods used were pro-active, anticipatory ones, designed more to assure compliance than to ascertain it. In four instances (studies 1, 3, 4 and 6) this involved crushed DSSD tablets being dispensed as a well-mixed suspension in water by the clinic staff. Since the studies were all out-patient ones, the patient had to visit the clinic to receive the medication. (Such dispensation of DSSD by someone other than the patient or the patient's relatives coincides with the policy recommendations of a Consensus Meeting organized by Sweden's National Board of Health and Welfare; see Socialstyrelsen, 1984.) In the remaining two instances (studies 2 and 7), assuring compliance involved self-administration by the patient with, however, the participation of the spouse or a significant other as a witness. This was coupled to a therapist-initiated manipulation of family dynamics so that the patient was positively reinforced by the spouse or significant other for not drinking. If the patient stopped being compliant, however, a time-out from such reinforcement would take place. This Disulfiram Assurance Program, as it is called, was developed by Azrin and coworkers. It is more closely examined in section 11.4.1.

11.4 DISULFIRAM THERAPY PARADIGMS

In discussing drug treatment generally, one can distinguish three possible regimens (Sereny *et al.*, 1986). The first involves voluntary acceptance of the therapy, the compliance to which is left to the discretion of the patient and is not supervised. This is the paradigm normally employed by physicians prescribing medication for out-patients. It is, however, a regimen which, in the vast majority of alcoholic patients placed on DSSD therapy, is not effective (section 11.4.2). The second regimen involves mandatory therapy, compliance to which is required and assured by being supervised. Except in cases of individuals committed to mental institutions, it is a paradigm rarely employed in medicine. It is not one applicable to DSSD therapy. The third regimen involves voluntary acceptance of therapy, but once therapy is accepted, compliance to it is required and some sort of supervision is employed to assure it. As pointed out by Brewer (1986), this is the regimen routinely used with those who are too young, too old, or too ill to take medicines reliably. When this paradigm is used in recidivist populations, a compliance failure is understood to set off into action agreed-upon negative contingencies. This understanding is frequently formalized by the signing of a contract between the patient and therapist. It is found that this paradigm is characteristic of all successful DSSD therapy. In this chapter, such therapy is discussed under three headings (sections 11.4.1, 11.4.3 and 11.4.4), depending on how compliance is assured.

11.4.1 Disulfiram Assurance Program

In the absence of daily, triweekly, or biweekly visits by the patient to the treatment facility, provision of DSSD therapy requires that the therapist organize the family environment so as to assure the patient's daily adherence to the therapy. This is the purpose of the Disulfiram Assurance Program developed by Azrin and coworkers (Azrin, 1976; Azrin et al., 1982; Sisson and Azrin, 1986). Its main elements are as follows.

1. The participation of a second individual, a significant other, preferably a spouse, whom the patient is encouraged to ask for assistance in remaining sober by monitoring daily compliance. The action is presented not as punitive, or one of surveillance, but rather as a caring one which is motivated by a wish to help.
2. The coupling of the performance of the act of DSSD ingestion to some daily routine, viz. mealtime, return home from work, or brushing one's teeth.

3. Anticipation, planning and rehearsal, between the patient and the significant other, of contingencies arising out of special situations likely to disrupt the daily routine, viz. sickness, vacations, running out of DSSD, etc.
4. Stipulation that the DSSD will only be ingested in the presence of the significant other; rehearsals of such a discussion as would be appropriate should either party propose to discontinue therapy; arrangements for prompt notification of the therapist, should failure of compliance occur, so that pre-crisis counseling can be scheduled.
5. Referral to a sympathetic physician for necessary medical examination and prescription of DSSD; formalization, in written form, of agreements between patient and therapist, specifying assignments each person agrees to complete, the target date, the reasons for following the procedure, and the actions that the patient and significant other will take in the event of deviation from the agreement.

In their studies, Azrin and coworkers coupled the Disulfiram Assurance Program to a second program that would create contingencies designed to motivate the patient not to drink. This was the Community-Reinforcement Behavioral Therapy (CRBT) 'designed to rearrange the vocational, family and social reinforcers of the alcoholic such that time-out from these would occur if he begun to drink' (Hunt, G.M. and Azrin, 1973). Where the drinking had affected the marital relationship, the CRBT involved marital counseling to maintain and improve the relationship, but also to make drinking of alcohol incompatible with it.

In the first of the studies employing the Disulfiram Assurance Program coupled to the CRBT (Table 11.1, study 2), Azrin (1976) found that during the 6 months of treatment, patients in the program achieved a high sobriety rate and had a very significant improvement in the days employed. Also, they were away from home far less often (Table 11.2). Furthermore, during the following 18 months the high sobriety rate was maintained: in the second, third and fourth 6-month periods only 3, 10 and 9% of the days, respectively, involved drinking.

In their second study (Table 11.1, study 7), Azrin *et al.* (1982) replicated the above investigation, extending it by the inclusion of a third group of patients who were randomized to the Disulfiram Assurance Program, but without this being coupled to the CRBT. By the sixth month, patients in the Disulfiram Assurance Program coupled with the CRBT did significantly better (on all three outcome measures) than those receiving the traditional treatment, thus replicating the earlier finding. Patients in the third, or freestanding Disulfiram Assurance Program group, did about as well on two outcome measures (days

Table 11.2 Comparison of various disulfiram treatments of alcoholism in terms of the percentage of days on which the stated behavior or condition occurred.

Patients	Azrin (1976)[a]			Azrin et al. (1982)[b]			
	Traditional disulfiram treatment	Disulfiram assurance + behaviour therapy	P	Traditional disulfiram treatment	Disulfiram assurance	Disulfiram assurance + behaviour therapy	P
Number	9	9		14	15	14	
drinking	55	2	<0.001	55	26	3	<0.01
unemployed	56	20	<0.001	36	11	7	<0.01
away from home	67	7	<0.001	15	0	0	<0.01

[a] 6 months of treatment.
[b] 6th month of treatment.

employed, days not away from home) as those whose program was coupled to the CRBT (Table 11.2). Nonetheless, the percentage of days that the patients in this group spent drinking during the sixth month was quite substantially higher than those whose program was coupled to the CRBT.

This study, however, yielded a crucially important finding when the role of marital status was examined (Azrin *et al.*, 1982). Patients in the Disulfiram Assurance Program remained totally abstinent, whether or not it was coupled to behavioral therapy (CRBT), provided they were married (Table 11.3). It is thus evident that DSSD becomes a very potent weapon in the family's fight against alcoholism, if it is sustained by a well-informed and appropriately counseled spouse.

Stimulated by this finding, Sisson and Azrin (1986) sought to determine whether women, rendered aware of the potential of DSSD therapy and provided with reinforcement training, could motivate their male, alcoholic, disinclined-to-seek-treatment close relatives (husband, brother, father) to enter such therapy. To this end, they randomly assigned a group of women, seeking help because of the severe alcoholic problems of close relatives, to either traditional counseling ($N=5$) or reinforcement counseling ($N=7$). The women in the latter group, were trained how to provide reinforcement for not drinking and withhold it during drinking. Additionally, the training focused on the effectiveness of DSSD therapy, on how to encourage the relative to take DSSD, on what common objections to DSSD he might raise, and how to identify moments when he would be most motivated to seek treatment, namely following 'specific occasions when their alcohol problems become especially severe.' If the drinker agreed at such a time to the suggested counseling, the woman was to contact the counselor and bring the drinker in immediately, regardless of time of day, or day of week.

Table 11.3 Outcome of various treatments of alcoholism as a function of marital status. Data of Azrin *et al.* (1982)

	Percentage of days spent drinking during 6th month of treatment[a]		
	Traditional disulfiram treatment	Disulfiram assurance	Disulfiram assurance + behaviour therapy
Single individuals	78	73	6
Married individuals	42	0	0

[a]By the 6th month, the mean compliances with disulfiram therapy in the three treatment groups dropped from first month levels of 72, 99 and 96% to 0, 64 and 83% respectively.

The goal of having the counseled woman's male alcoholic relative enter treatment was achieved in six of the seven cases in groups assigned to the reinforcement counseling (after a mean of 58 days). The male relatives of these women were drinking initially on an average of 81% of the days. By the third month after the alcoholics accepted counseling they were drinking on less than 6% of the days, were consuming about two drinks per episode and were taking DSSD on about two-thirds of the days. By the fifth month their drinking had decreased to 1% of days ($P < 0.001$). In contrast, in no instance did the alcoholic relatives of the women assigned to the traditional counseling enter treatment. They continued to drink at the same level throughout the 3 months for which data were available. Since this counseling was not proving helpful, the women assigned to it withdrew from the study at the end of 3 months.

11.4.2 Unsupervised compliance

Studies 5 and 9 in Table 11.1, i.e. those by Fuller and coworkers (Fuller and Roth, 1979; Fuller and Williford, 1980; Fuller *et al.*, 1983, 1986) are noteworthy for (a) the large number of subjects (128 and 606, respectively), (b) their duration (1 year in each instance), (c) their controlled double-blind design, and (d) the use of a compliance marker (riboflavin, Vit B_2). Patients in these studies were randomly assigned to one of three treatment groups prescribed, respectively, 250 mg, 1 mg and no DSSD. The patients in the first two of these groups were told they would be dispensed DSSD and were given a vivid description of the DER, though, in fact, a 1 mg dose is pharmacologically ineffective. The patients in the third group were advised they were being dispensed a vitamin medication and asked to take it. All patients were asked to return to the clinic for a series of scheduled appointments and to donate, when doing so, samples of urine. 'To allay possible suspicion by the patients that their adherence to the drug regimen was being tested,' the urines were checked for protein and glucose by a dipstick technique and the patients were told this was part of their health assessment. In fact, the urines were also used to determine compliance by being assayed for riboflavin, a 50 mg quantity of which had been incorporated in the medication dispensed to each group (i.e. in the vitamin pill and in the 250 and 1 mg DSSD capsules).

In the first of these studies (Fuller and Roth, 1979; Fuller and Williford, 1980; Fuller *et al.*, 1983), therapy with 250 mg of DSSD had no effect on the mean number of drinking days. The patients in each group drank on about one-third of the days (Table 11.1, study 5). In the second study (Fuller *et al.*, 1986), those who were prescribed the 250 mg rather than the 1 mg DSSD dose drank on significantly fewer days, according to the testimony of relatives and friends. The effect was, however, quite modest: a reduction from 30 to 19% of days (Table 11.1, study 9). Moreover, in neither study did the DSSD therapy increase the incidence of year-long abstinence, the criterion of treatment success used by the authors. (In the first study, the complete year-long abstinence rates for patients taking 250 mg, 1 mg, and no DSSD, were 21, 25 and 12%, respectively; in the second study they were 19, 23 and 16%, respectively.) In reporting on the results of the second study, Fuller *et al.* (1986) stated 'we did not find that disulfiram, *as it is conventionally used with outpatients*, enhanced the attainment of continuous abstinence more than counseling alone' (emphasis added).

Paradoxically, in spite of a nominal overall compliance rate of 58%, drinking occurred on about two-thirds of the days in the first of the two studies. Similarly, in the second study, 57% of those 'judged compliant' were not abstinent. The issue of compliance is an important one to focus on in evaluating these two studies. In both, compliance was monitored by collecting urine samples and assaying them for the riboflavin marker whenever the patients visited the treatment facility. Interpretation of the resulting figures is problematic. In the first study (Fuller and Roth, 1979; Fuller *et al.*, 1983), urines were to be collected on each of the 19 visits that the patients were prescheduled to make during the 1-year period. The average patient missed 37% of these appointments. Some patients scheduled additional visits, however, and the urines from these visits were also included in the analysis (Fuller, private communication), rendering it impossible to estimate on how many of the 19 prescheduled time points the patients were found to be compliant. In the second study (Fuller *et al.*, 1986), urines were to be obtained during the 39 prescheduled visits. If on ≥ 15 of these occasions the patient donated marker-positive urines, he was termed as 'compliant' or 'in good compliance'. Only 23% of the patients receiving the 250 mg DSSD therapy satisfied even this modest criterion (Table 11.1, study 9). Moreover, since the patients knew when they would be visiting the treatment facility, the degree to which their compliance behavior on these occasions corresponded to that during the rest of the treatment period, has been questioned (Cardwell, 1987). One might also seriously question whether a patient who takes a medication on only 15 of 39 occasions (38%) when this is tested, should be termed 'compliant'. In any event, no contingency was incorporated in the studies to motivate the patient to be compliant, in fact the patients remained unaware that compliance was being tested.

In a subsequent exchange of correspondence, Brewer (1987) challenged the 'apparent belief that simply giving patients a bottle of disulfiram and hoping they will take it regularly represents sound, conventional practice.' To make a point regarding what constitutes conventional practice in Britain, he cited a report of a Special Committee of the Royal College of Psychiatrists which states that it is advisable that 'a third person supervise the Antabuse, ... a relative or someone at work'. In Sweden, a Consensus Meeting organized by the National Board of Health and Welfare (Socialstyrelsen, 1984) went even further in its policy recommendation, stating that 'the treatment is best administered by other persons than the patient himself or his relatives.'

The marginal effectiveness of DSSD therapy as it is conventionally used in North America, that is with compliance being neither supervised nor otherwise assured, has been documented by the Rand Corporation study (Armor *et al.* 1976b). This analyzed the 6-month outcome of alcoholism treatment at 44 National Institute of Alcohol Abuse and Alcoholism (NIAAA) funded Alcoholism Treatment Centers (ATCs) and an 18-month follow-up at eight NIAAA-funded ATCs. Of the patients in the 44 ATC sample, 30% of the 2371 for whom outcome data was available (21% of those treated) had received DSSD at some point during treatment (manner of selection unspecified). In all treatment settings (hospital, intermediate care, or out-patient care) these patients had a marginally better 6-month outcome (those prescribed DSSD had, overall, a 77% remission rate; the rate for the others was 64%). The 18-month follow-up reached a greater proportion of those treated (62%), but failed to indicate any benefit of DSSD therapy.

11.4.3 Institutionally assured compliance

The majority of alcoholics who feel compelled to seek treatment do so because they find the alcohol-related problems they face to be overwhelming, yet, unaided, cannot control their cravings for ethanol. If they choose DSSD therapy and are told (a) that compliance with the therapy is essential to its success and (b) that to achieve compliance it is best for the DSSD to be dispensed to them three or more times a week under a contingency arrangement, they tend to find this acceptable. Although not controlled, a study by Sereny *et al.* (1986) illustrates this well. The program, which was made a prerequisite for continued treatment for patients who had relapsed ≥ 3 times, involved the taking of 500 mg of DSSD three times a week for a minimum of 6 months and doing so under supervision at the treatment facility. Missing of one dose occasioned a warning, missing two doses or drinking led to suspension from the clinic for $\geqslant 4$ months. Upon readmission a second failure led to a permanent discharge. The program was offered to 73 individuals and 68 accepted it. The difference in sobriety before and after induction into the program was termed 'remarkable' by the authors: 'Patients who could not remain sober from one visit to the next achieved many months of continuous sobriety.'

In the above study, Sereny *et al.* (1986) incorporated the therapist-initiated termination of the relationship as the contingency motivating the patient to be compliant. The rationale for doing so was that a therapeutic relationship in which a patient consistently fails to comply with therapy is unproductive and demoralizing. Liebson and Bigelow (1972) argued for a similar approach in the case of individuals dually addicted to ethanol and opiates. Noting that problem drinking is the most reliable predictor of therapeutic failure in methadone maintenance, they incorporated the therapist-initiated termination of methadone maintenance as the contingency designed to motivate patients to comply with DSSD therapy (Liebson *et al.*, 1973, 1978). They found that assignment to the therapy markedly decreased the incidence of drinking days (Table 11.1, studies 1 and 4).

Other examples of institutionally assured compliance are the study of Bigelow *et al.* (1976) in which the contingency set in motion by missing doses of DSSD was the loss of some predetermined fraction of a financial security deposit (Table 11.1, study 3), and that of Robichaud *et al.* (1979) in which the contingency involved notification of the employer (Table 11.1, study 6). An additional study, particularly worthy of note, is that of Gerrein *et al.* (1973). Although institutionally assured compliance was a feature of this study, it had no contingency or contractual arrangement components. Patients willing to be on DSSD therapy were randomized into four groups. Patients in one of the groups were dispensed 250 mg of DSSD twice weekly under supervision by the staff. Those in a second group were asked to come to the treatment facility weekly and at such time they were proffered a 7-day supply of 250 mg DSSD tablets. Those in the remaining two groups were simply asked to visit the facility on 1 or 2 days a week, respectively, but no DSSD was proffered. The outcome was quantitated in terms of the retention of patients in treatment after 8 weeks. The patients in the group receiving DSSD under supervision twice weekly remained in treatment more than twice as often as those dispensed DSSD to take on their own (85 vs 39%; $P < 0.05$) or those not receiving DSSD. In discussing these results, the authors of the study suggest that the frequent and close contact of the patients with the clinic over a period of weeks served to establish positive therapeutic relationships with staff members and that, being socially isolated, the patients found these reinforcing.

11.4.4 Probation-linked disulfiram treatment

A distinction needs to be drawn between the approaches outlined above and one where the DSSD ingestion is supervised directly by a probation officer and where the alternative to compliance is revocation of parole. Although participation in such programs can still be viewed, technically, as voluntary and so presented to the alcoholic, it is clearly further along the voluntary-coerced continuum than the studies discussed in previous sections. The institutional interest in such therapy may be directed more at alleviation of the societal problems attributable to ongoing alcohol abuse, than to effecting of a long-term cure. Such prioritizing of goals may seem at odds with the aspirations of the health professionals involved and may be challenged (Plant, 1983; Brewer and Smith, 1983b). Nonetheless, as discussed below, such treatments are found to be quite effective in achieving the sobriety of those treated. Accordingly, as in the case of methadone maintenance therapy of narcotic dependence, the approach may be acceptable to all parties concerned, because it relieves the patient's degradation and suffering and renders long-term rehabilitation more likely.

The effectiveness of this approach can be gauged from three studies. In the first of these, Bourne *et al.* (1966) reported on 132 offenders whose sentences were suspended by the court, provided they agreed to take DSSD for 30 or 60 days. During this period they were to come to the court daily to take the medication under the supervision of a probation officer. At the end of the study period, 59% of these individuals had either completed the stipulated treatment or were still actively taking the drug (the rest were lost to follow-up). Similarly, Haynes (1973) reported on 141 habitual offenders of whom 98%, given the choice between a 90-day jail sentence and one year of DSSD therapy, chose the latter. The subjects had to visit the probation office twice a week to take the DSSD under supervision; two or more failures to do so resulted in reinstatement of the sentence. Of the 73 individuals that remained in town (Colorado Springs, population 75 000), 19% broke probation and were returned to jail. The remaining 81% successfully completed the year of DSSD therapy. Moreover, the arrest rate during the year fell 13-fold for the group as a whole, i.e. from a mean of 3.8 arrests per individual during the preceding 12 months to 0.3 arrests per individual during the treatment year.

In the third of such studies, Brewer and Smith (1983a) reported on a population of 18 habitual offenders referred for probation reports pending trial for alcohol-related offenses. Told that DSSD therapy would help them remain abstinent until sentencing and that this would likely lead to their being given a suspended sentence, 16 agreed to enter into treatment and were followed for a minimum of 12 weeks. Nine of the 16 were compliant throughout, two others had a brief lapse and thereafter complied consistently. Three patients refused further treatment after some weeks in the program and were imprisoned. Only two committed additional offenses. Although in the preceding 2 years, the longest out-of-prison abstinence these men had averaged had been 6 weeks, while in treatment they averaged 30 weeks of abstinence, three with minor lapses.

11.5 ELECTION OF AND CONTINUATION IN TREATMENT

The behavioral impediments that prevent individuals from profiting from the benefits of DSSD therapy can be categorized under three headings. One of these, the lack of compliance with DSSD treatment, has been discussed above.

A second behavior that prevents alcoholics from accruing the advantages of DSSD therapy is their failure to continue with it. Drop-out rates reported by different studies vary markedly. For instance, while Azrin *et al.* (1982) reported a 6-month drop-out rate of zero, Kofoed (1987) reported a 12-month drop-out rate of 87%. In the latter study, the compliance of patients with DSSD therapy was monitored and, in the event of non-compliance, patients in one group were challenged while those in another group were not. The patients in the challenged group complied better (71 vs 44%; $P < 0.02$), however the drop-out rates for the two groups were the same. In other studies continuance rates as low as 7% have been reported (Ludwig *et al.*, 1970).

The third behavior which limits the number of alcoholics that can gain from DSSD therapy is their *a priori* refusal of it. Many alcoholics will request DSSD therapy, if they are given adequate information regarding it and an option to choose it. The extent to which this occurs varies markedly, however, with place and time by virtue of what appear to be culturally determined norms. Working in a hospital in Bridgeport, Massachusetts, Lubetkin *et al.* (1971) found only 10 individuals over a period of 4.5 months who were willing to participate in a DSSD program, although 200 to 300 alcoholics were referred to the hospital monthly. Not many miles away in a Boston hospital, Gerrein *et al.* (1973) found 40.5% of the patients willing to take DSSD.

Moreover, while this willingness was voiced by 64% of the black patients, only 38% of the white ones expressed it ($P<0.05$). More recent American figures for election of DSSD therapy are 27 and 38% (Brubaker *et al.*, 1987; Fuller *et al.*, 1986, respectively). In contrast, Öjehagen and Berglund (1986) have reported in a study from Sweden, that 91% of their patients, given the opportunity to choose their own treatment-program components, elected DSSD therapy. It is of interest, in this context, that the 70% increase in the use of DSSD in Sweden is considered to have significantly contributed to the 20–40% decrease in alcohol-related in-patient care that occurred in that country in the period 1978–84 (Romelsjö, 1987).

Brubaker *et al.* (1987) have sought to determine what beliefs and attitudes predict the alcoholic's request of DSSD therapy. They found that patients requesting DSSD therapy perceive it as allowing them to become more 'self-efficient' by (1) helping them resist the urge to drink, (2) enhancing their confidence in remaining sober and (3) helping them remain sober. Such patients also are more likely to believe that their significant others would want them to take DSSD and are also more motivated to comply with their physician or treatment counselor in this respect. The high motivating influence of significant others was noted earlier by Azrin *et al.* (1982) and was the method of induction of alcoholics into the study of Sisson and Azrin (1986).

Conversely, among individuals who reject DSSD therapy, Brubaker *et al.* (1987) noted a significantly stronger belief that DSSD would cause unpleasant side-effects. Lubetkin *et al.* (1971) had earlier come to a similar conclusion while investigating informally the strong resistance to DSSD therapy in a hospital setting. They found that rumors pervaded the hospital that (a) the mere ingestion of DSSD, even without ethanol, would cause a violent physical reaction, and that (b) the DER invariably leads to severe physical debilitation.

11.6 CHARACTERISTICS OF DISULFIRAM'S THERAPEUTIC EFFECTS

11.6.1 Time course of effect

The duration of the DSSD-induced sensitization to ethanol is a clinically important parameter. On the basis of self-experiments, the Danish investigators who originally suggested the use of DSSD in the treatment of alcoholism, reported that the duration of its action is related to dose (Hald *et al.*, 1948). They measured whether the ingestion of 40 ml of gin at various times following DSSD administration elicited one of the concomitants of the DER, namely the increase in facial skin temperature. On this basis they concluded that the effect persists for 3–4 days after a dose of 500 mg, and for 7–8 days following a dose of 1500 mg.

Using more moderate doses of DSSD (250 mg daily for 3 or more days), Iber and Chowdhury (1977) found that in patients free of liver disease the blood acetaldehyde response to a 5 g challenge dose of ethanol wanes rapidly (Table 11.4). The acetaldehyde blood levels these workers observed are only a fraction of those other investigators have reported for the DER (Table 10.4). This is not surprising since the ethanol challenge dose used by them was rather small and because the blood acetaldehyde was sampled 2 h after ethanol administration, i.e. well after it would have peaked (Fig. 10.1a). Nonetheless, their data make it evident that, in individuals with normal hepatic function, an ethanol challenge at 48 rather than at 24 h after the last dose of DSSD results in acetaldehyde levels that are only half as high. In patients with serious liver disease, the ethanol challenge elicits higher blood acetaldehyde levels. Even in such individuals, however, ethanol-challenge-induced increases in skin temperature were seldom observed if more than 3 days had passed since the last 250 mg dose of DSSD, and never if more than 4 days had elapsed.

Table 11.4 Duration of the ethanol sensitizing effect of disulfiram as shown by the response to a test dose of ethanol[a] in patients with and without liver disease. Data of Iber and Chowdhury (1977).

Hepatic status[b]	Bilirubin level	*Days since last dose of disulfiram*				
		1	*2*	*3*	*4*	*5*
		Incidence of detectable skin temperature reaction[c]				
Normal		3/47	0/27	0/12		
With liver disease	<2.5	9/9	6/8	1/7	0/4	0/2
With liver disease	>2.5[d]	6/6	5/5	4/4	1/3	0/3
		Blood acetaldehyde[e] (μg/100 ml)				
Normal		5.4±4.3 (18)[f]	2.8±3.1 (8)	0.8 (2)		
With liver disease		11.6±4.8 (8)	7.9±6.2 (7)	6.7±4.0 (7)		

[a]Ethanol test dose (5 g) administered following 3 or more days of treatment with disulfiram (250 mg/day).
[b]Biopsy proven.
[c]Number responding/number tested.
[d]All with active alcoholic hepatitis.
[e]At 120 min after the ethanol test dose.
[f]Number in parenthesis is the number of patients studied.

Additional evidence that the alcohol-sensitizing effects of DSSD are relatively short-lived, comes from studies of the DSSD-induced inactivation of leukocyte ALDH. This enzyme is similar, probably identical, to the hepatic mitochondrial enzyme E_2 which is considered to be responsible for metabolism of ethanol-generated acetaldehyde *in vivo* (section 9.5.2). Chronic therapy with 200–400 mg daily doses of DSSD results in a 40–60% inactivation of leukocyte ALDH. Within 2 days of cessation of the therapy, however, the inactivation of leukocyte ALDH wanes and reversion to control values occurs within 4–7 days (Helander *et al.*, 1988; Helander and Carlsson, 1990). Accordingly, to maintain an adequate inhibition of the E_2 enzyme and to protect the patient against ethanol imbibing, interadministration periods of more than 3–4 days should be avoided even when using a dose as high as 500 mg of DSSD. Unsupported statements that individuals receiving DSSD remain sensitized to ethanol for as long as 6 and 21 days (Peachey and Annis, 1984, 1985) require substantiation.

Another parameter of clinical interest is the time of onset of the ethanol-sensitizing effects of DSSD. Hald and Jacobsen (1948a) reported a marked elevation of blood acetaldehyde levels to occur following a challenge with 40 ml of gin 12 h after the administration of 1.5 g of DSSD. From the work of Brown *et al.* (1983) it is apparent that ALDH is already significantly inhibited by 8 h after the administration of a 500 mg dose of DSSD. When individuals who are given this dose consume 0.5 and 1.0 g/kg ethanol 8 and 8.5 h later, their breath acetaldehyde levels 15 min after the ethanol ingestions are clearly higher than those of DSSD-naive controls.

11.6.2 Dose–response relationships and therapeutic dosages

In the early days of DSSD therapy, the treatment paradigm called for much higher dosages of DSSD and for the patient to be challenged with test doses of ethanol as a form of aversion conditioning (section 10.2). Although the therapy was shown to be effective in controlled trials (Wallerstein, 1956, 1958; Wallerstein *et al.*, 1957), the high doses used caused the DER elicited to be frequently severe and some fatalities occurred (section 10.3.5). This resulted in the abandonment of the practice of inducing a DER as an aversive conditioning procedure. It also resulted in a general reluctance on the part of clinicians to test the pharmacological effectiveness of DSSD by administering ethanol. The introduction of a microcrystalline form of DSSD (Hald *et al.*, 1953) of greater effectiveness (Martensen-Larsen, 1950) contributed to the adoption of lower dosages (usually in the 250–500 mg/day range). Until recently, however, much of the information regarding DSSD effectiveness, in the doses currently employed, was anecdotal. A better understanding of the mechanism of the DER has since permitted the development of effective strategies for controlling, and if need be, treating this reaction (section 10.10). As a consequence, studies involving ethanol challenges begun to appear. In evaluating these there is a need to recognize that in Scandinavia an effervescent formulation of DSSD is marketed (sections 1.1 and 10.2) which has a 3-fold greater bioavailabilty than the non-effervescent form available in the United Kingdom (Andersen, 1991), and that *prima faciae* this likely also applies to the non-effervescent forms marketed in the United States and Australia.

How aversive is the DER depends of the levels of blood acetaldehyde. It, in turn, depends on the dose of ethanol (Brown *et al.*, 1983), and on the extent to which E_2 is inhibited, and thus on the dose of DSSD (section 9.2.1). Beyeler *et al.* (1985, 1987), who achieved a mean peak plasma acetaldehyde level of 5.1 µg/ml in the 12 patients in whom they observed a DER reaction (DSSD pretreatment: 400 mg/day for 3–6 days; ethanol challenge dose: 12.7 g/70 kg), reported that the patients all experienced dyspnea, the most unpleasant of the DER effects (section 10.3.2). On the other hand, Peachey *et al.* (1983), who achieved a peak mean blood acetaldehyde level of 2.0 µg/ml in six healthy volunteers (DSSD-pretreatment: 245 mg/70 kg/day for 3 days; ethanol challenge dose: 10.5 g/70 kg), reported an absence of aversive effects. They reported, however, that in a comparable group of volunteers in whom acetaldehyde metabolism was blocked with another agent (calcium carbimide) and a peak mean blood acetaldehyde level of 3 µg/ml was observed, significant dyspnea was observed and the subjects expressed significant discomfort. Thus, it appears that to achieve an aversive reaction, a level of 3–5 µg/ml blood acetaldehyde is required (cf. Table 10.4).

DER-related cardiovascular responses appear to occur at lower blood acetaldehyde levels than aversive symptoms such as dyspnea. This can be concluded from a Scandinavian study (Christensen *et al.*, 1991; Johansson *et al.*, 1991). In that study, non-alcoholic volunteers were challenged with ethanol (0.15 g/kg) after being maintained on various doses of DSSD for 14 days to determine what dose was sufficient to occasion a DER. In defining the DER, in addition to criteria for aversive symptoms, very low threshold cardiovascular response criteria were adopted. Specifically, subjects were deemed to have had a DER if they experienced a 20 mmHg decrease in diastolic blood pressure *or* an increase of 20 beats per min in pulse rate, *or* flushing plus a cumulative subjective score of $\geqslant 6$ on the following symptoms: heat sensation, nausea, vomiting, palpitations, breathlessness and headache, each scored on a 0–3 scale. As a consequence, while the aversive symptoms criteria were satisfied by only 10 of the 52 subject, the cardiovascular response criteria were fulfilled by 51 of the 52. It is telling, therefore, that the median blood acetaldehyde level observed at the time of the thus defined DER was 1.4 µg/ml (range 0.2—8.7) for 48 of these individuals and 2.0 µg/l for the remaining four.

The study by Christensen *et al.* (1991) was designed to determine, using non-alcoholic volunteers, the nature of the DSSD (effervescent formulation) dose-response relationship in a human population. After receiving a 100 mg maintenance dose of DSSD for 14 days, 21 of the 52 subjects (40%) satisfied the DER criteria upon challenge with ethanol. The dose of the remaining 31 subjects was increased to 200 mg DSSD per day. At the end of a further 14 days, all but 4 satisfied the DER criteria. After 14 days on a 300 mg DSSD dose the latter 4 also satisfied these criteria.

Although, in sum, 92% of the subjects satisfied the DER criteria after treatment for 14 days with a DSSD dose not exceeding 200 mg, for all but eight the aversive symptoms were not sufficiently strong to convince them to abstain from drinking. When the DSSD maintenance dose was increased by a further 100 mg, however, the DER reaction elicited by the same amount of ethanol was clearly aversive for most of the subjects. On the basis of these findings, Christensen *et al.* (1991) suggest a dose of 200 to 300 mg might be quite adequate for alcoholics, a suggestion given added weight by the study having been performed under the aegis of Dumex, Ltd., the Danish manufacturer of DSSD.

In a 1984 British study, Brewer reported that, of 63 out-patients maintained on a 200–300 mg/day dosage of DSSD for 1–2 weeks, only 52% had a flush reaction or showed other symptoms of a DER when challenged with 4—8 g of ethanol or when they consumed an alcoholic beverage. After the dose was raised to 400–500 mg/day, 21% still failed to react, and 11% failed to react when the dose was raised further to 600–700 mg/day, although all reacted when the dose was raised further, in one case to 1500 mg/day. These findings represent a non-response rate which is quite surprisingly greater than the data of Beyeler *et al.* (1985, 1987) and Christensen *et al.* (1991) would have suggested. The low response rate may have been due in part to the small ethanol challenge dose employed by Brewer (1984) and in part due the lower bioavailability of the British DSSD formulation. The patients were said by Brewer (1984) to have taken the DSSD in liquid form under 'reliable supervision', a matter of some importance because of the inclusion in the study of habitual offenders who elected the DSSD therapy as a condition of parole (Brewer and Smith, 1983a). In a subsequent publication, Brewer (1986) described how some patients sabotage supervised therapy by, for instance, inducing vomiting after swallowing the medication. When this sabotage technique was discovered, steps were taken to circumvent it (by asking such patients to remain with the supervisor for 30 min following administration). Nonetheless, it would be desirable that this important study be duplicated in a less sociopathic population.

11.6.3 Can disulfiram enhance ethanol-induced euphoria?

A concern that has sometimes been voiced is that alcoholics might find ethanol consumption more euphorogenic while on DSSD therapy (Chevens, 1953). In a double-blind study, Brown *et al.* (1983) asked a group of healthy non-alcoholic males ($n=23$) to consume 0.625 g/kg of ethanol (1.5 drinks per 70 kg) over a 2-h period starting 8 h after a 250 mg dose of DSSD. They observed a significantly greater euphoria in these subjects than in ones pretreated with placebo. They also analyzed, at 30-min intervals, their breath acetaldehyde and ethanol (for each of these substances the levels in breath and blood are proportional). Both the blood acetaldehyde and ethanol levels were higher in the DSSD-pretreated subjects, the ethanol levels by a mean of 20% (to a peak of 80 mg/dl), while the acetaldehyde levels rose to a high of 2.9 µg/ml, a level just below that necessary to elicit a DER (section 11.6.2). Concurrent increases in both acetaldehyde and ethanol blood levels are a common finding when ethanol administration follows DSSD pretreatment. They are due to the inhibition of ethanol elimination by acetaldehyde (section 10.7). Because the ethanol challenges were administered before the onset of maximum inhibition of E_2 by DSSD, the acetaldehyde levels observed were relatively low. Accordingly, the subjects did not experience a DER reaction and could enjoy the effects of the increased ethanol levels. Thus, while partial inhibition of E_2 by DSSD might cause consumption of small amounts of ethanol to have a more euphoriogenic effect than expected, consumption of larger amounts would negate this phenomenon.

11.6.4 Can disulfiram augment craving for ethanol?

A study by Nirenberg *et al.* (1983) is being cited as evidence that DSSD treatment enhances craving for ethanol (Liskow and Goodwin, 1987; Register *et al.* 1990). It therefore warrants closer scrutiny. In their study, Nirenberg *et al.*, (1983) asked alcoholics, who had been abstinent for at least 3 weeks (some on their own, others by using DSSD), to record their cravings daily for the subsequent 2 weeks. There was no significant difference between the frequency with which such cravings were recorded by the two sets of alcoholics during this period. When the second of the 2 weeks was considered separately, however, those using DSSD were seen to have recorded a significantly ($P < 0.05$) greater craving incidence. The authors provide no justification for the statistically problematic *a posteriori* subdivision of the period of observation. In any event, since the patients self-selected DSSD instead of being assigned to that treatment at random, any observed difference could have reflected pre-existing subject differences rather than the effects of DSSD. Nirenberg *et al.* (1983) recognized this and suggested the need for a controlled study. None, however, has been performed to date.

11.6.5 Can drinking through a reaction terminate the effect of disulfiram?

Yet another concern expressed occasionally is that, by drinking through the DER patients may 'burn off' the DSSD. In a double-blind, placebo-controlled study, Peachey *et al.*, (1981c, 1983) administered DSSD (245 mg/70 kg/day for 3 days) to six subjects and, starting 12 h after the last DSSD dose, repeatedly challenged them with very small ethanol doses. The first challenge was with 0.15 g/kg ethanol (equivalent to one third of a drink for a 70 kg person); blood acetaldehyde rose to a peak of 2 µg/ml (insufficient for a DER; section 11.4.2). Thereafter the subjects were challenged three times with 0.05 g/kg doses of ethanol. The first of these challenges occurred 90 min after the 0.15 g/kg challenge, the latter ones at 60-min intervals thereafter. The mean blood acetaldehyde levels in the 60-min periods following these challenges were 0.398, 0.285 and 0.246 µg/ml, respectively. Because the first of these was significantly higher ($P < 0.05$) than the second, Peachey *et al.* (1981c) concluded that 'the important implication of our findings is that, in man, disulfiram may not produce a completely irreversible inhibition.' They also reported, however, that the blood ethanol levels just prior to the first 0.05 g/kg ethanol challenge (but, since it is not mentioned, presumably not just prior to the second one) were significantly greater in the DSSD-pretreated than in the placebo group (as would be expected given that acetaldehyde inhibits ethanol metabolism: see section 10.7). This residual ethanol (from the preceding 0.15 g/kg dose), augmented by the 0.05 g/kg administered as the next challenge, would have led to a higher total body burden of ethanol at the start of the first 60-min period than at the start of the second one. The acetaldehyde levels would have been expected to reflect this and hence their mean values would have been higher. That this was so provided no support, therefore, for the premise that the inhibition of acetaldehyde metabolism by DSSD can be reversed by drinking.

Clinically, it is found that some patients on DSSD therapy try to drink. Bourne *et al.* (1966) reported this to be the case for 25% of a group of skid-row alcoholics. They experienced a reaction and subsequently became the most successful patients. Brewer and Smith (1983a) reported this to be also true of 56% of a group of habitual offenders. Most got 'a severe reaction and did not repeat the experiment.' When drinking does occur, the amounts involved are usually quite low. Thus, Liebson *et al.* (1978) reported that in 3497 DSSD treatment days of 25 patients dually addicted to opiates and alcohol, daily breathalyzer tests indicated positive blood ethanol to be rare and low (mean positive reading: 21 mg/dl). More frequently, if they can, patients discontinue taking DSSD 3 days before imbibing (Fuller and Roth, 1979).

In their DSSD-pretreated subjects, Peachey *et al.* (1981c, 1983) also observed a progressive and significant decline in the magnitude of the tachycardia and flushing responses to repeated ethanol challenges. Such decreases in the tachycardia elicited by an ethanol challenge need not signal a lessening of blood acetaldehyde levels. The tachycardia is a reaction to the acetaldehyde-induced peripheral vasodilation and fall in diastolic blood pressure (section 10.8.1). In DSSD-pretreated individuals, but not in ALDH-deficient DSSD-naive ones, the tachycardia peaks before the minimum of the diastolic pressure response is observed (Fig. 10.1), presumably because it is mediated by norepinephrine release. In DSSD-pretreated individuals, the DSSD-induced inhibition of dopamine β-hydroxylase (DBH) blocks norepinephrine synthesis (section 10.8). Accordingly, upon repeated ethanol challenge, the norepinephrine stores become depleted without a possibility of replenishment, and the response wanes. The mechanism of the flushing response is not understood, but it might similarly occur by a mechanism subject to exhaustion.

11.6.6 Interaction of disulfiram with skin lotions and after-shaves

The quantity of ethanol required to elicit a DER is small, 4–8 gm sufficing in the majority of patients receiving doses of 200–300 mg DSSD (section 11.2.2). Patients need to be warned, therefore, regarding sources of ethanol other than alcoholic beverages and the application of ethanol-containing after-shaves and gels to skin surfaces which might lead to the formation, inhalation, and pulmonary absorption of significant amounts of ethanol vapor. Mercurio (1952), for instance, reported that two patients receiving daily 500 mg DSSD doses for 2 weeks experienced a mild DER upon facial use of an after-shave containing 50% ethanol (1 oz would contain 15 g ethanol). Ellis *et al.* (1979) reported on the DER symptoms experienced by a patient receiving 125 mg of DSSD who, because of psoriasis, had to cover 20% of his body surface with a tar-gel containing one-third ethanol. Mercurio (1952) found that freely sponging the abdomen of DSSD-treated subjects with 70% ethanol elicited only a very mild and transient DER. When the 70% ethanol was dripped on the subjects hands and these were kept near their nares, however, a definite and persistent DER was observed. From this Mercurio concluded that the route of absorption was pulmonary rather than cutaneous.

An analogous reaction has been reported to take place when repeated topical applications are made of an alcoholic solution of monosulfiram, an acaricide with a thioether bridge replacing the disulfide one in DSSD (Burgess, 1990). Since administration of ethanol to rabbits orally pretreated with monosulfiram results in high acetaldehyde blood levels (Hald *et al.*, 1952) it appears that, like DSSD, this agent inhibits acetaldehyde metabolism. In humans, sufficient percutaneous absorption of monosulfiram can occur so that later ethanol ingestion can result in a DER-like syndrome (Gold, 1966; Plouvier *et al.*, 1982; Blanc and Deprez, 1990). Subsequent topical application of the acaricide itself can also have this effect, since its solution is an alcoholic one and inhalation of a sufficient amount of ethanol to cause DER-like symptoms can take place (Burgess, 1990).

Aliphatic alcohols such as ethanol, 1-propanol and 2-propanol (isopropyl alcohol) induce, when applied topically using patch tests, a dose-related cutaneous erythema in hydrated skin, though not in dry skin (Haddock and Wilkin, 1982). DSSD therapy (500 mg/day for 3 days followed by 250 mg/day for 11 days) has no effect on this phenomenon.

11.7 SIDE-EFFECTS OF DISULFIRAM THERAPY

For a physician, knowledge of the nature and incidence of side-effects is important for the rational institution of any therapy. In the case of DSSD, such knowledge is also essential for the patients. Partly this is so because they have to make an informed choice as to whether to request such therapy. In addition, however, the ambivalence that alcoholics feel towards their drinking manifests itself as a preoccupation with the side-effects of DSSD (Christensen *et al.*, 1984; Brubaker *et al.*, 1987) and can lead, in the absence of authentic information, to invention and the spreading of grossly exaggerated rumors regarding the toxicity of DSSD (Lubetkin *et al.*, 1971). A contributory factor in this respect is the difficulty in differentiating pathologies attributable to DSSD, since many of them 'could just as well be interpreted as symptoms caused by long standing alcohol abuse' (Christensen *et al.*, 1984).

DSSD therapy, in a 250 mg/day or a 400 mg thrice weekly dose, is remarkably free of side-effects. This is confirmed by a number of prospective, placebo-controlled, double-blind studies which are reviewed in section 11.7.1. In particular, these studies reveal that, contrary to supposition, DSSD use is not associated with the development of sexual problems, such problems being reported significantly more often by alcoholics receiving placebo medication.

DSSD has been used in the above-mentioned doses chronically and by large numbers of individuals since the mid-1950s. Although some instances of peripheral neuropathy (section 11.7.3) and hepatotoxicity (section 11.7.4) have been reported to result, they have been very few in number. At higher doses peripheral neuropathy, though still rare, if it occurs has an onset time of months rather than years. At such doses DSSD can also induce a reversible encephalopathy (section 11.7.2) and individuals with low pretreatment DBH levels are susceptible to this side-effect when taking DSSD doses of 500 mg/day. Also, concurrent treatment with metronidazole (Flagyl) and DSSD results in a high incidence (20%) of encephalopathies (Rothstein and Clancy, 1969a,b) and is therefore contraindicated.

The toxic interaction between DSSD and ethanol, that is the DER, is discussed separately (Chapter 10); information regarding its treatment is provided in section 10.10.

11.7.1 Controlled-trial studies of disulfiram side-effects

Chronic administration of DSSD to alcoholics in a dose of 200–250 mg/day or 400–500 mg every other day (or 3 times per week), appears to be free of major side-effects. The experience of Christensen *et al.* (1984) in this regard is instructive. Working with alcoholics, these workers found themselves 'constantly confronted with a flood of alleged side effects of disulfiram treatment.' Accordingly, they undertook a carefully designed, multicenter, double-blind, placebo-controlled, randomized study in which the patients ($n = 241$) were questioned regarding 27 expected and non-expected side-effects (the latter to mask the expected ones) during the 6 weeks on DSSD or placebo. Although many symptoms were reported, only one significant difference between the DSSD and placebo groups was observed. This, surprisingly, was the over-representation of sexual problems in the placebo group ($P=0.037$). The next largest difference between the two groups, unpleasant taste in those receiving DSSD, was not significant ($P=0.09$). The dose used by these Danish workers was not a large one (200 mg/day) but it corresponds, for instance, to the dosage recommended (200 mg/day or 400 mg every second day or Monday, Wednesday, Friday) by Sweden's National Board of Health and Welfare (Socialstyrelsen, 1984). Curiously, the greater incidence of sexual problems in the placebo group was also reported by Christensen (1973) and by Bliding *et al.* (1981) on the basis of double-blind cross-over studies ($n=30$ and 6, respectively).

In his cross-over study, Christensen (1973) found that patients on DSSD reported a higher incidence of tiredness, need for sleep, shortness of breath and muscular pains if the period of DSSD administration preceded that during which they received placebo, but not vice versa. These results suggest that these effects are DSSD-induced, but are of such low intensity that they are noticed only when subjects are particularly vigilant, as at the beginning of a clinical study. A similar phenomenon was reported by Silver *et al.* (1979) in another double-blind cross-over study of healthy young men ($n=30$). Those for whom the period of DSSD administration preceded the placebo one reported a higher incidence of drowsiness, difficulty remembering things, and being less excited and active while on DSSD. Conversely, those for whom the DSSD period followed that of placebo administration, failed to report any of these effects. Additionally, Silver *et al.* (1979) noted that the subjects had a higher incidence of abdominal discomfort while on DSSD, irrespective of whether the period of DSSD administration preceded or followed the placebo one. On the other hand, Christensen (1973) found that patients reported a higher incidence of dizziness during the placebo period, whether it preceded or followed that of DSSD administration. No side-effects attributable to DSSD were observed in the controlled studies of Bliding *et al.* (1981) or Sabreus *et al.* (1982), the latter involving 38 healthy young men. Peeke *et al.* (1979) studied the effect of a 2-week course of DSSD treatment (500 mg/day) on the scores of seven healthy volunteers on a battery of cognitive performance tasks. Only 3 of the 34 comparisons between experimental and control period scores showed significant differences. In two of these, the performance of the subjects was superior during the period of DSSD administration. Goyer *et al.* (1984) studied the effect of a 3-week course of DSSD therapy on the depression and anxiety scores of alcoholics. No differences were detected between the scores of a control group ($n = 12$), a group ($n = 13$) receiving a 250 mg/day dose and a group ($n = 12$) receiving a 500 mg/day dose of DSSD.

No side-effect other than drowsiness (Fuller *et al.*, 1986), was reported in the several clinical trials of DSSD therapy discussed in this chapter (section 11.4.2). The incidence of drowsiness was only greater in patients receiving DSSD when these were compared to open controls; there was no difference when the comparison was made with patients receiving a double-blind placebo.

In summary, therapy with moderate doses of DSSD is associated with drowsiness and some abdominal discomfort. The gastrointestinal symptoms tend to disappear if the drug is taken with some food. Drowsiness stops being an issue if the drug is taken last thing at night. It may then be even therapeutic (Lemere, 1953).

11.7.2 Encephalopathies

Psychotic reactions and other encephalopathies are associated with high-dose ($\geqslant 500$ mg/day) DSSD therapy (Bennett *et al.*, 1951; Martensen-Larsen, 1951) as are exacerbations of pre-existing psychoses (Heath et al., 1965; Nasrallah, 1979). No instance of such a reaction has been reported in any controlled therapeutic trials of DSSD (section 11.7.1) in which patients received doses lower than 500 mg/day. The condition is characterized by confusion and disorientation, sometimes by paranoid delusions and occasionally by hallucinations. Upon cessation of DSSD therapy it resolves itself in a few days to a couple of weeks. In 1967 Liddon and Satran reviewed the English language literature reports of these reactions. They found 20 papers reporting on a total of 52 cases. Most of these reports, however, dated from the earliest days of DSSD therapy (Fig. 11.2), that is from a period antedating the reduction of the clinically recommended dosage (section 10.2). Liddon and Satran (1967) stated that during this early period the figures that were published for the incidence of the reaction ranged from 2 to 20% of those receiving the drug, but they cautioned that these 'figures are misleading because they were published more than a decade ago ... and the present incidence is undoubtedly much lower.' This needs to be emphasized for these figures continue to be cited without the caveat (Goyer *et al.*, 1984). In this context it should be noted that in the large collaborative Veterans Administration study (Table 11.1, study 9), the incidence of psychiatric reactions among patients prescribed 250 mg/day of DSSD was not significantly higher than among controls (Branchey *et al.*, 1987).

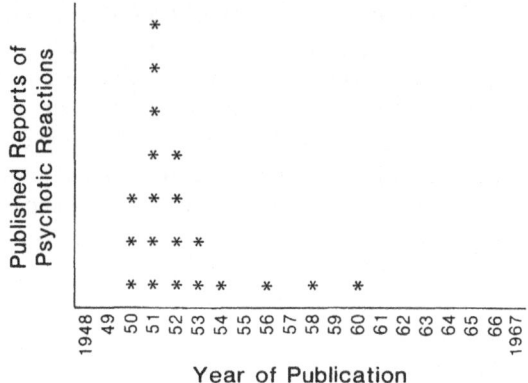

Figure 11.2   Year of publication of 20 reports of psychiatric reactions to disulfiram therapy identified by Liddon and Satran in their 1967 review of the topic. (Relevant dates: disulfiram was introduced for the treatment of alcoholism in 1948; the American Medical Association's Council on Pharmacy and Chemistry recommended dose reduction in 1952.)

Early manifestations of the encephalopathy are lethargy, behavioral withdrawal and depression, progressing to somnolence, ataxia and confusion. If the therapy is not interrupted, disorientation, possibly hallucinations and, rarely, convulsions may ensue (Liddon and Satran, 1967; Price and Silberfarb, 1976; Hotson and Langston, 1976; McConchie *et al.*, 1983). Once DSSD administration is discontinued, such patients make uneventful and full recoveries. In three reported instances, the encephalopathy resulted in the individuals becoming catatonic (Knee and Razani, 1974; Weddington *et al.*, 1980; Fisher, 1989); it is not clear whether this should be viewed as a separate diagnostic entity. In yet another case, the patient developed a bipolar affective disorder (Bakish and Lapierre, 1986).

The reaction appears to result from a derangement of brain catecholamine levels secondary, chiefly, to the inhibition of DBH by DSH through its chelation of the enzyme's copper. Hotson and Langston (1976) were the first to suggest catecholamine involvement upon finding abnormally low lumbar cerebrospinal fluid levels of 3-methoxy-4-hydroxyphenylacetic acid, a metabolite of norepinephrine (HVA Fig. 9.5). Major *et al.*, (1979a,b) were later able to measure the DBH levels in the cerebrospinal fluid of a group of alcoholics and to correlate the occurrence of the psychotic reaction in some of these individuals, to low pretreatment levels of the enzyme. This is particularly interesting because, though human cerebrospinal fluid DBH levels vary quite significantly from individual to individual, they remain remarkably constant in any one individual even when assayed months apart (Sternberg *et al.*, 1983). Major *et al.* (1979a,b) also found that such patients had low plasma amine oxidase, low platelet monoamine oxidase and high red blood cell catechol-*O*-methyl transferase levels. Combined, these latter three parameters were quite predictive of which individuals would develop a psychotic reaction to therapy with 500 mg/day doses of DSSD.

11.7.3 Peripheral neuropathy

Peripheral neuropathy is a rare though potentially severe side-effect of DSSD therapy. No instance of a DSSD-induced peripheral neuropathy has been reported in any of the controlled therapeutic trials. Clinical information regarding the syndrome derives, therefore, entirely from case reports. In an analysis of published reports for the period 1971–88, Frisoni and Di Monda (1989) were able to locate only eight case reports of patients who had developed this condition while on 250 mg/day, and in only one of these was the reaction severe (Table 11.5). Additionally, the mean onset at this dose was 4.6 years, a period more than twice as long as that which most patients require in therapy. Case reports published earlier were summarized by Gardner-Thorpe and Benjamin (1971) and by Mokri *et al.* (1981).

The initial clinical feature of the neuropathy is distal bilateral sensory impairment of the lower extremities (Moddel *et al.*, 1978; Olney and Miller, 1980; Mokri *et al.*, 1981). Patients present with numbness, burning or cramp-like pain and other paresthesias of the distal portions of the feet; later with absence of all modes of sensation to mid calf. Motor involvement is first observed as severe symmetrical weakness of the extensors and flexors of the toes, progressing proximally to foot drop and absence of ankle jerk, then to disturbances of gait, eventually resulting in difficulties in ambulation. Involvement of the upper extremities is a late development seldom observed. Typically, symptoms

Table 11.5 Analysis of case reports of disulfiram neuropathy. Relation of dose to severity and onset latency. From Frisoni and Di Monda (1989)

Daily dose (mg)	Number of case reports		Onset latency
	Total	Severe	
250	8	1 (13%)	4.6 years
400–600	19	13 (68%)	4.3 months
>750	5	3 (60%)	2.6 months

regress following cessation of DSSD therapy, though mild symptoms can persist for a long time.

Ultrastructurally, the condition is characterized by primary axonal degeneration with segmental axonal swellings produced by accumulation of masses of neurofilaments (Ansbacher *et al.*, 1982; Bilbao *et al.*, 1984). In this regard, the histopathology is similar to that seen in the peripheral nerves of animals exposed to CS_2 (Szendzikowski *et al.*, 1974). This correspondence has been advanced as evidence that this DSSD neurofilamentous axonopathy is mediated by the formation of CS_2.

The rarity of the condition suggests that factors other than dose are involved in its occurrence, though what these may be is not clear. In one individual, for instance, the condition developed only after 30 years, though he had taken the same 250 mg/day dose consistently throughout (Borrett *et al.*, 1985). Nonetheless, adjustment of the dose has been linked with changes in clinical status. Thus, a 35-year-old woman, who developed a neuropathy while on 500 mg/day, had no reappearance of the symptoms when, after 1 year's pause, the DSSD therapy was resumed with a 250 mg dose two to four times weekly (Mokri *et al.*, 1981). Likewise, paresthesia of both feet which developed in a 32-year-old man while on 250 mg/day, disappeared when the dose was reduced to 125 mg/day (Worner, 1982). On the other hand, increasing the dose from 750 to 1750 mg/day led to the appearance of neuropathy within a few days in an otherwise symptomless individual (Graveleau *et al.*, 1980).

The differential diagnosis of the DSSD-induced peripheral neuropathy from the ethanol-induced condition is rendered difficult by their considerable similarity (Table 11.6). To make the differentiation it is essential to establish (1) the occurrence of new symptoms during DSSD therapy, (2) abstinence from ethanol and (3) the presence of adequate nutrition.

11.7.4 Hepatotoxicity

Hepatotoxicity is a potentially serious but very rare reaction in patients on DSSD therapy. Berlin (1989) and Kahn *et al.* (1990) identified, respectively, 17 and 19 such cases in the English language literature to date. Reviews of the literature accompany some of the more recent case reports (Nässberger 1984a; Bartle *et al.*, 1985; Black and Richardson, 1985; Kahn *et al.*, 1990). In five cases, a DSSD challenge under controlled conditions resulted in prompt recurrence of the reaction (Ranek and Andreasen, 1977; Morris *et al.*, 1978; Kristensen, 1981;

Table 11.6 Similarities and differences between alcoholic and disulfiram neuropathy. Compiled by Frisoni and Di Monda (1989)

Aspects	Alcoholic neuropathy	Disulfiram neuropathy
History	Months or years of nutritional depletion	Usually a balanced diet
	Long-standing alcohol abuse	Usually no alcohol abuse since beginning of therapy
Onset	Usually insidious over months	Usually a matter of weeks
	Distally in the legs	Same
	Weakness, paresthesias, pain	Same
Progression	Usually slow	Somewhat faster
	More severe distally than proximally	Same
	Often limited to legs	Same
Signs	Symmetrical distribution	Same
	More severe distally than proximally	Same
	Often tenderness of muscles on pressure	Absent
	Constant depression or loss of ankle jerks	Same
	Sometimes disturbances or loss of sweating in the distal segments of limbs	Absent
	Glove and stocking sensory loss of input	Same
	Cranial nerves rarely involved	Same
Laboratory	Usually anaemia and/or macrocytosis	Usually absent
	Usually signs of liver disease	Sometimes sign of liver disease
Other	Sometimes signs of Wernicke disease (nystagmus lateral rectus muscle weakness or paralysis, palsies of horizontal and vertical gaze, postural hypotension, mental confusion)	Sometimes only mental confusion, memory disturbances and drowsiness
Biopsy	Usually axonal degeneration, rarely segmental demyelination	Same, but with axoplasmic neurofilamentous aggregates
EMG	Usually: mild to moderate slowing of motor and sensory conduction; marked decrease of SAP	Often: severe slowing to absence of motor and sensory conduction; marked signs of denervation

Bartle *et al.*, 1985). In two other instances resumption of therapy though not under controlled conditions, also resulted in renewed hepatotoxicity (Keeffe and Smith, 1974; Eisen and Ginsberg, 1975).

The occurrence of the reaction is not dose-dependent. The latency of the onset has varied from a few days to a few months. Typically, fatigue, malaise, nausea, anorexia and vomiting precede the development of jaundice. Serum bilirubin, serum alkaline phosphatase as well as aspartate and alanine aminotransaminases are all elevated. If the DSSD therapy is promptly discontinued, the condition clears in 2–3 weeks. If it is not discontinued massive necrosis can occur and several fatalities have been reported (Ranek and Andreasen, 1977; Schade *et al.*, 1983; Barth *et al.*, 1987).

No evidence of DSSD-induced hepatotoxicity has been reported in any controlled study. In a retrospective evaluation of the effects of DSSD treatment in a group of volunteers (either 250 or 500 mg/day for 3 weeks) no significant change were observed, *vis-à-vis* a control group, in the levels of serum chemistries indicative of hepatotoxicity, namely: serum glutamic oxaloacetic transaminase (SGOT), alkaline phosphatase (AP), lactate dehydrogenase (LDH) and total bilirubin (Goyer and Major, 1979).

Also of interest is the year-long investigation by Iber *et al.* (1987) of the hepatic status of 453 alcoholics who participated in the study of Fuller *et al.* (1986; Table 11.1, study 9). Although at some point elevations of serum bilirubin and aspartate aminotransferase (AST), were observed in 17 and 19% of the total study group respectively, no differences were observed in these indices of hepatotoxicity in the 160 patients prescribed 250 mg DSSD and the 293 controls. Instead significant correlations were observed between serum bilirubin ($P=0.004$) and aspartate aminotransferase ($P=0.004$) elevation and the failure of patients to remain abstinent from ethanol.

The etiology of the clinically reported cases of DSSD hepatotoxicity remains an important but unresolved question. Because of its rarity, its lack of dependence on dose, its variable latency of onset, and the absence of an animal model, it has been suggested that this is an instance of a drug hypersensitivity reaction (Keeffe and Smith, 1974). Yet, as pointed out by Nässberger (1984b) 'generally in drug-induced liver hypersensitivity reactions extrahepatic manifestations are often seen. The most common are fever, skin rashes, malaise and arthralgia. Peripheral eosinophilia is often present. However, in the reported cases of disulfiram induced hypersensitivity extrahepatic manifestations have been scanty.' Evidence at hand (section 8.3.5) suggests that DSSD, like its metabolite CS_2, is metabolized by the liver mixed function oxygenases (MFO) to carbonyl sulfide (COS), a more toxic metabolite. In the process atomic sulfur, a highly reactive form, is generated and becomes covalently bound to the endoplasmic reticulum (Dalvi *et al.*, 1974, 1975).

Although in normal rats CS_2 does not cause liver necrosis in any dose, in animals in whom MFO has been induced by phenobarbital pretreatment, the fraction of administered CS_2 that is oxidized is increased (De Matteis and Seawright, 1973). In such animals, administration of CS_2 causes centrilobular hepatic necrosis (Bond *et al.*, 1969). Workers exposed to CS_2 can also develop centrilobular necrosis (for review see Beauchamp *et al.*, 1983) and it has been suggested that liver damage in such individuals is the result of the combined exposure to CS_2 and to compounds which possess phenobarbital-like inducing activity (Dössing and Ranek, 1984). Exogenous chemical need not be the only factors involved. In rats, for instance, fasting also increases CS_2 liver toxicity (De Matteis and Seawright, 1973).

Hunter and Neal (1975) have reported that administration of DSH (5 mmol/kg in saline i.p.) to rats pretreated with phenobarbital (50 mg/kg i.p. for 5 days) also causes centrilobular necrosis, though administration of DSSD (2.5 mmol/kg in corn oil i.p.) failed to do so. Since DSSD is metabolized to DSH, this discrepancy could be due to the route, dose, or vehicle used. Given that in animal investigations and in controlled prospective clinical studies no evidence of DSSD hepatotoxicity has accrued, the above results suggest that some additional, and as yet unidentified, factor is involved in the rare instances when DSSD treatment leads to icteric changes. Evidently, this is an area that urgently requires further study.

11.7.5 Other side-effects

The DSH formed from DSSD is an inhibitor of DBH and accordingly DSSD therapy decreases synthesis of norepinephrine and thereby impairs sympathetic responses to extreme stress (section 10.8). Surgical anesthesia can present such a stress and Diaz and Hill (1979) reported four cases of serious acute hypotension in patients maintained on either halothane (1) or enflurane (3) and nitrous oxide. In all cases the hypotension responded to discontinuation of the anesthesia and fluid therapy in combination with vasopressors. Discontinuation of DSSD therapy before elective surgery might be indicated.

A case report has been published of hypertension associated with DSSD therapy (Volicer and Nelson 1984). The continued surreptitious consumption of alcohol by the patient renders interpretation problem-

atical. Other side-effects that have been reported include those resulting from the inhibition of drug metabolism (section 8.3.2).

11.7.6 Subclinical effects

Prospective studies of the effects of DSSD therapy on peripheral nerve
function have been undertaken by Palliyath and Schwartz (1988) and
Palliyath *et al.* (1990). In the first of these, 15 recovering alcoholics
were evaluated at 1 and 3 months while receiving 250 mg of DSSD
daily. In the second study, patients were evaluated at 1, 3 and 6 months
while receiving 250 mg ($n=33$) or 125 mg ($n=9$) DSSD daily. No
patient developed overt symptoms of a peripheral neuropathy and no
changes in peripheral nerve function were detected in patients receiving the 125 mg dose. A number of significant, though subclinical,
changes were observed at 6 months, however, in those on 250 mg of
DSSD. Thus there was a reduction in motor nerve (medial and peroneal) conduction velocities, a similar trend being also observed with
regard to the conduction velocities of the medial and sural sensory
nerves. Significant decreases were also observed in motor (median and
peroneal) latency and median sensory amplitude. Interestingly, in the
control patients, a significant improvement in nerve conduction velocities was observed over this same period. These patients, however, had
not been randomly assigned to control status and had baseline conduction velocity values lower than those in the experimental groups, a
possible indication of a greater initial ethanol-induced impairment.

Treatment with DSSD (500 mg/day for 3 weeks) results in an 18%
elevation of serum cholesterol levels (Table 8.1). After 6 weeks, a 37%
elevation is observed (Major and Goyer, 1978). No elevation is seen
during treatment with DSSD in a 250 mg/day dosage. Also, the elevation is not seen with the 500 mg/kg dosage if the patients are
additionally given pyridoxine in a 50 mg/day dosage. The rise in serum
cholesterol is attributable, in some part, to the inhibition of cholesterol
7α-hydroxylase, a specific P-450 hepatic enzyme (sections 8.3.2 and
8.3.4). In rats, the rise in blood cholesterol seen following administration of DSSD (15 mg/kg/day for 3 weeks) is accompanied by an
increased activity of hepatic hydroxy-β-methyl glutaryl coenzyme A
reductase, a rate-limiting step in cholesterol synthesis (Rogers and
Naseem, 1981).

DSSD therapy (800 mg/day for 5 days on withdrawal of ethanol,
followed by 400 mg/day for 3–4 weeks) retards the recovery of
alcoholics from alcohol-induced bone marrow damage (Casagrande
and Michot, 1989). The DSSD regimen was associated with significantly

slower fall in the sideroblast and ring sideroblast counts. The high dose of DSSD and the immediate institution of DSSD therapy upon withdrawal of ethanol are unusual, however, and may have contributed to the effect.

Van Thiel *et al.* (1979) have reported that administration of DSSD (500 mg/kg for 1 week) to healthy male volunteers significantly reduces basal thyroid-stimulating hormone (hTSH) levels and the hTSH response to administration of thyrotropin-releasing factor (TRH). Basal levels of follicle-stimulating hormone (FSH), luteinizing hormone (LH), growth hormone (hGH), prolactin (hProl), thyroxin (T_4), tri-iodothyronine (T_3), and testosterone remain normal, as do the FSH and LH responses to luteinizing hormone-releasing factor and the hTSH, hGH, hProl, T_3 and T_4 responses to TRH.

Gleerup *et al.* (1990) have examined the effect of DSSD administration (800 mg/day for 2 days followed by 400 mg/day for 12 days) to healthy volunteers on platelet function and fibrinolysis. They observed that the high DSSD dose brought about a transient platelet reactivity with collagen though not with adrenaline or ADP. Concurrently plasma β-thromboglobulin and Platelet Factor 4 (PF4) levels were higher. The 14-day treatment decreased euglobulin clot lysis time by 40% and plasma plasminogen activator inhibitor (PAI-1) activity by 30%.

DSH is a potent chelator of metal ions (Chapters 2 and 7). This has lead to the suggestion that DSSD therapy might increase the efficiency of gastric absorption and systemic retention of potentially harmful heavy metals. Hopfer *et al.* (1987) have reported that in alcoholics on DSSD (250 mg/day), serum and urinary nickel levels rise progressively with the duration of therapy. DSH has been used to lower body nickel burdens, and it is not clear what effect such DSSD therapy has on body nickel balance (section 7.2).

Although in experimental animals high doses (200 mg/kg, i.p.) of DSSD can cause inactivation of superoxide dismutase (section 8.4), Ohman and Marklund (1986) have reported that the activity of this enzyme is not significantly depressed in alcoholics receiving DSSD therapy (section 8.4.2).

11.7.7 Role of carbon disulfide

The metabolic formation of CS_2 from DSSD (section 5.6) and its excretion in breath was first shown by Merlevede and Casier (1961) and has been amply documented since (Kraml, 1973; Iber *et al.*, 1977, Paulson *et al.*, 1977; Rogers *et al.*, 1978; Rychtarik *et al.*, 1983; Faiman *et al.*, 1984). CS_2 is an important industrial chemical used in the production of rayon; exposure to it among industrial workers leads to various neuropathologies, including psychoses (Beauchamp *et al.*, 1983). It is not a normal constituent of breath or of intermediary metabolism. It is a highly volatile chemical (b.p. 46 °C) and inhalation of it in the workplace constitutes a continuing industrial hygiene concern, with maximum permissible exposure being set in the United States at 20 ppm (NIOSH, 1985). By way of comparison and based on the figures of Faiman *et al.* (1984), the peak CS_2 concentrations in breath seen during DSSD therapy average 2.7 ppm, and based on the figures of Phillips *et al.* (1986) those in alveolar air reach 14 ppm.

The neurotoxicity seen as the result of exposure to CS_2 has been postulated to be mediated by the formation of dithiocarbamates and chelation of copper and zinc (Bus, 1985). Conversely, the neuropathology seen with DSSD has been postulated to be mediated by the formation of CS_2 (Kane, 1970; Rainey, 1977). Neurofilamentous axonopathy can be observed in both instances (Ansbacher *et al.*, 1982), as already discussed in section 11.7.3.

11.8 CHEMICAL COMPLIANCE MONITORING

The two main methods of testing compliance rely on the excretion of end products of DSSD metabolism: CS_2 in breath and diethylamine (Et_2NH) in urine. CS_2 estimation in expired air is a non-invasive and potentially simple procedure which appears to have been underutilized. The bulk of the literature on the detection of this substance in gaseous samples has been concerned with monitoring CS_2 levels in ambient air as an industrial hygiene measure, using either a static or personal air sampler. The earlier methods all involved trapping of CS_2 in solutions containing diethylamine and copper, followed by evaluation of the chromophore formed (McKee, 1941; Hunt *et al.*, 1973). These methods provide real-time information regarding exposure and efforts have been made to apply them to expired air for the purposes of testing DSSD compliance (Kraml, 1973; Paulson *et al.*, 1977; Rogers *et al.*, 1978; Rychtarik *et al.*, 1983). Gas chromatographic methods have also been proposed for determination of CS_2 in breath, either directly in a sample of alveolar air (Phillips *et al.*, 1986), or by first trapping in Et_2NH solution, followed by chromatography of the methyl ester of diethyldithiocarbamic acid formed by the addition of methyl iodide (Wells and Koves, 1974). Compliance testing methods based on the presence of Et_2NH in the urine have been developed by Neiderhiser *et al.* (1976) and by Gordis and Peterson (1977). Fuller and Neiderhiser (1981) have reported on the clinical use of such a test.

An alternative more general methodology is the incorporation in the compounding of the medication of some indicator substance which is excreted in urine and easily identified therein. This method was employed by Fuller *et al.* (1983, 1986) who used 50 mg of riboflavin as a marker. Effective as such a method might be in a research setting, its wider use in treatment involving contingencies related to non-compliance would likely spur ingenious efforts at generating false positive urines.

11.9 DISULFIRAM IMPLANTS

For any drug which has to be taken daily on a chronic basis and for which compliance is a problem, administration in depot form as an implant is an obvious solution. Although the implanting of DSSD tablets was introduced early in DSSD's therapeutic history (Marie, 1955) and has been used extensively in some venues, all available evidence indicates that administered in this form, DSSD is not pharmacologically effective. Partly this may be due to the dose employed: Marie (1955) implanted up to 8×150 mg tablets, more recently it has been usual to implant 10×100 mg tablets. This is only two to four times the effective daily oral dose and it is difficult to envisage why it should cause inhibition of ALDH which lasts several months. The lack of pharmacological effectiveness may be also partly due to the low rate at which the DSSD is absorbed. When such tablets are implanted in the rat, in some experiments it takes in excess of 60 days for half the DSSD in the tablet to be absorbed (Hellström *et al.*, 1980), while in others very little absorption takes place at all (Fried, 1980), the differences being attributed by the experimenters to surgical technique. Lewis *et al.* (1975) measured levels of CS_2 (a metabolite of DSSD; Section 11.8) in the breath of patients following implantation of $1-3$ g of DSSD. They observed measurable levels in two-thirds of the patients in the period between 7 days and 12 weeks post implantation, suggesting that the dissolution rate of the tablets in humans is also slow. These workers also found that infusion of 5% ethanol $2-9$ weeks post implantation resulted in mild inebriation, but no DER reactions.

The lack of pharmacological effectiveness of 1 g implants of DSSD tablets has been reported in a number of studies. Bergström *et al.* (1982) reported that when patients implanted with 1 g of DSSD were challenged by the oral administration of 15 g of ethanol $4-6$ weeks later, none ($n = 11$) developed significant blood acetaldehyde levels and none experienced a significant DER, as judged by objective measures (changes in heart rate and blood pressure). Mörland *et al.*

(1984) and Johnsen *et al.* (1990), using sensitive assays of blood acetaldehyde levels, also failed to observe any significant differences in its levels following ethanol challenge of DSSD and placebo-implanted controls. In a double-blind study, Wilson *et al.* (1980) found that both DSSD- and placebo-implanted patients had more intense DERs, as judged by a number of subjective measures, than two groups of non-operated controls. This suggested that the subjective DER symptoms reported to occur following ethanol challenge of DSSD-implanted individuals in previous uncontrolled studies are ascribable to a placebo effect. In keeping with this, no differences have been found in relapse rates between DSSD- and placebo-implanted alcoholics (Borg *et al.*, 1984).

With the realization that DSSD tablet implants are ineffective, the use of other depot forms of DSSD is being explored. Phillips (1988) has administered to alcoholics ($n = 2$) finely powdered gamma-irradiation-sterilized DSSD (Phillips *et al.*, 1985) suspended in 15–25 ml normal saline. The drug was injected s.c. following infiltration of the site with local anesthetic. Upon challenge with ethanol (0.15 g/kg p.o.), at 7–28 days post administration of 1–2 g of this form of DSSD, Phillips observed significantly higher blood acetaldehyde levels and decreases in blood pressure (diastolic and systolic) than seen in the pretreatment period. Carey-Smith *et al.* (1988) also administered 1 g of the gamma-irradiation-sterilized DSSD, but in a 20% emulsion of soybean oil (4 ml) by deep i.m. injection. Mild to moderate liver function abnormalities were noted, as were local irritation, pain and some muscle spasms at the site of injection. Since no diethylamine, a DSSD metabolite, could be detected in urine, the authors concluded the side-effects might be vehicle-induced.

12

Immunomodulatory effects of diethyldithiocarbamate

12.1	INTRODUCTION	248
12.2	STIMULATON OF ANTIBODY RESPONSE TO SHEEP RED BLOOD CELLS	249
12.3	ENHANCEMENT OF MITOGEN-INDUCED LYMPHOPROLIFERATION	251
	12.3.1 Experimental animals	251
	12.3.2 Humans	254
12.4	EFFECT ON LYMPHOPROLIFERATIVE RESPONSE TO ALLOANTIGENS	255
12.5	INTERACTION WITH ASYMMETRICAL NEOCORTICAL LESIONS	256
12.6	EFFECTS ON CELL-MEDIATED CYTOTOXICITY	257
	12.6.1 Effects on T_c-cell-mediated activity	257
	12.6.2 Effects on natural killer cell activity	257
	12.6.3 Effects on antibody-mediated cellular cytotoxicity	260
12.7	EFFECT ON DELAYED-TYPE HYPERSENSITIVITY REACTION	261
12.8	INDUCTION OF T-CELL DIFFERENTIATION	261
	12.8.1 *In vivo* production of serum factors	261
	12.8.2 Hepatosin induction	264
	12.8.3 Direct *in vitro* induction of T-cell differentiation	265
	12.8.4 Effects on nuclear refringency	266
	12.8.5 Effect on lymphokine production	267
12.9	EFFECT ON LYMPHOCYTE POPULATIONS *IN VIVO*	267
	129.1 Experimental animals	267
	12.9.2 Humans	271
12.10	EFFECTS ON MONONUCLEAR PHAGOCYTIC CELLS	272
12.11	EXPERIMENTAL THERAPEUTICS	273
12.12	IMMUNOMODULATORY EFFECTS OF RELATED COMPOUNDS	275
12.13	CONCLUSIONS	275

12.1 INTRODUCTION

Diethyldithiocarbamate (DSH) has many interesting and potentially important immunomodulatory effects. Most of these were first described by Renoux and co-workers who, in their publications, referred to DSH as Imuthiol®. This body of work has remained little cited, likely due to lack of awareness of the equivalence of the two terms.

Imuthiol® is the trade name of the anhydrous sodium salt of diethyldithiocarbamic acid prepared by the Institut Mérieux of Lyon, France. It is obtained by dissolving commercial DSH in water, filtering it through a 150–250 µm membrane, then through a 0.2 µm membrane, and lyophilizing it at <40°C (De La Bastide *et al.*, 1986). It has been claimed that this brand of DSH is free of impurities said to comprise 10–12% of commercial samples of DSH (Renoux *et al.*, 1979; Renoux, 1981; Renoux and Renoux, 1981). Since much of the work on the immunostimulant properties of DSH has been performed using this anhydrous form of DSH rather than the trihydrate (section 2.1) the DSH doses and concentrations noted in this chapter are given in terms of the anhydrous material, unless otherwise specified. Imuthiol® has also been dispensed in the form of a gastroprotected pill suitable for oral administration (Renoux *et al.*, 1983b).

Many of the diverse immunostimulatory effects of DSH appear to be mediated indirectly by its effects on T-cell lineage. The primary evidence that has led to this conclusion falls under three rubrics. Firstly, administered concurrently with immunization against sheep red blood cells (SRBC), DSH increases the number of spleen cells producing IgG antibodies to this antigen, and later also the serum level of these antibodies. The production of such antibodies is considered to be a T-cell-dependent effect. Secondly, administered *in vivo*, DSH, though itself devoid of mitogenic activity, stimulates the lymphoproliferative response of mouse spleen cells and human peripheral blood mononuclear cells (PBMC) to phytohemagglutinin (PHA) and Concanavalin A (Con A), both T-cell mitogens. Thirdly, evidence has accrued of the induction of T-cell differentiation itself by DSH. Thus, *in vivo* administration of DSH to nude, athymic and thereby T-cell-deficient mice, results in the appearance in the spleen of these animals of cells bearing markers characteristic of T cells. Likewise, long-term culture of human PBMC with DSH results in the induction of CD3$^+$ and CD4$^+$ T cells from null cells.

The T-cell differentiation induced by DSH is not a direct effect. Thus, no differentiation occurs when DSH is incubated with human peripheral blood lymphocytes (PBL) depleted of monocytes or with nude mouse spleen cells *in vitro*. In mice, a T-cell differentiation-inducing factor, hepatosin, is produced by liver cells exposed to DSH. It remains to be fully characterized, as does the nature of the DSH-generated monocyte-produced signal that induces T-cell differentiation in PBMC cultures.

The other immunostimulatory effects of DSH that have been described all have the potential of being mediated, to various degrees, by the effects of DSH on T-cell lineage. These include lymphoproliferative responses to alloantigens, T-cell-mediated cytotoxicity, delayed-type hypersensitivity, antibody-dependent cell cytotoxicity, and even natural killer cell activity.

Given the low toxicity and short half-life of DSH, the diversity, uniqueness, and long duration of the immunomodulatory effects of relatively small single doses of this agent are little short of astonishing. Some special affinity of DSH, or its metabolites, for immune tissues may play a role (section 6.6.5). Although DSH itself is a metabolite of disulfiram (DSSD), a drug on the formulary of most countries, there has been virtually no work done to determine the degree to which the parent compound shares the immunomodulatory effects of DSH.

12.2 STIMULATION OF ANTIBODY RESPONSE TO SHEEP RED BLOOD CELLS

DSH, when administered s.c. to mice concurrently with i.v. immunization with 10^8 SRBC, can increase significantly the immunological response to this antigen. This is rendered apparent by an increase in the number of anti-SRBC (α-SRBC) IgM and IgG antibody-producing B lymphocytes in the spleen (Renoux and Renoux, 1974, 1977b; Renoux *et al.*, 1977) and by the appearance, 20 days after immunization, of a significant increase in the titers of α-SRBC IgG in blood (Renoux and Renoux, 1979). The antibody-producing cells are commonly referred to as the plaque-forming cells (PFC), an appellation that refers to the clear zones, or plaques, that appear around these cells when the surrounding SRBC, having been plated, incubated and sensitized by the α-SRBC antibodies are lysed. In the case of IgM-coated cells, the lysis occurs directly upon exposure to complement (hence direct PFC), while those coated with IgG have to be first exposed to α-IgG (hence indirect PFC).

Administration of DSH (0.5–25 mg/kg) concurrently with the SRBC immunization enhances both the direct and indirect PFC responses, i.e. both IgM- and IgG-PFC (Renoux *et al.*, 1977; H Renoux and Renoux, 1977b). Class switching by B lymphocytes from IgM to IgG is a T-lymphocyte-dependent phenomenon. Accordingly, this finding was one of considerable interest, since it indicated that the DSH effect was

T-cell-mediated. Also, the enhancement of the direct α-SRBC PFC response by administration of DSH concurrently with the immunization is not a non-specific polyclonal one, since DSH concurrently suppresses the normal direct non-specific response of mouse spleen cells to horse red blood cells (Renoux and Renoux, 1979; Renoux, 1984). Additionally, the enhancement of the α-SRBC response induced by *in vivo* DSH administration occurs without any concomitant alteration in the counts of viable spleen lymphocytes or changes in body, spleen, or liver weights, though a significant increase in the weight of the thymus takes place (Renoux *et al.*, 1979, 1987). DSH is not effective, however, *in vitro*: the secretion of α-SRBC IgM and IgG by spleen cells from mice immunized 4 days previously with 10^8 SRBC is uniformly inhibited by addition of DSH to the incubation medium (Renoux and Renoux, 1977b).

More surprisingly, administration of DSH to nude (*nu/nu*) mice concurrently with immunization with SRBC also results in a   splenic α-SRBC IgG-PFC response. The normal splenic PFC response of these athymic mice is characterized by the total absence of IgG-secreting cells (Renoux and Renoux, 1977a; Renoux, 1980). Accordingly, these results suggested not only that the DSH effect is T-cell-mediated, but also that DSH induces T-cell differentiation.

The enhancement of the IgG-PFC response induced by DSH administration concurrent to SRBC immunization peaks, in female BALB/c and C3H/He mice, after 2–3 days, though it persists for at least 7 days (Renoux and Renoux, 1981, 1984; Renoux, 1982). Other evidence suggests that in the C3H/He mice the effect persists for a month (Renoux, 1982). Also, in these mice co-administration of DSH with a SRBC priming challenge triples the α-SRBC PFC response observed following a second, or boosting, administration of 10^5 SRBC a month later. A further dose of DSH, this one concurrent with the SRBC boosting, increases the response 7-fold. Moreover, a single 25 mg/kg dose of DSH, administered a month after a priming dose of 10^8 SRBC, is as effective in enhancing the α-SRBC PFC response as a boosting with 10^5 SRBC (Renoux, 1982). On the basis of these findings, Renoux (1982) suggested that DSH administration increases considerably the number of memory T cells.

Efforts to ascertain the location of the genes controlling the DSH-induced enhancement of the α-SRBC PFC response have not been successful. DSH enhances uniformly the α-SRBC IgM- and IgG-PFC responses of mice of both the BALB/c [*H-2^d*] and   C3H/He [*H-2^k*] inbred strains. On the other hand, the enhancement of these responses in mice of the DBA/2 [*H-2^d*], C57BL/6 [*H-2^b*] and A/J [*H-2^a*] strains is class-, gender- and dose-specific (Renoux, 1982). Thus, the ability of DSH to enhance the response is not linked to the major histocompatibility complex (MHC) genes. Nor does it appear to be linked to the Qa locus, since in Qa-congenic mice (i.e. differing only by alleles at this locus) DSH enhances proportionately the α-SRBC IgM- and IgG-PFC responses of the Qa-1⁻ strain [*B6-H-2ᵏ*] and the Qa-1⁺ strain [*B6TL(+)*] (Renoux, 1984). Since the ability of DSH to enhance the response is, in some inbred strains, gender-specific, it has been suggested that the factors mediating the enhancement may be associated with the Y chromosome (Renoux, 1982; Guillaumin *et al.*, 1984).

Finally, DSH administration, unlike that of the immunostimulant levamisole, has never been found to inhibit the IgG-PFC response to SRBC immunization, though the effect of DSH administration on this response has been studied in many mouse strains and under a variety of experimental conditions (Renoux and Renoux, 1977a,b, 1979, 1980a, 1981, 1983, 1984; Renoux *et al.*, 1977, 1984; Renoux, 1982, 1984; Guillaumin *et al.*, 1984; Renoux and Biziere, 1987).

12.3 ENHANCEMENT OF MITOGEN-INDUCED LYMPHOPROLIFERATION

12.3.1 Experimental animals

In vivo pretreatment of mice with DSH can enhance the *in vitro* splenic lymphoproliferative response (S-LPR) of these animals to the mitogens PHA and Con A, given the right combination of pretreatment interval, strain, and mitogen (Fig. 12.1). Typically, the S-LPR is evaluated by preparing a suspension of spleen cells and culturing these with the mitogen. After 48 h of culture a 'pulse' of ³H-thymidine is added; the amount of the thymidine incorporated after a further 18 h of culture is a measure of DNA synthesis.

The *in vivo* administration of DSH itself is not mitogenic in mice (Renoux, 1982; Renoux *et al.*, 1984; M. Renoux *et al.*, 1986). At the same time, PHA and Con A specifically stimulate T-cell proliferation. Accordingly, it follows that the DSH-induced enhancement of the S-LPR to these mitogens is T-cell-mediated. In fact, the DSH-pretreatment-induced enhancement of the S-LPR to these mitogens is abrogated if Qa-1⁺ splenocytes are selectively removed by cytolysis with α-Qa-1 serum and complement (Renoux, 1984). The Qa-1 marker is characteristic of the T-cell subset mainly responsible for helper activity (Stanton *et al.*, 1978). Moreover, in nude mice, DSH pretreatment both markedly enhances the S-LPR to PHA and Con A and markedly increases the number of Thy-1⁺ splenocyte (Renoux and Renoux, 1983; Renoux *et al.*, 1984). The Thy-1 marker is considered characteristic of mature T cells, and nude mice, being athymic, are considered to lack T cells (Milich and Gershwin, 1977). Normally these mice have very few Thy-1$^+$ cells. Thus the DSH-induced stimulation of the S-LPR to mitogens is correlated in these animals with the induction of what appear to be T cells.

Although the ability of DSH to enhance the S-LPR to mitogens is clear, when the time course of the effect was investigated, DSH pretreatment times were found that result in the depression of S-LPR to one or both of these mitogens in all three strains studied (Renoux and Renoux, 1981, 1984). Fig. 12.1 shows the complexity of the time course of these phenomena; at certain pretreatment times, the effects of DSH are strain-determined and quite dissimilar. A 1 hr DSH pretreatment, for instance, enhances the S-LPR to Con A in C3H/He mice, but it depresses it in BALB/c mice. Yet, the time courses of the DSH enhancement of the splenic α-SRBC IgG-PFC response in these two strains are relatively parallel (Renoux and Renoux, 1981, 1984; Renoux, 1982). Beyond this, differences also exist between the effect of DSH on the LPR of spleen and lymph node cells (M. Renoux *et al.*, 1986).

Although DSH pretreatment also stimulates the S-LPR response to PHA and Con A in the guinea pig, the time course is quite different. Marked stimulation occurs on days 12 and 16, but not on days 4 and 8 post administration (Neveu *et al.*, 1982). Additionally, in the guinea pig, the concurrent S-LPR to pokeweed mitogen (PWM) and lipopolysaccharide (LPS) of *E. coli* are also enhanced by DSH pretreatment (Neveu *et al.*, 1982). In mice, DSH pretreatment consistently fails to enhance the S-LPR to PWM (Renoux and Renoux, 1980a, 1981, 1983, 1984; Renoux, 1982, 1984; Renoux *et al.*, 1984; Renoux and Biziere, 1987) or LPS (M. Renoux *et al.*, 1986).

DSH is a potent chelating agent. *In vivo*, zinc is one of the most abundant ions that it is known to chelate (sections 2.3 and 7.7). The enhancement of S-LPR by DSH pretreatment does not appear, however, to be mediated by the formation of the zinc chelate of DSH, $Zn(DS)_2$. Thus, pretreatment of female BALB/c mice with $Zn(DS)_2$, in doses of 0.1–5.0 mg/kg, s.c. administered 1–8 days previously, does not enhance the S-LPR to PHA or Con A. On the contrary, a 2.5 mg/kg dose of $Zn(DS)_2$ significantly ($P < 0.001$) depresses the response. On the other hand, a 1.0 mg/kg dose of the chelate significantly ($P < 0.01$) enhances the S-LPR to PWM (Renoux *et al.*, 1988b).

Chronic DSH treatment has particularly marked effects on the S-LPR to mitogens in mice. Thus, pretreatment of C3H/He mice with 25 mg/kg DSH 3 times per week for 4 weeks, enhances 2.0- and

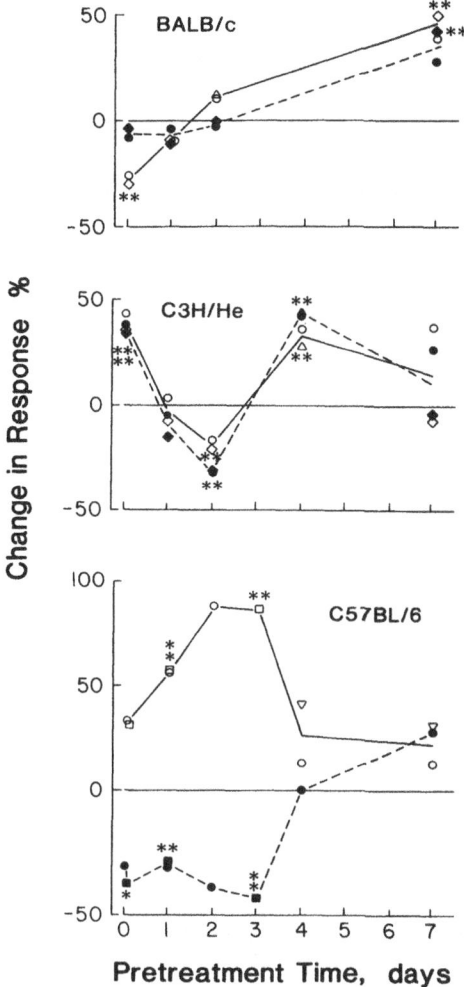

Figure 12.1 Composite summarizing graphically reports of the effects of *in vivo* diethyldithiocarbamate (DSH) pretreatment on the lymphoproliferative response to mitogens of mouse spleen cells from three inbred strains. Abscissa: pretreatment time relative to harvesting of spleen cells, first point at 1 h; ordinate: changes in magnitude of response relative to that of spleen cells from control mice. Closed symbols: phytohaemagglutinin; open symbols: Concanavalin A. The shape of the symbols identifies the source of the data. [Diamonds, data of Renoux *et al.* (1983b); circles, Renous and Renoux (1984); squares, M. Renoux *et al.* (1986); triangles, Mansour *et al.* (1986); inverted triangles, Renoux and Biziere (1987). DSH dose: Renoux and coworkers, 25 mg/kg; Mansour *et al.*, 125 mg/kg. For other experimental details see original publications.] Straight lines have no significance except as visual aids. $^*P<0.05$; $^{**}P<0.01$.

2.6-fold the day 4 S-LPR to PHA and Con A, respectively (Renoux and Renoux, 1980a). Except in nude mice, this level of enhancement is never observed following a single DSH dose (Fig. 12.1). In contrast, the effect of such chronic treatment on the α-SRBC IgG-PFC response 4 days post SRBC immunization is no greater than a single dose (Renoux and Renoux, 1980a).

The apparently profound effects of chronic DSH treatment are evident from the effects on the offspring of treated dams. The S-LPR to PHA of both male and female offspring at 20 days of age is significantly ($P<0.01$) enhanced by the administration of 25 mg/kg DSH to their C3H/HeJ dams twice a week for 3 weeks prior to mating and until birth, or alternatively from fecundation to birth (3 weeks). Maternal DSH pretreatment also enhances the S-LPR to Con A, but in a manner that is determined by the interaction of gender and treatment. If the treatment of the dams is begun prior to mating, then the enhancement in the male offspring is greater than in either the female or control pups. Conversely, if the dams are treated only after mating, then the enhancement in the female offspring is greater than in either the male or control pups (Renoux *et al.*, 1985).

The *in vitro*-induced S-LPR to mitogens is generally considered to mimic that induced *in vivo* by specific antigens (Roitt *et al.*, 1989). Renoux (1985a) has questioned, on the basis of the disparate responses illustrated in Fig. 12.1, the appropriateness of doing so with reference to the actions of DSH.

12.3.2 Humans

The human peripheral blood mononuclear cell lymphoproliferative response (PBMC-LPR) to mitogens is considered to be an indicator of functional immune status. Accordingly, its enhancement by *in vivo* pretreatment with a drug has potential clinical significance. Renoux *et al.* (1983b) have reported, in the context of a review article, that 5 days after DSH administration (5 mg/kg i.v.) to lung cancer patients in remission, a significant ($P<0.01$) stimulation of the PBMC-LPR to PHA and Con A was observed (see Fig. 12.2).

In vitro, 10^{-5} to 10^{-3} μg/ml (5.8×10^{-11} to 5.8×10^{-9} M) DSH enhances significantly the day 5 PBMC-LPR response to PHA (Mossalayi *et al.*, 1986). In slightly higher concentrations (17×10^{-3} μg/ml) DSH is without effect and at 43×10^{-3} to 86×10^{-3} μg/ml it massively inhibits (99%) the 4 day PBMC-LPR to both PHA and Con A under analogous conditions (Neveu *et al.*, 1980). Interestingly, depletion of

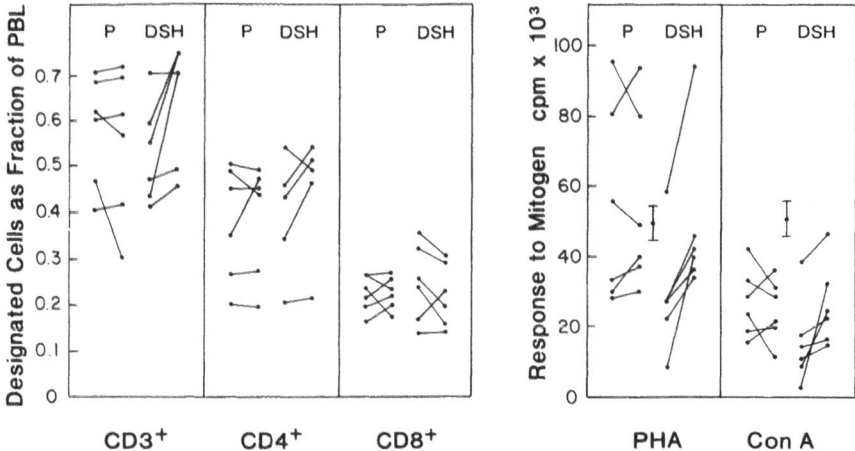

Figure 12.2 Diethyldithiocarbamate (DSH) associated changes in peripheral blood lymphocytes of lung cancer patients. Left: changes in surface markers. Right: changes in the lymphoproliferative responses to mitogen stimulation. Blood was sampled prior to and 5 days after i.v. administration of either 5 mg/kg DSH or placebo (P). Mitogens: PHA, phytohaemagglutinin; Con A, Concanavalin A. *P* values for DSH associated changes in CD3$^+$, CD4$^+$, and responses to PHA and Con A were all *P*<0.01; that in CD8$^+$ was *P*=0.06. Redrawn from Renoux *et al.* (1983b).

the PBMC culture of macrophages significantly decreases (to 29%; *P*<0.005) the inhibitory effect of DSH in the 43×10^{-3} µg/ml concentration on the PBMC-LPR to PHA. The effect of the higher DSH concentration is, however, undiminished by macrophage depletion. In the absence of DSH, macrophage depletion had no effect on the PBMC-LPR to PHA. Addition of 2-mercaptoethanol (2-ME) also reverses the inhibitory effect of DSH on the PBMC-LPR to PHA, but the significance of this is harder to determine, since 2-ME stimulates by 61% (*P*<0.001) the PBMC-LPR to PHA in control cultures (Neveu *et al.*, 1980). At higher concentrations yet (viz. 3 µg/ml) DSH inhibits the spontaneous incorporation of ^{3}H-thymidine by the Raji lymphoid cell line (Corke, 1984).

12.4 EFFECT ON LYMPHOPROLIFERATIVE RESPONSE TO ALLOANTIGENS

The effect of DSH pretreatment on the MHC-restricted response to alloantigens has been investigated using mixed lymphocyte culture

(MLC). The first step in the response is considered to be the recognition of class 2 MHC antigens by CD4$^+$ T cells; it leads to activation.

In vivo pretreatment of C3H/He mice with 25 mg/kg DSH 5 days prior to harvesting of spleen cells results in a marked enhancement of the LPR to the alloantigens of mitomycin-treated C57Bl/6 mouse spleen cells in a 5-day MLC (Renoux *et al.*, 1984; Renoux and Biziere, 1987).

12.5 INTERACTION WITH ASYMMETRICAL NEOCORTICAL LESIONS

Though this may be surprising, there is an increasing body of evidence that the immune system is under the lateralized influence of the brain's neocortex (Neveu, 1988). Renoux and co-workers (Renoux, 1980; Renoux *et al.*, 1982c, 1983c) reported that, in mice, large lesions of the left neocortex result in a depression of T-cell-mediated functions, while those of the right neocortex augment them. These findings were confirmed by Neveu's group (Neveu *et al.*, 1986a,b; Barneoud *et al.*, 1987) though almost diametrically opposite effects are obtained if smaller lateral lesions, confined to the dorsal part of the parieto-occipital cortex, are made (Barneoud *et al.*, 1987).

Obviously, much remains to be learned about these phenomena. Be that as it may, the effects of *in vivo* DSH administration on T-cell-dependent immunological events are markedly and asymmetrically affected by partial right and left neocortical ablations of the type used by Renoux and co-workers (for review see Renoux, 1988). For example, the stimulation of the α-SRBC PFC-IgG response and the S-LPR to PHA and Con A observed following *in vivo* pretreatment with DSH are either unaffected or enhanced by lesions of the left neocortex, but lesions of the right neocortex totally abrogate them (Renoux *et al.*, 1984; Renoux and Biziere, 1987). The same pattern is found for the effect of lateral neocortical lesions on several other immunomodulatory effects of DSH, namely on the *in vivo* production of serum factors that can induce T-cell differentiation (section 12.8.1). An almost complementary pattern has been reported for the effect of these lateral lesions on the immunomodulatory effects of DSH on natural killer cell activity (section 12.6.2). Likewise, lesions of the left neocortex abrogate the stimulation brought about by *in vivo* pretreatment with DSH of the C3H/He splenic lymphocyte response in MLC to the alloantigens of mitomycin-treated spleen cells from C57Bl/6 mice (section 12.4). Lesions of the right neocortex, on the other hand, enhance the stimulation (Renoux *et al.*, 1984; Renoux and Biziere, 1987).

12.6 EFFECTS ON CELL-MEDIATED CYTOTOXICITY

The effects of DSH on the three types of cell-mediated cytotoxicity which are recognized as possessing *in vivo* significance, namely those attributable to the MHC-restricted cytotoxic T (T_C) cells, to natural killer (NK) cells, and to the K cells involved in the antibody-dependent cellular cytotoxicity (ADCC), have each been investigated in a number of studies. The observations reported to date and discussed below present a complex, confusing, and incomplete array of significant effects which suggest complex time courses and dependence on the age of the animals used.

12.6.1 Effects on T_C-cell-mediated activity

Aging is associated with a decline in the splenic T_C responses. It is of some interest therefore that DSH, administered chronically (25 mg/kg/week s.c. for 16 weeks), markedly enhances the T_C cell activity in spleens of 16-month-old BALB/c [H-2^d] mice (Bruley-Rosset *et al.*, 1986). These workers assayed the cytotoxic activity upon harvesting the spleen cells 5 days after the last dose of DSH and culturing them with mitomycin-treated EL4 [H-2^b] lymphoma cells for 5 days. A follow-up report from the same laboratory (Florentin *et al.*, 1988) indicates that the response observed is a function of both the frequency with which DSH is administered and the amount of time allowed to pass between the last dose of DSH and the spleen cell harvest. Thus, significant ($P < 0.01$) enhancement results if the DSH is administered every 7 days, be it for 1, 4, or 16 weeks. If it is administered with either higher (3 times a week for 4 weeks) or lower (every 14 days for 16 weeks) frequency, the cytotoxic responses are depressed below those of controls. The length of time allowed to pass between the last DSH dose and spleen-cell harvest also has a decisive effect on the response observed. Thus in young BALB/c (Florentin *et al.*, 1988) and nude, athymic mice of BALB/c background (Florentin *et al.*, 1989) the T_C activity of spleen cells is most enhanced when these are harvested 7 days following DSH administration (be it as a single dose or the last of several weekly doses). Harvesting of BALB/c mouse spleen cells 3 days post the last dose of DSH gives the least enhacement, while the T_C activity of the spleen cells of the athymic mice harvested 2 or 5 days post DSH is actually inhibited.

12.6.2 Effects on natural killer cell activity

Renoux and co-workers have published a number of reports touching on the effects of *in vivo* DSH pretreatment on the NK activity of unfractionated mouse spleen cells. It is clear from reviewing the resulting complex, but sparsely filled data array (Table 12.1) that this agent enhances the splenic NK activity under a variety of specific conditions of age, pretreatment time, strain and DSH dosage. However, the DSH pretreatment can also inhibit splenic NK activity, given the right strain, age and pretreatment time (Table 12.1). The data permit few across-category comparisons and hence few, if any, generalizations about the effects of DSH on NK activity. Moreover, because the NK activity in question is that of unfractionated spleen cells, no information is available as to whether the DSH-induced enhancement of NK activity is due to NK cell proliferation, enhanced target binding or increased specific lytic activity. Finally, although NK cells constitute 2–5% of PBMC in humans, no information is available on the effect of DSH therapy on NK activity of human PBMC.

NK activity decreases naturally with age. Given the right pretreatment time, DSH stimulates NK activity in mice of both the C3H/He (Renoux *et al.*, 1982b, 1983b) and BALB/c strains (Florentin *et al.*, 1989) irrespective of age, but the extent of the stimulation is greater in young (8–10 weeks) mice (Bardos *et al.*, 1985; Florentin *et al.*, 1989). In nude, athymic mice of BALB/c background, animals which possess few T_C cells but high NK activity, DSH suppresses this activity (Florentin *et al.*, 1989), though again pretreatment time is crucial (greatest effect with a 7-day pretreatment, no effect with 2- or 5-day pretreatments). Since this represents a mirror image of the effect of DSH on T_C activity in these animals, it may be that DSH induces maturation of T_C cells from a prethymic subset of cells with NK activity.

NK cells lack both immunological memory and MHC restriction. Although these cells are stimulated by IL-2, the IL-2 effect could occur *via* a stimulation, in turn, of interferon (IFN) production, since IFN is known to also stimulate NK cells. This does not appear to be the case, however, since serum IFN titers in 8-week-old C3H/He mice and the 6- to 8-week old C57Bl/6 mice are not modified by DSH pretreatment at the times corresponding to or preceding changes in splenic NK activity (Renoux *et al.*, 1982b, 1983b; M. Renoux *et al.*, 1986)

Bardos *et al.* (1981) reported on the neocortical lateralization of NK activity in mice. Briefly, they found that lesions of the left neocortex severely depressed the splenic NK activity, but that right neocortical lesions were without effect. It is of interest, therefore, that 4 days following administration of DSH to mice with such lesions, NK activity of animals with lesions of the right neocortex is enhanced in a manner

Table 12.1 Modification of natural killer (NK) activity of mouse splenocytes induced by *in vivo* diethyldithiocarbamate (DSH) administration[a]

DSH Dose mg/kg	Animals Strain	age weeks	2 h	4 h	24 h	2 days	3 days	4 days	5 days[b]	7 days	References
2.5	C3H/He	4						2.54**			5
25	C3H/He	4						0.81			5
25	C3H/He	8	1.77**	1.09	0.79						3,5
25	C3H/He	14						1.58**			5
25	C3H/He	16[c]						1.68***			4,6
25	C3H/He	18						0.88			5
25	C3H/He	26	1.02	0.38*	0.26**	1.07				1.87*	3,5
25	C57BL/6	6–8			1.08		1.26*				7
25	BALB/c	8–10								2.03**	2
25	BALB/c	~78[d]								1.98**	1
400[e]	BALB/c	~70[f]							1.00		1

[a] in multiples of NK activity in control group; *: $P < 0.05$; **: $P < 0.01$; ***: $P < 0.001$; [b] following last dose; [c] nominal: 14 (per ref 3); 16–18 (per ref 6); [d] 18 months; [e] cumulative: 25 mg/kg per week from age 12 to 16 months; [f] 16 months.

References: 1. Bruley-Rosset *et al.* (1986); 2. Florentin *et al.* (1989); 3. Renoux *et al.* (1982b); 4. Renoux *et al.* (1982c); 5. Renoux *et al.* (1982b); 5. Renoux *et al.* (1983b); 6. Renoux and Biziere (1987); 7. M. Renoux *et al.* (1986).

analogous to that seen in the controls, but no enhancing effect is observed in animals with lesions of the left neocortex. The NK activity is severely depressed in both control and DSH treated mice with bilateral neocortical lesions (Renoux *et al.*, 1982c, 1984, 1987; Renoux and Biziere, 1987). The above pattern of asymmetrical neocortical control of splenic NK activity and its responses to DSH is almost exactly opposite to that described by Renoux and co-workers for T-cell-dependent immune phenomena (section 12.5). The pattern discerned is that of control by the left neocortex of the stimulation of NK activity, be it by the right neocortex or by DSH (Renoux *et al.*, 1982c)

Edwards *et al.* (1984) reported that 3×10^{-5} M DSH directly inhibits the NK activity of human PBL, that the effect appears to involve sulfhydryl groups and that it is blocked by preincubation with cysteine. Since these workers suspended the PBL in culture medium supplemented with fetal calf serum which contains high concentrations of Fe^{2+} ions, oxidation of DSH to DSSD likely took place (section 14.1) and the DSSD thus formed reacted with protein sulfhydryls to form mixed disulfides (section 5.2). Preincubation with cysteine would reduce the DSSD back to DSH and thus block the effect.

12.6.3 Effects on antibody-mediated cellular cytotoxicity

Although *in vivo* pretreatment with DSH can result in both a marked elevation and a marked depression of the ADCC (i.e. K-cell cytotoxicity) of mouse spleen, the available data so confound the variables of mouse age, strain, pretreatment schedule and time, and target cell, as to preclude any deduction regarding which factors may govern the observed response.

Acute 4-day *in vivo* pretreatment with DSH (25 mg/kg) is without effect in 16- to 18-week-old C3H/He mice on the ADCC to chicken red blood cells (CRBC) in the presence of α-CRBC serum (Renoux, 1982; Renoux *et al.*, 1984, 1987). On the other hand, 2-day pretreatment of 8- to 10-week-old C3H/HeJ mice with the same dose of DSH results in a markedly higher ($P<0.001$) spleen ADCC response to L1210 leukemia cells exposed to heat-inactivated rabbit α-L1210 serum, than that of controls (Florentin *et al.*, 1988).

Chronic administration of DSH (25 mg/kg/week for 16 weeks) to aged BALB/c mice (16 months old at harvest) depresses the spleen ADCC responses to CRBC in the presence of α-CRBC serum markedly below those of both young and aged controls (Bruley-Rosset *et al.*, 1986).

12.7 EFFECT ON DELAYED-TYPE HYPERSENSITIVITY REACTION

The delayed-type hypersensitivity (DTH) reaction is a T_H-cell-mediated phenomenon. It is therefore of interest that administration of DSH (0.5 mg/kg) concurrently with a suboptimal i.v. immunizing dose of SRBC (10^5) enhances the 24-h increase in footpad swelling following injection of an eliciting dose of SRBC (10^8) 2–30 days later. Somewhat surprisingly, in the dose range of 0.5–25 mg/kg, the enhancement of the DTH response appears to be inversely proportional to DSH dose (Renoux and Renoux, 1979). DSH pretreatment, in a dose of *ca* 25 mg/kg, can also augment the DTH reaction to a hapten-carrier complex in guinea pigs; whether it does so or not depends on the pretreatment interval used (Neveu, 1978).

Clinically, a delayed cutaneous hypersensitivity (DCH) test, employing the Multitest system (Institute Merieux, Lyon, France), is used to ascertain the effects of DSH therapy on patient immune status. Briefly, seven glycerinated antigens (tetanus toxoid, diphtheria toxoid, tuberculin, *Streptococcus, Candida, Trichophyton* and *Proteus*), as well as a glycerin control are applied using a plastic disposable multiple-puncture device. After 2 days, the DCH response is scored as the sum of the resulting indurations of 2 or more mm diameter; normal scores are greater than 10 mm, patients with scores of zero are considered anergic.

The use of the DCH test has only been marginally effective in documenting the immunostimulating effects of DSH. DSH therapy of HIV-positive (HIV^+) patients, whose DCH scores are frequently depressed and many of whom are anergic, has been consistently reported to be associated with increases in the DCH response (Lang *et al.*, 1985, 1986, 1987, 1988a,b,c; Pompidou *et al.*, 1985a; Hersh *et al.*, 1991), but in only one instance (Lang *et al.*, 1988c) was this found to be more than a trend ($P < 0.06$). DCH scores obtained following DSH treatment of patients having gastrointestinal surgery (Champault *et al.*, 1983) and in children afflicted with cancer (Renoux *et al.*, 1983b) show a similar tendency ($P = 0.07$) to increase.

12.8 INDUCTION OF T-CELL DIFFERENTIATION

12.8.1 *In vivo* production of serum factors

DSH administration results in the appearance in mouse serum of factor(s) that induce T-cell differentiation. Evidence that this is so came initially from the investigation of the effects of DSH administration on the splenic α-SRBC PFC response of nude mice. These mice are athymic and, normally, their immunization with SRBC elicits only a IgM-PFC response (Renoux and Renoux, 1977a). If DSH is administered concurrently with the immunization, however, a splenic α-SRBC IgG-PFC response is observed (Renoux and Renoux, 1977a; Renoux, 1980). Since IgG-PFC formation is T-cell-mediated, this suggests that DSH administration induces T-cell differentiation in these animals.

Seeking more direct *in vivo* evidence of the induction of T-cell differentiation by DSH, Renoux and Renoux (1977a) administered DSH (either 2.5 or 25 mg/kg s.c.) to female nude mice and 4 days later found a marked increase in the number of spleen cells bearing the Thy-1$^+$ marker characteristic for murine thymocytes and mature T cells. Though the increases associated with each dose were substantially the same, one can calculate that in each case they were significant ($P \leqslant 0.001$). Subsequently the experiment was repeated using DSH purified by the Institute Merieux, and the fraction of spleen cells bearing the CR marker of adult B cells also determined. No increase in CR$^+$ was observed, but the increase in Thy-1$^+$ cells was confirmed, with 25 mg/kg inducing a significantly ($P < 0.01$) greater number than 2.5 mg/kg (Renoux *et al.*, 1979; Renoux, 1980, 1982; Renoux and Renoux, 1981). Renoux *et al.* (1980a) have also reported that a 4-h incubation of human peripheral T-cell depleted lymphocytes with serum from female BALB/c mice administered DSH (25 mg/kg s.c.) 24 h previously, causes an increase in the number of lymphocytes bearing HTLA surface markers. In contrast, Hadden *et al.* (1989) using male nude mice, found no significant increase in Thy-1$^+$ spleen cells following chronic DSH administration (25 mg/kg i.p. five times a week for 3, 6 or 12 weeks). Further, these workers state that, in preliminary tests, no consistent or statistically significant induction was seen 4 days after DSH administration, the time interval used by Renoux and co-workers. In considering the inability of Hadden *et al.* to reproduce the findings of Renoux and co-workers, it should be noted that the route of administration and, more particularly, the gender of the mice Hadden *et al.* used differed from those employed by Renoux and co-workers (see sections 12.2 and 12.3.1 for the gender specificity of the immunomodulatory effects of DSH).

Addition of heat-treated serum of euthymic mice, though not that of athymic mice, to short-term (3.5-h) incubations of spleen cells from nude mice, leads to the *in vitro* acquisition of the Thy-1 marker by a fraction of spleen cells (Renoux and Renoux, 1980b). The degree to which this occurs is related in a complex way to the amount of the donor serum added to the incubation medium, and to mouse strain.

Pretreatment of the donor mice with DSH (25 mg/kg s.c.) affects the inducing activity of serum harvested 24 h after dosing in a complicated manner dependent on both strain and final serum concentration: different results are obtained when that concentration is 0.1–1% (low) or 2.5–10% (high) (Renoux and Renoux, 1980b). Briefly, the T-cell-inducing activity of C3H/He or C57BL/6 mouse serum in high concentration is depressed by DSH pretreatment. So is the activity of C57BL/6 serum in low concentration, but that of C3H/He serum in low concentration is enhanced, as is the activity of serum from nude mice, be it in low or high concentration (Renoux *et al.*, 1979; Renoux, 1980; Renoux and Renoux, 1980b). In nude mice, grafting of a syngeneic thymus much diminishes the ability of DSH to enhance the T-cell-inducing activity of serum in low concentration, and altogether prevents enhancement of the activity of serum in high concentration, though the grafting by itself induces the activity of serum in high concentration. Taken together these results led Renoux and Renoux (1980b) to conclude that mouse serum contains two heat-resistant factors, that each is active in a different concentration range, and that the transplanted thymus can inhibit the factor active at low serum concentration and can both synthesize and down-regulate the one active at high serum concentration.

Subsequently, Renoux *et al.* (1983a), using a 4-day rather than a 24-h DSH pretreatment interval, found DSH to enhance the T-cell-inducing activity of serum from female C3H/He mice in both low and high concentration, as did Pompidou *et al.* (1984a) using a 5-day pretreatment interval. However, these latter workers found that both shorter (1–4 days) or longer (6–7 days) pretreatment intervals result only in the enhancement of the activity of serum in high concentration, the activity of serum in low concentration being depressed. Pompidou *et al.* (1984a) also examined how the changes in the histology of the lymphoid organs correlate with the appearance of the differentiating activity in the serum of the DSH-treated mice. They reported prolonged hyperplasia of the thymus-dependent areas of the lymph nodes beginning on day 2 and those of the spleen on day 3 post DSH administration, with the changes becoming maximal on day 5 and persisting until day 15. No changes were detected in the thymus itself during the first 2 days; on the third day, however, the thymus was completely infiltrated by young thymocytes. No changes were observed in the B-cell areas of these organs at any time.

Lesions of the right neocortex elevate the serum T-cell-inducing activity of sera from control C3H/He mice. However, such lesions also abolish the enhancement of this activity induced by pretreatment with

DSH 4 days earlier. Lesions of the left neocortex, on the other hand decrease the activity of the sera from control mice and change the pattern of the increase observed in the sera of mice pretreated with DSH, increasing it at the lower concentrations (Renoux *et al.*, 1983a).

Gendre *et al.* (1983) have presented data that suggest that factors stimulating the PFC response may be transmitted from lactating mouse dams to their pups in the milk. DSH (25 mg/kg a week s.c.) was administered to the dams throughout the gestation period and in the first 6 weeks postpartum. The PFC response of dams receiving DSH and their pups was evaluated on a weekly basis in weeks 2–6 postpartum, as was that of controls. The response of the dams remained high throughout, on average 3.04 ± 0.86 times that of the controls ($P<0.01$). The response of their pups was also significantly ($P<0.01$) higher than that of the controls in weeks 2–5, rising to a maximum in week 4. The following week their response fell considerably and by week 6 was indistinguishable from that of the controls. This decline was presumably occasioned by the weaning of the pups which began in week 4.

12.8.2 Hepatosin induction

The heat-resistant (45 min at 56 °C) T-cell-inducing factor present in the serum of DSH-pretreated nude mice cannot be DSH itself, since incubation of nude mouse spleen cells with DSH (concentration and duration not given) is stated to have no T-cell-inducing effect (Renoux and Renoux, 1980b; Pompidou *et al.*, 1984a). Nor can it be a product of DSH metabolism in serum, since serum incubated with DSH *in vitro* is also without effect (Pompidou *et al.*, 1984a). Since the nude mice are athymic, it cannot be produced in the thymus. Therefore to identify the organ responsible for the production of the factor, Renoux and co-workers (Renoux *et al.*, 1982a, 1984; Renoux and Renoux, 1984) examined the T-cell-inducing activity of supernatants of DSH-conditioned and unconditioned cultures of C3H/He mouse lymph nodes, kidneys and liver cells. The culture media were harvested after 24 h incubation, heated at 100 °C for 1 h, centrifuged, the clear supernatant filtered through a UMO5, and then a UM1O membrane and lyophilized.

The lyophilized material obtained from both control liver cell cultures and those exposed to DSH (concentration specified only as being in the 10^{-3} to 10^{-10} mM/ml range), were active in bringing about Thy-1$^+$ cell induction in cultures of nude mouse spleen cells, when present in these cultures in concentrations of 10^{-7} to 10^2 µg/ml. The number of Thy-1$^+$ cells induced by the lyophilized material from the control cultures was always less than 50% of that found in normal

C3H/He spleens, but that induced by 10^{-6} to $10^{-1} \mu g/ml$ of the lyophilized material from the DSH-exposed cultures was nearly equal to that present in normal C3H/He spleens. Also, the lyophilized material from the control cultures was said to contain two active chromatographically separable fractions, but that from DSH-exposed cultures to contain only one (details not published). The latter was named hepatosin (Renoux *et al.*, 1982a, Renoux and Renoux, 1984; Renoux *et al.*, 1984). Although Thy-1 marker acquisition is induced by picogram quantities of hepatosin, concentrations even a thousand fold higher fail to modify the number of B cells (Renoux *et al.*, 1982a; Renoux and Renoux, 1984). Hepatosin is said (Renoux *et al.*, 1984) to be a peptide with a molecular weight of 2–5 kDa. Exposure of hepatocytes to rabbit α-hepatosin serum conjugated with fluorescein is said to produce an intracellular granular fluorescence (Renoux *et al.*, 1984).

To date hepatosin has not been identified with any other factor. Propranolol (10^{-5}M) is without any effect on the T-cell-inducing effect of all hepatosin concentrations. This leads to the conclusion (Renoux *et al.*, 1984) that hepatosin is distinct from ubiquitin, a substance that induces both T- and B-cell differentiation and is found in all tissues (Goldstein, G., 1974), but is antagonized by propranolol (Scheid *et al.*, 1978). Hepatosin appears to be distinct from the Facteur Thymique Serique (FTS) and TP5, two inducers of T-cell differentiation (Bach *et al.*, 1977; Goldstein *et al.*, 1979). Although in concentrations of 10^{-5} to $10^{1} \mu g/ml$ all three substances can induce such differentiation *in vitro*, only hepatosin induces T-cell differentiation also *in vivo*. Moreover, it does so when administered in doses of 1–100 ng/mouse, and without inducing any B-cell differentiation. FTS and TP5 have no effect on T-cell differentiation *in vivo* even in doses 100-fold higher than those of hepatosin (Renoux *et al.*, 1984).

Other properties ascribed to hepatosin include the ability to (1) induce T cells from mouse bone marrow cells, even in nude mice (Renoux *et al.*, 1982a), (2) reduce spleen weight and increase IgG responses in NZB mice, (3) increase the mean survival time and immune responses in syngeneic fibrosarcoma-bearing C57Bl/6 mice, and (4) induce HTLA$^+$ cells from human null cells (Renoux, 1984).

12.8.3 Direct *in vitro* induction of T-cell differentiation

Pompidou *et al.*, (1985b) found that DSH brings about T-cell differentiation in long-term (2–5 day) PBMC cultures (supplemented with 10% fetal calf serum, 200 mM glutamine, 50 $\mu g/ml$ gentamicin and 5×10^{-5} M

2-mercaptoethanol). The maximally active DSH concentration is 10^{-7} to 10^{-5} µg/ml (5.8×10^{-13} to 5.8×10^{-11}M). The *in vitro* cytotoxicity of DSH is quite low, and none would be expected at these concentrations (section 14.1). No cytotoxicity is seen during 4 h incubations of human PBMC with DSH in a 1.5×10^{-2} µg/ml concentration and after 24 or 48 h incubation it is only seen with DSH concentrations of 1.5×10^{-5} µg/ml or higher (Renoux, 1985b). Using monoclonal antibodies, Pompidou *et al.* (1986) observed that in long-term PBMC cultures exposed to DSH there is a significant ($P < 0.01$) increase, relative to controls, in the number of $CD3^+$ and $CD4^+$ T cells; however, the number of $CD8^+$ cells does not change. Also, the number of cells bearing the HLA-DR$^+$ marker characteristic of activated mature T cells almost doubles, most of this increase being accounted for by the increase in the number of $CD4^+DR^+$ and $CD8^+DR^+$ cells. These changes are accompanied by a total disappearance of null cells, but no changes are seen in the population of NK cells, B cells and monocytes. These results suggest that DSH has two actions, bringing about both the acquisition of the DR phenotype in null cells, and then, the acquisition by some of these cells of CD3 and CD4 molecules. Interestingly, exposure of PBMC from HIV$^+$ individuals to 10^{-5} µg/ml DSH for 4 days also results in a significant ($P < 0.01$) increase in the number of $CD4^+$ T cells, no change in the number of $CD8^+$ cells, and consequently in a increase in the CD4:CD8 ratio (Pompidou *et al.*, 1985b, 1986).

An important aspect of this work is the observation that some of the *in vitro* effects of DSH in long-term human PBMC culture require the presence of monocytes. Depletion of the cultures of monocytes (by adherence of the latter to plastic culture dishes during a 1-h preincubation) reduces very substantially the increase in $CD3^+$ and $CD4^+$ T-cell induction and in the number of activated $CD4^+$ and $CD8^+$ T cells (Pompidou *et al.*, 1986).

In a preliminary communication, Sanhadji *et al.* (1985) have reported that incubation of human bone marrow cells for 2–6 h with DSH (10^{-8} to 10^{-6} µg/ml) leads to an increase in $CD3^+$ and $CD4^+$ T cells relative to that observed in control cultures. No increase in IL-2 receptor expression is observed in these or the analogous PBMC cultures.

12.8.4 Effects on nuclear refringency

A rapid fall in nuclear refringency of human lymphocytes occurs upon their incubation for 20 min in the presence of DSH in a 10^{-5} µg/ml concentration (Pompidou *et al.*, 1985a). Nuclear refringency is measured as the brightness of cells when these are mounted in a medium of high refractive index and are viewed with a phase contrast microscope. It is a function of chromatin dispersion: the more condensed the chromatin, the greater the brightness of the cell. A reduction in natural refrigency is also a dose-dependent effect of incubating lymphocytes with PHA. It occurs within 20–30 min of exposure to the mitogen. It disappears after an hour, then reappears, reaches a maximum at 48 h, and persists for at least 72 h. Its magnitude is correlated with that of the lymphoproliferative effect of PHA (Pompidou *et al.*, 1980, 1984b). The effect of DSH on human lymphocytes has been found to be additive to that of PHA, and both the DSH effect and its additivity with that of PHA was reported to occur in lymphocytes from HIV[+] individuals (Pompidou *et al.*, 1985a, 1986).

12.8.5 Effect on lymphokine production

Chung *et al.* (1985) have stated, in a preliminary publication, that administration to mice of DSH in a 25 mg/kg s.c. dose 7 days prior to sacrifice increases both the Interleukin-2 (IL-2) production by spleen cells stimulated with Con A and the Interleukin-1 (IL-1) production by peritoneal macrophages stimulated with LPS. Mossalayi *et al.* (1986) have observed that while DSH in a $10^{-4}\,\mu g/ml$ ($5.8 \times 10^{-10}M$) concentration almost doubles ($P < 0.005$) the production of IL-2 in 2-day cultures of unfractionated human PBMC, it fails to do so in cultures of purified T cells ($> 96\%$ CD2^{+}) which have been depleted of monocytes (down to $< 2\%$ peroxidase positive cells) by adherence to fetal calf serum coated flasks. Although in such purified T-cell cultures IL-2 production is markedly stimulated by the addition of IL-1, DSH has no effect on this process (Mossalayi *et al.*, 1986). More recently, Mossalayi (private communication) has stated that the levels of prostaglandin E$_2$ (PGE$_2$), a substance known to be involved in the down-regulation of T lymphocytes by monocytes, are markedly lowered in unfractionated PBMC cultures by $1 \times 10^{-4}\,\mu g/ml$ DSH.

12.9 EFFECT ON LYMPHOCYTE POPULATIONS *IN VIVO*

12.9.1 Experimental animals

Very little information is available regarding the *in vivo* effects of DSH on mouse lymphocyte counts and the proportion of T and B lymphocytes, be it in peripheral blood or lymphoid organs. Some conclusions in this regard (Fig. 12.3) can be arrived at, however, from the data of M. Renoux *et al.* (1986) and Renoux and Biziere (1987). In the first of these studies, blood and spleen variables were determined at 2, 24 and 72 h after the administration of DSH (25 mg/kg s.c.) to 6- to 8-week old C57Bl/6 female mice. Two hours following DSH administration the blood leukocyte count fell (by 55%; *P*< 0.01), as did the blood lymphocyte count (to 56% of control; computed from Table 6 of M. Renoux *et al.*). Concurrently, the total spleen lymphocyte count rose rapidly and massively [Fig. 12.3: computed from total spleen count (Table 4 of M. Renoux *et al.*) and from the average sum of T and B cells in the spleen of control and DSH-treated mice (Table 1 of M. Renoux *et al.*)]. In particular, the spleen T-cell count rose quite substantially: by 56% at 2 h and by 99% at 24 h. The juxtaposition in time of the substantial fall in blood lymphocytes and the rise in the spleen lymphocyte population strongly bespeaks of the events being linked. *Prima faciae*, it suggests a DSH-induced migration of blood lymphocytes to the spleen.

Although the 1987 study of Renoux and Biziere involved mice of a different strain and age (16-week-old female C3H/HeJ mice, some with brain lesions), it is clear, from the data derived from mice without brain lesions, that administration of DSH (25 mg/kg s.c., 4 days prior) again resulted in a marked (48%; *P*< 0.01) elevation in the spleen T-cell

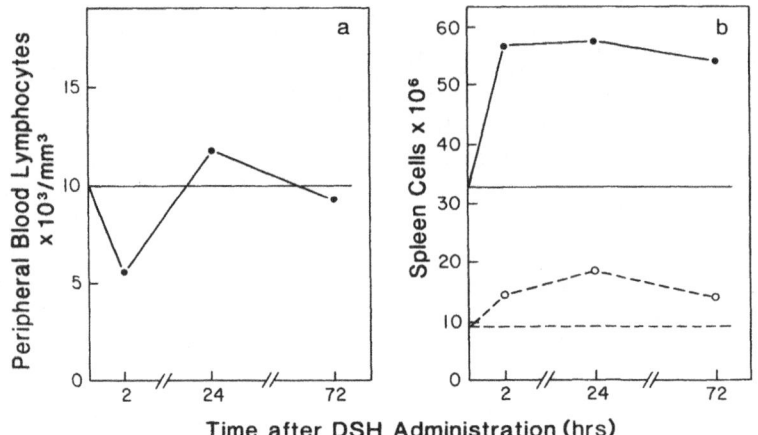

Time after DSH Administration (hrs)

Figure 12.3 Plots of peripheral blood and spleen lymphocyte counts at various times following s.c. administration of 25 mg/kg diethyldithiocarbamate (DSH) to C3H/He female mice. Constructed from the data of M. Renoux *et al.* (1986). (a) Solid circles: peripheral blood lymphocyte counts; horizontal line: counts in untreated mice. (b) Open circles: counts of Thy-1[+] cells; closed circles: sum of counts of Thy-1[+] and SIg[+] cells; horizontal lines: counts in untreated mice.

count as well as a 19% elevation ($P < 0.01$) in the total number of spleen cells.

Renoux and Biziere (1987) also measured, using monoclonal antibodies, the effects of DSH, administered to mice 4 days prior to sacrifice, on the phenotypic expression of surface MHC antigens by the spleen T cells. Specifically, they measured the expression of class 1(K) antigens and the class 2(I-A) and (I-E) antigens. They found that DSH increases the amount of spleen T-cell K and I-A antigens by 30 and 21%, respectively ($P < 0.001$), while the expression of I-E antigens is abrogated.

Since Renoux and Biziere (1987) also measured the S-LPR to PHA and Con A and the α-SRBC IgG-PFC responses in these animals and did so under six different conditions (involving various combinations of DSH pretreatment and lateral neocortical brain lesions) in each case, it is possible to evaluate the significance of the above-mentioned DSH-induced changes in the expression of MHC antigens on these responses. Turning first to the mitogen-derived data and applying multiple linear regression analysis to the resulting 12-point data set (6 conditions × 2 mitogens), we find that 79% of the variance in the data set can be accounted for by the following relationship:

$$\text{Con A-LPR} = 1.968K + 0.6061(\text{I-A}) \tag{12.1}$$

$$\text{PHA-LPR} = 1.968K - 0.0431(\text{I-A}) \tag{12.2}$$

where LPR is in units of ^{3}H-thymidine incorporation ($\text{cpm} \times 10^3$), and the expression of MHC surface antigens is given in terms of the percentage of the monoclonal antibody adsorbed (bound) to the T cells. It may be noted that the influence of K antigen appears to be more important than that of the I-A antigen for responses to both mitogens, but particularly so for those to PHA. Also, the parameter relating the K antigen to the LPR is the same for both Con A and PHA (the use of separate terms for the K antigen for each mitogen increased minimally the percentage of the variance that could be accounted for; also, introductions of terms relating LPR to the I-E antigen increased that percentage only slightly). Additionally, in equations (12.1) and (12.2) there is no constant term, indicating that, at zero K and I-A expression, no LPR would be expected. The ability of DSH pretreatment to stimulate the spleen T-cell response to mitogens is seen, therefore, as primarily correlated with its ability to increase the amount of K antigen expression.

Turning to the α-SRBC IgG-PFC response data generated by Renoux and Biziere (1987) and applying multiple linear regression analysis to the 6-point data set, we find that 92% of the variance can be accounted for by

$$IgG\text{-}PFC = -15\,096 + 464.8K - 58.20(I\text{-}A) + 96.18(I\text{-}E) \quad (12.3)$$

where IgG-PFC is the number of PFC per 10^6 splenocytes. In this instance, both the constant term and the I-E term have a sizable effect on the percentage of the variance that can be accounted for. The large negative value of the constant may be related to the conversion of IgM to IgG in this response. Here again, the ability of DSH pretreatment to stimulate the spleen T-cell response is, in large part, correlated with its ability to increase the amount of K antigen expression.

Class 1 antigens are considered to be expressed on all nucleated cells and the variation in the amount of K antigen being expressed must be regarded, therefore, as a measure of its cell surface concentration. The present finding suggests the magnitude of LPR and IgG-PFC responses is a function of this concentration. It also suggests that the role of class 2 antigens in determining the magnitude of the LPR may not be as important as that of the class 1(K) antigen, and that this may be more true for one mitogen than another.

The data of Renoux and Biziere (1987) regarding the twin effects of DSH and brain lesions on the expression MHC antigens on the T-cell surface was later amplified (Renoux *et al.*, 1988a) by inclusion of parallel lymph node T-cell data for C3H/HeJ mice. These reveal a dissimilar MHC antigen profile. For instance, whereas DSH pretreatment abrogates the expression of I-E antigens in spleen T cells, it markedly augments their expression in lymph node T cells. No information has been published, however, regarding the LPR of these cells to mitogen stimulation. Earlier M. Renoux *et al.* (1986) reported on the effect of DSH pretreatment on the LPR of C57BL/6 mouse spleen and lymph node T cells. Their data lead to the conclusion that the DSH effects on T cells in these two tissues are different.

More recently, the effect of chronic treatment with DSH (25 and 100 mg/kg/week for 6 weeks i.p.) on the fraction of cells bearing various T-cell and macrophage markers in the spleen, lymph nodes and thymus has been investigated by Yokum and co-workers (Halpern *et al.*, 1990, Halpern and Yokum, 1991) using BALB/c mice, MRL-$+/+$ mice and two strains of mice with immunological defects (MRL-*lpr/lpr* and NZB/W F_1 hybrid). The results obtained were strain- and tissue-dependent and so complex as to be characterized by the authors as 'capricious' (Halpern and Yokum, 1991). Briefly, in the MRL-*lpr/lpr* mice whose autoimmune disease is associated with the lymphoproliferation of Thy-1$^+$, Lyt-2$^-$, L3T4$^-$ null cells and a decline in Lyt-2$^+$ and L3T4$^+$ T cells, DSH treatment results in an increase in the percentage of cells bearing the Lyt-2$^+$ and L3T4$^+$ markers and a reduction in the fraction bearing the Thy-1$^+$ marker. It has no such effect in the MRL-+/+ mice, nor generally in the BALB/c mice (exception: elevation of Thy-1$^+$ and L3T4$^+$ cells in spleen, decrease in L3T4$^+$ cells in lymph nodes). In the NZB/W mice, DSH treatment increases the expression of Lyt-2$^+$ and L3T4$^+$ cells surface antigens in the spleen and lymph nodes, but not the thymus, and increases the expression of the Thy-1$^+$ cells surface antigens in lymph nodes. DSH also tends to increase the expression of Mac-1, Mac-2, and Mac-3 antigens in all the strains and tissues, but not consistently so. The latter finding is noteworthy, for although the mechanism of immunomodulating action of DSH is unknown, there is some evidence that it involves mononuclear phagocytic cells (section 12.10).

12.9.2 Humans

A number of investigators have reported that DSH treatment is clinically correlated with increased CD3$^+$ and CD4$^+$ T-cell counts, but with a decreased count of CD8$^+$ T cells. This was first reported by Renoux *et al.* (1983b) who, in a placebo-controlled study, observed a significant ($P<0.01$) increase in the CD3$^+$ and CD4$^+$ T-cell counts 5 days after i.v. administration of a 5 mg/kg dose of DSH to lung cancer patients in remission (Fig. 12.2). Concurrently, a trend ($P=0.06$) was noted for CD8$^+$ T-cell counts to decrease. Additionally, the LPR to PHA and Con A by the PBMC of these patients were significantly ($P<0.01$) enhanced by the DSH treatment (Fig. 12.2).

Subsequently, it has been found that DSH treatment is associated with increases in CD4$^+$ T-cell counts in patients with HIV infections. The first to report this were Lang *et al.* (1985) and Pompidou *et al.* (1986). These workers administered 8–10 mg/kg DSH as a chronic weekly treatment and reported that CD3$^+$ and CD4$^+$ T-cell counts increased in five of six patients treated with DSH for 3–6 months and in an overlapping four of five patients treated with DSH for 6 months. A significant ($P<0.01$) increase in the CD4$^+$ T-cell count was observed upon extension of this series to 11 patients, the number of CD4$^+$ cells rising from 265 ± 180 to 457 ± 254 cells/μl during the 3- to 6-month period of DSH therapy (Lang *et al.*, 1986, 1987). Similar findings have been reported in a number of subsequent clinical investigation of DSH therapy in patients with HIV infections (Table 13.1, studies 1, 2, 4 and 6).

12.10 EFFECTS ON MONONUCLEAR PHAGOCYTIC CELLS

The presence of monocytes appears to be required for a number of the *in vitro* effects of DSH on T lymphocytes. Thus, the T-cell differentiation induced in cultures of human PBMC by DSH in concentrations of 10^{-7} to $10^{-5}\,\mu g/ml$ (5.8×10^{-10} to $5.8 \times 10^{-8}M$) is very substantially diminished in cultures partially depleted of monocytes; these concentrations of DSH have no effect themselves on the number of monocytes found in such cultures following 2- to 5-day incubations (Pompidou *et al.*, 1985b). Also, monocytes are essential for the stimulation by DSH, in a $10^{-4}\,\mu g/ml$ concentration, of the *in vitro* elaboration of IL-2 by human PBMC (Mossalayi *et al.*, 1986). That the effects of DSH could, in some way, be mediated by monocytes was first suggested by Neveu *et al.* (1980), who found that the effects of a high concentration of DSH ($3.7 \times 10^{-2}\,\mu g/ml$) on the PBMC-LPR elicited by PHA are prevented by depletion of the PBMC of monocytes. Mossalayi (private communication) has since found that DSH ($10^{-4}\,\mu g/ml$) very markedly reduces PGE_2 titers in cultures that include monocytes without affecting the IL-1 production by monocytes. Since PGE_2 production by monocytes down-regulates T-cell activation, inhibition of PGE_2 elaboration would result in an activation of the T lymphocytes.

In a preliminary communication Chung *et al.* (1985) have reported that LPS stimulated IL-1 production by peritoneal macrophages of 8-week-old mice is enhanced by the s.c. administration of DSH (25 mg/kg s.c.) 7 days earlier. These authors also state that, in age-immunodepressed (16 month old) mice, DSH pretreatment enhances IL-1 production to the levels seen in young mice, irrespective of whether the DSH pretreatment consists of a single dose, or 4 weeks of treatment with either 1 or 3 doses a week. On the other hand, Schlick *et al.* (1984) have reported that incubation of BALB/c mouse peritoneal macrophages with DSH (50 µg/ml) has no significant effect on the production of granulocyte/monocyte colony stimulating factor (GM-CSF), and stated that DSH has also no effect on PGE_2 synthesis by macrophages.

One function of mononuclear phagocytes *in vivo* is the clearance of colloidal substances from the bloodstream. DSH administration (*ca* 25 mg/kg i.v. 13 days prior) increases the clearance of i.v. administered colloidal gold from the circulation of the guinea pig. Timing of the DSH adminstration is critical: administered concurrently, 6 h or 8 days earlier, DSH is without effect (Neveu and Vincendeau, 1983). DSH pretreatment also stimulates the removal of colloidal tin from the circulation. Again, timing is important: pretreatment of rats with DSH (5 or 25 mg/kg p.o.) 2–3 weeks earlier leads to significant enhancement of the clearance of i.v. administered ^{99m}Tc-labeled colloidal tin. DSH administration 1 week or 3 days earlier is without effect and administration 4 weeks earlier results in a significant impairment of the colloid's clearance (Corke *et al.*, 1984).

Efforts to discern the mechanism of the enhanced phagocytic activity induced by DSH pretreatment have been unavailing. *In vivo*, 6 and 14 day pretreatment of guinea pigs with 10 mg of DSH has no effect on the uptake of ^{99m}Tc-labelled colloidal sulfur by peritoneal macrophages (Neveu and Vincendeau, 1983). In the rat, peritoneal macrophage 'spreading' and the phagocytosis of latex particle by these cells is actually significantly inhibited ($P < 0.005$ and $P < 0.02$, respectively) by *in vitro* exposure to the admittedly high DSH concentrations of 0.16 and 0.31 µg/ml (Corke, 1984). The *in vitro* phagocytosis of *Listeria* by C3H/He mouse peritoneal macrophages is diminished by 50 µg/ml DSH significantly ($P = 0.01$) more so than by 500 µg/ml DSH. On the other hand, the Listericidal capacity of the macrophages is significantly ($P < 0.01$) enhanced by both these concentrations of DSH. This is not due to a direct effect of DSH on the *Listeria* since no changes are seen in the live *Listeria* count in the culture medium (Renoux and Renoux, 1979).

12.11 EXPERIMENTAL THERAPEUTICS

No animal model exists that is suitable for the investigation of the effects of therapeutic agents on the morbid process associated with HIV infection. DSH has, however, been shown to have therapeutic utility in murine infections with the LP-BM5 retrovirus (Hersh *et al.*, 1988). Inoculation of C57BL/6 mice with LP-BM5 causes T-cell deficiency, lymphadenopathy, hypergammaglobulinemia, and death with a median delay of 17.5 weeks. DSH administered i.p. in various doses on a 5 times per week schedule prolongs survival time in a dose related-manner. Thus, a 20-week survival was observed when a 20 mg/kg dose was used with this schedule, a 23-week survival when the dose was 200 mg/kg and a survival in excess of 26 weeks for 100% of the mice when the dose was 400 mg/kg (only 12.5% of the untreated controls had survived this long). After 26 weeks, T cells constituted 30.2% of spleen cells in the mice receiving the 400 mg/kg dose of DSH, but only 8.4% of spleen cells in the LP-BM5-infected controls. On the other hand, Mac + cells (macrophages and some B cells) constituted 43.6% of spleen cells in the controls, but only 14.3% in the DSH-treated mice, and spleen weight, which averaged 1 400 mg in the controls was only 200 mg in the treated group. Finally, the serum concentration of IgM, which was 12 000 µg/ml in the controls, was only 6 000 µg/ml in the treated mice.

In mice inoculated with encephalomyocarditis virus (in a dose lethal to 27 of 30 animals) DSH acts synergistically with IFN. Thus a 24-h pretreatment with DSH (20 mg/kg i.p) provides no protection (mortality = 27 of 30) and neither does treatment with IFN 1 h post inoculation (mortality = 22 of 30). When the inoculation of DSH-pretreated mice is followed an hour later by an injection of interferon, a reduced mortality (6 of 30) is observed (Cerutti and Chany, 1983).

The effect of treatment with DSH (25 or 100 mg/kg/week) on the spontaneous development in mice of autoimmune disease closely resembling human systemic lupus erythematosus has been investigated by Yocum and co-workers (Halpern *et al.*, 1990, Halpern and Yocum, 1991). In the MRL-*lpr/lpr* strain, in which the primary defect is one involving T-cell abnormalities, DSH treatment increased the survival period for 50% of the mice from the 20 weeks seen in the controls to 43 weeks. In addition, DSH treatment decreased lymphadenopathy, thymic atrophy and serum anti-DNA and anti-histoné   antibody levels (Halpern *et al.*, 1990). On the other hand, in the NZB/W strain, in which the primary defect is one involving B cell abnormalites, the DSH treatment had no significant effect on survival or on the serum anti-DNA and anti-histone antibody levels (Halpern and Yocum, 1991). It might be noted that DSH has been reported to have brought about a remission in a clinical case of lupus (section 13.4).

The effects of DSH on a number of other pathological conditions induced in mice have been investigated. The results obtained are reported below, but their interpretation is complex. DSH prevents a wasting disease induced in mice by a phenolic extract of *Brucella melitensis* cell wall fraction (Renoux and Renoux, 1979). In mice inoculated with an allogeneic sarcoma (10^6 180 TG Croker tumor cells), co-administration of DSH leads to a significant delay in tumor development, though there is no change in final survival rate (Cerutti and Chany, 1983).

Although DSH treatment does stimulate the S-LPR to Con A and PHA and the production of IL-2 by spleen cells depressed by cyclophosphamide administration, it does not restore these responses fully (Renoux and Renoux, 1980a, Rejas *et al.*, 1988). Likewise, it only partially restores the S-LPR to Con A in mice in which this response is depressed by azathioprine or hydrocortisone; it is, however, more effective in restoring in the same animals the S-LPR to PHA and IgG-PFC responses to control levels (Renoux and Renoux, 1980a).

M. Renoux *et al.* (1986) introduced a sterile suspension of calcium pyrophosphate microcrystals in the right pleural cavity of mice, and investigated the effects of DSH on the resultant pleurisy and the accompanying changes in immune parameters. The responses obtained, which were quite complex, were interpreted by these workers as indicating that DSH tended to restore towards normal the immune values affected by the pleurisy.

12.12 IMMUNOMODULATORY EFFECTS OF RELATED COMPOUNDS

Renoux and Renoux (1979) reported that the products of DSH hydrolysis, diethylamine and carbon disulfide, if administered concurrently but by separate s.c. injections, are not effective in enhancing the α-SRBC IgG-PFC response, although they do enhance this activity when administered together in the same syringe. This may simply reflect the rapidity with which the hydrolysis, given the right pH, is reversed (section 2.2). The hydrolysis is particularly rapid at acid pH (Fig. 2.1) and, given the potentially high acidity of stomach secretions, this needs to be kept in mind when DSH is reported as ineffective following oral administration, as, for instance, in enhancing vaccination against *S. typhimurium* (Luzy *et al.*, 1983).

Given that DSH is the principal known metabolite of DSSD *in vivo*, it would be anomalous if DSSD had no immunomodulating activity. Renoux (1982, 1984), however, injected various doses of DSSD, from 0.5 to 25 mg/kg, subcutaneously and reported that no enhancement of the α-SRBC IgG-PFC reaction occurred. The vehicle and manner of administration were not further described, but DSSD is very sparingly soluble in water (30 μg/ml, section 2.1). Accordingly, the suggestion (Renoux, 1984) that the absence of an effect may have been due to a lack of absorption may be correct. It is of interest in this context that Bihari *et al.* (1988) have reported that in AIDS and AIDS-related-complex (ARC) patients given DSSD, a considerable rise in T helper cells was observed, suggesting that DSSD does, indeed, have immunomodulatory activity.

12.13 CONCLUSIONS

In vivo, DSH administration has multiple immunomodulatory effects. The effects are often found to be dual, more frequently representing stimulation, but in some instances suppression. The direction of the effect is commonly found to be a function of the duration of time allowed to pass between DSH administration and sampling time (Fig.

12.1). Virtually all the immunomodulatory effects observed require the participation of CD4$^+$ helper T cells.

An important property of DSH is its ability to induce T-cell differentiation. This has been observed in mice following the *in vivo* administration of DSH. In humans in whom the peripheral blood CD4$^+$ T-cell population is depressed (viz. by disease), DSH administration tends to increase it back towards normal without inducing significant changes in the CD8$^+$ population (Fig. 12.2 and section 13.1). DSH also brings about induction and activation of CD4$^+$ T cells in cultures of human PBMC. For the effect to occur, however, the presence of monocytes is required (Pompidou *et al.*, 1986). This is also true of the DSH-induced stimulation of IL-2 production in such cultures (Mossalayi *et al.*, 1986).

Many of the effects of *in vivo* DSH administration become evident only after the passage of a significant amount of time (as much as 15 days in the case of the enhancement of the proliferative response of splenocytes to mitogens in guinea pigs), and are very much a function of both the species and strain used. It is difficult to envision these as direct effects, given that the half-life of DSH *in vivo* is rather short (about 10–11 min in mice; Table 6.1). Moreover, lymphocyte chromatin dispersion is evident within 20 min of exposure of PBMC to DSH (Pompidou *et al.*, 1985a). It is therefore likely that the effects observed at later times are sequelae of events that occur soon after DSH administration. It is known, for instance, that the antigen-initiated T-cell activation is a process that develops over a 7- to 10-day period (Crabtree, 1989). How DSH initiates this process remains to be determined. It could act as calcium ionophore, since it is an excellent chelator and its chelates have both a very high lipid/water partition coefficient and show a ready tendency to exchange the chelated metal for one of higher affinity (Table 2.1). It is of interest, in this context, that *in vivo* administration of Zn(DS)$_2$ does not enhance the S-LPR to PHA or Con A (Renoux *et al.*, 1988b). Alternatively, it could be that some of the effects of DSH are mediated by its metabolites. Such a role was suggested for the methyl ester of diethyldithiocarbamic acid by Guillaumin *et al.* (1986), who found significant quantities of it in the brain neocortex of animals dosed with DSH. DSH treatment has also been found to decrease PBL plasma membrane fluidity (Lehr *et al.*, 1989).

As shown in Fig. 12.3, DSH administration induces a relatively rapid and major shift of lymphocytes from blood to spleen. Whether parallel shifts occur in other lymphoid organs is an open but salient question. Investigations of the effects of DSH on lymphocyte number and function have been generally characterized by the implicit assumption that lymphocytes found at different sites are equivalent. Yet, the differing expression of MHC antigens on spleen and lymph node T cells, the dichotomous effects of DSH pretreatment thereon (Renoux *et al.*, 1988a), and the differences in the proliferative responses of these cells in control and DSH-pretreated animal (M. Renoux *et al.*, 1986), raise questions as to whether this assumption is a correct one. It follows from this, that the apparent sequestration of lymphocytes in the spleen 2 h after DSH administration (Fig. 12.3) could be the result of some DSH-induced alteration of the lymphocyte. The persistence of the splenic lymphocyte sequestration, in the face of a recovery in the number of lymphocytes in peripheral blood, raises questions regarding the provenance of the replacement cells and the possibility that these might be newly differentiated lymphocytes.

13

Clinical status of diethyldithiocarbamate as an immunostimulant

13.1 INTRODUCTION 279
13.2 IN THE TREATMENT OF HIV INFECTIONS AND AIDS 280
    13.2.1 Evaluation of side-effects 289
13.3 IN GASTROINTESTINAL SURGERY PATIENTS 290
13.4 AS A THERAPEUTIC AGENT IN AUTOIMMUNE DISEASE 290
13.5 IN PATIENTS WITH NEOPLASTIC DISEASE 291
13.6 AS AN ADJUVANT FOR INFLUENZA VACCINATION 292
13.7 SUMMARY 292

13.1 INTRODUCTION

Experimental studies in the laboratory clearly indicate that diethyl-dithiocarbamate (DSH) is a potent T-cell stimulant. These cells represent one of the body's main immunological mechanisms of defense against infection. Additionally, they play a crucial role in activating, when necessary, the B-cell antibody-mediated immune defense process. It follows, therefore, that an agent that can bring about their activation has a clear potential for reversing clinically encountered immunodepression.

While the mechanisms of immunosuppression are not well understood, its occurrence is correlated with infections, aging, autoimmune diseases, and exposure to toxicants. In particular, the principal feature of human immunodeficiency virus (HIV) infections is an immunosuppression characterized by a progressive destruction of CD4$^+$ helper cells and malfunctioning of the antibody-producing system. The public health emergency occasioned by the acquired immune deficiency syndrome (AIDS) and the absence of a curative treatment add to the urgency of the quest for an agent that might stop the progression of HIV infections to AIDS.

Controlled studies of DSH therapy suggest that it retards significantly the progression of HIV-positive (HIV$^+$) patients to AIDS and decreases the incidence of new opportunistic infections in patients with AIDS. Additionally, it appears to improve significantly the chances of early discharge for gastrointestinal surgery patients who present with infection. Both of these outcomes are found to be associated with a significant increase in the CD4$^+$ T-cell population. By contrast, in an autoimmune disease, rheumatoid arthritis, DSH therapy reduces significantly the patients' CD4$^+$/CD8$^+$ T-cell ratios, articular index, and pain scores. Also, a case report gives hope that it might prove useful in another autoimmune condition, juvenile lupus erythematosus. Finally, administered concurrently with influenza vaccination, DSH significantly enhances antibody titers in the aged. Its apparent lack of side-effects is buttressed by the 40-year-long therapeutic history of disulfiram (DSSD) in the treatment for alcoholism. The major toxicity associated with DSSD therapy has been the disulfiram-ethanol reaction (Chapter 8). Although it is appropriate to warn individuals receiving DSH immunotherapy of the possibility that ingestion of ethanol can precipitate such a reaction, no instances of severe reactions in patients on DSH have been reported to date.

Much of the clinical work on the immunostimulant effects of DSH has been performed using Imuthiol®, i.e. the anhydrous form of DSH. Accordingly, DSH doses are given in this chapter in terms of that material rather than of the trihydrate, unless otherwise specified (section 2.1).

13.2 IN THE TREATMENT OF HIV INFECTIONS AND AIDS

Six controlled studies of DSH treatment of HIV$^+$ patients have been published to date. In each instance, significant differences were found in favor of individuals receiving DSH (Table 13.1). The results of the most recent and largest of these studies (Hersh *et al.*, 1991) indicate that DSH therapy also benefits patients with AIDS. The six studies embody a variety of experimental designs and report a range of benefits that accrue to HIV$^+$ patients from the DSH therapy. They are, therefore, best discussed individually.

Early studies of the effects of DSH in HIV$^+$ patients were not controlled. The first report of such a study was a preliminary one by Lang *et al.* (1985), who administered DSH in an 8–10 mg/kg p.o. dose weekly for 3–6 months to 6 patients. They found that CD3$^+$ and CD4$^+$ T-cell counts rose in 5 of the 6 (on average 2.1- and 2.5-fold, respectively) and that the delayed cutaneous hypersensitivity (DCH) reaction clearly improved in 4, returning to normal in one of them. The likelihood that the rise in CD4$^+$ counts was associated with the DSH administration was enhanced by the observation that in 2 patients in whom these counts fell during a 3-month period without therapy, they rose again when therapy was reinstituted. The same was true of the number of rosette-forming cells (E-RFC) in these 2 patients. Later, as the DSH therapy was continued and the series of HIV$^+$ patients receiving it for 6 months had been expanded to 11, the CD4$^+$ T-cell count was found to have risen in all the patients. The increase was a significant one ($P<0.05$). The DCH reaction improved in 7 of the patients ($P<0.06$) and a slow improvement, including weight gain, was observed in all patients with initial general symptoms (Lang *et al.*, 1986, 1987). An analysis of the long-term (2–3 years) outcome of DSH therapy in the first 4 HIV$^+$ patients treated with it indicates that CD4$^+$ counts continued above entry levels for the whole period, and that weight gains of 6–10 kg were maintained, as were near-normal DCH scores in the 3 originally anergic patients. The only untoward effects were gastrointestinal irritation and a chemical odor on the breath (Lang *et al.*, 1988a).

Many of the above findings were confirmed by Lang *et al.* (1988b) in a placebo-controlled, double-blind study (Table 13.1, study 1). Its findings pointed to several other benefits of DSH therapy, and led to the suggestion that DSH forestalled the progression of the disease for at least the duration of the treatment. Patients were admitted to the study if they were HIV$^+$, had a CD4$^+$ count $<600/\mu$l, and belonged to Centers for Disease Control (CDC) categories II (asymptomatic infection), III (persistent generalized lymphadenopathy), or IV-A (constitutional disease: fever or diarrhea persisting over a month, involuntary weight loss $>10\%$ of baseline) as defined (Centers for Disease Control, 1986). Patients were excluded if any indication of AIDS was found. Patients in the treatment group received a 10 mg/kg/week oral dose of DSH for 16 weeks. None of the 38 patients in the DSH group progressed to AIDS or died, though in the control group 3 of 39 progressed to AIDS and 2 died. Scored on a scale of improved, stable, or worse, the clinical status of 42% of the patients in the DSH group was judged to have improved, though only 5% of the control group patients fell into this category ($P<0.05$). All 9 patients in the DSH group who had a history of weight loss, regained normal weight at 16 weeks. In 4 of the 7 patients in the DSH group who had splenomegaly at entry, the spleen became impalpable, while in the control group splenomegaly persisted in all 8 patients who had it at entry and developed in 2 others ($P<0.05$). Lymphadenopathy scores (based on

Table 13.1 Effects of diethyldithiocarbamate therapy in patients with HIV infections

| Patients[a] | | Treatments compared[b] | | CD4+ count | | | Progress to | | | Other significant benefits of DSH therapy |
	n	Drug	Dosage regimen	at entry per µl	change %	P	ARC	AIDS	death	
1. Lang et al. (1988b)										
HIV+, CDC group II, III or IV-A and CD4+ <660/µl	38	DSH	10 mg/kg qw po × 16w	405	+32	<0.05	–	0/38	0/38	Decreases in: splenomegaly (P<0.05) lymphadenopathy (P<0.05) symptoms[c] (P<0.001)
	39	Placebo		389	+18		–	3/39	2/39	
2. Lang et al. (1988c)										
HIV+ CDC group II, III, IV or IV–C2	26	DSH	10 mg/kg qw po × 1y	385	+25	<0.05	0/20	0/26	–	Increase in delayed hypersensitivity reaction (P<0.05)
	18	none		431	–24		4/16	1/18	–	
3. Brewton et al. (1987, 1989)										
AIDS or ARC and symptoms[d]	22	DSH	200 mg/m² qw iv × 16w	232	–25		–	2/16	–	Decrease in: lymphadenopathy (P<0.005) symptoms[d] (P<0.002)
	18	none		192	–30		–	5/16	–	
4. Hersh et al. (1987); Peterson et al. (1988); Kaplan et al. (1989)										
ARC and 2 symptoms[d] and 2 immune defects and CD4+ >200/µl	7	DSH	(200∫400∫800 mg/m² 800 mg/m² qw∫800 mg/m² qw/2 po) × 4w each	451	+29		–	0/7	–	Decrease in: lymphadenopathy (P=0.006)
	10	none		526	–26		–	3/10	–	

5. Reisinger et al. (1990)

Patient selection	n	Treatment	Regimen	CD4	CD4 change	P				Outcome
CDC groups II–IV	13	DSH	5 mg/kg qw iv × 24w ∫ 12m follow-up	318[e]	−21		2/13[f]	0/13[f]	—	Decreased CDC group progression during 12m follow-up (P<0.05)
	14	Placebo		422[e]	−36	<0.02	7/14[f]	4/14[f]	—	
	13	DSH	5 mg/kg qw po × 24w ∫ 12m follow-up	493[e]	−5		3/13[f]	0/13[f]	—	
	13	Placebo		467[e]	−6		3/13[f]	2/13[f]	—	

6. Hersh et al. (1991)

Patient selection	n	Treatment	Regimen	CD4	CD4 change	P				Outcome
HIV+ and 3 symptoms and 2 immune defects	137	DSH	400 mg/m² qw po × 24w	318	+18[g]			9/118	4/118	Decrease in opportunistic infections (P=0.032)
	140	Placebo		255	+1[g]			13/122	2/122	
AIDS: CDC groups IV–C1 or IV–K	53	DSH	400 mg/m² qw po × 24w	91	—			0/53	—	Decreases in opportunistic infections (P=0.046)
	56	Placebo		114	—			—	2/56	

[a] Nomenclature employed in patient selection description: HIV+, human immunodeficiency virus positive; AIDS, acquired immunodeficiency syndrome; ARC, AIDS related complex; CDC group definitions: Centers for Disease Control (1986). Symptoms: lymphadenopathy, fever, night sweats, weight loss, diarrhea, fatigue, thrush or hairy leukoplakia. Immune defects: CD4+ count of <500/µl, CD4+/CD8+ ratios of less than 0.5, hypergammaglobulinemia or positive cutaneous delayed hypersensitivity response to <3/7 antigens using Merieux Multitest.

[b] Convention and nomenclature employed in drug and dosage regimen description: DSH, diethyldithiocarbamate; qw, every week; qw/2, twice a week; iv, intravenous: po, orally; w, week; m, month; y, year; ∫, followed by.

[c] Persistent diarrhea, weight loss, persistent fever.

[d] Diarrhea, weight loss, fever, night sweats, fatigue, thrush, lymphadenopathy, hairy leukoplakia.

[e] CD4+ data at end of 24 weeks of treatment; exclusively from patients with entry CD4+ counts below 814/µl.

[f] During 24 weeks of treatment.

[g] CD4+ change computed jointly for HIV+ patients with and without AIDS.

lymph node size) diminished in the DSH group but progressed in the placebo group, the difference being significant ($P<0.05$). After 16 weeks of therapy, the CD4$^+$ cell counts of the patients in the DSH group were significantly ($P<0.05$) higher than those of the control group. Following a cross-over of 25 patients in the DSH group to placebo therapy for a further 16 weeks, a significant ($P<0.01$) fall in their CD4$^+$ cell counts was observed (Fig. 13.1). With regard to the DCH reaction, 3 of 29 patients in the DSH group remained anergic at 16 weeks as compared to 9 of 32 in the control group ($P<0.10$).

A second study by Lang *et al.* (1988c) was one of longer duration (Table 13.1, study 2). It involved a group of 44 HIV$^+$ patients who remained in the study for 1 year. At entry they fell into CDC categories

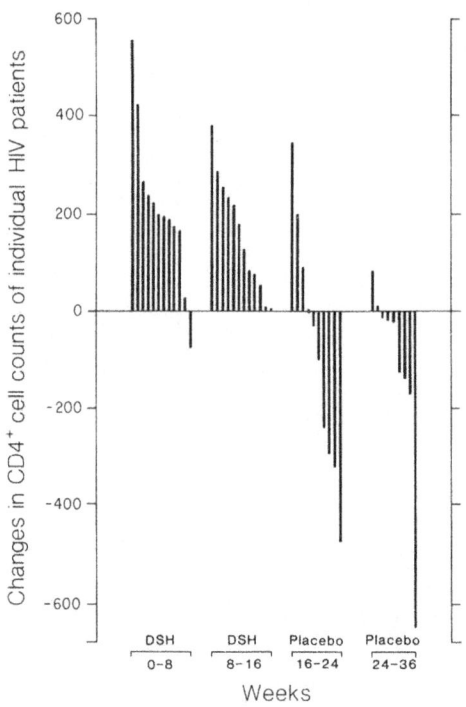

Figure 13.1 Effect of diethyldithiocarbamate (DSH) therapy on CD4$^+$ lymphocyte counts in patients with HIV infection. Patients were administered DSH (10 mg/kg once a week per os in an enterocoated capsule) and the number of CD4$^+$ lymphocytes per μl peripheral blood determined at 8-week intervals. After 16 weeks of DSH therapy the patients were switched to placebo for a further 16 weeks. Redrawn from Lang *et al.* (1988b).

II, III, IV and IVC2 (defined as presenting with any one of six other specified infectious diseases: Centers for Disease Control, 1986). Of the 44 patients, 26 were maintained on DSH (10 mg/kg/week) and 18 received no treatment. None of the 26 patients in the treated group progressed to AIDS and none of the 20 in categories II and III progressed to AIDS-related-complex (ARC), though in the untreated group one of the 18 patients progressed to AIDS and four progressed to ARC. The CD4$^+$ cell counts rose in the treated group from 385 to 483/µl, but fell in the control group from 431 to 326/µl, a significant ($P<0.05$) difference. Also a significant ($P<0.05$) increase in the DCH reaction was noted in the treated group, though in the controls it tended to diminish.

Brewton *et al.* (1987, 1989) have reported on 44 patients with ARC or AIDS (Table 13.1, study 3). Patients with no or limited symptoms were excluded as were four patients who progressed in the first 8 weeks of the study. Of the remaining patients, 48% had CD4$^+$ counts < 200/µl at entry. The patients were randomized to either treatment with a 200 mg/m^2/week i.v. dose of DSH (*ca* 5 mg/kg for a 70 kg man) for 16 weeks or no therapy. This was followed by a cross-over to the opposite arm for an equal period (that is, those initially randomized to DSH treatment received no therapy during the second 16-week period and vice versa). By 16 weeks a further 10 patients (18% of those on DSH, 33% of controls: $P=0.23$) progressed. Accordingly, except for life-table analyses which were inconclusive, outcome statistics were performed on the results from the first 16 weeks of the study only. During that period, 16 of the 22 receiving DSH but only 4 of the 18 receiving no treatment had one or more symptoms disappear ($P<0.002$). In particular, a 50% or greater reduction in the size of all lymph nodes was observed in 53% of those on DSH, but in only 7% of those receiving no treatment ($P<0.005$)

Some benefits of DSH therapy were also observed in a phase I study (Hersh *et al.*, 1987; Petersen *et al.*, 1988; Kaplan *et al.* 1989) designed to determine the tolerance, toxicity and maximally tolerated dose of DSH administered i.v. on a once a week basis (Table 13.1, study 4). It involved 25 patients with ARC and AIDS, though only the results from ARC patients with CD4$^+$ counts above 200/µl at entry are listed in Table 13.1. Patients randomized to DSH treatment were placed on a schedule whereby, over a period of 16 weeks, the i.v. dose of DSH escalated every 4 weeks from an original dose of 200 mg/m^2/week, to 400 mg/m^2/week, then to 800 mg/m^2/week and finally to 800 mg/m^2/0.5 weeks, respectively. Patients with CD4$^+$ counts below 200/µl at entry derived no benefit from the therapy, they all progressed; additionally, 2/7 in the DSH group and 4/6 controls died within 16 weeks. Among patients with CD4$^+$ counts above 200/μl at entry, those of the group receiving DSH rose during the 16-week treatment period (from 451 to 584/μl), while those of the controls fell (from 526 to 387/μl). Among these patients, those receiving DSH also experienced fewer symptoms and a significant ($P=0.006$) regression of lymphadenopathy, this being assessed in terms of the sum of the lymph node diameters.

Another study (Reisinger *et al.*, 1990) involved 60 CDC category II to IV patients who were matched in pairs and received placebo or DSH for 24 weeks (5 mg/kg/week i.v. or 10 mg/kg/week p.o.) and were followed for a further 12 months (Table 13.1, study 5). The progression to AIDS was significantly ($P<0.05$) less frequent (0/13) in the i.v. DSH group than in the i.v. placebo group (4/13). No deaths occurred among those who progressed to AIDS during the treatment period, but three of the four died in the follow-up period. The same trend with regard to progression to AIDS and subsequent mortality was seen in the groups receiving oral medication but it was not statistically significant. In contrast to the observations of Lang *et al.* (1988b), the CD4$^+$ cell levels did not increase during the 6-month treatment with DSH. However, among those with CD4$^+$ counts of less than 814/μl at entry, the fall during the treatment with i.v. DSH was significantly less ($P<0.02$) than in their matched controls. Also, at the end of the 6-month treatment period patients receiving i.v. DSH had a significantly ($P<0.05$) higher proportion of interleukin-2 (IL-2) receptor-positive monocytes than those in the i.v. placebo group (Reisinger *et al.*, 1990). Interleukin-1 (IL-1) production was also significantly different in the treated and placebo groups (M. Dietrich, private communication).

The multicenter, randomized, placebo-controlled, double-blind study by Hersh *et al.* (1991) is noteworthy because of the large number of patients involved and the finding that DSH therapy benefits both patients with symptomatic HIV infections and those with AIDS (Table 13.1, study 6). A total of 389 patients were admitted to eight study centers and randomized to a 400 mg/m^2 weekly i.v. dose of DSH or to placebo. During the 24 weeks of the study, the CD4$^+$ count of patients on DSH rose 18% while that of controls remained constant. Adverse reactions were minimal and more prevalent among placebo than DSH patients. Concurrently, of the patients who were anergic at entry (91%), seven of those receiving DSH, but only 1 on placebo developed a positive DCH reaction. Most impressively, however, the incidence of AIDS-defining opportunistic infections was significantly lower ($P<0.032$) among patients receiving DSH than among placebo controls. This reduction in opportunistic infections among patients

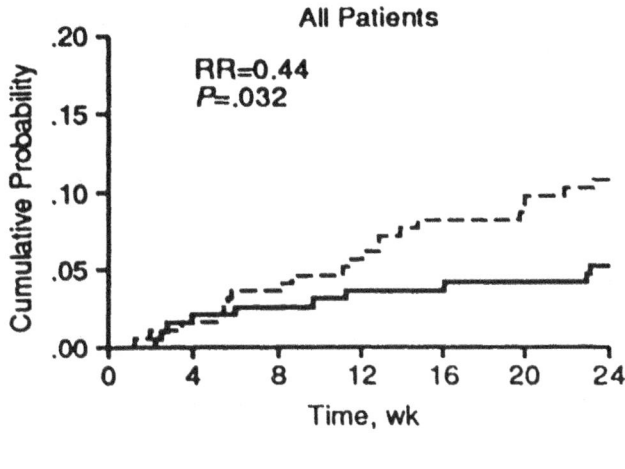

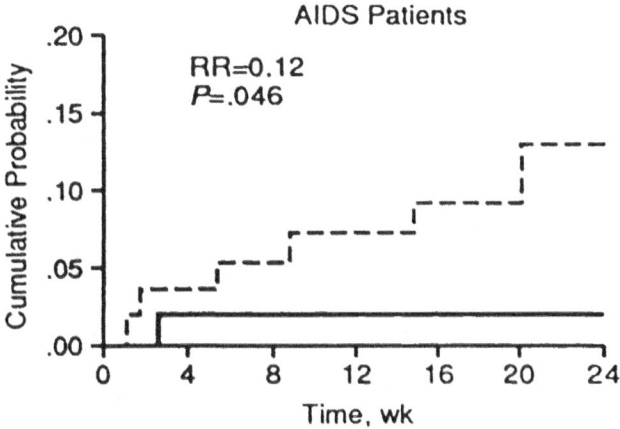

Figure 13.2 Effect of diethyldithiocarbamate (DSH) therapy on the cumulative probability of patients with HIV infection (top) and AIDS (bottom) progressing to a new opportunistic infection. Solid line, patients receiving DSH (400 mg/m² once a week per os for 24 weeks as enterocoated capsules). Dashed line, patients receiving placebo under double-blind conditions. *P* values are two-tailed. RR indicates relative risk. Reproduced with permission from Hersh *et al.* (1991).

receiving DSH was one seen, moreover, at each of the eight study centers. Furthermore, the DSH effect was a significant one ($P<0.042$) when the patients with AIDS were considered separately (Fig. 13.2). Analysis of the incidence of the opportunistic infections as a function of the patients' CD4⁺ counts at entry into the study, confirms an inverse relationship between these two variables. It also suggests, however, that DSH therapy is quite effective when the CD4$^+$ entry levels are quite low (less than 100/µl). Of special interest was the observation that concurrent therapy of 93 of the patients with zidovudine (azidothymidine, AZT), at the time of the study the only therapeutic agent licensed for the treatment of HIV infections, did not affect the outcome or cause an increase in adverse reactions, which were, in any event, fewer among the DSH than placebo patients.

Some concern has been expressed (Mariman, 1986) that, if the effect of DSH is simply to increase the number of CD4$^+$ T cells, then the increase would provide the HIV virus with extra target cells and relapse would occur when treatment was stopped. Indeed, in a cross-over trial (Lang *et al.* 1988b) the CD4$^+$ cell counts of patients returned to placebo resumed a decline. Combination of DSH therapy with an antiviral drug is a rational way of dealing with this problem. No benefit was found to accrue, however, from combined therapy with DSH and suramin, an effective HIV inhibitor *in vivo* (Taelman *et al.*, 1987). DSH does appear to possess some, albeit weak, direct anti-HIV activity. Added in a concentration of 2.5 or 7.5×10^{-2} µg/ml to 4-day cultures of HIV$^+$ human peripheral blood mononuclear cells (PBMC) or an HIV$^+$ H9 leukemic CD4$^+$ cell line, it inhibits the expression of reverse transcriptase, an HIV component, and of the HIV p15 and p24 proteins in a concentration-dependent fashion (Pompidou *et al.*, 1985c, 1986). Treatment of HIV$^+$ patients for 4 months with DSH had no effect, however, on the replicability of HIV in cultures of the PBMC of these patients (Escaich *et al.*, 1988). At the same time, PBMC from HIV$^+$ individuals, upon a 20-min exposure to 10^{-6} mg/ml DSH showed a decrease in nuclear refringency (a measure of chromatin dispersion) analogous to that seen with PBMC from normal individuals, and, when cultured for 4 days, showed a significant increase in the absolute number of CD4$^+$ T lymphocytes (Pompidou *et al.*, 1985a, 1986)

Since DSSD, which is metabolized to DSH *in vivo* (Chapter 6), is a Food and Drug Administration (FDA) approved drug in the United States, while DSH has only been approved in New Zealand, many physicians treating HIV$^+$ and AIDS patients in the States have started prescribing DSSD in the expectation that it would share the immuno-stimulant properties of DSH. Bihari *et al.* (1988) followed the CD4$^+$ T-cell counts in a group of 53 such patients who were maintained on DSSD (either 750 mg/week or 500 mg/0.5 weeks p.o.) for a mean of 3.3 months. In a preliminary communication they reported that in this group of patients, many of whom were also receiving other medications, the absolute number of CD4$^+$ T cells rose, on average, 36% during the course of therapy (from a mean of 191 to

259/µl; $P<0.05$). On the other hand, Hørding *et al.* (1990) have reported that in a 4-week double-blind study which involved three groups of HIV⁺ patients administered, respectively, placebo ($n=6$), 100 mg ($n=4$) and 400 mg ($n=5$) DSSD daily, no significant differences were observed in CD4⁺ or CD8⁺ counts, or responses of PBMC to mitogens. The study was, however, one of rather short duration and the dosing interval used was much shorter than in the studies involving DSH.

Overall, the results of the various clinical studies suggest that DSH therapy can inhibit the progression of HIV infection both in its early and late stages.

13.2.1 Evaluation of side-effects

No major adverse clinical or biological reactions have been reported in controlled studies of HIV⁺ patients receiving weekly dose of 5 mg/kg p.o. or i.v. to 400 mg/m² p.o. (Table 13.1, studies 1-3, 5 and 6). A metallic taste and abdominal discomfort were the most frequently observed minor side-effects (Reisinger *et al.*, 1990, however, noted that patients receiving placebo reported experiencing side-effects; the percentages of DSH and placebo patients reporting a metallic taste were 75 and 25 %, respectively, and those reporting abdominal discomfort were 42 and 24%, respectively). Less frequently mentioned were nausea, malaise, fatigue, difficulties of concentration and retrosternal burning chest pain.

One of the studies in Table 13.1 (study 4) was a Phase I study, that is a study in which the dose was progressively escalated to determine the maximally tolerated dose and the nature of the side-effects observed when this dose was exceeded. All but one of the 16 patients tolerated a weekly i.v. DSH infusion of 400 mg/m², and all but five tolerated a weekly 800 mg/m². Half of the patients tolerated the highest dosage used (twice weekly infusion of 800 mg/m²). Because of the nature of the Phase I study, it is not surprising that most of the patients in the study experienced side-effects. The incidence with which various side-effects occurred under these circumstances were: gastrointestinal upset (56% of patients), burning at the site of infusion (39%), metallic taste (28%), drowsiness or confusional states (22%), sneezing or watery eyes during the infusion (22%), hyperactivity (17%), delusional thinking or hallucinations (11%) and myoclonic jerks (6%). All these observed adverse effects resolved completely within one week of either the dose being reduced or DSH therapy being discontinued.

13.3 IN GASTROINTESTINAL SURGERY PATIENTS

Administration of DSH to patients undergoing gastrointestinal surgery has been reported in two controlled studies to be correlated with a decreased length of hospitalization and a decreased incidence of complications (Champault *et al.*, 1983; Chabal *et al.*, 1987). Specifically, in patients given one to three oral doses of 250 mg DSH 7 days apart (except in emergencies, the first dose was given pre-operatively), 71.7% had an uncomplicated recovery, as compared with only 26.7% of untreated controls ($P = 0.009$). In particular, significant benefits of DSH therapy were observed in patients with infections ($P = 0.04$) and those treated with antibiotics ($P = 0.01$). Although the number of doses received had no significant effect on these variables, it was significantly ($P < 0.011$) negatively correlated with the length of hospitalization. This averaged 22.7 days for the controls and 21.9, 18.7 and 18.1 days for those receiving 1, 2 and 3 doses of DSH, respectively. Also the $CD4^+$ T-cell counts of DSH-treated patients fell significantly less than those of controls (Champault *et al.*, 1983).

A second controlled study was conducted in patients requiring gastrointestinal surgery under general anesthesia of 1 h or less duration (Chabal *et al.*, 1987) Administration of 375 mg DSH by i.v. infusion on the eve of surgery, and again 5 days post-operatively, reduced the length of post-operative hospitalization from 17 to 11.6 days ($P < 0.002$). Prolonged post-operative hospitalization (more than 25 days) was necessary in 16 out of 92 controls, but only in 1 out of 95 patients receiving DSH ($P < 0.0001$). Additionally, although 27.4% of the controls experienced fever postoperatively, this was true for only 8.6% of the DSH-treated patients ($P = 0.004$).

13.4 AS A THERAPEUTIC AGENT IN AUTOIMMUNE DISEASE

Abnormalities of regulatory T cells are considered to be one of the primary causes of antibody production by B cells in autoimmune diseases (Stites *et al.*, 1987). It is therefore of interest that in a controlled study of patients with active rheumatoid arthritis and a $CD4^+/CD8^+$ ratio > 2, DSH has been found to decrease this ratio. Specifically, 7 days following a single 250 mg oral dose of DSH the $CD4^+/CD8^+$ ratio was reduced by 46% ($P < 0.05$) and both the absolute number and percentage of $CD8^+$ cells were increased significantly ($P < 0.05$), no change being observed in the number of $CD4^+$ cells (Corke *et al.*, 1986). A reduction of this ratio was also reported in a disseminated aspergillosis patient receiving DSH (Lemarié *et al.*, 1986).

Corke *et al.* (1986) performed a 6-month clinical trial in which 11 patients with active rheumatoid arthritis, who previously had failed to respond to D-penicillamine and who were taking non-steroidal anti-inflammatory drugs throughout the trial, received 250 mg of DSH p.o. every 7 days. A dramatic improvement in the clinical status was observed, as evaluated by a blinded observer (i.e. one unaware of what was the patient's treatment status). Specifically, significant improvements were noted in the articular index ($P<0.01$) and pain scores ($P<0.01$ at 3 months; $P<0.05$ at 6 months); a trend was also observed in favor of reduced morning stiffness, and in a fall in the erythrocyte sedimentation rate. A twelfth patient was dropped from the study upon developing a sensitivity reaction to the drug.

The possibility that DSH may also have a beneficial effect in juvenile systemic lupus erythematosus has been raised by a case report of a patient with this condition who had been previously treated with prednisone and developed a serious Cushingoid syndrome. Administration of DSH, in a 5 mg/kg/week p.o. dose, induced a long-lasting (1-year) remission (Delpine *et al.*, 1985).

13.5 IN PATIENTS WITH NEOPLASTIC DISEASE

Post-operative immunosuppression resultant from surgical intervention in the treatment of neoplastic disease is a cause of concern in that it might facilitate tumor cell dissemination as a consequence of surgical manipulation (Cochran *et al.*, 1972). Also, lymph nodes nearest to melanoma are known to be immunosuppressed (Hoon *et al.*, 1987), with more general immunosuppression being a feature of advanced neoplastic disease. Accordingly, a proven ability of DSH to reverse the immunosuppression would be of importance. Macrophages from individuals with progressive tumors are known to inhibit immune responses by secretion of prostaglandin. Mossalayi (private communication) reports DSH lowers prostaglandin E_2 titers in PBMC cultures. Thus, a potential exists for DSH as an immunostimulant in the treatment of neoplastic disease. The available information regarding its immunostimulant efficacy in such patients is, however, meager. Stimulation of the PBMC lymphoproliferative response (PBMC-LPR) to mitogens in lung cancer patients 7 days following i.v. administration of DSH in a 5 mg/kg dose was first reported in an uncontrolled study (Renoux *et al.*, 1980b; Renoux and Renoux, 1981). The majority of these patients underwent surgery and the DSH was first administered pre-operatively.

A subsequent controlled study, conducted on lung cancer patients prior to their receiving specific cancer therapy, was reported upon only in terms of its discussion in a review article (Renoux *et al.*, 1983b). However, it was noted that on the fifth day following administration of DSH in a 5 mg/kg i.v. dose, the recovery in the PBMC-LPR to PHA and Con A and the increase in the fraction of $CD3^+$ and $CD4^+$ T cells among the PBMC all reached the $P < 0.01$ level of significance (Fig. 12.2). Also while a trend ($P = 0.06$) was observed with regard to the decrease in the fraction of $CD8^+$ cells. No information was presented regarding the time course and duration of these effects. In the same article it was reported that the PBMC-LPR to both PHA and Con A increased in four out of four stage IV melanoma patients during a month-long period when these individuals received DSH in a 5 mg/kg i.v. dose weekly.

13.6 AS AN ADJUVANT FOR INFLUENZA VACCINATION

DSH appears to improve the influenza vaccine-induced antibody responses of age-immunodepressed, chronically hospitalized elderly patients (Lesourd *et al.*, 1988). Patients, in an aged (82.7 ± 7.9 years), previously unvaccinated, hospitalized population were given an influenza vaccine containing antigens from two A and two B influenza virus strains and, by random assignment, half were concurrently administered DSH (10 mg/kg). Thirty days later the antibody titers for three of the four antigens were significantly ($P < 0.05$) higher in the DSH-treated group than either in the control group or in a comparable group of vaccinated patients who had received yearly influenza vaccinations for several years. No difference was evident at 15 days post vaccination, at which time the titers in the control groups reached a plateau. The difference at 30 days can be ascribed to the continued rise in the titers of the DSH group, which was contributed to primarily by patients who had initially titers $\leqslant 20$ and were considered unprotected. Eight months after vaccination, the DSH group's antibody titers were still higher for each of the four antigens (significantly so in one instance) than those of the previously unvaccinated controls. Treatment with DSH appears to provide a potent adjuvant effect in this group of patients.

13.7 SUMMARY

The results of the six published controlled studies of DSH therapy all indicate that it benefits therapeutically patients with HIV infections. Possibly because of differences in experimental design, the results of these studies show a good deal of variability in the nature of the benefits reported, suggesting that the paradigm for the DSH treatment of these infections has not yet been optimized. To date DSH has been approved as a prescription drug for the treatment of HIV infections only in New Zealand. Though as yet no study has shown a significant DSH-therapy-induced decrease in mortality among HIV infected individuals, this is not surprising given the overall low mortality figures observed in these studies and their short duration relative to the time course of the disease.

Much of the other clinical data on the immunostimulant properties of DSH is preliminary. It has been tried and reported to be effective in so many conditions that it might be in danger of appearing to be a panacea. Replication and amplification of the findings reported to date are badly needed. On the other hand, the properties ascribed to DSH are quite unique and the agent appears to possess a low toxicity and an excellent safety record. Accordingly, further exploration of its clinical utility seems to be in order.

14

Modulation of various biological phenomena

14.1 CYTOTOXICITY 295
14.2 MODULATION OF THE EFFECTS OF OXIDATIVE STRESS 301
    14.2.1 Introduction 301
    14.2.2 Normobaric and quasinormobaric hyperoxia 302
    14.2.3 Hyperbaric hyperoxia 303
    14.2.4 Ozone toxicity 304
    14.2.5 Paraquat toxicity 304
    14.2.6 Pulmonary pathology 305
    14.2.7 Mechanisms 305
14.3 MODULATION OF THE EFFECTS OF RADIATION AND
    HYPERTHERMIA 306
    14.3.1 *In vivo* modulation of radiation effects 306
    14.3.2 Modulation of *in vitro* effects of radiation 310
    14.3.3 Modulation of *in vitro* effects of hyperthermia 311
    14.3.4 Summary 312

14.1 CYTOTOXICITY

The most striking aspect of the *in vitro* cytotoxicity of diethyldithiocarbamate (DSH) is that it is bimodal. This phenomenon was first described by Rigas *et al.* (1979), who reported on the effects of a range of DSH concentrations on human monocytes and polymorphonuclear granulocytes (PMN). While below 10^{-6}M DSH was not toxic, cytotoxicity rose to a maximum as the DSH concentration was increased to 2.5×10^{-5}M. Thereafter cytotoxicity decreased, reaching a minimum at 2.5×10^{-4}M (Fig. 14.1). Analogous results have been obtained (Table 14.1) for DSH cytotoxicity in exponentially growing cultures of Chinese hamster cells (Westman and Midander, 1984; Lin *et al.*, 1985) and mouse fibroblast cells (Maners *et al.*, 1985; Taylor *et al.*, 1986). In the latter, disulfiram (DSSD) cytotoxicity is similarly bimodal (Taylor *et al.*, 1986). The absolute concentrations reported by different workers to be associated with the cytotoxicity maximum and minimum differ

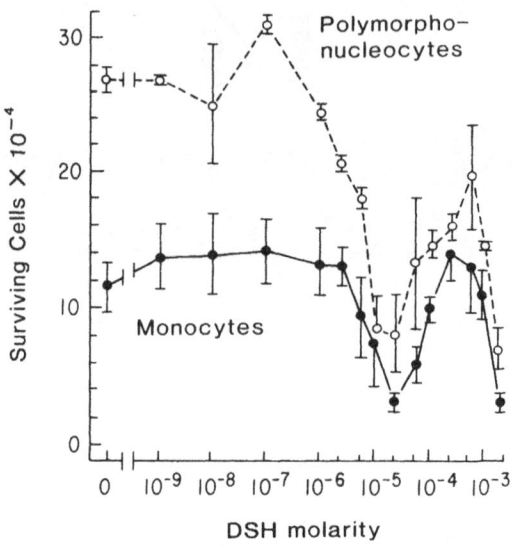

Figure 14.1 Survival of human peripheral blood mononuclear cells and polymorphonuclear granulocytes in culture following preincubation with diethyldithiocarbamate (DSH). Human defibrinated, platelet-depleted blood was preincubated for 2 h at 37 °C with DSH in the stated concentration. The blood was then diluted with two volumes of RPMI 1640 culture medium and incubated at 37 °C for 24 h. The viability of the cells was determined by Trypan Blue exclusion. Vertical bars indicate standard errors. Reproduced with permission from Rigas *et al.* (1979).

significantly, but the ratios of these concentrations remain more or less constant (range 9–20).

A DSH concentration-related bimodality also characterizes a variety of other *in vitro* cellular responses to DSH and its modulation of the effects of various agents (Table 14.2). Thus, bimodality characterizes the effect of DSH concentration on 5-^{3}H-uridine uptake, a measure of RNA synthesis, in both unstimulated and phytohemagglutinin (PHA)-stimulated lymphocytes (Rigas *et al.*, 1979). The unstimulated DSH-induced ^{3}H-uridine uptake is so highly correlated with DSH-induced cytotoxicity ($r=0.9864$; $n=70$) that it has been used as a measure of lymphocyte cytotoxicity in studying DSH radiosensitization (Rigas *et al.*, 1980). The radiosensitization proved to be also bimodally related to DSH concentration, with the concentrations for maximum and minimum sensitization coinciding with those for maximum and minimum cytotoxicity, respectively (Rigas *et al.*, 1979, 1980). Working with Chinese hamster cells in their exponential phase of growth, Lin *et al.* (1985) also observed a coincidence between the maximum and minimum radiosensitization- and cytotoxicity-inducing concentrations

Table 14.1 Parameters of bimodal *in vitro* diethyldithiocarbamate (DSH) and disulfiram (DSSD) cytotoxicity

Cell type	Agent	First maximum (M)	Subsequent minimum (M)	Max/Min conc. ratio	Incubation Medium	Incubation Supplement	Study
Human blood mono-nucleocytes	DSH	2.5×10^{-5}	2.5×10^{-4}	10	RPMI 1640	Human serum	Rigas et al. (1979)
Human blood PMNs	DSH	2.5×10^{-5}	5.0×10^{-4}	20	RPMI 1640	Human serum	Rigas et al. (1979)
Chinese hamster cells V79–379A	DSH	1.0×10^{-4}	2.0×10^{-3}	20	Earle's MEM	15% fetal calf serum	Westman and Midander (1984)
Chinese hamster cells V79	DSH	3.6×10^{-5}	3.4×10^{-4}	9	MEM	5% fetal, 5% new born calf serum	Lin et al. (1985)
Mouse fibroblast cells L-929	DSH	4.4×10^{-7}	4.4×10^{-6}	20	Earle's MEM	10% fetal calf serum	Maners et al. (1985) Taylor et al. (1986)
Mouse fibroblast cells L-929	DSSD	1.7×10^{-7}	3.4×10^{-7}	20	Earle's MEM	10% fetal calf serum	Taylor et al. (1986)

Table 14.2 Parameters of bimodal *in vitro* diethyldithiocarbamate (DSH) modulation of various phenomena

Phenomenon	DSH effect	Cell type	Maximum effect (M)	Subsequent minimum (M)	Study
Unstimulated ^{3}H-uridine uptake	Inhibition	Human blood mononucleocytes	2.0×10^{-5}	5.0×10^{-4}	Rigas *et al.* (1979)
PHA-stimulated ^{3}H-uridine uptake	Inhibition	Human blood lymphocytes	2.0×10^{-5}	5.0×10^{-4}	Rigas *et al.* (1979)
X-ray irradiation	Inhibition	Human blood lymphocytes	1.0×10^{-5}	1.0×10^{-4}	Rigas *et al.* (1979)
Beta (^{137}Cs) irradiation	Sensitization	Chinese hamster cells V79	4.4×10^{-5}	3.0×10^{-4}	Lin *et al.* (1985)
Heat exposure	Sensitization	Chinese hamster cells V79	3.4×10^{-5}	6.4×10^{-4}	Lin *et al.* (1985)
Bleomycin toxicity	Sensitization	Chinese hamster cells V79	2.9×10^{-5}	4.9×10^{-4}	Lin *et al* (1985)
Adriamycin toxicity	Sensitization	Chinese hamster cells V79	5.7×10^{-5}	5.0×10^{-4}	Lin *et al.* (1985)
Scheduled DNA synthesis	Inhibition	Rat thymocytes	4.4×10^{-5}	4.4×10^{-4}	Tempel *et al.* (1985) Spath and Tempel (1987)
Unscheduled DNA synthesis	Inhibition	Rat thymocytes	4.4×10^{-5}		Tempel *et al.* (1985) Spath and Tempel (1987)
Single-strand DNA breaks	Induction	Rat premeiotic male germ cells	1.0×10^{-3}	1.0×10^{-2}	Coogan *et al.* (1986)
NK cell-mediated cytotoxicity	Inhibition	Human blood lymphocytes	1.0×10^{-4}		Stacey and Craig (1989)
K cell-mediated cytotoxicity	Inhibition	Human blood lymphocytes	1.0×10^{-4}		Stacey and Craig (1989)
Antibody-dependent cytotoxicity	Inhibition	Human blood monocytes	1.0×10^{-4}		Conkling *et al.* (1982) Conkling *et al* (1985)

of DSH. Moreover analogous bimodal relationships were observed by these workers for DSH modulation of the cytotoxic effects of adriamycin, bleomycin and heat exposure. Other workers have reported (Table 14.2) scheduled and unscheduled DNA synthesis (Tempel *et al.*, 1985; Spath and Tempel, 1987), NK and K cell-mediated cytotoxicity (Stacey and Craig, 1989) and antibody-dependent cytotoxicity (Conkling *et al.*, 1982, 1985) to be all bimodally inhibited as a function of the DSH concentration. Likewise, induction of single-stranded DNA breaks has also been reported to be bimodally dependent on DSH concentration (Coogan *et al.*, 1986). These recurring findings of bimodality for the *in vitro* effect of DSH focus attention on the thiol–disulfide interconversion of DSH and on the possible relationship of these phenomena to the composition of the incubation media and supplements.

Analogous *in vitro* bimodality phenomena are also a feature of the cytotoxicity of a number of other thiols, thus glutathione (GSH), cysteine (Vergroesen *et al.*, 1967), cysteamine (Takagi *et al.*, 1974), ethofos (WR-2721: Mori *et al.*, 1983) and dithiothreitol (Held and Melder, 1987). Moreover, in common with these other thiols, DSH undergoes apparent autoxidation in serum-containing media under aerobic conditions (DSH half-life: 3.7 ± 0.8 h in 10% bovine calf serum-supplemented Eagle's minimal essential medium, 9.4 ± 4.0 h in McCoy's; Held and Melder, 1987). Such thiol 'autoxidations' are catalyzed by the transition metal ions: Cu^{2+} and Fe^{2+}. Cu^{2+} is more effective, for instance, in the oxidation of GSH, Fe^{2+} in that of cysteine (Jocelyn, 1972). Serum contains higher levels of such ions than do unsupplemented incubation media and addition of serum enhances both the rate of oxidation of the thiol (Tahsildar *et al.*, 1988) and its cytotoxicity (Held and Melder, 1987). Hydrogen peroxide is a product of thiol oxidation as rendered, overall, by

$$2RSH + O_2 \rightarrow RSSR + H_2O_2 \qquad (14.1)$$

Its formation, however, is a bimodal function of the thiol concentration, for at high thiol concentration the oxidation of the thiol by hydrogen peroxide itself is favored by a process rendered, overall, by

$$2RSH + H_2O_2 \rightarrow RSSR + 2H_2O \qquad (14.2)$$

Where this has been investigated, the thiol concentration resulting in the highest rate of hydrogen peroxide formation coincides with that for maximum cytotoxicity (Takagi *et al.*, 1974). Moreover, cytotoxicity is prevented by addition of catalase to the incubation medium (Takagi *et al.*, 1974; Held and Melder, 1987). Hydrogen peroxide is not sufficiently cytotoxic, however, to account wholly for the cytotoxicity that accompanies the oxidation of the thiol (Takagi *et al.*, 1974; Biaglow *et al.*, 1984); nor does formation of the superoxide radical play a significant role, since addition of superoxide dismutase (SOD) to the incubation medium has no effect on the cytotoxicity (Held and Melder, 1987). On the other hand, there is evidence that the very toxic hydroxyl free radicals are formed during thiol oxidation in the presence of Fe^{2+} (Searle and Tomasi, 1982), presumably by a Fenton-type reaction:

$$H_2O_2 + Fe^{2+}(RS^-)_2 \rightarrow OH^{\cdot} + OH^- + Fe^{3+}(RS^-)_2 \qquad (14.3)$$

Applied to DSH, this model suggests that, if neither the absence of trace metals has been assured nor an excess of catalase has been added, the observed bimodal cytotoxicity and other bimodal *in vivo* effects of DSH should be considered as resulting from the oxidation of DSH. A number of additional observations can be explained by the model. First, it provides a plausible explanation for the fact that the cytotoxicity of 2.5×10^{-5}M DSH is partially (57%) reversed by equimolar $ZnCl_2$. Zn^{2+} has long been known to inhibit the oxidation of cysteine (Mathews and Walker, 1909), and the formation of hydroxyl free radicals in a cysteine–Fe^{2+} system is inhibited by addition of Zn^{2+} (Searle and Tomasi, 1982). These effects occur because Zn^{2+} effectively competes with Fe^{2+} for binding to the thiol (Willson, 1987). Competition by Zn^{2+} for binding to DSH, likely inhibits its Fe^{2+} catalyzed oxidation.

Secondly, the model can be used to explain the apparent paradox that DSH enhances dithiothreitol cytotoxicity (Held and Melder, 1987), but that it inhibits cysteamine oxidation (Biaglow *et al.*, 1984). Cysteamine oxidation in incubation media is not stimulated by Fe^{2+}, suggesting that it is catalyzed by Cu^{2+}. Since DSH is an avid copper chelator, it follows that its inhibition of cysteamine oxidation is likely due to the removal of the Cu^{2+} ions catalyzing the reaction. On the other hand, dithiothreitol oxidation is inhibited by deferoxamine (Desferal), an iron chelator, and must, therefore, be catalyzed by Fe^{2+} (Held and Melder, 1987). So too is the 'autoxidation' of DSH, since it is observed to occur in the presence of the $Fe^{2+}O_2^-$ oxyhemoglobin complex (Kelner and Alexander, 1986). Accordingly, the cytotoxicity of dithiothreitol may be enhanced by the additional production of hydrogen peroxide due to DSH oxidation.

Thirdly, the model can explain the protection afforded by 10^{-2}M $CuCl_2$ against the cytotoxicity of 2.5×10^{-3}M DSH (Rigas *et al.*, 1979). At this DSH concentration the toxicity may be either due to DSH itself, or to the DSSD formed from it by oxidation. Since Cu^{2+} can bind either

DSH or DSSD to form Cu(DS)$_2$, it would lower the DSH and DSSD concentrations. Moreover, because of the high lipophilicity of Cu(DS)$_2$, there would be some expectation that the chelate would be translocated into the cell. Indeed, Trombetta *et al.* (private communication) have noted that incubation of cells in a serum-supplemented medium with DSH increases intracellular copper levels 4-fold.

Fourthly, the model can explain the observation that the cytotoxicity of a 1-h exposure to 2.4×10^{-4}M DSH cannot be reversed by the concurrent exposure of the cells to 10 mM GSH, though exposure to this concentration of GSH, subsequent to the removal of the DSH from the medium, does reverse the cytotoxicity (Trombetta *et al.*, private communication). In the former instance, GSH, by reducing any DSSD formed as a result of the oxidation of DSH (equation 14.1) back to DSH (Strömme, 1963a), would assure continued production of hydrogen peroxide via this reaction.

Finally, the model can help explain the decrease in the cytotoxicity of hydrogen peroxide occasioned by concurrent exposure of exponential phase Chinese hamster ovary cells to 1.0×10^{-4}M DSH (Harari *et al.*, 1989). At this DSH concentration the reaction represented by equation (14.2) likely helps to reduce the hydrogen peroxide levels. Additionally, in the presence of GSH, the DSH/DSSD redox pair can substitute for glutathione peroxidase and can couple the reduction of hydrogen peroxide to the hexose monophosphate pathway (Kumar *et al.*, 1986).

14.2 MODULATION OF THE EFFECTS OF OXIDATIVE STRESS

14.2.1 Introduction

Animals exposed to 100% oxygen at normobaric and quasinormobaric pressures (1–2.8 atm) exhibit primarily pulmonary toxicity, although some lymphoid effects are also evident. At higher partial pressure of oxygen the primary effect observed is central nervous system toxicity which manifests itself as generalized convulsions. DSH and DSSD can either protect or enhance each of these types of toxicity, depending on factors such as dose, the duration of the oxygen exposure and the time of their administration.

The oxidative stress induced by hyperoxia is mediated by the formation of the superoxide anion radical and other related reactive oxygen species. This is also considered to be the mechanism of the oxidative stress induced by a variety of other agents, including ozone, paraquat, and irradiation by ultraviolet light. Modulation by DSH and

DSSD of the oxidative stress caused by these latter treatments is also discussed in this section. The abilities of DSH and DSSD to alter the effects of ionizing radiation and hyperthermia, phenomena thought to be mediated by a similar mechanism, are discussed separately in section 14.3.

14.2.2 Normobaric and quasinormobaric hyperoxia

Continuous exposure to 100% oxygen leads to biphasic toxicity in rats: a number of the animals die within the first 24 h, while the remainder survive until 72 h, at which point mortality begins to rise again and progresses to 100%. Administered to rodents in sufficient dosage at the start of oxygen exposure, both DSH and DSSD increase the early (24–48 h) mortality, as detailed below. Paradoxically, if the dose of DSH is kept relatively low, it can also protect the animal against late (87–96 h) oxygen mortality. Additionally, yet lower DSH doses, if administered some days before oxygen exposure, protect animals from late pulmonary and lymphoid oxygen toxicity.

Administered in doses of 250–500 mg/kg at the start of oxygen exposure, DSH increases the 24-h mortality in adult rats, though doses of 100–200 mg/kg are ineffective in this respect (Deneke *et al.*, 1979; Deneke and Fanburg, 1980). Likewise, administration of 250 or 500 mg/kg, both at the beginning and again at 24 h of oxygen exposure, increases the 48-h mortality in 3- to 5-day-old rats; the effect is not observed, however, if a 125 mg/kg dose is used instead (Frank *et al.*, 1978). The effects of the 250 mg/kg DSH dose in adult rats are specially noteworthy since this dose of DSH has opposite effects on the 24- and 96-h oxygen mortality, significantly increasing the early and significantly decreasing the late mortality (Deneke and Fanburg, 1980). The latter phenomenon suggests that DSH renders the organism better able to resist oxidative stress, but that the effect takes a long time to develop. It is therefore of interest that pretreatment of mice with a 125 mg/kg dose of DSH 2, 4 or 7 days prior to oxygen exposure (though not 14 days prior, or at the start of the exposure) protects the animals against the toxic effects of the exposure. The protection is a marked one, the 4-day pretreatment, for instance, reduces the 87-h mortality from 59% to zero (Mansour *et al.* 1986). Such pretreatment also protects animals against various toxic effects of hyperoxia on the lymphoid system. Thus it significantly decreases the oxygen-induced spleen and thymic cell involution, the oxygen-induced impairment in the ability of the animal to produce anti-sheep red blood cell (α-SRBC) antibodies in response to SRBC immunization, and the impairment of spleen cell proliferative response to the mitogen Con A (Mansour *et al.*, 1986). Using shorter pretreatment times might have the opposite effect. This is suggested by the fact that a 1-h pretreatment with 200 mg/kg DSH shortens significantly the survival of rats exposed to 2 atm of oxygen (Forman *et al.*, 1980); the elevation in oxygen pressure could also contribute, however, to the shortened survival.

Overall, the modulation of oxygen toxicity by DSSD bears many similarities to that of DSH. Thus 20, 50 and 200 mg/kg doses of DSSD administered i.p. in aqueous suspension to rats at the beginning of exposure to normobaric oxygen significantly increase the 24- and 48-h mortality, though doses of 5 and 10 mg/kg are without effect (Deneke *et al.*, 1979). Also, in rats exposed to oxygen at 2 atm pressure, a 1-h pretreatment with 200 mg/kg DSSD administered in a similar manner enhances the 12- and 16-h mortality (Forman *et al.*, 1980).

14.2.3 Hyperbaric hyperoxia

Pretreatment with DSH or DSSD is generally observed to delay the toxic effects of exposure to hyperbaric oxygen. However, under some conditions DSH has also been found to shorten seizure time. From the available data it is not clear whether dose, pretreatment time, or species differences determine which effect is observed.

In mice exposed to oxygen at 6 atm pressure, pretreatment with 500 mg/kg DSH is effective in doubling survival time (43 min in controls), if the DSH is administered 16 or 40 min prior to oxygen exposure, but not if 5- or 63-min pretreatment times are employed (Gerschman *et al.*, 1958). Likewise, a 400 mg/kg dose of DSH doubles the onset time of convulsions (9 min in controls) in mice exposed to 6 atm oxygen if it is administered 1 h prior, but is ineffective if pretreatment times of 0.5, 1.5, 2 or 3 h are used (Faiman *et al.*, 1971a).

DSSD, in a 400 mg/kg dose, also increases the seizure onset times in mice exposed to 4 or 6 atm of oxygen, if administered 1–4 h prior (by factors of 2 and 10 times, respectively). With the 1- to 4-h pretreatment time, a 200 mg/kg DSSD dose is also effective in delaying the onset of seizures in mice exposed to 6 atm of oxygen (lengthening the onset times by factors of 2–4 times, respectively), but is ineffective if administered 8, 16 or 24 h prior to exposure (Faiman *et al.*, 1971a,b). The yet lower DSSD dose of 120 mg/kg is effective in delaying the onset of convulsion in mice exposed to 4 atm of oxygen (174 min in controls) if administered 4 h prior, but not 1 h prior

(Faiman *et al.*, 1971a); it is also ineffective when administered 30 min prior to mice exposed to 5 atm of oxygen (Jamieson and van den Brenk, 1964).

Rats and dogs are similarly protected against hyperbaric oxygen toxicity by DSSD. Thus in a 200 mg/kg dose, administered i.p. in corn oil 60 min prior to a 90-min exposure to 5 atm of oxygen, DSSD has been reported to prevent seizures in 8 out of 8 animals, though seizures were observed in 15 of 23 controls (Alderman *et al.*, 1974). Likewise in dogs, pretreatment with 100 mg/kg DSSD i.p. in aqueous suspension 1 h prior to exposure to oxygen at 4.5 atm was found to delay the onset time for convulsions (10 min in controls) by a factor of 4 (Currie *et al.*, 1973).

In contrast, DSH has been reported to enhance the toxicity of hyperbaric (4 atm) oxygen in rats. Thus a 500 mg/kg dose administered 1 or 2 h prior has been reported to shorten the convulsion onset time (137 min in controls) by 14 and 55%, respectively. A 1000 mg/kg dose administered 2 h prior was found to enhance hyperbaric oxygen toxicity even more: it shortened the seizure onset time by 75% (Puglia and Loeb, 1984).

14.2.4 Ozone toxicity

DSH enhances the toxicity of ozone when this is present in inhaled air at a concentration of *ca* 4 ppm. Under such circumstances a 30-min pretreatment with 1.2 g/kg DSH shortens the survival of mice from 6.8 to 5.5 h (Goldstein *et al.*, 1979).

14.2.5 Paraquat toxicity

Paraquat toxicity is mediated by the formation of reactive oxygen species. The compound undergoes a one electron reduction by the action of various flavoprotein reductases. The paraquat radical produced is rapidly oxidized by molecular oxygen with the formation of the superoxide radical. In biological systems, the formation of hydroxyl radical in the presence of paraquat and oxygen is increased by ferric complexes possessing low dissociation constants. In mice, DSH, administered either shortly before or concurrently with paraquat, enhances its toxicity. Thus 1.2 g/kg DSH, administered 30 min prior to 25 mg/kg paraquat, increases day 7 mortality from 15 to 90% (Goldstein *et al.*, 1979), while concurrent administration of 200 mg/kg DSH and 120 mg/kg paraquat increases the 48-h mortality from 50 to 100% (Matkovics *et al.*, 1982).

14.2.6 Pulmonary pathology

The effects of DSSD and DSH on the pulmonary pathology induced by hyperoxia parallel those on the whole animal. A 200 mg/kg dose of DSSD which, when given at the beginning of exposure of rats to normobaric oxygen increases early mortality, results at 24 h in a degree of marked peribronchial, perivascular and intra-alveolar pulmonary edema similar to that seen in control animals after 72 h of exposure to oxygen. Also, after 24 h of exposure to oxygen, the weight of the lungs from DSSD-administered animals is significantly higher than that in the controls (Deneke *et al.*, 1979). On the other hand, pretreatment of mice with the same dose of DSSD 4 h prior to a 2-h exposure to hyperbaric oxygen (3 atm) significantly protects against lung damage (Faiman *et al.*, 1971a). Likewise, 4 and 7 day pretreatment with 125 mg/kg DSH lowers significantly the pulmonary edema observed after 87 h of exposure to normobaric oxygen (Mansour *et al.*, 1986)

14.2.7 Mechanisms

Oxygen toxicity is thought to be mediated, in the first instance, by the increased formation of the toxic superoxide anion radical, O_2^- . Upon dismutation, this radical yields hydrogen peroxide with which it can then undergo a Fenton-type reaction to give the hydroxyl radical, ˙OH. The latter is extremely reactive and initiates free radical chain reactions. DSH is an efficient free radical scavenger even when present in only μM concentrations (Zanocco *et al.*, 1989) and it could, therefore, delay the onset of tissue damage during the short period of time associated with toxicity development during highly hyperbaric oxygen exposure. However, in considering what mechanisms might explain the *in vivo* modulation of oxygen toxicity by DSH over periods of many hours, even days, cognizance must be taken of the short half-life of DSH in rodents (about 10 min; see Table 6.1). This raises the possibility that the modulation could be mediated by enzyme inactivation. One enzyme known to be inhibited by DSH is dopamine *β*-hydroxylase, a copper enzyme (section 8.3). Its possible mediation of the DSH-induced delay in the onset of hyperbaric oxygen seizures has been considered, but since other dopamine *β*-hydroxylase inhibitors are ineffective in delaying such seizures (Faiman *et al.*, 1971a,b) such mediation appears unlikely.

Administration of either DSH or DSSD in doses of 200 mg/kg or more results in the *in vivo* inhibition of SOD, a CuZn enzyme that catalyzes the reduction of superoxide anion to hydrogen peroxide (section 8.4). Recovery from DSH-induced inhibition of SOD is relatively rapid.

Nonetheless, the interim rise in superoxide radical levels that is brought about by SOD inhibition, leads in turn to the irreversible inactivation of glutathione peroxidase (GSHPx, section 8.5). GSHPx is the primary enzyme responsible for the removal of the hydrogen peroxide that is formed in the dismutation of the superoxide. As a result, the DSH-induced inactivation peak-times for these two enzymes are staggered. Thus in control mice exposed to room air, for instance, peak inactivation of lung SOD occurs within 1 h of the i.m. administration of 1.2 g/kg DSH, whereas 6.5 h elapse before the inactivation of lung GSHPx reaches its peak (Goldstein *et al.*, 1979). This chain of events can therefore extend the modulation of oxidative stress by DSH for the longer periods of time associated with normobaric oxygen, ozone and paraquat toxicity, since it creates conditions favoring the production of hydroxy radicals by Fenton-type reactions.

The ability of an intermediate dose of DSH (250 mg/kg) to decrease the 96-h mortality during long-term normobaric oxygen exposure is correlated with the ability of such a dose to bring about an elevation in the levels of enzymes involved in the removal of hydrogen peroxide, namely, GSHPx, glutathione reductase and glucose-6-phosphate dehydrogenase (Deneke and Fanburg, 1980). This is also the mechanism which Mansour *et al.* (1986) have suggested may be responsible for the protective effect of DSH against pulmonary and lymphoid oxygen toxicity when administered 4–7 days prior to oxygen exposure. Although this increase in the levels of the enzymes of the glutathione cycle can be viewed as compensatory to an earlier inactivation of GSHPx, it should be noted that no parallel enhancement of SOD is observed (Deneke and Fanburg, 1980).

14.3 MODULATION OF THE EFFECTS OF RADIATION AND HYPERTHERMIA

14.3.1 *In vivo* modulation of radiation effects

The discovery that DSH can act as a radioprotective agent *in vivo* dates back to the early 1950s when it was reported that in mice the i.p. administration of 300–335 mg/kg DSH just prior to exposure to a lethal dose of radiation resulted in the survival of all 10 animals tested (Bacq and Herve, 1953; Alexander *et al.*, 1955). Subsequent investigators have confirmed the radioprotective effect of DSH pretreatment (Table 14.3).

Using ^{35}S-DSH, Strömme and Eldjarn (1966) found that DSH distributes rapidly to most tissues, including those most vulnerable to radiation: bone marrow, spleen and intestinal mucosa. At 10 min post

Table 14.3 *In vivo* radioprotective effects of diethyldithiocarbamate (DSH) in mice

DSH dose (mg/kg)	Pretreatment interval (min)	Dose modifying factor[a]	Study
400	30	1.2	Milas *et al.* (1984)
500	30	1.0	Evans *et al.* (1983a)
ca 700	5	1.7	Van Bekkum (1956)
1000	30	1.6	Milas *et al.* (1984)
1000	30	1.8	Evans *et al.* (1983a)
1000	120	1.9	Evans *et al.* (1983a)
1400	30	1.7	Evans *et al.* (1983a)
1000	−60[b]	1.1	Evans *et al.* (1983a)

[a] Ratio of the 30-day irradiation LD_{50} values in control and DSH-treated animals.
[b] DSH administered 1 h post irradiation.

administration the ^{35}S levels in these tissues were about half of those in blood.

As a radioprotector DSH is somewhat less potent than ethofos (WR-2721), the compound currently considered to be the most effective in this regard (Landauer *et al.*, 1988). Nonetheless, DSH is one of the more potent radioprotective agents and its low toxicity renders it an attractive alternative to the more toxic ethofos (Evans *et al.*, 1983a; Evans, 1985).

A puzzling aspect of the protective action of DSH against radiation-induced mortality is that this agent is equally protective whether it is administered 120 or 5 min prior to irradiation (Table 14.3). Given that the half-life of DSH in mice is 10–24 min (Table 6.1), the fraction of administered DSH remaining unmetabolized at 120 min would be expected to be between 0.02 and 3%. Consideration of the radio-protective effects of DSH on hematopoietic tissue renders clear the probable cause of this paradox.

Hematopoietic tissue is particularly sensitive to irradiation. One technique used to determine what effects various pretreatments have on it is the spleen colony assay of Till and McCulloch (1961). Briefly, the animals are killed immediately following exposure to various doses of radiation and marrow cells are flushed from their excised femurs. An appropriate number of these cells are injected into isologous hosts previously exposed to supralethal levels of radiation; 8 days later the number of colonies of proliferating cells in the host spleen is determined. Using this technique, Evans *et al.* (1983a) found that, at each radiation dose tested, a larger number of colonies were formed by marrow cells from mice administered 1000 mg/kg DSH 30 min prior than from controls (Fig. 14.2a), giving a dose modifying factor (DMF) of 1.5. Using the same technique and a DSH dose of 15 mg/mouse (*ca* 750 mg/kg) administered 15 min prior to irradiation, Allalunis-Turner and Chapman (1984) reported an apparent DMF of 1.7. They also noted, however, that DSH administration increased by 31% the number of colonies formed by marrow cells from non-irradiated animals (their Fig. 1). If, based on this finding, the data of Evans *et al.* (1983a) are re-examined it becomes evident that these authors assumed that marrow cells from non-irradiated mice would form the same number of colonies whether the animals received DSH or not, and forced the regression for data obtained in animals administered DSH through the same intercept as that for the controls (Fig. 14.2a). If no such assumption is made, however, and the best-fit regression line for the points generated from DSH-treated animals is computed (Fig. 14.2b), it indicates that DSH administration would increase by 37% the number of colonies formed by marrow cells from non-irradiated animals.

The data of Evans *et al.* (1983a) appear, according to this analysis, to corroborate the inference made by Allalunis-Turner and Chapman (1984) that DSH has the ability to stimulate stem cell proliferation independently of any radiation exposure. The same inference was made independently by Milas *et al.* (1984) based on their finding that DSH increases marrow-cell colony formation, if its administration precedes irradiation (by 5 days, 1 day or 30 min), but not if it follows it (by 30 min). The latter observation dovetails with the finding (Table 14.3) that DSH is ineffective in modifying the radiation $LD_{50/30}$ dose if it is administered 60 min post irradiation. The saliency of this conclusion becomes evident in the context of the marked immuno-stimulant properties of DSH (Chapter 12), since many of the attendant phenomena might be explicable in terms of the stimulation of stem cell proliferation. Even after allowances are made for this stimulation, DSH appears to possess a residual radioprotective effect. Thus, for instance, Allalunis-Turner and Chapman (1984) calculated the corrected DMF to be 1.3. The same figure is obtained if a corrected DMF is calculated from the data of Evans *et al.* (1983a) as presented in Figure 14.2b.

Other tissues, such as the jejunum, the stem cells in the testes, and hair follicles, are protected *in vivo* from radiation damage by DSH pretreatment (Milas *et al.*, 1984). Strangely, the DSH dose that protects the jejunum (400 mg/kg) does not protect the testes, while the dose that protects the testes (1000 mg/kg) fails to protect the jejunum.

Attempts to utilize DSH in conjunction with radiation therapy of cancer in animal models have produced mixed results. Administered i.p.,

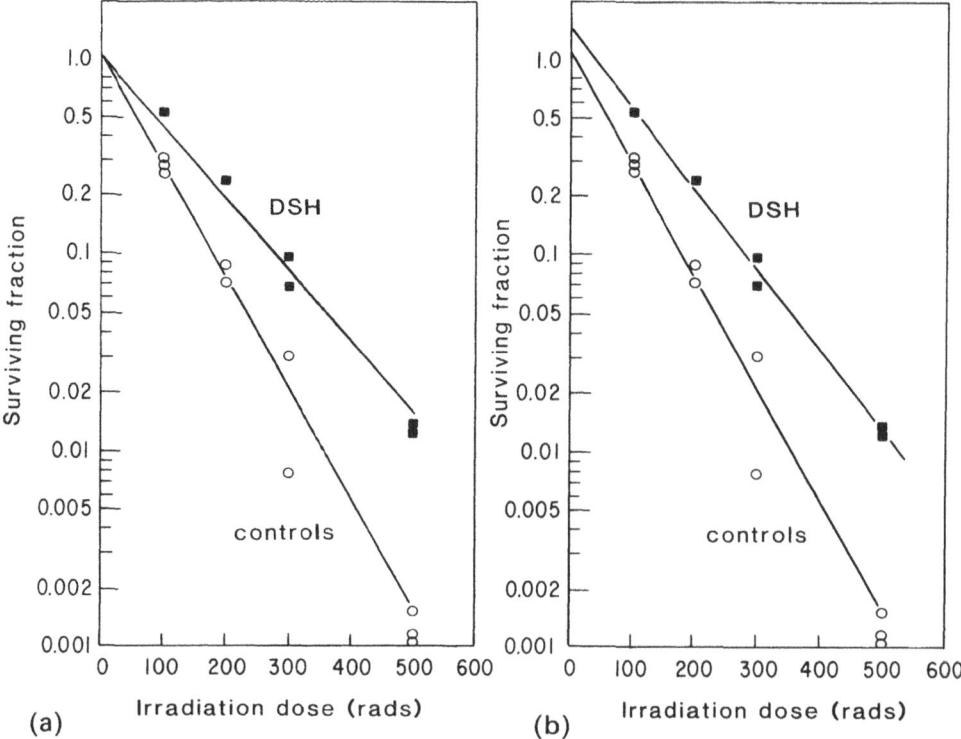

Figure 14.2 Protection by diethyldithiocarbamate (DSH) against radiation-induced bone marrow cytotoxicity. Closed squares: mice administered 1000 mg/kg DSH, i.v., 30 min prior to irradiation. Open circles: control mice. Upon receiving the stated radiation dose the mice were killed and the marrow cells flushed from their excised femurs. A known number of these cells were injected i.v. into host mice pretreated with 950 rads of total body irradiation, 10 host animals being used per point. The number of colonies formed by the injected cells in the spleens of the host mice was determined 8 days later. That number, divided by the number of colonies formed when unirradiated donor mice were used, is reported as the surviving fraction. In panel (a) the regression line for cells from DSH-treated animals is constrained to intercept ordinate at a survival fraction value of unity. In panel (b) the same data are presented as in (a) but the best-fit regression line for cells from DSH-treated mice is calculated without any restrictions. (Panel (a) redrawn with permission from Evans *et al.* (1983a)).

DSH induces moderate radiosensitization of a tumor (RIF sarcoma) following whole body irradiation (Evans, 1985), as it does under some conditions of intratumoral (rhabdomyosarcoma) administration (Kent and Blekkenhorst, 1988). On the other hand, its i.p. administration to mice protects fibrosarcomas located in their legs from single doses of local irradiation (Milas *et al.*, 1984).

14.3.2 Modulation of *in vitro* effects of radiation

Paradoxically, although *in vivo* investigations have amply demonstrated the radioprotective effects of DSH treatment, the bulk of *in
vitro* investigations on the modulation of radiation injury by DSH have
focused on its enhancement of the cytotoxic effects of ionizing
radiation.

The *in vitro* cytotoxicity induced by irradiation is considered to be
mediated by the radiolysis of water and the resulting formation of the
toxic superoxide anion radical, $O_2^{\cdot-}$. DSH is an effective inhibitor of the
CuZn SOD, the primary enzyme responsible for the detoxication of
$O_2^{\cdot-}$ (section 8.4). Accordingly, the study of the radiation modulating
effects of DSH on cells *in vitro* has been spurred by the concept that
by inhibiting SOD, DSH would render cells more susceptible to the
effects of radiation. Indeed, exposure of either lymphocyte or exponential phase cultures to DSH and radiation results in greater
cytotoxicity than is seen in cultures exposed to radiation alone (Lin *et
al.*, 1979; Rigas *et al.*, 1980; Westman and Marklund, 1980; Westman
and Midander, 1984). Nonetheless, several lines of evidence indicated
that the SOD inhibition model for DSH-induced radiosensitization is
not a tenable one. Firstly, under some conditions the exposure of
plateau phase cultures to DSH and radiation results in radioprotection
(DMF values of 1.18 and 1.17, respectively) rather than radiosensitization (Evans *et al.*, 1982). Secondly, the DSH-induced enhancement of
radiation cytotoxicity in lymphocyte and exponential phase cultures is
observed regardless of whether or not the DSH concentration used
results in SOD inhibition (Lin *et al.*, 1979; Rigas *et al.*, 1980). Thirdly,
in such cultures the radiosensitizing effect of DSH (measured as
inhibition of ³H-uridine uptake) is bimodal and greater following
exposure to 10^{-5}M than to 10^{-4}M DSH. In these latter particulars the
effect is wholly coincident with the bimodality of the cytotoxic effects
of DSH itself in these cultures (Rigas *et al.*, 1980). This suggests that
the observed 'radiosensitization' by DSH is best considered as a sum-
mation of independent DSH- and irradiation-induced cytotoxicities.
This by itself, however, does not account for the fact that under some
conditions the 'radiosensitization' is not observed.

As discussed in section 14.1, the cytotoxicity induced by DSH in cell
cultures incubated in medium supplemented with fetal calf serum
(FCS) is most likely due to the Fe^{2+}-catalyzed autoxidation of the thiol.
This process results in the generation of hydrogen peroxide and
hydroxyl free radicals. The sensitivity of cells to such reactive oxygen
species (ROS) is markedly enhanced by trypsinization, this enhancement dissipating after 16 h (Held and Melder, 1987). Herein appears to

lie the reason for the reported sensitivity of exponential phase cultures to DSH cytotoxicity since, in the studies reviewed, such cultures are routinely trypsinized at the beginning of each experiment to assure disaggregation. In contrast, in the reviewed studies, trypsinization was not routinely performed in experiments involving plateau phase cultures.

The model derived from the above considerations is one of an independent but additive DSH cytotoxicity which affects trypsin-sensitized cells and is mediated by the formations of ROS resulting from the autoxidation of DSH in Fe^{2+}-containing media. This model can be used to explain the otherwise puzzling finding of Westman and Midander (1984), that exponential phase cultures, if exposed to DSH at 2 h post irradiation, show 'radiosensitization', but fail to do so if exposed to DSH at 16 or 24 h post irradiation. These cultures were trypsinized just prior to irradiation and hence at 2 h post irradiation would have still been sensitive to the ROS derived from DSH autoxidation, but would have lost this sensitivity by 16 h.

The model can also be used to explain the observations of Evans *et al.* (1982). Working with plateau phase cultures, these workers observed incubation of the culture with DSH for 60 min had no 'radiosensitizing' effect, if the DSH was washed out just prior to irradiation. On the other hand concurrent exposure to DSH and irradiation did result in 'radiosensitization,' but only if the culture was maintained in Eagle's minimum essential medium (MEM), those maintained in Hank's balanced salt solution (HBSS) failing to show this effect. In these experiments cultures were trypsinized immediately following irradiation. Accordingly, cultures exposed to DSH only prior to irradiation were, in fact, exposed to DSH only prior to trypsinization and thus not sensitized to ROS. In contrast those exposed concurrently to DSH and irradiation were trypsinized while still exposed to DSH. They were thereby sensitized to ROS generated from DSH in Fe^{2+}-containing medium. In particular, this would have been true of cultures maintained in MEM, since it was supplemented with 15% FCS, a source of Fe^{2+}. On the other hand, cultures maintained in HBSS, a Fe^{2+}- free medium, would not be exposed to ROS.

14.3.3 Modulation of *in vitro* effects of hyperthermia

DSH has been reported to increase the cytotoxicity of hyperthermia (Lin *et al.*, 1979, 1985; Evans *et al.*, 1983b) and hyperthermia in combination with irradiation (Wagner *et al.*, 1984) in cell cultures. Using exponential phase cultures, Lin *et al.* (1979, 1985) found that the hyperthermia cytotoxicity enhancement by DSH is bimodal and greater following exposure to 10^{-5}M than to 10^{-4}M DSH (Table 14.2). The bimodality of this effect is wholly coincident with that of DSH-induced cytotoxicity (Table 14.1) and is very likely attributable, as is the *in vitro* 'radiosensitization' (section 14.3.2), to the autoxidation of DSH in Fe^{2+}-containing media, and the generation thereby of ROS. From the observations of Evans *et al.* (1983b) it appears, moreover, that the DSH-mediated enhancement of hyperthermia cytotoxicity coincides with exposure of the cells to trypsin. These workers trypsinized the cultures immediately following exposure to heat. No enhancement of hyperthermia cytotoxicity was observed in cultures which were exposed to DSH for 60 min and from which the DSH was washed out just prior to the heat treatment, and trypsinization. On the other hand, the hyperthermia cytotoxicity was enhanced in cultures which were exposed concurrently to DSH and heat, and which were therefore trypsinized in the presence of DSH. Trypsinization is known to render cells sensitive to the effects of ROS produced during thiol autoxidation (Held and Melder, 1987).

14.3.4 Summary

DSH is an effective *in vivo* radioprotector. Evans *et al.* (1983a) have calculated, based on mouse data, that a 4–5 g dose would be radio-protective in humans, possibly without the toxicity attendant upon the use of ethofos (WR-2721). Doses as high as 4 g have been used in humans in the treatment of acute nickel-carbonyl toxicity.

The radioprotective action of DSH *in vivo* appears to be due, in part, to its ability to stimulate stem cell proliferation. While this action of DSH counters the effects of radiation on bone marrow, it is independent of it. Not all the *in vivo* radioprotective action of DSH can be explained on this basis and, moreover, DSH is also an effective plateau phase cell culture radioprotector *in vitro*. Many other thiols share these latter radioprotective properties and their mechanism continues to be the subject of intensive study, free radical scavenging, hydrogen atom donation, formation of mixed disulfides, metal chelation, and production of hypoxia being some of the postulated mechanisms.

The apparent DSH-induced radio- and hyperthermia sensitization observed in lymphocytes and exponential phase cultures is due, in all likelihood, to the cytotoxic effects of hydrogen peroxide and hydroxyl free radicals generated by Fe^{2+}-catalyzed autoxidation of DSH. The principal source of Fe^{2+} ions in cultures are the blood serum supplements of the media.

15

Modulation of cancer chemotherapy

15.1 INTRODUCTION 313
15.2 PRECLINICAL STUDIES 315
    15.2.1 Effect on mortality induced by chemotherapeutic agents . . . 315
    15.2.2 Effect on cisplatin nephrotoxicity 317
    15.2.3 Effect on chemotherapeutic agent-induced gastrointestinal
        toxicity 319
    15.2.4 Efffect on chemotherapeutic agent-induced bone marrow
        toxicity 320
    15.2.5 Effect on the tumoricidal action of chemotherapeutic agents . 323
    15.2.6 Nature of the effect on bone marrow cells 325
    15.2.7 Potentiation of tumoricidal action of oxazaphosphorines . . . 327
15.3 CLINICAL STUDIES 328
    15.3.1 Dose conversion to humans 329
    15.3.2 Toxic effects associated with diethyldithiocarbamate infusion 329
    15.3.3 Effect on cisplatin nephrotoxicity 331
    15.3.4 Effect on nausea and vomiting 331
    15.3.5 Effect on hematological toxicity 332
    15.3.6 Effect on neuropathy and ototoxicity 333
    15.3.7 Effect on cisplatin pharmacokinetics 333
    15.3.8 Effect on antitumor responses 333
15.4 CONCLUSIONS 334

15.1 INTRODUCTION

A common characteristic of most chemotherapeutic drugs is their low therapeutic ratio. Accordingly, supplementary agents which hold the promise of improving the ratio, by either reducing the toxicity of the chemotherapeutic drug towards normal tissue or increasing its toxicity towards neoplastic tissue, are the focus of considerable interest. Animal studies render it clear that, under appropriate circumstances, diethyl-dithiocarbamate (DSH) can protect normal tissues from the toxic effects of a variety of chemotherapeutic drugs. Moreover, DSH achieves this without compromising the tumoricidal effectiveness of the drugs in question. Additionally, such studies indicate that both DSH and disulfiram (DSSD) have the ability to increase the toxicity of some chemotherapeutic agents towards neoplastic tissue while either not affecting or reducing their toxicity towards normal tissue. Some of the advantages and benefits observed in animals have proved transferable to the clinical situation. The conditions under which other benefits of such therapy accrue have not been sufficiently clearly defined in animal studies and identifying these conditions clinically is proving difficult.

By far the most explored chemoprotective activity of DSH is its ability to act as a rescue agent for the nephrotoxicity induced by cisplatin [*cis*-dichlorodiammineplatinum(II)], one of the most important chemotherapeutic agents introduced in the last two decades. Its use is limited clinically by the development of several toxicities; of these the renal toxicity is the most severe and thus potentially dose-limiting (Borch and Markman, 1989; Gandara *et al.*, 1990). The nephrotoxicity can be controlled by a program of diuresis, but there is a limit to the degree to which it can be prevented by these means and, with the introduction of high-dose cisplatin therapy, nephrotoxicity has again become a problem. Chemically, in some respects Pt(II) resembles Hg(II) and, like the latter, it has a tendency to become bound to sulfhydryl groups in the kidney. The resulting renal histopathologies are strikingly similar. Not only can the administration of DSH prevent the development of platinum nephrotoxicity, but DSH is unique in that it will do so even when administered 2 hrs following cisplatin. It is therefore a true rescue agent. This property of DSH is all the more remarkable given that the plasma half-life of cisplatin is only 30 min. As discussed in section 7.9, this property is due to the ability of DSH to remove platinum from intracellular targets to which it becomes bound.

The development of carboplatin [*cis*-diammine(1,1-cyclobutanedicarboxylato)platinum(II); Paraplatin] has helped shift attention to the ability of DSH to moderate the bone marrow toxicity which carboplatin, an agent free of renal toxicity, shares with cisplatin and many other chemotherapeutic agents. Since for carboplatin, and a number of other agents, this toxicity is dose-limiting, the ability of DSH to prevent it has been explored more generally. The results indicate a generic ability of DSH to prevent the myelosuppression caused by the majority of anti-neoplastic agents against which it has been tested.

The ability of DSSD to potentiate the tumoricidal effect and to decrease the bladder toxicity of cyclophosphamide, 2-bis[(2-chloroethyl)amino]-tetrahydro-2-H-1,3,2-oxazaphosphorine 2-oxide, an important anti-neoplastic and immunosuppressive drug of the oxazaphosphorine series, is a less well-explored property which nonetheless holds some promise of improving chemotherapy (section 15.2.7)

15.2 PRECLINICAL STUDIES

15.2.1 Effect on mortality induced by chemotherapeutic agents

DSH administration can antagonize the lethal effect of a number of chemotherapeutic agents. As shown in the LD_{50} isobologram for combinations of cisplatin and DSH in mice (Fig. 15.1), the 9 day LD_{50} for cisplatin increases from 10.8 to 24 mg/kg, if DSH (1000 mg/kg) is administered 30 min following cisplatin (Evans *et al.*, 1984). This LD_{50} dose for the combination is a much higher one than would have been

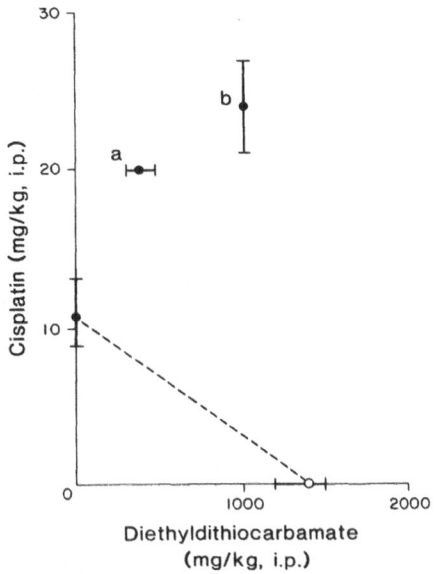

Figure 15.1 Antagonism of cisplatin toxicity by diethyldithiocarbamate (DSH) in mice: isobologram for the interaction between i.p.-administered cisplatin and DSH. Dashed diagonal: locus of expected LD_{50} points for mixtures of the two agents given a simple additivity of their toxic effects. Closed circles: LD_{50} points with their 95% confidence limits for cisplatin and its combinations wth DSH; point (a) obtained by administering DSH 2 h after cisplatin, point (b) by administering DSH 0.5 h after cisplatin (from Evans *et al.*, 1984). Note the much larger dose of cisplatin necessary to elicit the same toxic endpoint when followed by DSH rescue. Open circle: mean and range of LD_{50} values for i.p.-administered DSH as calculated from Table 16.1.

predicted on the basis of a simple additivity of the toxic effects of the two agents (represented by the dashed diagonal in Fig. 15.1). Likewise, it is found that in mice dosed with 20 mg/kg of cisplatin and administered DSH 2 h later, the dose of DSH necessary to reduce the mortality to 50% is 375 mg/kg. DSH administration also counteracts the toxic effects of more chronic cisplatin treatment in this species. Thus, the 60% mortality observed when cisplatin (6 mg/kg i.p.) is administered 4 times per day for 3 days, is reduced to 7–12% if DSH is administered i.p. 2 h after each cisplatin treatment (Khandekar, 1983). The reduction in cisplatin toxicity observed is much the same regardless of whether the DSH dose is 250, 500, or 1000 mg/kg. DSH administration (500 mg/kg i.p.) 1 h post cisplatin is also effective in decreasing toxicity of intermittent cisplatin dosing (8 mg/kg i.v. 3 times at 5-day intervals), the 15-day mortality falling from 100 to 0% as a consequence of the DSH treatment (Murthy *et al.*, 1987).

A DSH-mediated reduction in cisplatin toxicity is also observed in rats. Treatment with DSH (750 mg/kg i.p.) 2 h after i.p. cisplatin, raises the 15-day LD_{50} from 8.5 to 10.8 mg/kg (Khandekar, 1983).

DSH also protects rodents against the mortality induced by lethal doses of carboplatin. Rats administered 60 mg/kg carboplatin i.v. experience 100% mortality by day 11. Administration of DSH concurrently (750 mg/kg i.p.) with carboplatin prevents the lethality as does administration of multiple DSH doses (300 mg/kg i.p.) at 0, 2 and 4 h after carboplatin (Dible *et al.*, 1987). The same DSH dosing schedules prevent the lethality of a 150 mg/kg i.v. dose of carboplatin in mice and raise the 14-day i.v. carboplatin LD_{50} in ADJ/PC6A tumor-bearing mice from 115 to 216 mg/kg (Dible *et al.*, 1987).

Tetraplatin   [tetrachloro(*dl-trans*)1,2-diaminocyclohexaneplatinum (IV)] is yet another platinum chemotherapeutic agent the toxicity of which is antagonized by DSH. Thus, in rats, treatment with a 16.5 mg/kg i.v. dose of tetraplatin results in a 67% 5-day mortality, but administration of DSH (750 mg/kg i.p.) 30 min following the tetraplatin results in the survival of all the animals (Carfagna *et al.*, 1990).

DSH reduces the toxicity of cyclophosphamide, a non-platinum chemotherapeutic agent. Thus, the 20-day LD_{50} of cyclophosphamide in ddY mice is increased from 520 to *ca* 650 mg/kg by administration of a 100 mg/kg dose of DSH 30 min earlier (Furusawa *et al.*, 1988). In contrast, Cox *et al.* (1976) have reported that pretreatment of mice with DSSD (100 mg/kg p.o.) 2 h prior to cyclophosphamide decreases the LD_{50} from 335 to 238 mg/kg. Likewise, pretreatment of rats with DSSD (1000 mg/kg) 2 h prior to cyclophosphamide lowers the LD_{50} from 254 to 77 mg/kg (Habs *et al.*, 1984).

15.2.2 Effect on cisplatin nephrotoxicity

Cisplatin nephrotoxicity is characterized by histopathological changes and destruction of the proximal tubular epithelial cells of the kidney. DSH protects against this destruction. For instance, by day 4 following treatment of mice with cisplatin (18 mg/kg i.p.) 57% of the proximal tubules are destroyed. However, if the animals are treated with DSH (500 mg/kg i.p.), either 0.5 h prior or 2 h following the cisplatin, only 17 or 30% of the tubules, respectively, are affected (Gale *et al.*, 1982a); similar findings were reported by Murthy *et al.* (1987). Timing appears to be important: a 4-h delay in the administration of DSH renders it ineffective.

When cisplatin is administered to rats in a moderately nephrotoxic dose (7.5 mg/kg i.v., for instance) the renal lesions and the accompanying rise in blood urea nitrogen (BUN) levels peak on day 5. The ability of DSH to counter this cisplatin-induced rise in BUN is used as a measure of its effectiveness in reducing cisplatin nephrotoxicity. From the accumulated body of experimental information (Table 15.1) it is apparent that to be effective in this respect, DSH has to be administered between 0.5 and 4 h post cisplatin and that it is less effective if administered i.p. rather than either i.v. or s.c. (Borch and Pleasants, 1979; Borch *et al.*, 1980). The latter phenomenon is likely due to the high proportion (about 50%) of the i.p. administered DSH that undergoes first pass metabolism (section 6.6.2) and, consequently, the smaller amount of it reaching the kidney. This has been documented by Borch *et al.* (1980) who compared the amount of free DSH excreted in the urine following i.v. and i.p. injection. They found that, though the fraction of administered DSH thus excreted is very small (0.3% or less), nonetheless, in absolute terms, three times as much DSH appears in the urine in the first 120 min following a 100 mg/kg i.v. dose than following a 500 mg/kg i.p. dose The reversal of cisplatin nephrotoxicity appears to be due to chelation by DSH of platinum bound to tissue without displacement of that which, by that time, has formed platinum-bisguanosine adducts (section 7.9); the latter binding mediates the antitumor effects of cisplatin.

Administered to rats 30 min following tetraplatin (16.5 mg/kg i.v.), DSH (750 mg/kg i.p.) reduces by 60% the day 5 tetraplatin-induced increase in BUN. It also protects these animals from the coagulative necrosis which is observed upon histological examination of their kidneys (Carfagna *et al.*, 1990).

Since DSSD is metabolized *in vivo* to DSH, its administration could, theoretically, also lead to a reversal of cisplatin nephrotoxicity. When the effectiveness of DSSD and DSH in this regard was compared

Table 15.1 Effect of diethyldithiocarbamate (DSH) on blood urea nitrogen (BUN) following dosing with cisplatin

Cisplatin Dose (mg/kg)	Route	DSH Dose (mg/kg)	Route	Hours post cisplatin	Day post cisplatin	Change from cisplatin control (%)	P	Reference
Mouse								
10	i.p.	250	s.c.	2	~4	−58	<0.05	Bodenner et al. (1986b)
14	i.p.	250	s.c.	2	~4	−59	<0.05	Bodenner et al. (1986b)
		500	s.c.	2	~4	−79	<0.05	
		750	s.c.	2	~4	−72	<0.05	
		1000	s.c.	2	~4	−71	<0.05	
Rat								
7.5	i.v.	750	i.p.	−0.5	5	+79	<0.001	Borch and Pleasants (1979)
				0	5	−9	>0.25	
				0.75	5	−76	<0.001	
				1	5	−73	<0.001	
				1.5	5	−74	<0.001	
				2	5	−41	<0.001	
				3	5	−67	<0.001	
				4	5	−55	<0.005	
				6	5	−11	>0.3	
7.5	i.v.	500	i.p.	0.5	5	−35	<0.05	Borch and Pleasants (1979)
				1	5	−62	<0.001	
				2	5	−69	<0.001	
7.5	i.v.	100	i.v.	2	5	−53		Borch et al. (1980)
		750	i.p.	2	5	−21		
7.5	i.v.	100	i.v.	2	5	−73	<0.05	Bodenner et al. (1986b)
				5	5	−27	>0.05	
				10	5	+25	>0.05	
6.5	i.v.	750	i.p.	?	3	−73		Dible et al. (1987)
Dog								
1 × 5 days	i.v.	200 × 5 days	i.v.	2	10	−67		Bodenner et al. (1986b)

directly in rats, DSSD proved much less effective than DSH in reversing the cisplatin-induced rise in BUN levels, although it evidenced a similar trend (Borch *et al.*, 1983; Bodenner *et al.*, 1986b). This contrasts with the effectiveness of DSSD in minimizing in mice the cisplatin-induced tubular necrosis and reducing BUN levels to normal (Wysor *et al.*, 1982) when, combined with hydration, it is administered in a 250 mg/kg p.o. dose 4 h after each dose of cisplatin (3 mg/kg/day for 7 days, i.p.).

15.2.3 Effect on chemotherapeutic agent-induced gastrointestinal toxicity

A major problem encountered in the study of gastrointestinal toxicity of chemotherapeutic agents, and particularly their clinically trouble-some ability to induce severe and persistent nausea and vomiting, is that rodents do not possess the vomiting reflex. This forces inves-tigators, wishing to study the possible reversal of these symptoms by DSH, to either use a species that does possess this reflex (viz. dogs), or to select indices of gastrointestinal toxicity other than emesis.

In rodents, diarrhea and an unusual cisplatin-induced stomach engor-gement have been studied to this end. In mice, administration of cisplatin (18 mg/kg i.p.) causes the stomach/body weight ratio to increase 4.75-fold by day 4. Treatment of mice with DSH (500 mg/kg i.p.) reduces this phenomenon by 69%, if administered 0.5 h prior to cisplatin. If the DSH is administered 2 or 4 h after the cisplatin, the reduction is 43 and 37%, respectively (Gale *et al.*, 1982a). In rats, the incidence of cisplatin-induced diarrhea is 95, 100 and 100%, respect-ively, following 7.5, 10 and 14 mg/kg i.v. doses of this agent. The incidence falls to zero in each instance, however, if DSH (250 mg/kg i.p.) is administered 2 h later (Borch and Pleasants, 1979; Bodenner *et al.*, 1986b). In an analogous fashion, the administration to rats of DSH (750 mg/kg i.p.) 30 minutes following a 16.5 mg/kg i.v. dose of tetra-platin reduces to zero the 95% incidence of diarrhea otherwise seen in these animals (Carfagna *et al.*, 1990).

Gylys *et al.* (1979) established the dog as an appropriate model for the investigation of cisplatin-induced emetic effects. Administration of cisplatin (1 mg/kg i.v.) causes, in this species, multiple episodes of emesis. These start 120 min following the administration of cisplatin, but the majority of the episodes (74%) occur after 3 or more hours. Administration of DSH (25 mg/kg i.v.) 3 hrs after cisplatin decreases the number of emesis episodes occurring thereafter by 89% (Bodenner *et al.*, 1986b). DSSD (25 mg/kg p.o.), administered 1 h post cisplatin, is less effective, the observed 25% reduction in emesis episodes is not significant ($P > 0.05$).

15.2.4 Effect on chemotherapeutic agent-induced bone marrow toxicity

Cisplatin (6.5 mg/kg i.v.) causes anemia, leukopenia and thrombocytopenia in the rat. DSH administered in multiple doses (300 mg/kg i.p. at 0, 2 and 4 h post cisplatin) can prevent all these three manifestations of bone marrow toxicity (Dible *et al.*, 1987). Likewise, in mice administration of DSH (300 mg/kg s.c.) 2 h after each dose of a more chronic cisplatin treatment (5 mg/kg/day for 5 days i.p.) reduces by 39% the magnitude of the leukopenia nadir. Such DSH treatment also prevents the day 7 cisplatin-induced 65% decrease in bone marrow lymphocytes and the 45% decrease in bone marrow granulocytes (Bodenner *et al.*, 1986b). Gringeri *et al.* (1988) have reported a similar finding concerning the effect of DSH (300 mg/kg i.v.) administered 2 h after a single dose of cisplatin (10 mg/kg i.v.). In dogs, dosed in a like manner with cisplatin (1 mg/kg/day for 5 days, i.v.), administration of DSH (300 mg/kg s.c.) 2 h after each cisplatin dose prevents the bone marrow from becoming hypocellular, though the leukopenia induced by the cisplatin is not affected by the DSH (Bodenner *et al.*, 1986b).

DSH also protects animals to a degree against bone marrow toxicity induced by other platinum derivatives. Thus, in mice it reduces the day 17 anemia induced by carboplatin (150 mg/kg i.v) if the DSH (750 mg/kg i.p.) administration occurs concurrently with that of carboplatin, but not if it takes place 2, 4 or 24 h later (Dible *et al.*, 1987). In rats injected with carboplatin (60 mg/kg i.v.), it reduces the resulting anemia and leukopenia, though not the thrombocytopenia, when administered i.p. as multiple 300 mg/kg doses 0, 2 and 4 h after the carboplatin (Dible *et al.*, 1987). Given as a 30-min post-treatment, DSH (750 mg/kg i.p.) also reduces the day 5 leukopenia and thrombocytopenia induced in rats by a 16.5 mg/kg i.v. dose of tetraplatin (Carfagna *et al.*, 1990).

Leukopenia, anemia and thrombocytopenia are all evidence of hemopoietic toxicity. The effect of toxic agents on mouse bone marrow stem cells can be also studied directly by killing the animals some time after treatment with the agent in question and flushing the bone marrow cells from the femur. The ability of these cells to give rise to colonies either *in vivo* in the spleen of immunosuppressed host animals or *in vitro*, in cultures exposed to appropriate colony stimulating factors (CSF), is determined. Since not all cells able to form colonies in host spleens are able to do so in culture and *vice versa*, these two assays of hematological function are complementary. The spleen colony assay has been described in section 14.3.1. It involves injection of a known number of donor bone marrow cells into the host animals and counting the number of colonies on the surface of the spleen some 8–12 days later. These are referred to as colony forming units (CFU). The number of CFU is compared with that observed when control animals are used as donors. The result is usually reported as the ratio of the two, this being termed the surviving fraction (SF). The *in vitro* assay involves plating of a known number of cells, diluted with medium conditioned so as to contain CSF, incubating them for 7 days and comparing the number of colonies formed by cells from treated and control animals to obtain a SF. Since the cells that proliferate under these circumstances are predominantly precursors of (neutrophilic) granulocytes and macrophages the assay is referred to as that of granulocyte–macrophage colony forming cells (GM-CFC).

The cytotoxicity of administered cisplatin against CFU results in a SF smaller than unity. The relationship between the cisplatin dose and the logarithm of the CFU SF is linear (Evans *et al.*, 1984; Gringeri *et al.*, 1988). The same is true of carboplatin. Administration of DSH (300 mg/kg i.v.) 2 h after that of carboplatin, for example, protects the CFU against carboplatin cytotoxicity and increases the CFU SF at each carboplatin dose; these data can be fitted with a second regression line (Fig. 15.2). Assuming the two regression lines have the same intercept on the ordinate, the ratio of their slopes is the factor by which any dose of carboplatin would have to be increased to have the same effect in animals administered DSH as it has when administered alone. This is a measure of the protective effect of DSH and is called the dose modification factor (DMF). Gringeri *et al.* (1988) computed the DMF for the 300 mg/kg i.v. dose of DSH *vis-à-vis* carboplatin cytotoxicity and reported its value to be 3.3. They found the parallel DMF for cisplatin to be 3.3. The DMF value obtained for cisplatin by Evans *et al.* (1984), who used a 1000 mg/kg i.p. dose of DSH, was 3.2. The assumption mentioned above, that both regression lines have the same intercept on the ordinate, presupposes that in animals not pretreated with platinum drugs DSH treatment has no effect on CFU SF. The validity of this assumption is discussed in section 15.2.6.

Investigation of the effect of varying DSH dose on its modulation of carboplatin cytotoxicity against CFU, reveals a remarkable lack of dose-dependence over a range of DSH doses encompassing three orders of magnitude. Thus, although DSH, administered i.v. 3 h after carboplatin, is ineffective when doses of 0.0003–0.03 mg/kg are used, doses in the range of 0.3–300 mg/kg provide significant protection, and

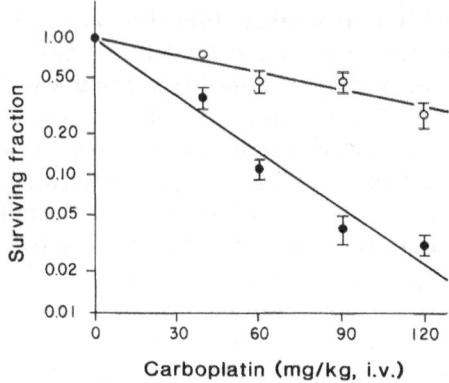

Carboplatin (mg/kg, i.v.)

Figure 15.2 Protection by diethyldithiocarbamate (DSH) against carboplatin bone marrow cytotoxicity. Mice were administered the stated dose of carboplatin, killed 24 h later the marrow cells flushed from their excised femurs. A known number of these cells were injected i.v. into host mice pretreated with 950 rads of total body irradiation, 15 host mice being used per point. The number of colonies formed by the injected cells in the spleens of the host mice was determined 12 days later. That number, divided by the number of colonies formed when untreated mice were used, is reported as the surviving fraction. Open circles: mice administered 300 mg/kg DSH, i.v., 3 h after the stated dose of carboplatin. Closed circles: control mice treated with carboplatin only. Redrawn from Gringeri *et al.* (1988).

there is no difference in the effectiveness of doses in the latter range (Schmalbach and Borch, 1989b). It should be noted that, over this complete range of doses, there is a close correspondence between the DSH-induced reduction in carboplatin cytotoxicity against the CFU and the DSH augmentation of carboplatin-depressed *in vivo* bone marrow DNA synthesis rates (Schmalbach and Borch, 1989b). With regard to the modulation of the cytotoxicity of cisplatin against CFU, all doses of DSH tested to date [100–750 mg/kg i.v. (Gringeri *et al.*, 1988); 1000 mg/kg i.p. (Evans *et al.*, 1984)] have proved effective. Also, given the short half-life of DSH *in vivo* (10 min) its ability to modulate the cisplatin cytotoxicity against the CFU exhibits a marked tolerance regarding the time of its administration *vis-à-vis* that of cisplatin. Thus, Gringeri *et al.* (1988) using a 300 mg/kg i.v. dose, detected no difference in the effectiveness of DSH, whether it is administered 30 min before cisplatin or 3 or 5 h after it. Although the effectiveness of DSH is somewhat less if the administration occurs 1.5 h before cisplatin, it still is substantial. Taken together, these findings indicate that very low DSH doses reduce at least some aspects of the bone marrow toxicity of platinum drugs. The doses in question are some 2 to 3 orders of magnitude lower that those necessary for reduction of cisplatin nephrotoxicity.

DSH has been reported to be much less effective in modulating the cytotoxicity of platinum drugs towards GM-CFC. Administered in a 300 mg/kg i.v. dose 3 h after carboplatin it has no effect on the GM-CFC SF reduction induced by the latter. Given in the same dose 2 h after cisplatin it partly reverses the SF reduction (Gringeri *et al.*, 1988).

Doxorubicin (Adriamycin), 1,3-bis(2-chloroethyl)-1-nitrosourea (carmustine, BCNU), cyclophosphamide and mitomycin C are other chemotherapeutic agents that are cytotoxic against both mouse CFU and GM-CFC. Treatment with DSH 2–3 h following doxorubicin, BCNU, or cyclophosphamide can significantly lower this toxicity (Pannacciulli *et al.*, 1989; Schmalbach and Borch, 1989a). With mitomycin C, DSH is effective if administered 30 min but not 3 h following the chemotherapeutic agent (Schmalbach and Borch, 1989a).

Nitrogen mustard (mechlorethamine, HN_2) is yet another chemotherapeutic agent whose cytotoxicity against mouse CFU is antagonized by DSH. Administration of DSH (20 mg/mouse, $\simeq 910$ mg/kg, i.p.) 15 or 30 min prior to HN_2 (0.15 mg/mouse, $\simeq 6.8$ mg/kg, i.v.) increases the CFU SF 16- and 5-fold, respectively, relative to that obtained using HN_2 only; treatment with DSH 4 h prior to HN_2 is without effect (Valeriote and Grates, 1989). Pretreatment of such animals with DSSD (3 mg/mouse, $\simeq 136$ mg/kg, i.p.) 15 min, 1 h or 4 h prior to HN_2 has no protective effect against the cytotoxic effect of the latter against the CFU. DSH and DSSD have the opposite effect relative to the cytotoxicity of HN_2 against leukemic cells; this is discussed in section 15.2.6.

15.2.5 Effect on the tumoricidal action of chemotherapeutic agents

In doses that provide protection from many of the toxic effects of cisplatin and carboplatin, DSH produces no inhibition of their antitumor effects.

The tumoricidal actions of chemotherapeutic agents are frequently evaluated by determining, in mice inoculated with a given tumor, how much longer is their survival if treated with the agent in question. The results are expressed in terms of T/C, defined as

$$T/C = \frac{\text{survival time of treated mice}}{\text{survival time of control mice}} \times 100$$

The effect of DSH administration on T/C provides a measure of its modification of the tumoricidal action of the chemotherapeutic agent.

In mice bearing a variety of tumors (all those tested to date), administration of DSH 1–4 h following the injection of moderate doses of cisplatin (3–12 mg/kg) has minimal effects on T/C (Gale *et al.*, 1982a; Khandekar, 1983; Bodenner *et al.*, 1986b). Similarly, administration of DSH 2 h following 40–90 mg/kg doses of carboplatin or a 16 mg/kg dose of CHIP [(*cis*-diisopropylamine-*cis*-dichloro-*trans*-dihydroxylato)platinum(IV)] has little effect on T/C (Bodenner *et al.*, 1986b). Following toxic doses of cisplatin in the range of 16–21 mg/kg, administration of DSH (dose range 50–500 mg/kg) increases T/C as a linear function of dose (Gale *et al.*, 1982a). In considering these latter results, it should be borne in mind that a DSH-induced increase in T/C can be due either to its enhancement of tumoricidal action of the chemotherapeutic agent or to its antagonism of the latter's toxic effects.

In rats bearing mammary tumor 13762, administration of DSH (750 mg/kg i.p.) 2 h after cisplatin (2–8 mg/kg i.v.) leads, during the first 21 days, to a response identical to that seen following cisplatin alone. Nonetheless, thereafter the onset of the relapse occurs sooner and the tumor grows more rapidly. When the DSH dose is decreased to 100 mg/kg and administered i.v., however, the effect on the tumor is indistinguishable from that of cisplatin alone (Borch *et al.*, 1980). The same is true of ADJ/PC6A tumor-bearing mice administered 300 mg/kg DSH at 0, 2 and 4 h following a 0.6 mg/kg i.v. dose of cisplatin (Dible *et al.*, 1987). On the other hand, administration of DSH concurrently with carboplatin to these mice (be it as a single 750 mg/kg dose or the first of several smaller doses) nullifies the carboplatin effect. Yet, if the 750 mg/kg DSH dose is injected 2 h after carboplatin, it has no effect on the tumoricidal action of carboplatin at all (Dible *et al.*, 1987). This suggests that antagonism by DSH of the tumoricidal and myelotoxic effects can be separated by appropriate timing. It would be interesting, in view of the ability of DSH to antagonize the myelosuppressive effects of some platinum drugs, even when administered before them, to determine whether pretreatment with DSH had any effect on carboplatin toxicity.

A different method has been used to study the effects of DSSD and DSH on the tumoricidal actions of HN_2. It depends on the ability of leukemic murine bone marrow cells to form spleen colonies when injected into immunosuppressed host animals. These are counted on the surface of the host spleen in the same manner as CFU and are referred to as LCFU. Using this method, Valeriote and Grates (1986) found that administration of DSSD (6 mg/mouse, ≈ 272 mg/kg, i.p.) to AKR leukemic mice 15 min prior to HN_2 (0.3 mg/mouse, ≈ 14 mg/kg, i.p.) enhances the cytotoxicity of HN_2 against the LCFU, decreasing the SF 1700-fold. Yet, it does not affect the HN_2-induced decrease in the

CFU SF in normal mice. Using similar doses (3 mg/mouse DSSD i.p. and 0.15 mg/mouse HN_2 i.v.) these authors subsequently reported (Valeriote and Grates, 1989) that the enhancement of the HN_2 cytotoxicity against LCFU is greatest (a 4000-fold decrease in the SF) when the DSSD administration precedes that of HN 2 by 15–30 min. Under those conditions the DMF for DSSD *vis-à-vis* HN_2 cytotoxicity against CFU is 3.0.

In the experiment just described, Valeriote and Grates (1989) administered DSSD as a colloidal suspension having the composition, ethanol:POE 40 (Tween 40):normal saline in the proportion 0.5:0.5:9. Suspended in either ethanol or saline, DSSD has little activity. Suspended in 1% POE in saline its activity is similar to that seen with the complete vehicle. The vehicle alone causes an enhancement of the cytotoxicity of HN_2 against LCFU, decreasing the SF 4- to 16-fold. With pretreatment periods longer than 15–30 min, the effect of DSSD wanes rapidly; by 6 h little difference from controls is observed (Valeriote and Grates, 1989). The rapid waning may be tumor-type specific, however, since no such waning is observed when L1210 leukemic mice are used (Valeriote and Grates, 1986).

Administration of DSH (20 mg/mouse, $\simeq 910$ mg/kg, i.p.) 15 min prior to HN_2 also enhanced the cytotoxicity of HN_2 against LCFU, although for DSH the enhancement (a 5000-fold decrease in the SF) is maximal when the DSH is administered 2–4 h prior to HN_2. No explanation is available why the effect of DSH is so much delayed relative to that of DSSD since *in vivo* the two are interconvertible (Chapter 5).

15.2.6 Nature of the effect on bone marrow cells

DSH antagonizes the cytotoxic action on CFU or GM-CFC of so many diverse agents that it is hard to envisage a unitary mechanism whereby it could interfere with their actions. Yet the parallelism in the DSH antagonism of carboplatin's cytotoxic action on CFU and of carboplatin's depression of *in vivo* DNA synthesis by bone marrow cells, strongly suggests the former is not due to some sort of *ex vivo* event. This leads to the supposition, already discussed in relation to the ability of DSH to antagonize the effects of radiation (section 14.3.1), that DSH, through some *in vivo* action, can stimulate CFU and GM-CFC independently of the cytotoxic action of chemotherapeutic agents. Although various investigators have looked for such stimulation and have reported that they were unable to observe it (Gringeri *et al.*, 1988; Schmalbach and Borch, 1989a; Pannacciulli *et al.*, 1989), an analysis of the available CFU and GM-CFC data appears, *prima faciae* to support this supposition.

Reference needs to be first made to the work of Allalunis-Turner and Chapman (1984) who treated control mice with DSH (15 mg/kg i.p.) 15 min before harvesting the bone marrow. In their Fig. 1 they report the CFU SF from such mice to have been 31% higher than that of untreated controls. In their Fig. 2 they report analogous results for the GM-CFC. In their Fig. 3, moreover, they report that the increase in GM-CFC SF, seen following treatment of the mice with DSH, is a function of the time at which the marrow cells were harvested. Thus, it is maximal when the cells are harvested 1 h after DSH injection, but not evident if the cells are harvested 6 h after DSH administration. Secondly, the work of Evans *et al.* (1983a, 1984) on the effect of DSH (1000 mg/kg i.p.) on the cytotoxicity of radiation and cisplatin against the CFU in mice is congruent with the premise that DSH independently stimulates the CFU. If one fits regression lines to their DSH data (Fig. 5 of Evans *et al.*, 1983a; Chart 1 of Evans *et al.*, 1984) without forcing them through the SF $= 1$ point on the ordinate, then the zero radiation (Fig. 14.2) and zero cisplatin intercepts give values 37 and 31% higher, respectively, than those of controls not treated with DSH. Employment of an analogous approach for the CFU data obtained by Gringeri *et al.* (1988), in mice administered DSH (300 mg/kg i.v.) 3 h after carboplatin (Fig. 15.2), yields at zero carboplatin an SF value 21% higher than that of control animals.

From the work of Allalunis-Turner and Chapman (1984) it appears that the DSH effect is a transient one, requiring, for it to be observed, that the marrow cells be harvested relatively soon after DSH administration. When Gringeri *et al.* (1988), Schmalbach and Borch (1989a) and Pannacciulli *et al.* (1989) looked for DSH-induced stimulation of CFU, the time periods allowed to elapse between DSH administration and harvesting were 21, 22 and 22 h, respectively. While this may provide an explanation as to why they did not observe DSH-induced enhancement of the CFU SF, it raises the corollary of why they did observe DSH to antagonize the cisplatin cytotoxicity against CFU in such animals, given that the time of harvest was the same. Possibly DSH causes an activation of hemopoietic stem cells whereby they become better able to respond to a challenge, be this harvesting or the myelosuppressive effect of a chemotherapeutic agent, but that the activation is transient and that in the absence of a challenge, there is a reversion to the *status quo ante*.

The GM-CFC assay depends on the ability of granulocytes and macrophage progenitor cells to proliferate in culture when exposed to medium appropriately conditioned so as to contain CSF. Conditioning of the media is achieved by incubating it for some days with, for instance, the lungs of mice previously injected with endotoxin or, alternatively, spleen cells exposed to pokeweed mitogen. Multi-CSF (interleukin-3, IL-3) is the factor produced, for instance, under the latter conditions (Metcalf, 1984; Pimentel, 1990). The possibility that DSH causes bone marrow cells to elaborate a CSF has been explored by Schmalbach and Borch (1990), who established, to this end, long-term bone marrow cultures (LTBMC) using 25% horse serum supplemented medium. They observed that exposure of the LTBMC to 300 μM DSH in unsupplemented medium for 1 h results, over the period of the subsequent 24 h, in the appearance of a CSF in the medium such that incubation of fresh bone marrow cells with it causes enhanced GM-CFC formation. The effect is seen when 100–1000 μM DSH is used, although the greatest effect is observed with the 300 μM concentration. In an additional effort to discern which bone marrow cells might be responsible for the elaboration of this CSF, Schmalbach and Borch (1990) replaced the 25% horse serum, supplementing the LTBMC, with 20% bovine serum. Under these latter conditions the LTBMC is limited to stromal cells. Nonetheless, exposure of these cells to 300 μM DSH for 1 h results in the elaboration of the CSF which begins within 8 h of exposure to DSH and ends in less than 24 h. Interestingly, treatment of the LTBMC with 300 μM carboplatin by itself or concurrently with DSH neither enhances nor inhibits GM-CFC.

15.2.7 Potentiation of tumoricidal action of oxazaphosphorines

DSSD is able to restore the sensitivity to oxazaphosphorines of tumors that become resistant to these agents. A critical protective mechanism against the cytotoxicity of cyclophosphamide is the deactivation of its active metabolite. Briefly, cyclophosphamide is a prodrug which requires bioactivation via cytochrome P-450 mixed function oxidation to the active metabolite, 4-hydroxycyclophosphamide, which in turn in its tautomeric form as aldophosphamide is deactivated by aldehyde dehydrogenase (ALDH) to carboxyphosphamide (Sladek, 1988; Sladek *et al.*, 1989). Resistant L1210 murine leukemia cells possess 200 times higher ALDH activity than do the sensitive cells and 2.3 times the ALDH activity of murine liver (Hilton, 1984a). The resistance of these cells to 4-hydroxycyclophosphamide can be overcome by their pretreatment for 60 min with 10 μM DSSD (Hilton, 1984b). These findings were confirmed and extended to both mafosfamide, another oxazaphosphorine, and to a second leukemia cell line, P388, by Sladek and

Landkamer (1985). DSSD also increases the sensitivity of human hematopoietic progenitor cells to mafosfamide, but has little effect on its toxicity *vis-à-vis* a number of human malignant cell lines with low NAD-linked ALDH activity (Kohn *et al.*, 1987). Oxazaphosphorine resistance in leukemic cells is associated with elevation of a cytosolic ALDH which is very sensitive to DSSD. Thus Russo *et al.* (1988), upon partial purification of a low K_m cytosolic ALDH from resistant L1210 murine cells found that its K_i for DSSD is 6µM. It may be noted that the most efficient isozyme for detoxication of aldophosphamide in mouse liver is AHD-2, the low K_m cytosolic form, equivalent to human E 1 enzyme (Manthey *et al.*, 1990) which is very sensitive to DSSD inhibition *in vitro* (section 9.2.2).

In vivo, DSSD pretreatment (80 mg/kg i.p.), administered 24 h before cyclophosphamide (80 mg/kg i.v.) to mice bearing mammary carcinoma, results in prolonged serum half-lives of both cyclophosphamide and its alkylating metabolites (Donelli *et al.*, 1976). These workers observed that tumor weights in DSSD-pretreated animals increase at a 59% slower rate. They also reported that, in mice bearing Lewis lung carcinoma, DSSD pretreatment resulted in significantly lower tumor weights (by 45%), 50% fewer metastases, and significantly longer survival. Likewise, Hacker *et al.* (1982b) reported that administration of DSSD (200 mg/kg i.p.) to L1210 inoculated mice 30 min prior to cyclophosphamide (150 mg/kg, i.p.) results in a dramatic increase in the incidence of long-term (>60 days) survivors, 70% versus 5% in cyclophosphamide-treated controls.

DSSD protects against bladder toxicity occasioned by therapeutic doses of cyclophosphamide. In a 125 mg/kg p.o. dose, DSSD significantly reduces bladder toxicity if administered within 1 h of the cyclophosphamide (100 mg/kg, i.p.) treatment (Hacker *et al.*, 1982a,b). DSSD is not effective in preventing cystitis, however, if administered 2 h prior to cyclophosphamide (Hacker *et al.*, 1982a,b; Habs *et al.*, 1984).

15.3 CLINICAL STUDIES

The ability of DSH, demonstrated by preclinical studies, to inhibit the undesired effects of cisplatin, particularly its kidney and gastrointestinal toxicity, gave rise to the expectation that DSH might prove useful clinically (Borch, 1986a,b). As a first step, several Phase I clinical studies of DSH, administered in conjunction with cisplatin chemotherapy, were undertaken to determine the nature of its dose-limiting toxicities. In the process, efforts were made to establish whether normal tissues were protected by DSH rescue against cisplatin toxicity (Qazi *et al.*,

1988; Gandara *et al.*, 1988b, 1989, 1990; Berry *et al.*, 1990). Phase II studies have been undertaken to address specifically the question whether DSH can protect against the toxicity of high-dose therapy with cisplatin (Paredes *et al.*, 1988) or carboplatin (Rothenberg *et al.*, 1988). Some of the studies have been also concerned with investigation of the pharmacokinetics of DSH (Qazi *et al.*, 1988; DeGregorio *et al.*, 1989), or alternatively with the effect of DSH on the pharmacokinetics of cisplatin (Paredes *et al.*, 1988; DeGregorio *et al.*, 1989). Finally, although the preclinical evidence that DSSD inhibits the toxic effects of cisplatin is marginal at best, its ready availability as a drug and the fact that it is well tolerated led to both Phase I (Stewart *et al.*, 1987) and Phase II (Verma *et al.*, 1990) studies of DSSD in conjunction with cisplatin chemotherapy. In the course of the latter study it became apparent that in the dose employed (mean 3 g) DSSD augments cisplatin toxicity.

15.3.1 Dose conversion to humans

Using the approach of Freireich *et al.* (1966) that proportionality between different species is based on an idealized body surface area (actually the body weight to the 2/3 power times a species unique constant), Gale *et al.* (1982a) have calculated that the human equivalent of a 500 mg/kg dose in the mouse would be 2.43 g/60 kg person. Paredes *et al.* (1988), using the same concepts of proportionality, calculated the preclinical dose range of 100–750 mg/kg to be equivalent in humans to doses of 528–3700 mg/m².

15.3.2 Toxic effects associated with diethyldithiocarbamate infusion

In all the clinical studies mentioned in this chapter, DSH was administered i.v. by infusion over periods varying from 30 min to 3.5 h and in doses of 600 mg/m² (~ 1 g/70 kg) to 4000 mg/m² (~ 11 g/70 kg). The DSH infusions were started 30–45 min and 3 h after the termination of those of cisplatin and carboplatin, respectively. Within 5 min or so of starting of the infusion generalized peripheral vasodilation is evident, the skin is flushed, the patients report feeling warm and conjunctival injection is observed. Soon thereafter chest tightness and anxiety are experienced. At their worst, the toxic symptoms include anxiety and apprehension severe enough to give the impression of acute psychosis, burning sensation in the mucous membranes of the eyes, the eyelids, and the palate, burning chest pain, severe diaphoresis, moderate to severe abdominal cramps and numbness of the infusion arm. The toxic effects are said to be independent of dose (Qazi *et al.*, 1988) or speed of infusion (Borch *et al.*, 1987) and that doses as high as 7.5 g/m^2 ($\sim 13 \text{ g/70 kg}$) have been given without serious side-effects (Borch *et al.*, 1987). The symptoms can be turned on and off by starting and stopping the infusion (Borch, private communication), are said to ameliorate 'with time and transient slowing of the infusion' (Qazi *et al.*, 1988), and they dissipate rapidly with the end of the infusion. With the lowest dose (600 mg/m^2), a burning sensation of the head and neck was the only discomfort reported (Paredes *et al.*, 1988) though the pain could be severe (Newman *et al.*, 1988). It was abrogated by pretreatment of the patients with hydromorphone (4 mg, i.v.). At the higher doses the adverse effects are severe, sufficiently so to cause termination of the infusion in four instances, to 'hamper further patient recruitment' (Qazi *et al.*, 1988), to require 'generous amounts of sedation' (Berry *et al.*, 1990) with benzodiazepines and barbiturates, and to occasion the administration of ephedrine to decrease the parasympathetic component (Rothenberg *et al.*, 1988). Moreover, in the one study in which 4 g/m^2 was infused in 30 min, all patients experienced severe toxic effects and a 'degree of distress' that 'cannot be overemphasized' (Rothenberg *et al.*, 1988). Also, the planned 1-h infusion of the same dose in another study (DeGregorio *et al.*, 1989) resulted, in the event, in infusion durations from 1 to 3.5 h 'related to the constitutional side effects.' Hypertension (increases in systolic blood pressure of 60–75 mmHg) observed initially can be followed several hours later by hypotension (decreases in blood pressure of up to 60 mmHg) necessitating fluid resuscitation.

No information is available regarding the mechanism of this toxic reaction. In many ways the symptomatology associated with it is similar to that of the disulfiram–ethanol reaction (DER) as described in Chapter 9. Some of the investigators involved (Rothenberg *et al.*, 1988; Borch, private communication) have described the similarity as 'striking.' The DER is occasioned by the inhibition of aldehyde dehydrogenase and the resulting accumulation of ethanol-derived acetaldehyde. The inhibition of dopamine β-hydroxylase and the depletion of norepinephrine stores modulate the effects of the acetaldehyde. In the absence of ethanol ingestion, the blood acetaldehyde levels are normally very low, at the limit of detection, and certainly well below the $5 \, \mu\text{M}$ concentration associated with the DER. DSH administration, like that of DSSD, will result in the inhibition of aldehyde dehydrogenase and the DSH doses used in cisplatin rescue are massive, relative to the dose of DSSD employed to achieve a therapeutic level of ALDH inhibition (250–500 mg p.o.). What effect these doses of DSH have on the level of ALDH inhibition and blood acetaldehyde has not been explored. It is also not clear to what extent the course and nature of the observed DSH toxicity was influenced by the high-dose chemotherapy these patients had received.

15.3.3 Effect on cisplatin nephrotoxicity

Preclinical studies indicate that the antagonism by DSH of cisplatin's nephrotoxicity stands apart in requiring the use of high doses of DSH. The failure of the study by Paredes *et al.* (1988) to detect any effect of DSH infusion (600 mg/m^2) in a prospective randomized Phase II study of cancer patients treated with cisplatin (120 mg/m^2) and 5-fluorouracil (1000 mg/m^2) has been ascribed to the DSH dose used being suboptimal (Gandara *et al.*, 1988a; Qazi *et al.*, 1988; Berry *et al.*, 1990). The studies of Qazi *et al.* (1988) and Berry *et al.* (1990) were Phase I studies and thus lacked comparison groups. These workers used much higher DSH doses and reported minimal nephrotoxicity; Berry *et al.* (1990) concluded the absence of any nephrotoxicity was 'remarkable.' A third Phase I study, which to date has not been published except in abstract and review format (Gandara *et al.*, 1988a, 1989, 1990), has compared patients receiving DSH (4 g/m^2) in conjunction with high-dose cisplatin therapy with a historical control group of 79 patients who received the identical cisplatin therapy but no DSH. In the latter group 49% had creatinine levels in excess of 1.5 mg%, while in the group receiving DSH only 19% did. While these latter results are encouraging, this treatment needs to be further evaluated. Additionally, for 'use of this drug as a chemoprotector in the community setting' its toxicity 'needs to be ameliorated' (Berry *et al.*, 1990).

15.3.4 Effect on nausea and vomiting

Although in preclinical studies DSH has been found to antagonize cisplatin-induced gastrointestinal toxicity and, more particularly, to markedly decrease the incidence of vomiting in dogs (section 15.2.3), clinical results to date are disappointing. In controlled studies by Paredes *et al.* (1988) no difference was observed in the incidence of nausea and vomiting in the DSH and control groups beyond that induced by the administration of standard antiemetic medication. In the Phase I study of Berry *et al.* (1990) about half the patients who received cisplatin doses ≤140 mg/m^2 followed by DSH (4 g/m^2) experienced intractable vomiting, 36% of these individuals requiring hospitalization because of this toxicity. Likewise, Rothenberg *et al.* (1988) reported that in their study of carboplatin (800 mg/m²) followed by DSH (4 g/m²) all the patients experienced severe nausea and vomiting (at least 6 episodes/24 h). The only exception to this dismal litany is the statement by Qazi *et al.* (1988) that 3/10 in their study had a 'significant amelioration of typical platinum-induced nausea and vomiting' following treatment with the cisplatin–DSH combination compared to previous experience with cisplatin alone. Unfortunately, the preclinical base of empirical knowledge regarding the control of platinum-induced vomiting is limited to information derived from just three dogs (section 12.2.3), a number dwarfed by that of the patients ($n=81$) from whom the above information is derived. In this context, it should be noted that the antagonism of the emetic effects of cisplatin were achieved in dogs by administration of a 25 mg/kg dose of DSH [equivalent, on a (body weight)$^{0.73}$ basis, to a 950 mg dose in a 62.5 kg person], while the doses administered to patients were as high as 4 g/m² (11 g/70 kg person). Such large doses of DSH provoke a syndrome which in many respects is similar to the DER. Though the similarity may be spurious, it should be noted that nausea and vomiting are also prominent components of the DER. This raises the possibility that infusion with high doses of DSH may itself cause or augment these symptoms. In the case of cisplatin, the use of such high DSH levels is considered necessary to counteract the drug's nephrotoxicity. This does not apply, however, to carboplatin and lower doses of DSH could prove more effective in counteracting the nausea and vomiting induced by the latter chemotherapeutic agent.

15.3.5 Effect on hematological toxicity

Myelosuppression is a dose-limiting toxicity for high-dose carboplatin therapy. The effect of DSH (4 g/m²), administered 3 h after high-dose carboplatin, on this toxicity was explored by Rothenberg *et al.* (1988) on the basis of a historical comparison with patients receiving carboplatin alone for the treatment of the same neoplasm (ovarian cancer). Treatment with DSH was associated with leukopenia which though shorter (on average 34%) was also more intense (nadirs lower by 20%, on average). This, Rothenberg *et al.* (1988) associate with a statistically significantly ($P=0.02$) greater tendency for patients treated with DSH to develop fever than was true of those who received carboplatin alone (risk factors of 0.28 and 0.12, respectively). They also advanced the possibility that the lower white blood cell count nadirs might have been a factor in the death from infectious complications of three of the patients treated with DSH (none of the patients in the comparison study died). The DSH administration was also associated with episodes of thrombocytopenia which, like the leukopenia episodes, were on average shorter in duration (by 54%), but reached lower nadirs (on average by 21%). It should be noted that since carboplatin is much less nephrotoxic than cisplatin, its dose-limiting toxicity is myelosuppression, and that preclinical data suggest this might be preventable by much lower doses of DSH, if optimally timed. Such doses would likely be free of the above complications.

Myelosuppression was not significant in the Phase I studies of Qazi *et al.* (1988) and Berry *et al.* (1990) of combined cisplatin–DSH treatment. Also, no differences in hematological toxicity were observed in the Phase II study by Paredes *et al.* (1988) in patients administered a cisplatin–fluorouracil combination with and without DSH. On the other hand, Gandara *et al.* (1989) reported that, in a historical comparison of studies of high-dose cisplatin with and without DSH, the former had a 3 times lower incidence of leukopenia (<3000 cells/μl: 6 and 18%, respectively) and a 4 times lower incidence of thrombocytopenia ($<130\,000$ cells/μl: 6 and 24%, respectively).

15.3.6 Effect on neuropathy and ototoxicity

High-dose cisplatin therapy is associated with a significant incidence of neuropathy (moderate to marked paresthesias) and ototoxicity. Comparing two groups of patients who received high-dose cisplatin, Gandara *et al.* (1990) reported that while those not treated with DSH had a neuropathy and ototoxicity incidence of 38 and 37%, respectively, those administered DSH ($4\,g/m^2$) had an incidence of 2 and 0%, respectively.

15.3.7 Effect on cisplatin pharmacokinetics

In clinical studies, infusion of DSH 30–45 min after termination of that of cisplatin is reported to be without effect on cisplatin pharmacokinetics in terms of total body clearance, volume of distribution, area under the plasma curve (Paredes *et al.*, 1988) or the platinum in plasma ultrafiltrate (DeGregorio *et al.*, 1989).

15.3.8 Effect on antitumor responses

No adequate conclusion can be reached, on the basis of clinical studies published to date, regarding the influence of DSH on the tumor response to either high-dose cisplatin or high-dose carboplatin chemo-therapy. All but one of the clinical investigations in which tumor responses were noted and in which high-dose cisplatin and DSH were used, have been Phase I studies lacking comparison groups. The exception, the randomized prospective study by Paredes *et al.* (1988), involved administration of both cisplatin and fluorouracil and relatively low doses of DSH. No difference in either tumor response rates, or median patient survival time were observed in the group administered DSH. In the high-dose carboplatin ovarian cancer study of Rothenberg *et al.* (1988), in which patients received DSH, the 19% overall tumor response rate observed was within the 95% confidence limits of the 27% response rate previously reported for high-dose carboplatin in patients with this tumor.

15.4 CONCLUSIONS

The mechanisms whereby DSH antagonizes cisplatin induced neph-rotoxicity and the myelotoxicity of this and other chemotherapeutic agents are necessarily different. The former involves the chelation of platinum bound to tissues and its removal. For this effect to take place it may be necessary to achieve *in vivo* DSH concentrations of 400 μM or more and thus high doses of the agent may have to be given. Also, the DSH has to be administered after cisplatin. Preclinical studies indicate much lower doses of DSH are effective in counteracting the myelotoxicity of cisplatin and other agents. No low-dose DSH clinical studies specifically designed to test for protection from myelosuppression have been reported to date. Preclinical studies indicate that DSH can be effective in this regard even if administered as much as 90 min before or 2–3 hrs after the chemotherapeutic agent, a factor of possible importance with agents such as carboplatin the tumoricidal action of which may be compromised if it is administered concurrently with DSH. A striking feature of the actions of DSH, both with respect to antagonism of lethality and myelotoxicity, is the absence of a clear dose dependence. Another feature worthy of note is the importance of timing. Both of these features echo some of the immunomodulatory actions of DSH and raise interesting questions regarding the mechan-isms involved.

16

Toxicology

16.1 INTRODUCTION 335
16.2 ACUTE TOXICITY 336
    16.2.1 Determination of lethal doses 336
    16.2.2 Problems of administration: local toxicity and absorption . . . 337
    16.2.3 Acute disulfiram intoxication 340
16.3 CHRONIC TOXICITY 341
16.4 EFFECTS ON LIVER 342
16.5 TESTING FOR MUTAGENICITY 343
16.6 TESTING FOR CARCINOGENICITY 344
16.7 TESTING FOR TERATOGENIC AND REPRODUCTIVE TOXICITY . . 345

16.1 INTRODUCTION

The context for any discussion of the toxicology of disulfiram (DSSD) and diethyldithiocarbamate (DSH) is the dosages used therapeutically. For disulfiram these have been 250 to 500 mg/day since the mid-1950s, 250 mg/day being the prevalent dose in North America (Table 11.1). A 400 mg trice weekly dosage is extensively employed in Scandinavia. In these two latter dosages DSSD has proved remarkably free of side-effects (Section 11.7).

For DSH, the doses that have proved effective in the experimental treatment of HIV infections (Table 13.1) have ranged (with the exception of a Phase I study: see below) from weekly doses of 5 mg/kg, p.o. or i.v., to 400 mg/m^2 p.o. (equivalent in a 70 kg person to weekly doses of 350 and 700 mg, respectively). In these doses, DSH did not induce any major adverse clinical or biological reactions (section 13.2.1). Among the minor side-effects most frequently observed were a metallic taste and abdominal discomfort. Transient nausea and fatigue were also reported. Higher doses have been employed in the treatment of nickel carbonyl intoxication (section 7.6.3) where as much as 4 g/day has been used without significant toxicity. High doses have also been administered in Phase I studies, that is studies designed to determine the tolerance, toxicity and maximally tolerated dose of the

335

agent. In one of these, performed in patients with HIV infections, $800 \, mg/m^2$ was administered twice weekly for 4 weeks (section 13.2.1). Other Phase I studies, involving acute infusions, have been performed in patients undergoing cancer chemotherapy where DSH was used as a rescue agent. In the latter studies the infused DSH dose was escalated as high as $7.5 \, g/m^2$ (equivalent 13 g in a 70 kg person). The acute toxic manifestations observed during infusions of such high DSH doses are not insignificant (section 15.3.2), but dissipate rapidly when the infusion is terminated.

Animal studies have found no evidence that either DSSD or DSH have teratogenic effects (section 16.7), *in vivo* mutagenic effects (section 16.5), or that they have any carcinogenic activity (section 16.6). Studies of the lethal doses of these agents in animals (section 16.2.1) indicate consistently that the p.o. LD_{50} of DSSD and the i.p. LD_{50} of DSH in rodents are above $1.2 \, g/kg$. The very low solubility of DSSD in water renders determination of its toxicity problematic if large oral doses or i.p. administration of the powder as a slurry is employed (section 16.2.2). Animal studies of the acute toxic effects of high doses of DSSD are supplemented by clinical information gleaned from case reports of suicidal attempts and accidental ingestion (section 16.2.3). Chronic toxicity studies in animals have focused on neuropathy associated with DSSD administration (section 16.3); efforts to identify a dosing paradigm that would result in DSSD-induced hepatoxicity have been less successful (16.4). It should be added that DSSD is remarkable in that, in spite of many years of clinical use in thousands of patients, there are relatively few reports of toxic side-effects subsequent to the dose reduction which occurred in the mid-1950s.

16.2 ACUTE TOXICITY

16.2.1 Determination of lethal doses

In mice and rats, the LD_{50} for i.p.-administered diethyldithiocarbamate (DSH) is consistently reported to be in the $1.2-1.5 \, g/kg$ range (Table 16.1). The dose–response curve is quite sharp, the LD_{10} and LD_{90} values being 1.35 ± 0.07 and $2.00 \pm 0.10 \, g/kg$, respectively (Bodenner *et al.*, 1986b). The LD_{50} values for p.o.-administered DSH are slightly higher; the possibility of stomach-acid-catalyzed decomposition of the DSH to carbon disulfide (CS_2) and diethylamine (sections 2.2 and 7.6.1) has to be kept in mind in evaluating these figures. If disulfiram (DSSD) is administered p.o. to rats as a solution in oil, its LD_{50} is comparable to that for i.p.-administered DSH. The LD_{50} values obtained following the administration of aqueous slurries of DSSD are harder to interpret because of the very limited solubility of DSSD in aqueous media and the local tissue injury induced by the agent (section 16.2.2). Renoux (1982) ascribed the particularly high figure (2.83 g/kg) for the LD_{50} of p.o.-administered Imuthiol brand of DSH to its higher purity. The toxicity of DSH salts other than the sodium one has been little explored.

Thallium diethyldithiocarbamate has a toxicity (Table 16.1) very similar, on an equimolar basis, to that of thallium nitrate, suggesting that the chelate dissociates readily. This is in accord with the extraction constant for the reaction of thallium ions with DSH being relatively low (Table 2.1).

16.2.2 Problems of administration: local toxicity and absorption

In undertaking to evaluate DSSD toxicity, very high doses of DSSD are sometimes administered. The very low solubility of DSSD and the tendency for such high doses not to be absorbed from the site of administration render interpretation of the results problematical. Rats administered 3.5 g/kg p.o., for instance, exhibit only moderate toxicity from which they recover in 4 days, yet upon autopsy on day 7 following administration of the DSSD the stomachs of about half of these animals are found to contain DSSD bezoars covered with green mucous (Child and Crump, 1952). Accordingly, the 8.6 g/kg p.o. LD_{50} for DSSD obtained under such conditions has little practical significance. When, to obviate absorption difficulties, DSSD is administered in divided doses (350 mg/kg every 15 min) or in a lipid solvent (cottonseed oil) the acute LD_{50} is several-fold lower (Table 16.1). Incomplete absorption is also evident when large doses of DSSD in aqueous suspension are administered parenterally. Granules of DSSD are observed *in situ* 3 days following i.p. administration of a 7.2 g/kg dose of the compound in water to mice (Child and Crump, 1952). Likewise, following s.c. administration of large doses (1.5 and 4 g/kg) of DSSD in 50% aqueous suspension or 8% sesame seed oil, the material is found to persist for as long as 8 weeks in the form of DSSD 'tumors' (typical foreign body granulomas) at the site of injection (Child and Crump, 1952).

Tissue injury at the site of administration or instillation of large doses of DSSD is another complicating factor. In rats administered such doses p.o., a generalized visceral hyperemia, and a distended, edematous gastrointestinal tract are observed, with gastric ulceration as a common finding (Child and Crump, 1952). Also, following i.p. administration of

Table 16.1 Acute toxicity of disulfiram, diethyldithiocarbamate salts and methyl ester

Substance	Species	LD50 g/kg				Reference	Remarks
		p.o.	i.p.	s.c.	i.v.		
Disulfiram	mouse		0.65			Hald et al., 1952	
		1.98				Hazard et al., 1957	
	rat	8.6±0.4	0.58±0.09			Child and Crump, 1952	in divided doses
		2.5±0.4				Child and Crump, 1952	in cottonseed oil
		1.3±0.4				Child and Crump, 1952	
	rabbit	2.05				Brieger, 1947	
		1.8±0.1				Child and Crump, 1952	
Sodium diethyldithiocarbamate	mouse		1.5			Hald et al., 1952	
			~1.5			West and Sunderman, 1958	
			~1.75			Scholler et al., 1961	
			(0.95–1.40)			Maj and Vetulani, 1970	
			1.50			Schönenberger and Lippert, 1972	
			1.40			Cantilena and Klaassen, 1981	
		1.87				Renoux, 1982	
			1.30			Domingo et al., 1985	
					1.7±0.1	Bodenner et al., 1986b	

Compound	Species			Reference	Notes
	rat	~1.50	~1.50	West and Sunderman, 1958	
			1.25	Scholler et al., 1961	
			1.25	Schönenberger and Lippert, 1972	
			1.23	Frank et al., 1978	20–24 day old rats
			1.30	Frank et al., 1978	3–5 day old rats
			1.08	Frank et al., 1978	as Imuthiol brand
				Renoux, 1982	
	rabbit	2.83	0.5	Hald et al. 1952	
	dog	3.5		Child et al., 1951	
			~1.0	Scholler et al., 1961	
Cadmium diethyldithiocarbamate	mice	0.65		Gale et al., 1981	
Tin diethyldithiocarbarmate	mice	2.60		Carrara et al., 1988	
Thallium diethyldithiocarbamate	rat	0.031		Rauws et al., 1969	3 weeks LD50
Zinc diethyldithiocarbamate	rabbit	0.57		Brieger, 1947	
Diethyldithiocarbamic acid methyl ester	mouse	0.26 (0.24–0.29)		Faiman et al., 1983	
	rat	0.17 (0.12–0.22)		Faiman et al., 1983	

large doses, inflammation of the peritoneal cavity and extensive visceral adhesions are observed (Child and Crump, 1952). In a human injected s.c. with a 2 g dose of sterile DSSD powder in 10 ml normal saline as a slurry (Phillips *et al.*, 1985), local redness and swelling were observed in the first 2 days after administration, these manifestations subsiding spontaneously thereafter. In both this and another individual, administered a 1 g dose of DSSD powder, a diminishing s.c. lump could be detected for the 4 weeks of the study (Phillips, 1988). Experiments in rats indicate that when DSSD is administered s.c. in an aqueous slurry, absorption is quite slow. Following administration of a 0.5–1.0 g/kg dose of radiolabeled DSSD in this manner, the excretion of the radiolabel occurs by a first-order process with a half-life of 7.53 days (Phillips and Gresser, 1984). At 88 days post injection, the site of administration is grossly and microscopically normal, and no tissue necrosis is evident.

16.2.3 Acute disulfiram intoxication

Animals given toxic doses of DSSD p.o. develop first a mucous diarrhea, anorexia, emesis (observed in dogs, rodents do not possess the reflex), and lethargy. With larger doses ataxia and hypothermia are noted, as well as a flaccid paralysis that begins in the hind limbs and progresses to encompass the trunk, the forelegs, the neck, and finally the respiratory muscles. Patchy demyelinization of the medulla and cerebellum, and in chronic studies, of the spinal cord are observed (Child and Crump, 1952). Other histological changes observed in rats are toxic necrosis of the spleen and degeneration of the proximal convoluted tubules of the kidney, while in livers of dogs and rabbits numerous regions of focal necrosis and cord dissociation are seen.

Several instances of ingestion of large quantities of DSSD with suicidal intent provide the information, discussed below, regarding its acute toxicity in humans. In one case ingestion of approximately 25 g of disulfiram resulted in somnolence, with coma developing on the third day. By the fifth day flaccid tetraparesis developed. In the third week the patient became oriented and could move the proximal parts of her upper limbs. For 14 weeks no compound muscle action potential or sensory action potential could be detected after stimulation of the peroneal nerve. The patient improved gradually thereafter, but at 15 months bilateral paralysis of the flexor and extensor muscles of the foot and complete sensory loss were still present (Hirschberg *et al.*, 1987). In an analogous case (Schütz *et al.*, 1983) suicidal ingestion of 22.5 g resulted in stupor that progressed to coma and severe tetraparesis. Recovery lasted 2 years. In both of these cases, sural nerve biopsy revealed axonal degeneration. Two successful suicide attempts with DSSD which came to the attention of a telephone hotline service are mentioned by Fournier *et al.* (1967). These were said to have involved 10 and 20 g of DSSD and to have a fatal outcome after 2 and 3 days, respectively. The authors were unable, however, to obtain additional details. Pediatric DSSD intoxications have been reported by Wokittel (1960) and Buskowicz (1962). In those cases ingestion of 3 g and 20 tablets, respectively, lead to vomiting and somnolence. In the latter case the child became flaccid. With time she improved, but still showed discoordination of gait at 1, 2 and 4 years.

16.3 CHRONIC TOXICITY

Rats maintained on a 1% DSSD feed look healthy and gain weight but after 10 weeks on the diet some develop a progressive neuropathy, first observable as a disturbance of gait, then foot drop progressing eventually to complete paralysis of the hind limbs; no involvement of the fore limbs is seen (Anzil, 1985). Alternatively, the neuropathy can be produced experimentally by implanting i.p. or s.c. about 1.7 g/kg DSSD powder weekly for 3–5 weeks (Anzil, 1980) or 2.5 g/kg for 3 weeks (Anzil and Dozic, 1978). Administration of DSSD to rats (220-580 mg/kg daily for 1–3 weeks) also has a neurotoxic effect on the autonomic system, the rat ileum becoming unresponsive to 5-hydroxytryptamine stimulation (Mansner *et al.*, 1968; Savolainen *et al.*, 1984). Chronic DSH administration to rabbits (Mur, 1964; Edington and Howell, 1969; Rasul and Howell, 1973b), sheep (Mur, 1964) and hens (Howell and Edington, 1968; Rasul and Howell, 1973a, 1974) is also neurotoxic, leading to demyelinization lesions. The pattern of lesions is somewhat different, however, from that seen with DSSD, marked involvement of long spinal pathways is noted.

Clinically, peripheral neuropathies attributable to DSSD are seldom seen (section 9.3.2). When observed, they follow a pattern similar to that seen in rats. Nerve biopsies reveal distal axonopathies, be it in humans or rats. More recently, it has been reported, on the basis of nerve biopsies of affected humans, that the axons are distended with filaments, and thus that the axonopathy is a neurofilamentous one (Ansbacher *et al.*, 1982). Although the point has been debated (Anzil, 1985), the publication of micrographs provides morphological evidence for this conclusion (Bilbao *et al.*, 1984; Bergouignan *et al.*, 1988).

The mechanism of action whereby DSSD induces the neuropathy remains unclear. DSSD has been found to inhibit *in vitro* tubulin polymerization in a dose-dependent manner (Potchoo *et al.*, 1986) and this too has been advanced as a possible mechanism of the neuropathy. However, the inhibition, which requires DSSD concentrations of 10^{-6} M, is only observed following a preincubation of the microtubular protein with DSSD. Another possibility that has been advanced is that the neuropathy is caused by CS_2, a metabolite of DSSD, which itself also causes a peripheral neuropathy (Rainey, 1977). The finding that the DSSD-induced lesion, like that induced by CS_2, is a neurofilamentous axonopathy has strengthened this theory (Bilbao *et al.*, 1984). Then again, DSH, another metabolite of DSSD, is a potent copper chelator and low levels of copper have been linked to neuropathy (Mills and Fell, 1960). Since *in vivo* CS_2 forms dithiocarbamates (section 6.7), its effects could also be mediated by copper chelation. The possibility that some individuals in the population metabolize DSSD differently and are thereby more susceptible to CS_2 neurotoxicity has been raised by Djurić *et al.* (1973). These workers reported that following DSSD dosing the urine of individuals sensitive to CS_2 contains significantly less DSH than that of controls. Since DSH decomposes spontaneously in solution to CS_2 as a function of pH (section 2.2) the ratio of these two compounds in urine would depend on its acidity. The failure of Djurić *et al.* (1973) to acknowledge this, or to indicate that they safeguarded their urine samples against it raises the possibility that their findings were artefactual.

Chronic DSH toxicity has been investigated by Sunderman *et al.* (1967) who administered DSH in doses of 30, 100 and 300 mg/kg/day p.o. for 90 days to groups of 25 male and 25 female rats and to pairs of male and female beagle dogs and compared them to control groups of a like size. The rats in the two higher dose groups gained weight significantly more slowly, at 90 days the body weights of those in the 300 mg/kg/day group being some 18% below those of the controls. Female rats in the 300 mg/kg/day group also had significantly reduced hematocrit values, hemoglobin concentration and red blood counts at 90 days. When the rats were sacrificed at the end of the 90-day period, kidney weights of the 300 mg/kg group were significantly lower than those of the controls and glomerular congestion was noted. No noteworthy changes were found in the livers, gonads, skeleton or gastrointestinal tract. During the entire period of observation, dogs administered DSH in doses of 30 and 100 mg/kg/day were comparable in appearance, behavior, appetite and maintenance of body weight to the control animals. Emesis was observed in several of the test dogs. Dogs in the 300 mg/kg/day group had slight losses in body weight and one of the female dogs died on day 70.

16.4 EFFECTS ON LIVER

Milandri *et al.* (1980) found no histological damage of the liver in rats administered 100 mg/kg DSSD twice weekly for 90 days. Kirchmeyer *et al.* (1979) found weakly expressed histological and ultrastructural changes in rats administered 600 mg/kg DSSD daily for 3 days. At this dosage, DSSD significantly increased serum alkaline phosphatase (AP) and blood ATP. Also, it exacerbated the hepatic damage induced by D-galactosamine pretreatment (Mach, 1986). Hunter and Neal (1975) found that the i.p. administration of DSH in a dose of 5 mmol/kg (1126 mg/kg) did not induce hepatic damage in rats. If the rats were pretreated with 50 mg/kg phenobarbital daily for 5 days, however, this dose of DSH caused centrilobular necrosis. In this the action of DSH resembles that of CS_2 and likely results from induction of a cytochrome P-450 isozyme capable of metabolizing CS_2 oxidatively to carbonyl sulfide (COS) with the formation of extremely reactive atomic sulfur (section 8.3.5). No analogous hepatic damage was obtained when 2.5 mmol/kg (740 mg/ kg) DSSD was administered to rats pretreated for 5 days with 50 mg/kg phenobarbital daily (Hunter and Neal, 1975), or upon administration of 100 mg/kg DSSD concurrently with 50 mg/kg phenobarbital daily for 8 days (Milandri *et al.*, 1980).

Hepatotoxicity is a very uncommon clinical reaction to DSSD (section 11.7.4). When observed, such reactions do not present as typical drug hypersensitivity reactions. At the same time, the dose of DSSD taken does not appear to be a determinant. Thus the precipitating factors remain unknown. In individuals receiving therapeutic doses of DSSD (250 and 500 mg/day for 3 weeks), blood chemistries indicative of hepatotoxicity, namely serum glutamic oxaloacetic transaminase (SGOT), AP, lactate dehydrogenase (LDH) and total bilirubin do not change significantly (Goyer and Major, 1979). A dual elevation of SGOT and AP was noted by these workers to occur significantly ($P=0.028$) more frequently in DSSD patients than controls, but the absence of dose-dependence, the relatively low P value and the use of multiple statistical comparisons, all render any conclusion that might be drawn from them, prior to confirmation, tenuous.

16.5 TESTING FOR MUTAGENICITY

When DSSD is tested *in vivo*, no evidence of mutagenicity is found. Thus, it does not bring about induction of micronuclei in the bone marrow of Chinese hamsters injected with it; also neither DSSD nor ZnDS increase the sex-linked recessive lethals in *Drosophila* (Donner *et al.*, 1983). On the other hand, results obtained in various *in vitro* tests have been interpreted as indicating that DSSD and the salts of DSH have mutagenic properties (Levinson *et al.*, 1978; Donner *et al.*, 1983; Rannug *et al.*, 1984). Both these compounds are found to cause mutations in the *Salmonella typhimurium/* microsome assay (Rannug *et al.*, 1984). DSSD is also found to induce sister chromatid exchanges in Chinese hamster ovary cells (Donner *et al.*, 1983). Since DSSD and DSH cannot, chemically, be classified as alkylating, these findings are considered 'confusing' (Rannug *et al.*, 1984). As discussed in section 14.1, DSH and DSSD exhibit a bimodal cytotoxicity *in vitro*. This is ascribable to their ability to act, in the presence of oxygen and iron, as a hydrogen peroxide generating system. It is of interest therefore that the mutagenicity of DSSD in the *Salmonella typhimurium*/microsome assay is enhanced by oxygen (Rannug and Rannug, 1984). The above suggest that re-evaluation of the possible role of hydrogen peroxide generation in the observed *in vitro* mutagenic effects of these agents is in order.

16.6 TESTING FOR CARCINOGENICITY

All available evidence suggests that DSSD and DSH are not carcinogenic. Administration of DSH in feed (1250 and 2500 ppm) to rats of either sex for 104 weeks fails to result in a greater incidence of tumors than is seen in matched controls. Likewise, administration of this compound in feed (500 and 4000 ppm) to mice of either sex for 108–109 weeks also fails to result in a greater number of tumors than is seen in control groups (National Cancer Institute, 1979). The interpretation of these and an earlier inconclusive study (Innes *et al.*, 1969) is rendered difficult because of the use of the oral route and the instability of DSH when exposed to an acid milieu such as would likely be present in the stomach.

With respect to DSSD, although many patients have taken the drug continuously for extended periods of time, in some instances for as long as 30 years (Borrett *et al.*, 1985), no evidence of any associated neoplasms has emerged. On the contrary, the drug has been investigated as an anticarcinogen in animal studies (for review see Fiala, 1981; Bertram, 1988).

16.7 TESTING FOR TERATOGENIC AND REPRODUCTIVE TOXICITY

While administration of DSSD in sufficient dose will cause maternal and fetal mortality, no dose has been found that will induce teratogenic effects. Thus, administration of single oral doses of 125–500 mg/kg of DSSD in carboxymethyl cellulose to golden Syrian hamsters on day 7 or 8 of gestation is not teratogenic (Robens, 1969). At 500 mg/kg, significant maternal mortality is observed, and with a 1000 mg/kg dose, the maternal mortality is 100%.

In rats, administration of DSSD (100 mg/kg/day, p.o.) from day 3 through day 12 or 13 of gestation results in 83% fetal resorption (Salgo and Oster, 1974). At this dose the DSSD induces significant maternal toxicity, coma or death being observed in one third of the animals after 8 days of treatment. Delaying the start of DSSD administration to day 8 results in an absence of resorptions; no gross malformations are observed. Reduction of the DSSD dose to 50 mg/kg/day greatly reduces maternal toxicity. Continuation of this regimen to Day 21 of gestation has no effect on the viability of the fetuses and no teratological effects visible on gross examination.

In rabbits, i.v. administration of either 0.5 or 1.0 g/kg DSH daily, 5 days a week from day 0 of gestation to day 20 results in complete resorption, although the dams appeared well throughout the course of the experiment (Howell, 1964).

In chicken embryos, cadmium and zinc diethyldithiocarbamates are powerful embryotoxic agents, with LD_{50} values of 2.4 and 3.6 nmol/egg, respectively (Korhonen *et al.*, 1983).

Appendix–The road to Antabuse*

Professor Erick Jacobsen

As some will remember Denmark managed surprisingly well during the occupation and the second world war – and so did Medicinalco. General manager Lucassen had wisely taken care that not much was lacking, not even in what was then known as Medicinalco's Biological–Chemical laboratory. We were about twenty people there, plus a couple of doctors working on a thesis as unpaid volunteers. We each had our special responsibility. M.Sc. (Pharm.) Valdemar Larsen worked as a pharmacologist, M.Sc. (Pharm) Jens Hald and Ph.D. Inger Gad took care of analysis and control, Jorgen Tind Christensen was a fine synthesist etc. It was a small family where you could have no secrets from each other. We occupied the third and fourth floor of building 14 and a quarter of the third floor of building 13 and because of the small quarters communication was very easy. Dr. Larsen's pharmacological laboratory was situated just above Dr. Hald's and if we were in a hurry for the analysis of a blood sample, Larsen would simply knock in the floor with a stick brought for that purpose.

In these surroundings Hald, on an early March day came into my office. He had with him six tablets and as agreed I ate the tablets. That day was the turning point, though on the face of it nothing happened.

It all began as far back as the International Conference of Physiology in Russia in 1935. I had the opportunity to hear Szent Gyorgyi, Nobel prize winner for his discovery of ascorbic acid, give a lecture on cell metabolism. This was not a part of the biochemistry syllabus for doctors and pharmacists at the time but it was an important and very

---

*This, previously unpublished, historical account of the discovery of the therapeutic properties of disulfiram was written by one of the co-discoverers, since deceased.

347

interesting subject and so I wrote a small book about it. 'Cellernes Anding' (The Mechanism of Cell Respiration) aroused flattering interest among specialists, so much even, that I was later asked to direct a seminar for about twenty young researchers, some of whom would later hold high academic positions. As in other seminars each participant had to prepare a talk on a particular aspect for later discussion. Hald, who had worked on the metabolism of amphetamine (Medicinalco's Mecodrin) and similar substances was naturally included in the seminar, and was to speak on the importance of copper in the metabolism and of how it is vital to lower animals.

At the time the war and hence the isolation of Denmark was in its fifth year and there were shortages of a number of things. Soap was lacking and that of course affected the general standard of hygiene which again meant that scabies now appeared even in good families. An ointment for scabies might be a profitable idea. A Swedish ointment, containing a sulphur compound called disulfiram, was available and might also do for the Danish market.

Even in those days products were not marketed without careful safety studies. Hald and Gad found that disulfiram would bind copper very effectively and this fact inspired Hald to expand the indication for disulfiram to be used also against other parasites. Copper is also necessary in the metabolism of intestinal worms; in addition disulfiram is very sparingly soluble, making intestinal absorption limited. All in all it seemed an ideal remedy for worms. We found a couple of laboratory rabbits that excreted worms' eggs, fed them doses of disulfiram and discovered that the eggs disappeared. Encouraged by this result we decided to launch the product as an anthelminthic.

Of course it would have been irresponsible to launch it without further biological studies so we proceeded to give rats and rabbits large doses which were tolerated well. To be on the safe side we decided to test the substance on ourselves as well. We took several doses and felt none the worse even after several days treatment. We then provided a hospital department with some tablets, but to our disappointment they found no anthelminthic effect on their patients and the brilliant idea would have been shelved along with all the other disappointments so common in our business. If not for ...

Four sandwiches washed down with a beer was what I usually had for lunch. The others stuck to milk or water. One day I suddenly felt sick after lunch. I was blushing and had slight palpitations and nausea. The symptoms soon disappeared but came back after lunch next day. It could be allergy to something in my food but a few days later I was really taken back. On 21 March I was visiting some friends who offered me fruitwine. I had a few glasses, an amount that would not usually bother me, and became really sick. A few months earlier I had published a small book 'Omgang mod Alkohol' (How to Enjoy Alcohol), meant to teach people how to deal sensibly with alcohol. The book was humoristic and not too popular with abstainers. Now I got my just deserts. Now I could not hold alcohol myself. I told Hald the story, more as a joke, but he had experienced the same problems; a friend had visited him with a rare expensive bottle. We looked at each other and realized: 'the pills'.

In order to make sure we persuaded a third person from the laboratory to take some of the tablets, promising him a beer for lunch the next day as a reward. He too became sick and now it was clear. Disulfiram somehow reacted with even small amounts of alcohol in the body. Naturally, the idea of trying the substance in the treatment of alcoholics immediately suggested itself. But during my years of studying and through the work on the book on alcohol I had learned that there were only a few alcoholics in Denmark. After the price of alcoholic beverages had been raised drastically in 1917 the number of alcoholics had fallen to almost none. Denmark obviously would not be big market for such a product.

Nevertheless, we were intrigued by the strange effect of disulfiram and continued research. As it could not be tested on animals, we used ourselves as guinea pigs. We did not get much further though. We found that even less than 1/4 permille alcohol in the blood gave a reaction and that the reaction would disappear when the alcohol had been broken down. Seemingly the same effect could also be produced by other substances such as the fertilizer calcium cyanamide or the mushroom ink cap, but still we had not an explanation.

In the autumn of 1947 came the breakthrough. The student association asked me to give a lecture on alcohol; owing to my book I was considered an expert in the field. The lecture turned out to be one of those big Saturday nights, a full house, the press and everything. In order to make clear to the young people that alcohol was not always pleasant I started speaking about the 'aversion cure'. The idea was to put an emetic in the drink and when the patient had tried this a sufficient number of times he would throw up at the mere sight of a drink. The papers brought the story the next day and the letters started coming, 'Doctor, please let me try this cure, it is my last chance' or something to that effect. It seemed that there were after all alcoholics in Denmark; and they were very much in need of help. We certainly did not want to neglect them but we lacked the experience and the place for the treatment.

Some way or other we came in contact with Dr. Martensen-Larsen, probably the only doctor in Denmark specialized in the treatment of alcoholics. He had actually used the aversion cure but had given it up as non-effective. In the course of our talks I told him about the tablets. 'The only thing we know for sure is that it has not killed neither us or our rabbits' – 'Let me have them, I guess it does not make much difference which kills my patients, the alcohol or the pills', he answered.

We heard nothing from him for a couple of months but after the New Year he called and told us that because of the tablets ten of his patients had managed to keep from drinking during the holidays – and that had not happened for years – so he wanted more tablets, he had even taken on more patients. Apparently, Denmark had more alcoholics than we had imagined.

Now we really had to work on disulfiram. Showing an effect was not enough, if we did not know more about what caused the reaction we might seriously endanger the patients. Our first idea was allergy provoked by disulfiram in connection with alcohol. This was supported by the fact that injection of histamine, a substance released from the cells in allergy, produced symptoms similar to our reaction. We could not determine an increase in the histamine level in the blood during a reaction but we still saw allergy as the most likely cause.

Hald rightly objected that it was hardly probable that as little or less than 1/4 permille could have an effect on body cells; an intestinal reaction was more likely since the concentration of alcohol in the intestine would be at least 10 times higher. If that was true, then alcohol given direct into the blood stream should produce no reaction. The question had to be settled and it was my turn to play the guinea pig. I took the tablet a day before and Larsen rigged up a syringe by which he, with the aid of a crank, could infuse a saline solution with an alcohol concentration corresponding to that of a normal beer over half an hour. It worked marvellously. At first I became a little drunk, then so ill that I had to get a car home to bed. The answer was plain to see, but even more exciting results would come of our experiments.

In the middle of the test Hald came into the room to look. He told us that the room reeked of acetaldehyde. Being in the room we had not noticed the smell as it gradually appeared but here was the key to understanding.

We knew that alcohol metabolises step by step in the body. The first step is acetaldehyde which under normal circumstances is broken down so quickly that it does not accumulate. However this seemed to happen with disulfiram. Another experiment confirmed it. After consuming disulfiram and four cl of gin we led the expired air through a solution which would absorb acetaldehyde and allow a chemical determination. Four cl of gin without disulfiram produced nothing but gin whereas disulfiram gave a result and an accumulation of acetaldehyde was also found in blood. We proved it on ourselves and on rabbits – and now we could use rabbits instead of submitting ourselves to the rather unpleasant experiments.

However, this did not solve all the questions. Was the reaction caused by acetaldehyde or by something else? We had to carry out more detailed pharmacological investigations and managed to get the assistance of the kind and interested Professor Erling Asmussen of the Institute of Theoretical Gymnastics at the University. He was examining the heart and lung function of athletes, exactly what we needed. Two students volunteered and we went there with our equipment. We found that if we injected acetaldehyde in an amount similar to that which disulfiram and alcohol would produce, the volunteer would get the typical symptoms: blushing, higher pulse rate and heavier breathing. Histamine did not have quite the same effect. The guilty party had been found.

We were later told that also in test tubes disulfiram would inhibit the catabolism of acetaldehyde in liver cells. This was established in the University's Coll Physiological Institute by Professor N.O. Kjeldgaard who was inspired by our investigations. Popularly speaking disulfiram causes alcohol to 'browse' in the body during the down-breaking so that the bad acetaldehyde accumulates in the body.

In the meantime Dr. Martensen-Larsen had continued his work and by now had more than a hundred patients, all recruited by ear-to-mouth method. Large quantities of disulfiram was now required to meet the demand and synthesis was given over to the factory.

Once they were unlucky. The preparation came out black and stayed black despite a number of re-crystallizations. The laboratory was asked for help. Dr. Gad who had done a lot of work on analyses of copper knew that a coloured compound might be cleared with carbon tetrachloride. The copper came from a brass tap on the vat the factory had used. We re-crystallized with carbon tetrachloride and quite unexpectedly were rewarded with beautifully snow white crystals which after drying became a fine powder consisting of virtually single molecules. The powder was used in the production of tablets and shortly afterwards Dr. Martensen-Larsen phoned to ask what we had done, the tablets were suddenly twice as strong as before.

Seemingly the absorption in the intestine was faster and better with the very fine powder. The 'accident' in combination with the experience of our laboratory had given us a product with a much more certain effect than that of the many copies which were soon on the market – and what was more, the method could be patented. A name had to be found. We decided on ANTABUS, a contracted form of the greek word anti = against and the latin abusus = abuse. As it happened the preparation came to be known under that name all over the world.

What later happened is a story in itself. We made one of the first announcements at the Physiology Congress in Oslo in 1948 and through the Swedish newspapers the story spread to the international press, attracting quite a lot of attention. We received congratulations from Canada and India, a telegram which offered us 1 million dollars for the 'invention' and countless letters of 'please, send enough for a cure' with enclosed dollar bills (which we of course returned). An official delegation came from Sweden and a private delegation from France. However, most important was that the Danish pharmacist Kaj Rothmar, at the time president of the Canadian-American company Ayerst, secured his company Antabuse for America. They treated the matter splendidly, and we owe to them that the whole thing did not drown in inappropriate sensation. Neither could we complain that it was silenced to death. One reason for the ready acceptance of Antabuse was that through our experiments we had shown that Antabuse in itself, even together with alcohol, is not toxic, but it was a substance which changed the effect of alcohol by changing the body's metabolism of alcohol.

In Denmark Martensen-Larsen had not only established clinical use but also shown how side-effects could be avoided. Even Hald and I took on patients so as to see treatment in practice. We found rather quickly that Antabuse is not a cure by itself, however it will prevent patients from impulsive drinking. But leading a happy life without alcohol is not easy as all that, and cannot be managed on Antabuse alone. Patients need help also from their doctors, social workers, psychologists, their own families, or even from former patients who themselves have overcome their alcoholism.

Antabuse never became a very profitable business. Sales in Denmark are reasonable but hardly enormous. Export and licences still pay some but this had decreased after the expiry of the patents. On the other hand Antabuse did start something which otherwise would have taken many years. Patients who formerly had been invisible simply because there was no help to get now came forward. A public commission, giving recognition to alcoholism as a disease, was established and state funded clinics where all treatment is free were opened – there are now 54 of them in Denmark. And this is something after all, as Hans Christian Andersen says.

References and further reading

References are listed alphabetically by first author, then chronologically by year. For any one first author and year, two-author references follow single-author ones and precede those with more than two authors.

Aarnio, M. and Koivula, T. (1986) Aldehyde dehydrogenase of rat stomach and intestinal mucosa. *Prog. Clin. Biol. Res.*, **232**, 103–9.

Aaseth, J., Søli, N.E. and Førre, O. (1979) Increased brain uptake of copper and zinc in mice caused by diethyldithiocarbamate. *Acta Pharmacol. Toxicol.*, **45**, 41–4.

Aaseth, J., Alexander, J. and Wannag, A. (1981) Effect of thiocarbamate derivatives on copper, zinc, and mercury distribution in rats and mice. *Arch. Toxicol.*, **48**, 29–39.

Adachi, J., Mizoi, Y., Fukunaga, T., Ogawa, Y. and Imamichi, H. (1990) Comparative study on ethanol elimination and blood acetaldehyde between alcoholics and control subjects. *Alcohol. Clin. Exp. Res.*, **13**, 601–4.

Adachi, T. and Marklund, S.L. (1989) Interactions between human extracellular superoxide dismutase C and sulfated polysaccharides. *J. Biol. Chem.*, **264**, 8537–41.

Agarwal, D.P. and Goedde, H.W. (1986) Pharmacogenetics and ecogenetics. *Experientia*, **42**, 1148–54.

Agarwal, D.P. and Goedde, H.W. (1987) Human aldehyde dehydrogenase isozymes and alcohol sensitivity. *Isozymes*, **16**, 21–48.

Agarwal, D.P. and Goedde, H.W. (1989) Human aldehyde dehydrogenases: Their role in alcoholism. *Alcohol*, **6**, 517–23.

Agarwal, D.P., Cohn, P., Goedde, W.H. and Hempel, J. (1989) Aldehyde dehydrogenase from human erythrocytes: Structural relationship to the liver cytosolic isozyme. *Enzyme*, **42**, 47–52.

Agarwal, R.P., McPherson, R.A. and Phillips, M. (1983) Rapid degradation of disulfiram by serum albumin. *Res. Commun. Chem. Pathol. Pharmacol.*, **42**, 293–310.

Agarwal, R.P., Phillips, M., McPherson, R.A. and Hensley, P. (1986) Serum albumin and the metabolism of disulfiram. *Biochem. Pharmacol.*, **235**, 3341–47.

Akabane, J.S. Nakanishi, H., Kohei, R., Matsumara, R. and Ogata, H. (1964) Studies on sympathomimetic action of acetaldehyde. I. Experiments with blood pressure and nictitating membrane response. *Jap. J. Pharmacol.*, **14**, 295–307.

Akerboom, T.P.M. and Sies, H. (1981) Assay of glutathione, glutathione disulfide, and glutathione mixed disulfides in biological samples. *Methods Enzymol.*, **77**, 373–82.

Åkerström, S. (1956) The cuprous salts of *N,N*-disubstituted dithiocarbamic acids and their degree of polymerization. *Acta Chem. Scand.*, **10**, 699–701.

Alderman, J.L., Culver, B.W. and Shellenberger, M.K. (1974) An examination of the role of γ-aminobutyric acid (GABA) in hyperbaric oxygen-induced convulsions in the rat. I. Effects of increased γ-aminobutyric acid and protective agents. *J. Pharmacol. Exp. Ther.*, 190, 334–40.

Alexander, P., Bacq, Z.M., Cousens, S.F., Fox, M., Herve, A. and Lazar, J. (1955) Mode of action of some substances which protect against the lethal effects of X-rays. *Radiat. Res.*, 2, 392–415.

Allain, P. and Krari, N. (1991) Diethyldithiocarbamate, copper and neurological disorders. *Life Sci.*, 48, 291–9.

Allalunis-Turner, M.J. and Chapman, J.D. (1984) Evaluation of diethyldithiocarbamate as a radioprotector of bone marrow. *Int. J. Radiat. Oncol. Biol. Phys.*, 10, 1569–73.

Allerberg, F., Roberts, G., Reisinger, E. and Dierich, M.P. (1991) Spectrum of *in vitro* antifungal activity of ditiocarb sodium. *Arzneimittleforschung*, 41, 443–8.

Altura, B.M., Carella, A. and Altura, B.T. (1978) Acetaldehyde on vascular smooth-muscle: possible role in vasodilator action of ethanol. *Europ. J. Pharmacol.*, 52, 73–83.

Amaral, D., Kelly-Falcoz, F. and Horecker, B.L. (1966) Galactose oxidase of *Polyporus circinatus. Methods Enzym.*, 9, 87–92.

Andersen, M.P. (1991) Comparison of the bioavailability of disulfiram given as effervescent tablets and tablets. *Alcohol Alcohol.* 26, 233.

Andersen, O. (1984) Chelation of cadmium. *Envir. Health Persp.*, 54, 249–66.

Andersen, O., Nielsen, J.B. and Svendsen, P. (1988) Oral cadmium chloride intoxication in mice: diethyldithiocarbamate enhances rather than alleviates acute toxicity. *Toxicology*, 52, 331–42.

Andersen, O. and Nielsen, J.B. (1989) Effects of diethyldithiocarbamate on the toxicokinetics of cadmium chloride in mice. *Toxicology*, 55, 1–14.

Andersen, O., Nielsen, J.B. and Jones, M.M. (1989) Effects of dithiocarbamates on intestinal absorption and organ distribution of cadmium chloride in mice. *Pharmacol. Toxicol.*, 64, 239–43.

Andersson, S. and Bostrøm, H. (1984) Effect of disulfiram on rat liver cholesterol 7α-hydrolase. *Biochem. Pharmacol.*, 33, 2930–32.

Ansbacher, L.E., Bosch, E.P. and Cancilla, P.A. (1982) Disulfiram neuropathy: a neurofilamentous distal axonopathy. *Neurology*, 32, 424–28.

Anzil, A.P and Dožić, S. (1978) Disulfiram neuropathy: An experimental study in the rat. *J. Neuropathol. Exp. Neurol.*, 37, 585.

Anzil, A.P. (1980) Selected aspects of experimental disulfiram neuromyopathy. In *Advances in Neurotoxicology* (ed. L. Manzo), Pergamon Press, Oxford, pp.359–66.

Anzil, A.P. (1985) Morphological assessment of neurotoxicity: Disulfiram neuropathy as an animal model of human toxic axonopathies. In *Neurotoxicology* (eds K. Blum and L. Manzo), Marcel Dekker, New York, pp.535–58.

Armor, D.J., Polich, J.M. and Stambul, H.B. (1976a) Alcoholism and Treatment. Rand Corporation, Santa Monica, USA, p. 70.

Armor, D.J., Polich, J.M. and Stambul, H.B. (1976b) Alcoholism and Treatment. Rand Corporation, Santa Monica, USA, pp. 120–1.

Armstrong, J.D. (1957) The protective drugs in the treatment of alcoholism. *Can. Med. Assoc. J.*, 77, 228–32.

Arthur, J.R., Morrice, P.C., Nicol, F., Beddows, S.E., Boyd, R., Hayes, J.D. and Beckett, G.J. (1987) The effects of selenium and copper deficiencies on glutathione *S*-transferase and glutathione peroxidase in rat liver. *Biochem. J.*, 248, 539–44.

Asmussen, E., Hald, J., Jacobsen, E. and Jorgensen, G. (1948a) Studies on the effect of tetraethylthiuramdisulphide (Antabuse) and alcohol on respiration and circulation in normal human subjects. *Acta Pharmacol.*, 4, 297–304.

Asmussen, E., Hald, J. and Larsen, V. (1948b) The pharmacological action of acetaldehyde on the human organism. *Acta Pharmacol.*, **4**, 311–20.

Aspila, K.I., Chakrabarti, C.L. and Sastri, V.S. (1975) Studies on solvent extraction of some substituted dithiocarbamic acids. *Anal. Chem.*, **47**, 945–6.

Azrin, N.H. (1976) Improvements in the community-reinforcement approach to alcoholism. *Behav. Res. Ther.*, **14**, 339–48.

Azrin, N.H., Sisson, R.W., Meyers, R. and Godley, M. (1982) Alcoholism treatment by disulfiram and community reinforcement therapy. *J. Behav. Ther. Exp. Psychiatry*, **13**, 105–12.

Bach, J.F., Dardenne, M., Pleau, J.M. and Rosa, J. (1977) Biochemical characterization of a serum thymic factor. *Nature*, **266**, 55.

Bacq, Z.M. and Herve, A. (1953) Action radioprotectrice des bloqueurs de cuivre (agents de chelation). *Arch. Int. Physiol.*, **61**, 433–4.

Baekeland, F., Lundwann, K.L. and Kissin, B. (1975) Methods for the treatment of chronic alcoholism: A critical appraisal. In *Research Advances in Alcohol and Drug Problems*, Vol. 2 (eds R.J. Gibbins, Y. Israel, H. Kalant *et al.*), John Wiley, New York, pp. 247–327.

Baekeland, F. and Lundwann, K.L. (1977) Engaging the alcoholic in treatment and keeping him there. In *The Biology of Alcoholism*, Vol. 5. *Treatment and Rehabilitation of the Chronic Alcoholic* (eds B. Kissin and H. Begleiter), Plenum, New York, pp. 161–95.

Bakish, D. and Lapierre, Y.D. (1986) Disulfiram and bipolar affective disorder: a case report. *J. Clin. Psychopharmacol.*, **6**, 178–80.

Bandow, G.T., Afonso, S. and Rowe, G.G. (1977) The acute systemic and coronary hemodynamic effects of acetaldehyde. *Arch. Int. Pharmacodyn. Ther.*, **230**, 120–30.

Bannister, J.V. and Calabrese, L. (1987) Assays for superoxide dismutase. *Methods Biochem. Anal.*, **32**, 279–312.

Bannister, J.V., Bannister, W.H. and Rotilio, G. (1987) Aspects of the structure, function, and applications of superoxide dismutase. *CRC Crit. Rev. Biochem.*, **22**, 111–80.

Bannister, S.J., Sternson, L.A. and Repta, A.J. (1979) Urine analysis of platinum species derived from *cis*-dichlorodiammineplatinum(II) by high-performance liquid chromatography following derivatization with sodium diethyldithiocarbamate. *J. Chromatogr.*, **173**, 333–342.

Bardos, P., Degenne, D., Lebranchu, Y., Biziere, K. and Renoux, G. (1981) Neocortical lateralization of NK activity in mice. *Scand. J. Immunol.*, **13**, 609–11.

Bardos, P., Degenne, D., Florentin, I., Guillaumin, J.M. and Renoux, M. (1985) Modulation of NK activity by Imuthiol®. *Int. J. Immunopharmacol.*, **7**, 335, 1985.

Bardsley, W.G., Crabbe, J.C. and Scott, I.V. (1974) The amine oxidases of human placenta and pregnancy plasma. *Biochem. J.*, **139**, 169–81.

Barneoud, P., Neveu, P.J., Vitiello, S. and Le Moal, M. (1987) Functional heterogeneity of the right and left cerebral neocortex in the modulation of the immune system. *Physiol. Behav.*, **41**, 525–30.

Barth, R., Resnick, R.H. and Smoller, B. (1987) Disulfiram and fulminant hepatitis. *Dig. Dis. Sci.*, **32**, 1059.

Bartkowiak, A., Grzelinska, E. and Bartosz, G. (1983) Aging of the erythrocyte. XVII. Changes in the properties of superoxide dismutase. *Int. J. Biochem.*, **5**, 763–5.

Bartle, W.R., Fisher, M.M. and Kerenyi, N. (1985) Disulfiram-induced hepatitis: Report of two cases and review of the literature. *Dig. Dis. Sci.*, **30**, 834–7.

Baselt, R.C., Sunderman, F.W., Jr, Mitchell, J. and Horak, E. (1977) Comparisons of antidotal efficacy of sodium diethyldithiocarbamate, D-penicillamine upon acute toxicity of nickel carbonyl in rats. *Res. Commun. Chem. Pathol. Pharmacol.*, **18**, 677–88.

Basinger, M.A., Jones, M.M., Gilbreath, S.G., IV, Walker, E.M., Jr., Fody, E.P. and Mayhue, M.A. (1989) Dithiocarbamate-induced biliary excretion and the control of *cis*-platinum nephrotoxicity. *Toxicol. App. Pharmacol.*, **97**, 279–88.

Bass, M. (1963) Thallium poisoning: A preliminary report. *J. Am. Osteopath. Assoc.*, **63**, 229–35.

Beach, C.A., Mays, D.C., Guiler, R.C., Jacober, C.H. and Gerber, N. (1986) Inhibition of elimination of caffeine by disulfiram in normal subjects and recovering alcoholics. *Clin. Pharmacol. Ther.*, **39**, 265–70.

Beauchamp, R.O., Jr, Bus, J.S., Popp, J.A., Boreiko, J.C. and Goldberg, L. (1983) A critical review of the literature on carbon disulfide toxicity. *CRC Crit. Rev. Toxicol.*, **11**, 169–278.

Beck, O., Eriksson, C.J.P., Kiianmaa, K. and Lundman, A. (1986) 5-Hydroxyindole-acetic acid and 5-hydroxytryptophol levels in rat brain: Effects of ethanol, pyrazole, cyanamide and disulfiram treatment. *Drug, Alcohol Dep.*, **16**, 303–8.

Becker, M.C. and Sugarman, G. (1952) Death following 'test drink' of alcohol in patients receiving Antabuse. *J. Am. Med. Assoc.*, **149**, 568–71.

Beedham, C. (1987) Molybdenum hydroxylases: Biological distribution and substrate-inhibitor specificity. *Prog. Med. Chem.*, **24**, 85–127.

Bell, R.G. and Smith, H.W. (1949) Preliminary report on clinical trials of Antabuse. *Can. Med. Assoc. J.*, **60**, 286–8.

Belliveau, J.F., O'Leary, G.P., Jr, Cadwell, L. and Sunderman, F.W., Jr (1985) Effect of diethyldithiocarbamate on nickel concentrations in tissues of NiCl$_2$-treated rats. *Ann. Clin. Lab. Sci.*, **15**, 349–50.

Bennett, A.E., McKeever, L.G. and Turk, R.E. (1951) Psychotic reactions during tetraethylthiuramdisulfide (Antabuse) therapy. *J. Am. Med. Assoc.*, **145**, 483–4.

Benson, A.M. and Barretto, P.M. (1985) Effects of disulfiram, diethyldithiocarbamate, bisethylxanthogen, and benzyl isothiocyanate on glutathione transferase activities in mouse organs. *Cancer Res.*, **45**, 4219–23.

Berger, D. and Weiner, H. (1977) Effects of disulfiram and chloral hydrate on the metabolism of catecholamines in rat liver and brain. *Biochem. Pharmacol.*, **26**, 741–7.

Bergouignan, F.X., Vital, C., Henry, P. and Eschapasse, P. (1988) Disulfiram neuropathy. *J. Neurol.*, **238**, 382–3.

Bergström, B., Öhlin, H., Lindblom, P.E. and Wadstein, J. (1982) Is disulfiram implantation effective? *Lancet*, **i**, 49–50.

Berlin, R.G. (1989) Disulfiram hepatotoxicity: A consideration of its mechanism and clinical spectrum. *Alcohol Alcohol.*, **24**, 241–6.

Berry, J.M., Jacobs, C., Sikic, B., Halsey, J. and Borch, R.F. (1990) Modification of cisplatin toxicity with diethyldithiocarbamate. *J. Clin. Oncol.*, **8**, 1585–90.

Bertram, B., Frei, E., Scherf, H.R., Schuhmacher, J., Tacchi, A.M. and Wiessler, M. (1985) Influence of a prolonged treatment with disulfiram and D(-)penicillamine on nitrosodiethylamine-induced biological and biochemical effects in rats. *J. Cancer Res. Clin. Oncol.*, **109**, 9–15.

Bertram, B. (1988) The modifying effect of disulfiram on the carcinogenicity of some *N*-nitrosamines: Mechanistic investigations. In *Combined Effects in Chemical Carcinogenesis* (ed. D. Schmahl), Verlagsgesellschaft, Weinheim, pp. 193–229.

Beyeler, C., Fisch, H.-U. and Preisig, R. (1985) The disulfiram-alcohol reaction: factors determining and potential tests predicting severity. *Alcohol. Clin. Exp. Res.*, 9, 118–24.

Beyeler, C., Fisch, H.U. and Preisig, R. (1987) Kardiovaskulare und metabolische Veranderungen wahrend der Antabus-Alkohol-Reaktion: Grundlagen zur Erfassung des Schweregrades. *Schweiz. Med. Wochenschr.*, 117, 52–60.

Bhagat, B., Gray, L. and Dhalla, N.S. (1966) Restoration of the response of the isolated atria of guinea-pigs to tyramine and possible significance of β-hydroxylation. *Nature*, 210, 823–4.

Biaglow, J.E., Issels, R.W., Gerweck, L.E. *et al.* (1984) Factors influencing the oxidation of cysteamine and other thiols: Implications for hyperthermic sensitization and radiation protection. *Radiat. Res.*, 100, 298–312.

Bigelow, G., Strickler, D., Liebson, I. and Griffiths, R. (1976) Maintaining disulfiram ingestion among outpatient alcoholics: a security-deposit contingency contracting procedure. *Behav. Res. Ther.*, 14, 378–81.

Bihari, B., Martin, J. and Seaman, D. (1988) The use of disulfiram as an immunomodulating agent. Fourth International Conference on AIDS, Abstract volume I, Stockholm, p. 230, Abstract 3042.

Bilbao, J.M., Briggs, S.J. and Gray, T.A. (1984) Filamentous axonopathy in disulfiram neuropathy. *Ultrastruct. Pathol.*, 7, 295–300.

Black, J.L. and Richardson, J.W. (1985) Disulfiram hepatotoxicity: Case Report. *J. Clin. Psychiatry*, 46, 67–8.

Black, S.D. and Coon, M.J. (1989) P-450 cytochromes: Structure and function. *Adv. Enzymol.*, 60, 35–87.

Bláha, K., Tichý, M., Cikrt, M., Havrdová, J. and Horáková, L. (1985) Effect of chelating agents on Cd distribution: QSAR study. *Toxicol. Xenobiochem.*, 1985, 183–93.

Bláha, K., Cikrt, M., Kašparová, L. and Jones, M.M. (1988) Synergistic enhancement of biliary excretion of cadmium by the simultaneous administration of two dithiocarbamates. *Toxicol. Lett.*, 42, 207–13.

Blair, A.H and Bodley, F.H. (1969) Human liver aldehyde dehydrogenase: partial purification and properties. *Can. J. Biochem.*, 47, 265–72.

Blanc, D. and Deprez, P. (1990) Unusual adverse reaction to a acaricide. *Lancet*, 335, 1290–1.

Blaustein, J.D., Brown, T.J. and McElroy, J.F. (1986) Some catecholamine inhibitors do not cause accumulation of nuclear estrogen receptors in rat hypothalamus and anterior pituitary gland. *Neuroendocrinology*, 43, 143–9.

Bliding, A., Dahilof, L.G. and Olsson, A.M. (1981) Antabus ger patienterna impotens skarck – utan anledning. *Acta Soc. Med. Svec. Hyg.*, 90, 278.

Bloom, A.S., Quinton, E.E. and Carr, L.A. (1977) Effects of cycloheximide, diethyldithiocarbamate and D-amphetamine on protein and catecholamine biosynthesis in mouse brain. *Neuropharmacology*, 16, 411–18.

Blum, J. and Fridovich, I. (1983) Superoxide, hydrogen peroxide, and oxygen toxicity in two free-living nematode species. *Arch. Bioch. Biophys.*, 222, 35–43.

Blum, J. and Fridovich, I. (1985) Inactivation of glutathione peroxidase by superoxide radical. *Arch. Bioch. Biophys.*, 240, 500–8.

Bode, H. (1954) Systematische Untersuchungen uber die Anwendbarkeit der Diathyldithiocarbaminate in der Analyse. Die Bestandigkeit des Natrium-Diathyldithiocarbaminates und seine Extrahierbarkeit in Abhangigkeit vom pH-Wert der Losung. *Z. Anal. Chem.*, 142, 414–23.

Bodenner, D.L., Dedon, P.C., Keng, P.C. and Borch, R.F. (1986a) Effect of diethyl-dithiocarbamate on *cis*-diamminedichloroplatinum(II)-induced cytotoxicity, DNA cross-liking, and γ-glutamyl transpeptidase inhibition. *Cancer Res.*, **46**, 2745–50.

Bodenner, D.L. Dedon, P.C., Keng, P.C., Katz, J.C. and Borch, R.F. (1986b) Selective protection against *cis*-diamminedichloroplatinum(II)-induced toxicity in kidney, gut, and bone marrow by diethyldithiocarbamate. *Cancer Res.*, **46**, 2751–55.

Bond, E.J., Butler, W.H., De Matteis, F. and Barnes, J.M. (1969) Effects of carbon disulphide on the liver of rats. *Br. J. Ind. Med.*, **26**, 335–7.

Borch, R.F. and Pleasants, M.E. (1979) Inhibition of *cis*-platinum nephrotoxicity by diethyldithiocarbamate rescue in a rat model. *Proc. Natl. Acad. Sci. USA*, **76**, 6611–4.

Borch, R.F., Katz, J.C., Lieder, P.H. and Pleasants, M.E. (1980) Effect of diethyl-dithiocarbamate rescue on tumor response to *cis*-platinum in a rat model. *Proc. Natl. Acad. Sci. USA*, **77**, 5441–4.

Borch, R.F., Bodenner, D.L. and Katz, J.C. (1983) Diethyldithiocarbamate and *cis*-platinum toxicity. In *Platinum Coordination Complexes in Cancer Chemotherapy* (eds M.P. Hacker, E.B. Douple and I.H. Krakoff), Martinus Nijhoff Publishing, Boston, pp. 154–64.

Borch, R.F. (1986a) Compositions for the inhibition of undesired effects of platinum (II) compounds. Canadian Patent, CA 1,200,490, 11 February 1986 (cf. *Chem. Abstr.*, **105**, 30097r, 1986).

Borch, R.F. (1986b) Inhibition of undesired effects of platinum compounds. US Patent, U.S. 4,581,224, 8 April 1986 (cf. *Chem. Abstr.*, **105**, 35630u).

Borch, R.F., Dedon, P.C., Gringeri, A. and Montine, T.J. (1987) Inhibition of platinum drug toxicity by diethyldithiocarbamate. In *Platinum and Other Metal Coordination Compounds in Cancer Chemotherapy* (ed. M. Nicolini), Martinus Nijhoff Publishing, Boston, pp. 216–27.

Borch, R.F. and Markman, M. (1989) Biochemical modulation of cisplatin toxicity. *Pharmacol. Ther.*, **41**, 371–80.

Borg, S., Halldin, J., Kyhlhorn, E., Mannerfelt, M. and Strandberg, K. (1984) Implantation of disulfiram: Results from a placebo-controlled multicenter study. In *Pharmacological Treatment of Alcoholism: Withdrawal and Aversion Therapy*. Socialstyrelsens Lakemedelsavdelning, 75125 Uppsala, Sweden, 1985/2 pp. 65–88.

Borrett, D., Ashby, P., Bilbao, J. and Carlen, P. (1985) Reversible, late-onset disulfiram-induced neuropathy and encephalopathy. *Ann. Neurol.*, **17**, 396–9.

Bosron, W.F. and Li, T.K. (1986) Genetic polymorphism of human liver alcohol and aldehyde dehydrogenases, and their relationship to alcohol metabolism and alcoholism. *Hepatology*, **6**, 502–10.

Bourne, P.G., Alford, J.A. and Bowcock, J.Z. (1966) Treatment of skid-row alcoholics with disulfiram. *Q. J. Stud. Alcohol*, **27**, 42–8.

Bowman, K.M., Simon, A., Hine, C.H. *et al.* (1951) A clinical evaluation of tetraethylthiuramdisulphide (Antabuse) in the treatment of problem drinkers. *Am. J. Psychiatry*, **107**, 832–8.

Branchey, L., Davis, W., Lee, K.K. and Fuller, R.K. (1987) Psychiatric complications of disulfiram treatment. *Am. J. Psychiatry*, **144**, 1310–2.

Brewer, C. and Smith, J. (1983a) Probation linked supervised disulfiram in the treatment of habitual drunken offenders: results of a pilot study. *Br. Med. J.*, **287**, 1282–3.

Brewer, C. and Smith, J. (1983b) Probation linked disulfiram treatment. *Br. Med. J.*, **287**, 1795.

Brewer, C. (1984) How effective is the standard dose of disulfiram? A review of the alcohol-disulfiram reaction in practice. *Br. J. Psychiatry*, **144**, 200–2.

Brewer, C. (1986) Patterns of compliance and evasion in treatment programmes which include supervised disulfiram. *Alcohol Alcohol.*, **21**, 385–8.

Brewer, C. (1987) Disulfiram treatment of alcoholism. *J. Am. Med. Assoc.*, **257**, 926.

Brewton, G.W., Hersh, E.M., Mansell, P., Rios, A., and Reuben, J. (1987) Use of Imuthiol (diethyldithiocarbamate, DTC) in symptomatic HIV infection. *Third International Conference on AIDS*, Abstract volume, National Institute of Health, Bethesda, MD, p. 98, Abstract TP.218.

Brewton, G.W., Hersh, E.M., Rios, A., Mansell, P.W.A., Hollinger, B and Reuben, J.M. (1989) A pilot study of diethyldithiocarbamate in patients with acquired immune deficiency syndrome (AIDS) and the AIDS-Related Complex. *Life Sci.*, **45**, 2509–20.

Brieger, H. (1947) Toxicity and toxicology of several accelerators used in the rubber industry. *Ind. Med.*, **16**, 473–4.

Brien, J.F. and Loomis, C.W. (1983a) Chemical assays for disulfiram and carbimide (cyanamide) in biological fluids. *Alcohol. Clin. Exp. Res.*, **7**, 256–63.

Brien, J.F. and Loomis, C.W. (1983b) Disposition and pharmacokinetics of disulfiram and calcium carbimide (calcium cyanamide). *Drug Metab. Rev.*, **14**, 113–26.

Brien, J.F. and Loomis, C.W.(1983c) Pharmacology of acetaldehyde. *Can. J. Physiol. Pharmacol.*, **61**, 1–22.

Brien, J.F. and Loomis, C.W. (1985) Aldehyde dehydrogenase inhibitors as alcohol-sensitizing drugs: a pharmacological perspective. *Trends Pharmacol. Sci.*, **6**, 477–80.

Brien, J.F., Tam, G.S., Cameron, R.J., Steenaart, N.A.E. and Loomis, C.W. (1985) A comparative study of the inhibition of hepatic aldehyde dehydrogenases in the rat by methyltetrazolethiol, calcium carbimide, and disulfiram. *Can. J. Physiol. Pharmacol.*, **63**, 438–43.

Brown, C.T. and Knoblock, E.C. (1951) Antabuse therapy in the army: a preliminary report of fifty cases. *U.S. Arm. Forces Med. J.*, **2**, 191–202.

Brown, M.W., Porter, G.S. and Williams, A.E. (1974) The determination of disulfiram in blood, and of exhaled carbon disulphide using cathode ray polarography. *J. Pharm. Pharmacol.*, **26** S, 95P–96P.

Brown, Z.W., Amit, Z., Smith, B.R., Sutherland, E.A. and Selvaggi, N. (1983) Alcohol-induced euphoria enhanced by disulfiram and calcium carbimide. *Alcohol. Clin. Exp. Res.*, **7**, 276–8.

Brubaker, R.G., Prue, D.M. and Rychtarik, R.G. (1987) Determinants of disulfiram acceptance among alcohol patients: a test of the theory of reasoned action. *Addict. Behav.*, **12**, 43–51.

Brugere, S., Saavedra, A. and Penna, M. (1986) Cardiorespiratory inhibitory reflex induced by intravenous administration of acetaldehyde in rats. *Alcohol*, **3**, 317–22.

Bruley-Rosset, M., Vergnon, I. and Renoux, G. (1986) Influences of sodium diethyldithiocarbamate, DTC (Imuthiol)® on T cell defective responses of aged BALB/c mice. *Int. J. Immunopharmac.*, **8**, 287–97.

Burgess, I. (1990) Adverse reactions to monosulfiram. *Lancet*, **336**, 873.

Bus, J.S. (1985) The relationship of carbon disulfide metabolism to development of toxicity. *Neurotoxicology*, **6**, 73–80.

360   References

Buskowicz, C. (1962) Zespól mózgowy u dziecka w nastepstwie ostrego zatrucia Antabusem. *Neurol. Neuroch. Psychiat. Polska,* **12,** 293–5.

Busse, S., Mulloy, C.T. and Weise, C.E. (1978) *Disulfiram in the Treatment of Alcoholism: An Annotated Bibliography.* Addiction Research Foundation, Toronto, 346 pp.

Byczkowski, J.Z. and Gessner, T. (1988) Biological role of superoxide ion-radical. *Int. J. Biochem.,* **20,** 569–80.

Canellakis, E.S. and Tarver, H. (1953) The metabolism of methyl mercaptan in intact animal. *Arch. Bioch. Biophys.,* **42,** 446–55.

Cantilena, L.R., Jr and Klaassen, C.D. (1981) Comparison of the effectiveness of several chelators after single administration of cadmium. *Toxicol. App. Pharmacol.,* **58,** 452–60.

Cantilena, L.R., Jr, Irwin, G., Preskorn, S. and Klaassen, C.D. (1982) The effect of diethyldithiocarbamate on brain uptake of cadmium. *Toxicol. App. Pharmacol.,* **63,** 338–43.

Cao, Q.-N., Tu, G.-C. and Weiner, H. (1989) Presence of cytosolic aldehyde dehydrogenase isozymes in adult and fetal rat liver. *Biochem Pharmacol.,* **38,** 77–83.

Cardwell, M. (1987) Disulfiram treatment of alcoholism. *J. Am. Med. Assoc.,* **257,** 926.

Carey-Smith, K.A., Joll, T.A., Nyoni, V.S. and Irvine, B.L. (1988) Assessment of intramuscular emulsified disulfiram in alcoholics by estimation of urinary diethylamine. *J. Stud. Alcohol,* **49,** 571–5.

Carfagna, P.F., Chaney, S.G., Chang, J and Holbrook, D.J. (1990) Reduction of tetrachoro(*dl-trans*)1,2-diaminocyclohexaneplatinum(IV) (tetraplatin) toxicity by the administration of diethyldithiocarbamate (DDTC), S-2(3-aminopropylamino)ethylphosphorothioic acid (WR-2721), or sodium selenite in the Fisher 344 rat. *Fund. Appl. Toxicol.,* **14,** 706–19.

Carlsson, A., Lindqvist, M., Fuxe, K. and Hökflet, T. (1966) Histochemical and biochemical effects of diethyldithiocarbamate on tissue catecholamines. *J. Pharm. Pharmacol.,* **18,** 60–2.

Carlsson, A., Fuxe, K. and Hökfelt, T. (1967) Failure of dopamine to accumulate in cerebral noradrenaline neurons after depletion with diethyldithiocarbamate. *J. Pharm. Pharmacol.,* **19,** 481–3.

Carmichael, F.J., Israel, Y., Saldivia, V., Giles, H.G., Meggiorini, S. and Orrego, H. (1987) Blood acetaldehyde and the ethanol-induced increase in splanchnic circulation. *Biochem. Pharmacol.,* **36,** 2673–8.

Carmichael, F.J., Saldivia, V., Varghese, G.A., Israel, Y. and Orrego, H. (1988) Ethanol-induced increase in portal blood flow: role of acetate and A_1 and A_2-adenosine receptors. *Am. J. Physiol.,* **255,** G417–G423.

Carper, W.R., Dorey, R.C. and Beber, J.H. (1987) Inhibitory effect of disulfiram (Antabuse) on alcohol dehydrogenase activity. *Clin. Chem.,* **33,** 1906–8.

Carrara, M., Zampiron, S., Cima, L., Sindellari, L., Trincia, L. and Voltarel, G. (1988) Inhibitory properties of tin(IV) diethyldithiocarbamates on tumoral cells growth. *Pharmacol. Res. Commun.,* **20,** 611–12.

Casagrande, G. and Michot, F. (1989) Alcohol-induced bone marrow damage: Status before and after a 4-week period of abstinence from alcohol with and without disulfiram. *Blut,* **59,** 231–6.

Catignani, G.L. and Neal, R.A. (1975) Evidence for the formation of a protein bound hydrodisulfide resulting from the microsomal mixed function oxidase catalyzed desulfuration of carbon disulfide. *Biochem. Biophys. Res. Commun.,* **65,** 629–36.

Cavanagh, J.B. and Barnes, J.M. (1973) Peripheral neuropathy caused by chemical agents. *CRC Crit. Rev. Toxicol.*, **2**, 365–417.

Cederbaum, A.I. and Dicker, E. (1979) The effect of pargyline on the metabolism of ethanol and acetaldehyde by isolated rat liver cells. *Arch. Bioch. Biophys.*, **193**, 551–9.

Cederbaum, A.I. and Dicker, E. (1981) Effect of cyanamide on the metabolism of ethanol and acetaldehyde and on gluconeogenesis by isolated rat hepatocytes. *Biochem. Pharmacol.*, **30**, 3079–88.

Centers for Disease Control (1986) Classification system for human T-lymphotropic virus type III/lymphoadenopathy-associated virus infections. *Morb. Mort. Week. Rep.*, **35**, 334–9.

Cerutti, I. and Chany, C. (1983) Coordinated therapeutic effects of immune modulators and interferon. *Infect. Immun.*, **42**, 728–32.

Cha, Y.-N., Heine, H.S. and Moldéus, P. (1982) Differential effects of dietary and intraperitoneal administration of antioxidants on the activities of several hepatic enzymes of mice. *Drug Metab. Dispos.*, **10**, 434–5.

Cha, Y-N., Heine, H.S. and Ansher, S. (1983) Comparative effects of dietary administration of antioxidants and inducers on the activities of several hepatic enzymes in mice. *Drug-Nutr. Interact.*, **2**, 35–45.

Chabal, J., Boulez, J., Clement, G. and Defayolle, M. (1987) Reduction du cout de l'hospitalisation en chirurgie digestive apres traitement par immuno-stimulant. *Press Med.*, **16**, 1244.

Champault, G., Biron, G., Bouthelier, P. and Defayolle, M. (1983) L'immuno-stimulation en chirurgie viscerale. *Med. Chir. Dig.*, **12**, 537–43.

Chengelis, C.P. and Neal, R.A. (1979) Hepatic carbonyl sulfide metabolism. *Biochem. Biophy. Res. Commun.*, **90**, 993–9.

Chevens, L.C.F. (1953) Antabuse addiction. *Br. Med. J.*, **1**, 1450–1.

Child, G.P., Barbera, E., Osinski, W., Russ, Z. and Hemsted, G. (1950) Studies on pharmacology of tetraethylthiuramdisulfide (Antabuse) and the 'Antabuse-alcohol' syndrome in animals and man. *Fed. Proc.*, **9**, 22.

Child, G.P., Osinski, W., Bennett, R.E. and Davidoff, E. (1951) Therapeutic results and clinical manifestations following the use of tetraethylthiuram disulfide (Antabuse). *Am. J. Psychiatry*, **107**, 774–80.

Child, G.P. and Crump, M. (1952) The toxicity of tetraethylthiuram disulphide (Antabuse) to mouse, rat, rabbit and dog. *Acta Pharmacol. Toxicol.*, **8**, 305–14.

Child, G.P., Crump, M. and Leonard, P. (1952) Studies of the disulfiram-ethanol reaction. *Q. J. Stud. Alcohol*, **13**, 571–82.

Choo, L.Y. and Riendeau, D. (1987) Disulfiram is a potent inhibitor of rat 5-lipooxygenase activity. *Can. J. Physiol. Pharmacol.*, **65**, 2503–6.

Christensen, J.K. (1973) Bivirninger efter disulfiram. *Ugeskr. Laeger*, **135**, 1457–9.

Christensen, J.K., Rønsted, P. and Vaag, U.H. (1984) Side effects after disulfiram. *Acta Psychiatr. Scand.*, **69**, 265–73.

Christensen, J.K., Moller, I.W., Rønsted, P., Angelo, H.R and Johansson, B. (1991) Dose-effect relationship of disulfiram in human volunteers. I. Clinical Studies. *Pharmacol. Toxicol.*, **68**, 163–5.

Christensen, O.B. and Kristensen, M. (1982) Treatment with disulfiram in chronic nickel dermatitis. *Contact Dermatitis*, **8**, 59–63.

Chung, V., Florentin, I. and Renoux, G. (1985) Effect of Imuthiol administration to normal or immunodeficient mice on IL1 and IL2 production and immune responses regulated by these mediators. *J. Immunopharmacol.*, **7**, 335.

Ciarulo, D.A., Barnhill, J. and Boxenbaum, H. (1985) Pharmacokinetic interaction of disulfiram and antidepressants. *Am. J. Psychiatry*, **142**, 1373–4.

Cikrt, M., Lepši, P., Bitterová, D. and Jones, M.M. (1984) The effect of sodium diethanolamine dithiocarbamate on distribution and excretion of Cd in rats drinking Cd-containing water. *Res. Commun. Chem. Path. Pharmacol.*, **43**, 497–505.

Cikrt, M., Lepši, P., Horáková, L, Bláha, K., Bitterová, D. and Jones, M.M. (1986a) Effects of dithiocarbamates on cadmium distribution and excretion in chronically exposed rats. *J. Toxicol. Environ. Health*, **17**, 419–27.

Cikrt, M., Basinger, M.A., Jones, S.G. and Jones, M.M. (1986b) Structural effects in the dithiocarbamate-enhanced biliary excretion of cadmium. *J. Toxicol. Environ. Health*, **17**, 429–39.

Cobby, J., Mayersohn, M. and Selliah, S. (1977a) Methyl diethyldithiocarbamate, a metabolite of disulfiram in man. *Life Sci.*, **21**, 937–42.

Cobby, J., Mayersohn, M. and Selliah, S. (1977b) The rapid reduction of disulfiram in blood and plasma. *J. Pharmacol. Exp. Ther.*, **202**, 724–31.

Cobby, J., Mayersohn, M. and Selliah, S. (1978) Disposition kinetics in dogs of diethyldithiocarbamate, a metabolite of disulfiram. *J. Pharmacokinet. Biopharm.*, **6**, 369–87.

Cocco, D., Calabrese, L., Rigo, A., Argese, E. and Rotilio, G. (1981a) Re-examination of the reaction of diethyldithiocarbamate with the copper of superoxide dismutase. *J. Biol. Chem.*, **256**, 8983–6.

Cocco, D., Calabrese, L., Rigo, A., Marmocchi, F. and Rotilio, G. (1981b) Preparation of selectively metal-free and metal-substituted derivatives by reaction of Cu-Zn superoxide dismutase with diethyldithiocarbamate. *Biochem. J.*, **199**, 675–80.

Cochran, A.J., Splig, W.G.S., Mackie, R.M. and Thomas, C.E. (1972) Postoperative depression of tumour-directed cell-mediated immunity in patients with malignant disease. *Br. Med. J.*, **4**, 67–70.

Collins, G.G.S. (1965) Inhibition of dopamine-β-hydroxylase by diethyldithiocarbamate. *J. Pharm. Pharmacol.*, **17**, 526–7.

Committee on Medical and Biologic effects of Environmental Pollution, National Research Council (1975) *Nickel*. National Academy of Sciences, Washington, D.C., pp. 106–28.

Conkling, P., Papermaster-Bender, G., Whitcomb, M. and Sagone, A.L. (1982) Oxygen dependence of human alveolar macrophage-mediated antibody-dependent cytotoxicity. *Infec. Immun.*, **38**, 114–21.

Conkling, P., Cornwell, D.G. and Sagone, A.L., Jr (1985) Effect of diethyldithiocarbamate (DDC) on human monocyte function and metabolism. *Inflammation*, **9**, 149–61.

Coogan, T.P., Stump, D.G., Barsotti, D.A. and Rosenblum, I.Y. (1986) Superoxide dismutase modification and genotoxicity of transition-metal chelators. *Adv. Exp. Med. Biol.*, **197**, 284–90.

Cooper, A.J.L. (1983) Biochemistry of sulfur-containing amino acids. *Annu. Rev. Biochem.*, **52**, 187–222.

Corke, C.F. (1984) The influence of diethyl-dithiocarbamate ('Imuthiol') on mononuclear cells *in vitro*. *Int. J. Immunopharmacol.*, **6**, 245–7.

Corke, C.F., Sedgwick, A.D., MacKay, A.R., Bates, M.B. and Willoughby, D.A. (1984) Enhancement of colloidal clearance in normal rats by sodium diethyl dithiocarbamate (DTC). *Int. J. Immunopharmacol.*, **6**, 535–7, 1984.

Corke, C.F., Gul, V., Huckisson, H.C., Holborow, E.J. and Renoux, G. (1986) Imuthiol (sodium diethyldithiocarbamate) and rheumatoid arthritis. *Int. J. Immunotherap.*, **2**, 163–9.

Council on Pharmacy and Chemistry (1952) Antabuse (disulfiram) in the treatment of alcoholism. *J. Am. Med. Assoc.*, **149**, 275–77.

Cox, P.J., Phillips, B.J. and Thomas, P. (1976) Studies on the selective action of cyclophosphamide (NSC-26271) inactivation of the hydroxylated metabolite by tissue-soluble enzymes. *Cancer Treat. Rep.*, **60**, 321–26.

Crabtree, G.R. (1989) Contingent genetic regulatory events in T lymphocyte activation. *Science*, **243**, 355–61.

Cramer, J.A., Mattson, R.H., Prevey, M.L., Scheyer, R.D. and Ouellette, V.L. (1989) How often is medication taken as prescribed? A novel assessment technique. *J. Am. Med. Assoc.*, **261**, 3273–7.

Cronholm, T. (1985) Hydrogen transfer between ethanol molecules during oxidoreduction *in vivo*. *Biochem. J.*, **229**, 315–22.

Crow, K.E., Kitson, T.M., MacGivvon, K.H. and Batt, R.D. (1974) Intracellular localisation and properties of aldehyde dehydrogenases from sheep liver. *Bioch. Biophys. Acta*, **350**, 121–8.

Crow, K.E., Cornell, N.W. and Veech, R.L. (1977) The rate of ethanol metabolism in isolated rat hepatocytes. *Alcohol. Clin. Exp. Res.*, **1**, 43–7.

Currie, W.D., Gelein, R.M., Sanders, A.P. (1973) Comparison of protective agents against hyperbaric oxygen in large animals. *Aerosp. Med.*, **44**, 996–8.

Dalvi, R.R., Poore, R.E. and Neal, R.A. (1974) Studies of the metabolism of carbon disulfide by rat liver microsomes. *Life Sci.*, **14**, 1785–96.

Dalvi, R.R., Hunter, A.L. and Neal, R.A. (1975) Toxicological implications of the mixed-function oxidase catalyzed metabolism of carbon disulfide. *Chem. Biol. Interact.*, **10**, 347–61.

Danielsson, B.R.G. (1984) Placental transfer and fetal distribution of cadmium and mercury after treatment with dithiocarbamates. *Arch. Toxicol.*, **55**, 161–7.

Danielsson, B.R.G., Oskarsson, A. and Dencker, L. (1984) Placental transfer and fetal distribution of lead in mice after treatment with dithiocarbamates. *Arch. Toxicol.*, **55**, 27–33.

Danscher, G., Haug, F-M.Š. and Fredens, K. (1973) Effect of diethyldithiocarbamate (DEDTC) on sulphide silver stained boutons: reversible blocking of Timm's sulphide silver stain for 'Heavy' metals in DEDTC treated rats (light microscopy). *Exp. Brain Res.*, **16**, 521–32.

Danscher, G., Shipley, M.T. and Andersen, P. (1975) Persistent function of mossy fibre synapses after metal chelation with DEDTC (Antabuse). *Brain Res.*, **85**, 522–6.

Davidson, W.J. and Wilson, A. (1979) Determination of nanogram quantities of disulfiram in human and rat plasma by gas-liquid chromatography. *J. Stud. Alcohol*, **40**, 1073–7.

Dawson, A.G. (1981) Inhibitory effect of acetaldehyde on the oxidation of ethanol by a high-speed supernatant fraction of rat liver. *Biochem. Pharmacol.*, **30**, 2349–52.

Dawson, A.G. (1983) Ethanol oxidation in systems containing soluble and mitochondrial fractions of rat liver: Regulation by acetaldehyde. *Biochem. Pharmacol.*, **32**, 2157–65.

de Bruine, J.F., van Royen, E.A., Vyth, A., de Jong, J.M.B.V. and van der Schoot, J.B. (1985) Thallium-201 diethyldithiocarbamate: An alternative to iodine-123 *N*-isopropyl-*p*-iodoamphetamine. *J. Nucl. Med.*, **26**, 925–30.

de Bruïne, J.F. (1988) *Brain SPECT with Tl-201 DDC*. Amsterdam, Radopi, 147 pp.

de Bruïne, J.F., Limburg, M., van Royen, E.A., Hijdra, A., Hill, T.C. and van der Schoot, J.B. (1990) SPET brain imaging with 201 diethyldithiocarbamate in acute ischaemic stroke. *Europ. J. Nucl. Med.*, **17**, 248–51.

Dedon, P.C. and Borch, R.F. (1987) Characterization of the reactions of platinum antitumor agents with biologic and non-biologic sulfur-containing nucleophiles. *Biochem. Pharmacol.*, **36**, 1955–64.

DeGregorio, M.W., Gandara, D.R., Holleran, W.M., Perez, E.A., King, C.C., Wold, H.G., Montine, T.J. and Borch, R.F. (1989) High-dose cisplatin with diethyldithiocarbamate (DDTC) rescue therapy: preliminary pharmacologic observations. *Canc. Chemother. Pharmacol.*, **23**, 276–8.

Deitrich, R.A. (1966) Tissue and subcellular distribution of mammalian aldehyde-oxidizing capacity. *Bioch. Pharmacol.*, **15**, 1911–22.

Deitrich, R.A. and Erwin, V.G. (1971) Mechanism of the inhibition of aldehyde dehydrogenase *in vivo* by disulfiram and diethyldithiocarbamate. *Mol. Pharmacol.*, **7**, 301–7.

De La Bastide, B., Rene, M., Charbonnier, C.J. and Mircea, M. (1986) Immunity modulating drugs. Europ. Patent Appl., EP 179,694 30 April, 1986 (cf. *Chem. Abstr.*, **105**, 85204d, 1986).

Delepine, N., Desbois, J.-C., Taillard, F., Allaneau, C. and Renoux, G. (1985) Sodium diethyldithiocarbamate inducing long-lasting remission in case of juvenile systemic lupus erythematosus. *Lancet*, **2**, 1246.

De Matteis, F. and Seawright, A.A. (1973) Oxidative metabolism of carbon disulfide in the rat: Effect of treatments which modify the liver toxicity of carbon disulfide. *Chem. Biol. Interact.*, **7**, 375–88.

De Matteis, F. (1974) Covalent binding of sulfur to microsomes and loss of cytochrome P-450 during the oxidative desulfuration of several chemicals. *Molec. Pharmacol.*, **10**, 849–54.

Deneke, S.M., Bernstein, S. P. and Fanburg, B.L. (1979) Enhancement by disulfiram (Antabuse) of toxic effects of 95 to 97% O_2 on the rat lung. *J. Pharmacol. Exp. Ther.*, **208**, 377–80.

Deneke, S.M. and Fanburg, B.L. (1980) Involvement of glutathione enzymes in O_2 tolerance development by diethyldithiocarbamate. *Biochem. Pharmacol.*, **29**, 1367–73.

Derr, R.F. and Draves, K. (1983) Methanethiol metabolism in the rat. *Res. Commun. Chem. Pathol. Pharmacol.*, **39**, 503–6.

Derr, R.F. and Draves, K. (1984) The time course of methanethiol in the rat. *Res. Commun. Chem. Pathol. Pharmacol.*, **46**, 363–70.

Diaz, J.H. and Hill, G.E. (1979) Hypotension with anesthesia in disulfiram-treated patients. *Anesthesiology*, **51**, 366–8.

Dible, S.E., Siddik, Z.H., Boxall, F.E. and Harrap, K.R. (1987) The effect of diethyldithiocarbamate on haematological toxicity and antitumor activity of carboplatin. *Europ. J. Canc. Clin. Oncol.*, **23**, 813–8.

Dickinson, F.M. and Berrieman, S. (1979) The separation of sheep liver cytoplasmic and mitochondrial aldehyde dehydrogenases by isoelectric focusing, and observations on the purity of preparations of the cytoplasmic enzyme, and their sensitivity towards inhibition by disulfiram. *Biochem. J.*, **179**, 709–12.

Dickinson, F.M., Hart, G.J. and Kitson, T.M. (1981) The use of pH-gradient ion-exchange chromatography to separate sheep liver cytoplasmic aldehyde dehydrogenase from mitochondrial enzyme contamination, and observations on the interaction between the pure cytoplasmic enzyme and disulfiram. *Biochem. J.*, **199**, 573–9.

Dierickx, P.J. (1984) *In vitro* interaction of dithiocarb with rat liver glutathione S-transferases. *Pharmacol. Res. Commun.*, **16**, 135–43.

Diquet, B., Gujadhur, L., Lamiable, D., Warot, D., Hayoun, H. and Choisy, H. (1990) Lack of interaction between disulfiram and alprazolam in alcoholic patients. *Europ. J. Clin. Pharmacol.*, **38**, 157–60.

Divatia, K.J., Hine, C.H. and Burbridge, T.N. (1952) A simple method for the determination of tetraethylthiuramdisulfide (Antabus) and blood levels obtained experimentally in animals and clinically in man. *J. Lab. Clin. Med.*, **39**, 974–82.

Djurić, D., Postić-Grujin, A., Graovac-Leposavić, L. and Delić, V. (1973) Disulfiram as an indicator of human susceptibility to carbon disulfide: Excretion of diethyl-dithiocarbamate sodium in the urine of workers exposed to CS_2 after oral administration of disulfiram. *Arch. Environ. Health*, **26**, 287–9.

Domar, G., Fredga, A. and Linderholm, H. (1949) A method for quantitative determination of tetraethylthiuram disulphide (Antabuse, Abstinyl) and its reduced form, diethyldithiocarbamic acid, as found in excreta. *Acta Clin. Scand.*, **3**, 1441–2.

Domingo, J.L., Llobet, J.M. and Corbella, J (1985) Protection of mice against the lethal effects of sodium metavanadate: A quantitative comparison of a number of chelating agents. *Toxicol. Lett.*, **26**, 95–9.

Donelli, M.G., Bartošek, I., Guaitani, A., Martini, A., Colombo, T., Pacciarini, M.A. and Modica, R. (1976) Importance of pharmacokinetic studies on cyclophosphamide (NSC-26271) in understanding its cytotoxic effect. *Cancer Treat. Rep.*, **60**, 395–401.

Donner, M., Husgafvel-Pursiainen, K., Jenssen, D. and Rannug, A. (1983) Mutagenicity of rubber additives and curing fumes: Results from five short-term bioassays. *Scand. J. Work Environ. Health*, **9**, **Suppl. 2**, 27–37.

Dössing, M. and Ranek, L. (1984) Isolated liver damage in chemical workers. *Br. J. Ind. Med.*, **41**, 142–4.

Doucette, S.R. and Willoughby, A. (1980) Relevance of caffeine symptomatology to alcohol rehabilitation efforts. *US Navy Med.*, **71**, 6–13.

Drum, D.E., Li, T.-K. and Vallee, B.L. (1969a) Considerations in evaluating the zinc content of horse liver alcohol dehydrogenase preparations. *Biochemistry*, **8**, 3783–91

Drum, D.E., Li, T.-K. and Vallee, B.L. (1969b) Zinc isotope exchange in horse liver alcohol dehydrogenase. *Biochemistry*, **8**, 3792–7.

Drum, D.E. and Vallee, B.L. (1970) Differential chemical reactivities of zinc in horse liver alcohol dehydrogenase. *Biochemistry*, **9**, 4078–86.

Dry, J. and Pradalier, A. (1973) Intoxication par la phenytoine au course d'une association therapeutique avec le disulfirame. *Therapie*, **28**, 799–802.

Dunlap, C.E., III, and Leslie, F.M. (1985) Effect of ascorbate on the toxicity of morphine in mice. *Neuropharmacology*, **8**, 797–804.

Duritz, G. and Truitt, E.B. (1964) A rapid method for the simultaneous determination of acetaldehyde and ethanol in blood using gas chromatography. *Q. J. Stud. Alcohol*, **25**, 498–510.

Dutton, G.J. and Illing, H.P.A. (1972) Mechanism of biosynthesis of thio-β-D-glucuronides and thio-β-D-glucosides. *Biochem. J.* **129**, 539–50.

Eade, N.R. (1959) Mechanism of sympathomimetic action of aldehydes. *J. Pharmacol. Exp. Ther.*, **127**, 29–34.

Eckert, G. (1957) Ein Beitrag zur Anwendung disubstituierter Dithiocarbaminat-Verbindungen für analytische Trennungen. *Z. Anal. Chem.*, **155**, 22–35.

Eckfeldt, J., Mope, L., Takio, K. and Yonetani, T. (1976) Horse liver aldehyde dehydrogenase: Purification and characterization of two isozymes. *J. Biol. Chem.*, **251**, 236–40.

Edington, N. and Howell, J.M. (1969) The neurotoxicity of sodium diethyldithiocarbamate in the rabbit. *Acta Neuropath.*, **12**, 339–47.

Edwards, B.S., Merritt, J.A., Jelen, P.A. and Borden, E.C. (1984) Effects of diethyldithiocarbamate, an inhibitor of interferon antiviral activity, upon human natural killer cells. *J. Immunol.*, **132**, 2868–75.

Egle, J.L., Jr, Hudgins, P.M. and Lai, F.M. (1973) Cardiovascular effects of intravenous acetaldehyde and propionaldehyde in the anesthetized rat. *Toxicol. App. Pharmacol.*, **24**, 636–44.

Eisen, H.J. and Ginsberg, A.L. (1975) Disulfiram hepatotoxicity. *Ann. Intern. Med.*, **83**, 673–5.

Eldjarn, L. (1950a) The metabolism of tetraethyl thiuramdisulphide (Antabus, Aversan) in the rat, investigated by means of radioactive sulphur. *Scand. J. Clin. Lab. Invest.*, **2**, 198–201.

Eldjarn, L. (1950b) The metabolism of tetraethyl thiuramdisulphide (Antabus, Aversan) in man, investigated by means of radioactive sulphur. *Scand. J. Clin. Lab. Invest.*, **2**, 202–8.

Ellis, C.N., Mitchell, A.J. and Beardsley, G.R. (1979) Tar gel interaction with disulfiram. *Arch. Dermatol.*, **115**, 1367–8.

Eneanya, D.I., Bianchine, J.R., Duran, D.O. and Andresen, B.D. (1981) The actions and metabolic fate of disulfiram. *Annu. Rev. Pharmacol. Toxicol.*, **21**, 575–96.

Eneanya, D.I., Andresen, B.D., Gerber, N. and Bianchine, J.R. (1983) Identification and characterization of the glucuronide metabolite of diethyldithiocarbamic acid in the bile from the isolated perfused rat liver by gas chromatography and mass spectrometry. *Res. Commun. Chem. Pathol. Pharmacol.*, **41**, 441–54.

Eriksson, C.J.P., Sippel, H.W. and Forsander, O.A. (1977) The determination of acetaldehyde in biological sample by headspace gas chromatography. *Anal. Biochem.*, **80**, 116–24.

Eriksson, C.J.P., Mizoi, Y. and Fukunaga, T. (1982) The determination of acetaldehyde in human blood by the perchloric acid precipitation method: The characterization and elimination of artefactual acetaldehyde formation. *Anal. Biochem.*, **125**, 259–63.

Eriksson, C.J.P. (1983) Human blood acetaldehyde concentration during ethanol oxidation (update 1982). *Pharmacol. Biochem. Behav.*, **18, Suppl. 1**, 141–50.

Eriksson, C.J.P. (1985) Endogenous acetaldehyde in rats: Effects of exogenous ethanol, pyrazole, cyanamide and disulfiram. *Biochem. Pharmacol.*, **34**, 3979–82.

Escaich, S., Ritter, J., Retornaz, G. *et al.* (1988) Comparison of the effects of therapy with suramin 3′azidothymidine (AZT) and diethyldithiocarbamate (DTC) on HIV replication. *Fourth International Conference on AIDS, Abstract Volume I*, Stockholm, p. 258, Abstract 3155.

Etzioni, A. and Remp, R. (1973) Antabuse. In *Technological Shortcuts to Social Change,* Russell Sage, New York, pp. 53–77.

Evans, R.G., Engel, C., Wheatley, C. and Nielsen, J. (1982) Modification of the sensitivity and repair of potentially lethal damage by diethyldithiocarbamate during and following exposure of plateau-phase cultures of mammalian cells to radiation and cis-diamminedichlorplatinum(II). *Cancer Res.*, **42**, 3074–8.

Evans, R.G., Engel, C.R., Wheatley, C.L., Nielsen, J.R. and Ciborowski, L.J. (1983a) An *in vivo* study of the radioprotective effect of diethyldithiocarbamate (DDC). *Int. J. Rad. Oncol.*, **9**, 1635–40.

Evans, R.G., Nielsen, J., Engel, C. and Wheatley, C. (1983b) Enhancement of heat sensitivity and modification of repair of potentially lethal heat damage in plateau-phase cultures of mammalian cells by diethyldithiocarbamate. *Radiat. Res.*, **93**, 319–25.

Evans, R.G., Wheatley, C., Engel, C. Nielsen, J. and Ciborowski, L.J. (1984) Modification of the bone marrow toxicity of *cis*-diamminedichloroplatinum(II) in mice by diethyldithiocarbamate. *Cancer Res.*, **44**, 3686–90.

Evans, R.G. (1985) Tumor radiosensitization with concomitant bone marrow radioprotection: a study in mice using diethyldithiocarbamate (DDC) under oxygenated and hypoxic conditions. *Int. J. Rad. Oncol.*, **11**, 1163–9.

Ewing, S.P., Lockshon, D. and Jencks, W.P. (1980) Mechanism of cleavage of carbamate anions. *J. Am. Chem. Soc.*, **102**, 3072–84.

Eybl, Y., Jones, M.M., Koutenská, M., Koutenský, J., Sýkora, J., Drobnik, J. and Švec, F. (1988) Comparison of the effects of sodium *N*-benzyl-D-glucamine dithiocarbamate and Ditripentat on the toxicity, excretion, and tissue distribution of cadmium in mice. *Arch. Toxicol.*, **Suppl. 12**, 438–40.

Ezrielev, G.I. (1973) Acetaldehyde and alcoholism. Pharmacogenesis of a disulfiram-alcohol reaction and its management by binding acetaldehyde with sodium metabisulfite. *Zhurn. Nevropat. Psikiat.*, **73**, 238–43.

Fackler, J.P., Jr, Seidel, W.C. and Fetchin, J.A. (1968) Five-coordinate complexes of platinum(II) and palladium(II). *J. Am. Chem. Soc.*, **90**, 2707–9.

Faiman, M.D., Mehl, R.G. and Oehme, F.W. (1971a) Protection with disulfiram from central and pulmonary oxygen toxicity. *Biochem. Pharmacol.*, **20**, 3059–67.

Faiman, M.D., Mehl, R.G. and Myers, M.B. (1971b) Brain norepinephrine and serotonin in central oxygen toxicity. *Life Sci. Part II*, **10**, 21–34.

Faiman, M.D., Dodd, D.E., Nolan, R.J., Artman, L. and Hanzlik, R.E. (1977) A rapid and simple radioactive method for the determination of disulfiram and its metabolites from a single sample of biological fluid or tissue. *Res. Commun. Chem. Pathol. Pharmacol.*, **17**, 481–96.

Faiman, M.D., Dodd, D.E. and Hanzlik, R.E. (1978a) Distribution of S^{35} disulfiram and metabolites in mice, and metabolism of S^{35} disulfiram in the dog. *Res. Commun. Chem. Pathol. Pharmacol.*, **21**, 543–67.

Faiman, M.D., Dodd, D.E., Minor, S.S. and Hanzlik, R. (1978b) Radioactive and nonradioactive methods for the *in vivo* determination of disulfiram, diethyldithiocarbamate, and diethyldithiocarbamate-methyl ester. *Alcohol. Clin. Exp. Res.*, **2**, 366–9.

Faiman, M.D. (1979) Biochemical Pharmacology of Disulfiram. In *Biochemistry and Pharmacology of Ethanol*, Vol. 2 (eds E. Majchrowicz and E.P. Noble), Plenum, New York, pp. 325–48.

Faiman, M.D. Artman, L. and Haja, K. (1980) Disulfiram distribution and elimination in the rat after oral and intraperitoneal administration. *Alcohol. Clin. Exp. Res.*, **4**, 412–19.

Faiman, M.D., Artman, L. and Maziasz, T. (1983) Diethyldithiocarbamic acid-methyl ester distribution, elimination, and LD_{50} in the rat after intraperitoneal administration. *Alcohol. Clin. Exp. Res.*, **7**, 307–11.

Faiman, M.D., Jensen, J.C. and Lacoursiere, R.B. (1984) Elimination kinetics of disulfiram in alcoholics after single and repeated doses. *Clin. Pharmacol. Ther.*, **36**, 520–6.

Fairfield, A.S., Meshnick, S.R. and Eaton, J.W. (1983) Malaria parasites adopt host cell superoxide dismutase. *Science*, **221**, 764–6.

Farrés, J., Julià, P. and Parés, X. (1988) Aldehyde oxidation in human placenta: Purification and properties of 1-pyrroline-5-carboxylate dehydrogenase. *Biochem. J.*, **256**, 461–7.

Farrés, J., Guan, K.-L. and Weiner, H. (1989) Primary structures of rat and bovine liver mitochondrial aldehyde dehydrogenase deduced from cDNA sequences. *Eur. J. Biochem.*, **180**, 67–74.

Feldman, R.I and Weiner, H. (1972) Horse liver aldehyde dehydrogenase. II. Kinetics and mechanistic implications of the dehydrogenase and esterase activity. *J. Biol. Chem.*, **247**, 267–72.

Ferencz-Biro, K. and Pietruszko, R. (1984) Human aldehyde dehydrogenase: catalytic activity in oriental liver. *Biochem. Biophys. Res. Commun.*, **118**, 97–102.

Ferguson, J.K.W. (1949) Antabuse. *Can. Med. Assoc. J.*, **60**, 295–6.

Fiala, E.S. (1981) Inhibition of carcinogen metabolism and action by disulfiram, pyrazole, and related compounds. In *Inhibition of Tumor Induction and Development* (eds M.S. Zedeck and M. Lipkin), Plenum, New York, pp. 23–69.

Fisher, C.M. (1989) 'Catatonia' due to disulfiram toxicity. *Arch. Neurol.*, **46**, 798–804.

Flohe, L. (1982) Glutathione peroxidase brought into focus. In *Free Radicals in Biology.*, Vol. **5**, (ed W.A. Pryor), Academic Press, New York, pp. 223–54.

Flood, J.F., Smith, G.E., Bennett, E.L., Alberti, M.H., Orme, A.E. and Jarvik, M.E. (1986) Neurochemical and behavioral effects on catecholamine and protein synthesis inhibitors in mice. *Pharmacol. Biochem. Behav.*, **24**, 631–45.

Florentin, I., Chung, V., Degenne, D., Bardos, P., Guillaumin, J.-M., Renoux, M. and Renoux, G. (1988) An immunostimulant, imuthiol, amplifies the cytotoxic responses to tumor cells in young and aged mice. *Int. J. Immunotherap.*, **4**, 5–11.

Florentin, I., Chung, V., Renoux, M. and Renoux, G. (1989) Imuthiol influences on cytotoxic T cells and NK activity in +/+ and athymic nude BALB/c mice. *Immunopharmacol. Immunotoxicol.*, **11**, 645–55.

Ford, D.B. and Benson, A.M. (1988) Differential responses of mouse UDP-glucuronyltransferases and beta-glucuronidase to disulfiram and related compounds. *Biochem. Biophys. Res. Commun.*, **153**, 149–55.

Forman, H.J., York, J.L. and Fisher, A.B. (1980) Mechanism for the potentiation of oxygen toxicity by disulfiram. *J. Pharmacol. Exp. Ther.*, **212**, 452–5.

Forte-McRobbie, C.M. and Pietruszko, R. (1985) Aldehyde dehydrogenase content and composition of human liver. *Alcohol*, **2**, 375–81.

Forte-McRobbie, C.M. and Pietruszko, R. (1986) Purification and characterization of human liver 'high K_m' aldehyde dehydrogenase and its identification as glutamic γ-semialdehyde dehydrogenase. *J. Biol. Chem.*, **261**, 2154–63.

Fournier, E., Fournier, A., Rochefort, K, Efthymiou, M.-L. and Mellerio, F. (1967) Incidents et accidents du traitement par le disulfiram (antabuse): Revue générale et observations personnelles. *Thérapie*, **22**, 559–600.

Fox, R. (1958) Antabuse as an adjunct to psychotherapy in alcoholism. *N.Y. State J. Med.*, **58**, 1540–4.

Frank, L., Wood, D.L. and Roberts, R.J. (1978) Effect of diethyldithiocarbamate on oxygen toxicity and lung enzyme activity in immature and adult rats. *Biochem. Pharmacol.*, **27**, 251–4.

Frederickson, R.E., Frederickson, C.J. and Danscher, G. (1990) *In situ* binding of bouton zinc reversibly disrupts performance on spatial memory task. *Behav. Brain Res.*, **38**, 25–33.

Freireich, E.J., Gehan, E.A., Rall, D.P., Schmidt, L.H. and Skipper, H.E. (1966) Quantitative comparison of toxicity of anticancer agents in mouse, rat, hamster, dog, monkey, and man. *Cancer Chemother.*, **50**, 219–44.

Freund, G. (1973) Hypothermia after acute ethanol and benzyl alcohol administration. *Life Sci.*, **13**, 345–9.

Freundt, K.J. (1978) Variable inhibition of human hepatic drug metabolizing enzymes by disulfiram. *Int. J. Clin. Pharmacol.*, **16**, 323–30.

Fridovich, I. (1983) Superoxide radical: an endogenous toxicant. *Annu. Rev. Pharmacol. Toxicol.*, **23**, 239–57.

Fridovich, I. (1989) Superoxide dismutases: An adaptation to a paramagnetic gas. *J. Biol. Chem.*, **264**, 7761–4.

Fried, R. (1980) Biochemical actions of anti-alcoholic agents. *Substance Abuse Alc. Actions/Misuse*, **1**, 5–27.

Friedman, H., Matsuzaki, S., Choe, S. *et al.* (1979) Demonstration of dissimilar acute heamodynamic effects of ethanol and acetaldehyde. *Cardiovasc. Res.*, **13**, 477–87.

Friedman, S. and Kaufman, S. (1965) 3,4-Dihydroxyphenylethylamine β-hydroxylase: Physical properties, copper content, and role of copper in the catalytic activity. *J. Biol. Chem.*, **240**, 4763–73.

Frisoni, G.B. and Di Monda, V. (1989) Disulfiram neuropathy: A review (1971–1988) and report of a case. *Alcohol Alcohol.*, **24**, 429–37.

Fukumori, R., Minegishi, A., Satoh, T., Kitagawa, H. and Yanura, S. (1979) Effects of disulfiram on turnover of 5-hydroxytryptamine in rat brain. *Life Sci.*, **25**, 123–30.

Fuller, R.K. and Roth, H.P. (1979) Disulfiram for the treatment of alcoholism: an evaluation of 128 men. *Ann. Intern. Med.*, **90**, 901–4.

Fuller, R.K. and Williford, W.O. (1980) Life-table analysis of abstinence in a study evaluating the efficacy of disulfiram. *Alcohol. Clin. Exp. Res.*, **4**, 298–301.

Fuller, R.K. and Neiderhiser, D.H. (1981) Evaluation and application of a urinary diethylamine method to measure compliance with disulfiram therapy. *J. Stud. Alcohol*, **42**, 202–7.

Fuller, R.K., Roth, H. and Long, S. (1983) Compliance with disulfiram treatment of alcoholism. *J. Chron. Dis.*, **36**, 161–70.

Fuller, R.K., Branchey, L, Brightwell, D.R. *et al.* (1986) Disulfiram treatment of alcoholism: A Veterans Administration Cooperative Study. *J. Am. Med. Assoc.*, **256**, 1449–55.

Furusawa, S., Saski, K. and Takayanagi, G. (1988) Reduction of cyclophosphamide-induced toxicity by diethyldithiocarbamate and carbon disulfide and its possible mechanism. *J. Pharmacobio. Dyn.*, **11**, 284–7.

Gale, G.R. (1981) Diethyldithiocarbamic acid sodium salt. *Drugs of the Future*, **6**, 225–7.

Gale, G.R., Smith, A.B. and Walker, E.M., Jr (1981) Diethyldithiocarbamate in treatment of acute cadmium poisoning. *Ann. Clin. Lab. Sci.*, **11**, 476–83.

Gale, G.R., Atkins, L.M. and Walker, E.M., Jr. (1982a) Further evaluation of diethyldithiocarbamate as an antagonist of cisplatin toxicity. *Ann. Clin. Lab. Sci.*, **12**, 345–55.

Gale, G.R., Atkins, L.M. and Walker, E.M., Jr. (1982b) Effects of diethyldithiocarbamate on organ distribution and excretion of cadmium. *Ann. Clin. Lab. Sci.*, **12**, 463–70.

Gale, G.R., Atkins, L.M., Walker, E.M., Jr and Smith, A.B. (1983a) Comparative effects of diethyldithiocarbamte, dimercaptosuccinate, and diethylenetriaminepentaacetate on organ distribution and excretion of cadmium. *Ann. Clin. Lab. Sci.*, **13**, 33–44.

Gale, G.R., Atkins, L.M., Walker, E.M., Jr, Smith, A.B. and Hynes, J.B. (1983b) Comparative effects of three dialkyldithiocarbamates on acute toxicity, organ distribution, and excretion of cadmium. *Ann. Clin. Lab. Sci.*, **13**, 207–16.

Gale, G.R., Atkins, L.M., Walker, E.M., Jr, Smith, A.B. and Jones, M.M. (1983c) Mechanism of diethyldithiocarbamate, dihydroxyethyldithiocarbamate, and dicarboxymethyldithiocarbamate action on distribution and excretion of cadmium. *Ann. Clin. Lab. Sci.*, **13**, 474–81.

Gale, G.R., Walker, E.M., Jr and Smith, A.B. (1983d) Effects of combined treatment with diethyldithiocarbamate and dihydroxyethyldithiocarbamate on distribution and excretion of cadmium. *Res. Commun. Chem. Pathol. Pharmacol.*, **41**, 293–302.

Gale, G.R., Atkins, L.M., Walker, E.M., Jr, Smith, A.B. and Jones, M.M. (1984a) Dithiocarbamates and cadmium metabolism: further correlations of cadmium chelate partition coefficients and pharmacological activity. *Ann. Clin. Lab. Sci.*, **14**, 137–45.

Gale, G.R., Atkins, L.M., Smith, A.B., Walker, E.M., Jr and Jones, M.M. (1984b) Comparative effects of *N,N*-disubstituted dithiocarbamates and dimercaptosuccinate on mobilization of methylmercury in mice. *Res. Commun. Chem. Pathol. Pharmacol.*, **45**, 119–35.

Gale, G.R., Shinobu, L.A., Jones, M.M., Atkins, L.M. and Smith, A.B. (1984c) Effects of sodium *N*-methyl-*N*-dithiocarboxyglucamine on cadmium distribution and excretion. *Life Sci.*, **35**, 2571–8.

Gale, G.R., Atkins, L.M. and Smith, A.B. (1985a) Effects of diethyldithiocarbamate and selected analogs on cadmium metabolism following chronic cadmium ingestion. *Res. Commun. Chem. Pathol. Pharmacol.*, **47**, 107–14.

Gale, G.R., Smith, A.B., Atkins, L.M. and Jones, M.M. (1985b) Effects of diethyldithiocarbamate and *N*-methyl-*N*-dithiocarboxyglucamine on murine hepatic cadmium-metallothionein *in vitro. Res. Commun. Chem. Pathol. Pharmacol.*, **49**, 423–34.

Gale, G.R., Atkins, L.M., Smith, A.B. and Jones, M.M (1986a) Effects of diethyldithiocarbamate and selected analogs on lead metabolism in mice. *Res. Commun. Chem. Pathol. Pharmacol.*, **52**, 29–44.

Gale, G.R., Atkins, L.M., Smith, A.B. and Jones, M.M (1986b) Comparative effects of parenteral and oral administration of selected dithiocarbamates on body burdens and organ distribution of cadmium in mice. *Res. Commun. Chem. Pathol. Pharmacol.*, **53**, 129–32.

Gale, G.R., Atkins, L.M., Smith, A.B., Jones, S.G. and Jones, M.M. (1987) Amphipathic dithiocarbamates as cadmium antagonists: *N*-cyclohexyl-*N*-sulfonatoalkyl derivatives. *Res. Commun. Chem. Pathol. Pharmacol.*, **58**, 371–91.

Gale, G.R., Atkins, L.M., Smith, A.B., Jones, S.G. and Jones, M.M. (1988) Dithiocarbamate treatment of chronic cadmium intoxication in mice. *Toxicol. Let.*, **44**, 77–84.

Gale, G.R., Smith, A.B. and Atkins, L.M. (1989a) Comparative effects of disulfiram and diethyldithiocarbamate on cadmium distribution in mice. *Res. Commun. Chem. Pathol. Pharmacol.*, **63**, 395–410.

Gale, G.R., Atkins, L.M., Smith, A.B., Singh, P.K. and Jones, M.M. (1989b) *N,N*-disubstituted dithiocarbamates as cadmium antagonists: *N*-(4-methoxybenzyl)-*N*-dithiocarboxy-D-glucamine. *Toxicol. Let.*, **48**, 105–15.

Gallagher, C.H. and Reeve, V.E. (1976) Interrelationships of copper, cytochrome oxidase, phospholipid synthesis and adenine nucleotide binding. *Aust. J. Exp. Biol. Med. Sci.*, **54**, 593–600.

Gandara, D.R., Perez, E.A., DeGregorio, M.W. and Borch, R. (1988a) Cisplatin and Fluorouracil with and without sodium diethyldithiocarbamate rescue. *J. Clin. Oncol.*, **6**, 1785–6.

Gandara, D., DeGregorio, M. Perez, E., Holleran, W., Denham, A. and Lawrence, H.J., (1988b) Diethyldithiocarbamate (DDTC) rescue following very high-dose cisplatin (200 mg/m²/cycle): Preliminary results of a Phase I trial and pharmacokinetic observations. *Proc. Am. Soc. Clin. Oncol.*, 7, 69.

Gandara, D.R., Perez, E.A., Lawrence, H.J. and DeGregorio, M.W. (1989) Phase I trial of high dose cisplatin plus diethyldithiocarbamate rescue: Toxicity profile compared to patients receiving high dose cisplatin rescue alone. *Proc. Am. Ass. Cancer Res.*, 30, 241.

Gandara, D.R., Wiebe, V.J., Perez, E.A., Makuch, R.W. and DeGregorio, M.W. (1990) Cisplatin rescue therapy: Experience with sodium thiosulfate, WR2721, and diethyldithiocarbamate. *Crit. Rev. Oncol. Hematol.*, 10, 353–65.

Gardner-Thorpe, C. and Benjamin, S. (1971) Peripheral neuropathy after disulfiram administration. *J. Neurol. Neurosurg. Psychiatry*, 34, 253–59.

Gendre, F., Huart, B., Deschaux, P. and Fontanges, R. (1983) Étude du transfer de l'immunostimulation de la mère au Souriceau à l'aide de deux immunostimulants et du test 'PFC'. *Compt. Rend. Acad. Sc. Paris*, 296 Serie III, 15–8.

Gerrein, J.R. Rosenberg, C.M. and Manohar, V. (1973) Disulfiram maintenance in outpatient treatment of alcoholism. *Arch. Gen. Psychiatry*, 28, 798–802.

Gerschman, R., Gilbert, D.L. and Caccamise, D. (1958) Effect of various substances on survival times of mice exposed to different high oxygen tensions. *Am. J. Physiol.*, 192, 563–71.

Gessner, P.K. (1973) *In vivo* ethanol metabolism: kinetics of inhibition. In *Proceeding of First Annual Alcoholism Conference of the National Institute of Alcohol Abuse and Alcoholism* (ed. M.E. Chafetz), US Government Printing Office, Washington, DC, pp. 79–99.

Gessner, P.K. (1974) The isobolographic method applied to drug interactions. In *Drug Interactions* (eds P.L. Morselli, S. Garattini and S.N. Cohen), Raven Press, New York, pp. 349–62.

Gessner, P.K. and Hasan, M.M. (1987) Freundlich and Langmuir isotherms as models for the adsorption of toxicants on activated charcoal. *J. Pharm. Sci.*, 76, 319–27.

Gessner, P.K. (1988) A straightforward method for the study of drug interactions: An isobolographic analysis primer. *J. Am. Coll. Toxicol.*, 7, 987–1012.

Gessner, T. and Jakubowski, M. (1972) Diethyldithiocarbamic acid methyl ester a metabolite of disulfiram. *Biochem. Pharmacol.*, 21, 219–30.

Gigon, P.L., Gram, T.E. and Gillette, J.R. (1968) Effect of drug substrates on the reduction of hepatic microsomal cytochrome P-450 by NADPH. *Biochem. Biophys. Res. Com.*, 31, 558–62.

Giles, H.G., Au, J. and Sellers, E.M. (1982) Analysis of plasma diethyldithiocarbamate: A metabolite of disulfiram. *J. Liq. Chromat.*, 5, 945–51.

Gleerup, G., Boström, S., Hansson, G., Teger-Nilsson, A.-C., Sjöquist, P.-O. and Winther, K. (1990) Effect of disulfiram on the platelet function and fibrinolysis in healthy volunteers. *Haemostasis*, 20, 215–8.

Glud, E. (1949) The treatment of alcoholic patients in Denmark with 'Antabuse': with suggestions for its trial in the United States. *Q. J. Stud. Alcohol*, 10, 185–97.

Goedde, H.W., Harada, S. and Agarwal, D.P. (1979) Racial differences in alcohol sensitivity: A new hypothesis. *Hum. Genet.*, 51, 331–4.

Goedde, H.W., Agarwal, D.P., Harada, S., Rothhammer, F.M. Whittaker, J.O. and Lisker, R. (1986) Aldehyde dehydrogenase polymorphism in North American, South American, and Mexican Indian populations. *Am. J. Hum. Genet.*, 38, 395–9.

Goedde, H.W. and Agarwal, D.P. (1990) Pharmacogenetics of aldehyde dehydrogenase (ALDH). *Pharmacol. Ther.*, **45**, 345–71.

Goering, P.L., Tandon, S.K. and Klaassen, C.D. (1985) Induction of hepatic metallothionein in mouse liver following administration of chelating agents. *Toxicol. App. Pharmacol.*, **80**, 467–72.

Gold, S. (1966) A skinful of alcohol. *Lancet*, **ii**, 1417.

Goldstein, B.D., Rozen, M.G., Quintavalla, J.C. and Amoruso, M.A. (1979) Decrease in mouse lung and liver glutathione peroxidase activity and potentiation of the lethal effects of ozone and paraquat by the superoxide dismutase inhibitor diethyldithiocarbamate. *Biochem. Pharmacol.*, **28**, 27–30.

Goldstein, G. (1974) Isolation of bovine thymin; a polypeptide hormone of the thymus. *Nature*, **147**, 11.

Goldstein, M., Anagnoste, B., Lauber, E. and McKereghan, M.R. (1964) Inhibition of dopamine β-hydroxylase by disulfiram. *Life Sci.*, **3**, 763–7.

Goldstein, M., Lauber, E. and McKereghan, M.R. (1965) Studies on the purification and characterization of 3,4-dihydroxyphenylethylamine β-hydroxylase. *J. Biol. Chem.*, **240**, 2066–72.

Goldstein, M. and Nakajima, K. (1966) The effects of disulfiram on the replition of brain catecholamine stores. *Life Sci.*, **5**, 1133–8.

Goldstein, M. and Nakajima, K. (1967) The effect of disulfiram on catecholamine levels in the brain. *J. Pharmacol. Exp. Ther.*, **157**, 96–102.

Gonias, S.L., Oakley, A.C., Walther, P.J. and Pizzo, S.V. (1984) Effects of diethyldithiocarbamate and nine other nucleophiles on the intersubunit protein cross-linking and inactivation of purified human α_2-macroglobulin by *cis*-diamminedichloroplatinum(II). *Cancer Res.*, **44**, 5764–70.

Goodchild, M. (1969) The non-specificity of diethyldithiocarbamate. *J. Pharm. Pharmacol.*, **21**, 54.

Gordis, E. and Peterson, K. (1977) Disulfiram therapy in alcoholism: Patient compliance studied with a urine-detection procedure. *Alcohol. Clin. Exp. Res.*, **1**, 213–6.

Gosselin, R.E., Smith, R.P. and Hodge, H.C. (1984) *Clinical Toxicology of Commercial Products*, 5th edn., Williams and Wilkins, Baltimore, pp. III-159–III-163.

Goyer, P.F. and Major, L.F. (1979) Hepatotoxicity in disulfiram-treated patients. *J. Stud. Alcohol*, **40**, 133–7.

Goyer, P.F., Brown, G.L., Minichiello, M.D. and Major, L.F. (1984) Mood altering effects of disulfiram in alcoholics. *J. Stud. Alcohol*, **45**, 209–13.

Grafström, R. and Greene, F.E. (1980) Differential effects of disulfiram and diethyldithiocarbamate on small intestinal and liver microsomal benzo[*a*]pyrene metabolism. *Biochem. Pharmacol.*, **29**, 1517–23.

Grafström, R. and Holmberg, B. (1980) The effect of long term treatment with disulfiram on content of cytochrome P-450 and on benzo(a)pyrene mono-oxygenase activity in microsomes isolated from the rat small intestinal mucosa. *Toxicol. Lett.*, **7**, 79–85.

Graham, W.D. (1951) *In vitro* inhibition of liver aldehyde dehydrogenase by tetraethylthiuram disulphide. *J. Pharm. Pharmacol.*, **3**, 160–8.

Grandjean, P., Kristensen, K., Jørgensen, P.J., Nielsen, G.D. and Andersen, O. (1990) Trace element status in alcoholism before and during disulfiram treatment. *Ann. Clin. Lab. Sci.*, **20**, 28–35.

Graveleau, J., Ecoffet, M. and Villard, A. (1980) Les neuropathies périphériques dues au disulfirame. *Nouv. Presse Med.*, **9**, 2905–7.

Green, A.L. (1964) The inhibition of dopamine-β-oxidase by chelating agents. *Biochim. Biophys. Acta*, **81**, 394–7.

Greenblatt, D.J., Abernethy, D.R., Divoll, M.M Smith, R.B. and Shader, R.I. (1983) Old age, cimetidine, and disposition of alprazolam and triazolam. *Clin. Pharmacol. Ther.*, **33**, 253.

Greenfield, N.J. and Pietruszko, R. (1977) Two aldehyde dehydrogenases from human liver: Isolation via affinity chromatography and characterization of the isozymes. *Biochim. Biophys. Acta*, **483**, 35–45.

Griffiths, D.E. and Wharton, D.C. (1961) Studies of the electron transport system. XXXV. Purification and properties of cytochrome oxidase. *J. Biol. Chem.*, **236**, 1850–6.

Gringeri, A., Keng, P.C. and Borch, R.F. (1988) Diethyldithiocarbamate inhibition of murine bone marrow toxicity caused by *cis*-diamminedichloroplatinum(II) or diammine-(1,1-cyclobutanedicarboxylato)platinum(II). *Cancer Res.*, **48**, 5708–12.

Guan, K.L., Pak, Y.K., Tu, G.C., Cao, Q.N. and Weiner, H. (1988) Purification and characterization of beef and pig liver aldehyde dehydrogenases. *Alcohol. Clin. Exp. Res.*, **12**, 713–9.

Guarnieri, C., Flamigni, F., Ventura, C. and Rossoni-Caldarera, C. (1981) Inhibition of rat heart superoxide dismutase activity by diethyldithiocarbamate and its effect on mitochondrial function. *Biochem. Pharmacol.*, **30**, 2174–6.

Guillaumin, J.M., Renoux, M. and Renoux, G. (1984) Influence de la race, de l'âge et du sexe sur l'immunomodulation par deux composés soufrés. *Reprod. Nutr. Develop.*, **24**, 208.

Guillaumin, J.-M., Lepape, A. and Renoux, G. (1986) Fate and distribution of radioactive sodium diethyldithiocarbamate (Imuthiol) in the mouse. *Int. J. Immunopharmac.*, **8**, 859–65.

Gylys, J.A., Doran, K.M. and Buyniski, J.P. (1979) Antagonism of cisplatin induced emesis in the dog. *Res. Commun. Chem. Pathol. Pharmacol.*, **23**, 61–8.

Habs, M., Hebebrand, J. and Schmähl, D. (1984) Influence of sulfur-containing compounds on the acute toxicity of cyclophosphamide in male Sprague-Dawley rats. *Arzneimittelforschung*, **34**, 792–3.

Hacker, M.P., Newman, R.A. and Ershler, W.B. (1982a) The prevention of cyclophosphamide cystitis in mice by disulfiram. *Res. Commun. Chem. Pathol. Pharmacol.*, **35**, 145–54.

Hacker, M.P., Ershler, W.B., Newman, R.A. and Gamelli, R.L. (1982b) Effect of disulfiram (tetraethylthiuram disulfide) and diethyldithiocarbamate on the bladder toxicity and antitumor activity of cyclophosphamide in mice. *Cancer Res.*, **42**, 4490–4.

Hadden, J.W., Caspritz, G., Zheng, Q.-Y., Chen, H., Wolstencroft, R. and Hadden, E.M. (1989) Thymosin, interleukins, isoprinosine and imuthiol do not reconstitute T-cells in athymic nude mice. *Int. J. Immunopharmacol.*, **11**, 13–9.

Haddock, N.F. and Wilkin, J.K. (1982) Cutaneous reactions to lower aliphatic alcohols before and during disulfiram therapy. *Arch. Dermatol.*, **118**, 157–9.

Hald, J. and Jacobsen, E. (1948a) The formation of acetaldehyde in the organism after ingestion of Antabuse (tetraethylthiuramdisulphide) and alcohol. *Acta Pharmacol.*, **4**, 305–10.

Hald, J. and Jacobsen, E. (1948b) A drug sensitising the organism to ethyl alcohol. *Lancet*, **ii**, 1001–5.

Hald, J., Jacobsen, E. and Larsen, V. (1948) The sensitizing effect of tetraethylthiuramdisulphide (Antabuse) to ethyl alcohol. *Acta Pharmacol.*, **4**, 285–96.

Hald, J. and Larsen, V. (1949) The rate of acetaldehyde metabolism in rabbits treated with Antabuse (tetraethylthiuramdisulphide). *Acta Pharmacol.*, **5**, 292–7.

Hald, J., Jacobsen, E. and Larsen, V. (1949a) Formation of acetaldehyde in the organism in relation to dosage of Antabuse (tetraethylthiuramdisulphide) and to alcohol-concentration in blood. *Acta Pharmacol.*, **5**, 179–88.

Hald, J., Jacobsen, E. and Larsen, V. (1949b) The rate of acetaldehyde metabolism in isolated livers and hind limbs of rabbits treated with Antabuse (tetraethylthiuramdisulphide). *Acta Pharmacol.*, **5**, 298–308.

Hald, J., Jacobsen, E. and Larsen, V. (1952) The antabuse effect of compound related to antabuse and cyanamide. *Acta Pharmacol. Toxicol.*, **8**, 329–37.

Hald, J.G., Gad, I.G. and Deans, A.A.V. (1953) Tetraethylthiuram disulfide. U.S. Patent. U.S. 2,647,15 July 28, 1953 (cf. *Chem. Abstr.*, **48**, 8257i, 1954).

Haley, T.J. (1979) Disulfiram (tetraethyldithioperoxydicarbonic diamide): a reappraisal of its toxicity and therapeutic application. *Drug Metab. Rev.*, **9**, 319–35.

Hallaway, M. (1959) The stability of sodium diethyldithiocarbamate in biochemical experiments. *Biochem. Biophys. Acta*, **36**, 538–40.

Halls, D.J. (1969) The properties of dithiocarbamates: A review. *Mikrochim. Acta (Wien)*, **1969**, 62–77.

Halpern, M.D., Hersh, E. and Yocum, D.E. (1990) Diethyldithiocarbamate, a novel immunomodulator, prolongs survival in autoimmune MRL-*lpr/lpr* mice. *Clin. Immunol. Immunopathol.*, **55**, 242–54.

Halpern, M.D. and Yocum, D.E. (1991) The paradoxical effects of diethyldithiocarbamate: Comparison between New Zeland black/white F_1 hybrid and Balb/c mice. *Clin. Immunol. Immunopathol.*, **58**, 69–79.

Hanes, C.S., Bronskill, P.M., Gurr, P.A. and Wong, J. T.-F. (1972) Kinetic mechanism for the major isoenzyme of horse liver alcohol dehydrogenase. *Can. J. Biochem.*, **50**, 1385–413.

Harada, S., Agarwal, D.P. and Goedde, H.W. (1980) Electrophoretic and biochemical studies of human aldehyde dehydrogenase isozymes in various tissues. *Life Sci.*, **26**, 1773–80.

Harada, S., Agarwal, D.P. and Goedde, H.W. (1982) Mechanism of alcohol sensitivity and disulfiram-ethanol reaction. *Sub. Alc. Act./Mis.*, **3**, 107–15.

Harari, P.M., Tome, M.E., Fuller, D.J.M., Carper, S.W. and Gerner, E.W. (1989) Effects of diethyldithiocarbamate and endogenous polyamine content on cellular responses to hydrogen peroxide cytotoxicity. *Biochem. J.*, **260**, 487–90.

Häring, N. and Ballschmiter, K. (1980) Chromatographie von Metallchelaten-IX: Adsorptive Voranreicherung für Bestimmungen von Kobalt, Kupfer und Nickel im Mikrogramm/liter-bereich nach Umkehrphasen-chromatographie der Diäethyldithiocarbamate. *Talanta*, **27**, 873–9.

Harrington, M.C., Henehan, G.T.M. and Tipton, K.F. (1988) The interrelationship of alcohol dehydrogenase and aldehyde dehydrogenase in the metabolism of ethanol in the liver. *Biochem. Soc. Trans.*, **16**, 239–41.

Hart, B.W., Yourick, J.J. and Faiman, M.D. (1990) *S*-Methyl-*N,N*-diethylthiolcarbamate: A disulfiram metabolite and potent rat liver mitochondrial low K_m aldehyde dehydrogenase inhibitor. *Alcohol*, **7**, 165–9.

Haycock, J.W., van Buskirk, R. and McGaugh, J.L. (1977) Effects of catecholaminergic drugs upon memory storage processes in mice. *Behavior. Biol.*, **20**, 281–310.

Haynes, S.N. (1973) Contingency management in a municipally-administered Antabuse program for alcoholics. *J. Behav. Ther. Exp. Psychiatry*, **4**, 31–2.

Hazard, R., Cheymol, J., Chabrier, P. and Giudicelli, R. (1957) Structure chimique et activité pharmacologique de sels d'amines tertiaires. *Arch. Inter. Pharmacodyn.*, **112**, 36–49.

Heath, R.G., Nesselhof, W., Bishop, M.P. and Byers, L.W. (1965) Behavioral and metabolic changes associated with administration of tetraethylthiuram disulfide (Antabuse). *Dis. Nerv. System*, **26**, 99–105.

Heikkila, R.E., Cabbat, F.S. and Cohen, G. (1976) *In vivo* inhibition of superoxide dismutase in mice by diethyldithiocarbamate. *J. Biol. Chem.*, **252**, 2182–5.

Helander, A. and Tottmar, O. (1986) Cellular distribution of human blood aldehyde dehydrogenase. *Alcohol. Clin. Exp. Res.*, **10**, 71–6.

Helander, A. and Tottmar, O. (1987a) Metabolism of biogenic aldehydes in isolated human blood cells, platelets and in plasma. *Bioch. Pharmacol.*, **36**, 1077–82.

Helander, A. and Tottmar, O. (1987b) Effects of ethanol, acetaldehyde and disulfiram on the metabolism of biogenic aldehydes in isolated human blood cells and platelets. *Bioch. Pharmacol.*, **36**, 3981–5.

Helander, A. and Tottmar, O. (1988) Effects of disulfiram, cyanamide and 1-aminocyclopropanol on the aldehyde dehydrogenase activity in human erythrocytes and leukocytes. *Pharmacol. Toxicol.*, **63**, 262–5.

Helander, A., Carlsson, S. and Tottmar, O. (1988) Effects of disulfiram therapy on aldehyde dehydrogenase activity in human leukocytes and erythrocytes. *Biochem. Pharmacol.*, **37**, 3360–3.

Helander, A. and Johansson, B. (1989) Inhibition of human erythrocyte and leukocyte aldehyde dehydrogenase activities by diethylthiocarbamic acid methyl ester: An *in vivo* metabolite of disulfiram. *Biochem. Pharmacol.*, **38**, 2195–8.

Helander, A. and Carlsson, S. (1990) Use of leukocyte aldehyde dehydrogenase activity to monitor inhibitory effect of disulfiram treatment. *Alcohol. Clin. Exp. Res.*, **14**, 48–52.

Held, K.D. and Melder, D.C. (1987) Toxicity of the sulfhydryl-containing radioprotector dithiothreitol. *Radiat. Res.*, **112**, 544–54.

Hellström, E., Tottmar, O. and Fried, R. (1980) Implantation of disulfiram in rats. *Pharmacol. Biochem. Behav.*, **13: S1**, 73–82.

Hellström, E. and Tottmar, O. (1982a) Acute effect of ethanol and acetaldehyde on blood pressure and heart rate in disulfiram-treated and control rats. *Pharmacol. Biochem. Behav.*, **17**, 1103–9.

Hellström, E. and Tottmar, O. (1982b) Effects of aldehyde dehydrogenase inhibitors on enzymes involved in the metabolism of biogenic aldehydes in rat liver and brain. *Biochem. Pharmacol.*, **31**, 3899–905.

Hellström, E., Tottmar, O. and Widerlöv, E. (1983) Effects of oral administration or implantation of disulfiram on aldehyde dehydrogenase activity of human blood. *Alcohol. Clin. Exp. Res.*, **7**, 231–6.

Hellström-Lindahl, E. and Oskarsson , A. (1989a) Increased availability of mercury in rat hepatocytes by complex formation with diethyldithiocarbamate. *Toxicol. Lett.*, **49**, 87–98.

Hellström-Lindahl, E. and Oskarsson, A. (1989b) Response of rat hepatocyte cultures to cadmium chloride and cadmium-diethyldithiocarbamate. *Toxicology*, **56**, 9–21.

Hempel, J.D. and Pietruszko, R. (1981) Selective chemical modification of human aldehyde dehydrogenases E_1 and E_2 by iodoacetamide. *J. Biol. Chem.*, **256**, 10889–96.

Hempel, J., Pietruszko, R., Fietzek, P. and Jörnvall, H. (1982) Identification of a segment containing a reactive cysteine residue in human liver cytoplasmic aldehyde dehydrogenase (isoenzyme E_1). *Biochemistry*, **21**, 6834–8.

Hempel, J., von Bahr-Lindström, H. and Jörnvall, H. (1984) Aldehyde dehydrogenase from human liver: Primary structure of the cytoplasmic isoenzyme. *Eur. J. Biochem.*, **141**, 21–35.

Hempel, J., Keiser, R. and Jörnvall, H. (1985) Mitochondrial aldehyde dehydrogenase from human liver: Primary structure, differences in relation to the cytosolic enzyme, and functional correlations. *Eur. J. Biochem.*, **153**, 13–28.

Hempel, J. and Jörnvall, H. (1986) Functional topology of aldehyde dehydrogenase structures. *Prog. Clin. Biol. Res.*, **232**, 1–14.

Hempel, J., Harper, K. and Lindahl, R. (1989) Inducible (Class 3) aldehyde dehydrogenase from rat hepatocellular carcinoma and 2,3,7,8-tetrachlorodibenzo-*p*-dioxin-treated liver: Distant relationship to the Class 1 and 2 enzymes from mammalian liver cytosol/mitochondria. *Biochemistry*, **28**, 1160–7.

Henehan, G.T.M., Ward, K., Kennedy, N.P., Weir, D.G. and Tipton, K.F. (1985) Subcellular distribution of aldehyde dehydrogenase activities in human liver. *Alcohol*, **2**, 107–10.

Hepner, G.W. and Vesell, E. (1974) Assessment of aminopyrine metabolism in man by breath analysis after oral administration of ^{14}C-aminopyrine. *N. Engl. J. Med.*, **291**, 1384–8.

Hersh, E.M., Petersen, E.A., Yocum, D.E., Gorman, R.S. and Darragh, J.M. (1987) Dose response study of diethyldithiocarbamate (DTC or Imuthiol) in patients (PTS) with ARC and AIDS. *Third International Conference on AIDS*, Abstract volume, National Institute of Health, Bethesda, MD, p. 47, Abstract MP.225.

Hersh, E.M., Mosier, D., Funk, C. and Petersen, E.A. (1988) Effective therapy of murine AIDS model (LP-BM5) retrovirus infection of C57BL6 mice with diethyldithiocarbamate (DTC). *Fourth International Conference on AIDS*, Abstract volume I, Stockholm, p. 228, Abstract 3035.

Hersh, E.W., Brewton, G. Abrams, D. *et al.* (1991) Ditiocarb sodium (diethyldithiocarbamate) therapy in patients with symptomatic HIV infection and AIDS: A randomized, double-blind, placebo-controlled, multicenter study. *J. Am. Med. Assoc.*, **265**, 1538–44.

Heubusch, P. and DiStefano, V. (1978) Activation of brain tyrosine hydroxylase in rats exposed to carbon disulfide and sodium diethyldithiocarbamate. *Tox. App. Pharmacol.*, **46**, 143–9.

Hidaka, H., Asano, T. and Takemoto, N. (1973) Analogues of fusaric (5-butylpicolinic) acid as potent inhibitors of dopamine β-hydroxylase. *Mol. Pharmacol.*, **9**, 172–7.

Hilton, J. (1984a) Deoxyribonucleic acid crosslinking by 4-hydroperoxycyclophosphamide in cyclophosphamide-sensitive and -resistant L1210 cells. *Biochem. Pharmacol.*, **33**, 1867–72.

Hilton, J. (1984b) Role of aldehyde dehydrogenase in cyclophosphamide-resistant L1210 leukemia. *Cancer Res.*, **44**, 5156–60.

Hine, C.H., Anderson, H.H., Macklin, A., Burbridge, T.N., Simon, A. and Bowman, K.M. (1950) Some observations of the effects of small doses of alcohol in patients receiving tetraethylthiuramdisulfide (Antabuse). *J. Pharmacol. Exp. Ther.*, **98**, 13–4.

Hine, C.H., Burbridge, T.N., Macklin, E.A., Anderson, H.H. and Simon, A. (1952) Some aspects of the human pharmacology of tetraethylthiuramdisulphide (Antabus)-alcohol reactions. *J. Clin. Invest.*, **31**, 317–25.

Hirschberg, M., Ludolph, A., Grotemeyer, K.H. and Gullotta, F. (1987) Development of a subacute tetraparesis after disulfiram intoxication. *Eur. Neurol.*, **26**, 222–8.

Ho, B.T., Khan, M.M., Major, L.F., Fang, V.S. and Estevez, V.S. (1985) Trace elements and disulfiram. In *Metal Ions in Neurology and Psychiatry* (eds), Alan Liss, New York, pp. 139–49.

Ho, S.B., DeMaster, E.G., Shafer, R.B., Levine, A.S., Morley, J.E., Go, V.L.W. and Allen, J.I. (1988) Opiate antagonist nalmefene inhibits ethanol-induced flushing in Asians: A preliminary study. *Alcohol. Clin. Exp. Res.*, **12**, 705–12.

Hoeldtke, R. and Kaufman, S. (1978) A tritium-release *in vivo* assay of dopamine-β-hydroxylase activity in sympathetic neurons. *Biochem. Pharmacol.*, **27**, 2499–506.

Hoeldtke, R.D. and Stetson, P.L. (1980) An *in vivo* tritium release assay of human dopamine B-hydroxylase. *J. Clin. Endocrinol. Metab.*, **51**, 810–5.

Honjo, T. and Netter, K.J. (1969) Inhibition of drug demethylation by disulfiram *in vivo* and *in vitro*. *Biochem. Pharmacol.*, **18**, 2681–3.

Hoon, D.S.B., Bowker, R. and Cochran, A.J. (1987) Suppressor cell activity in melanoma-draining lymph nodes. *Cancer Res.*, **47**, 1529–33.

Hopfer, S.M., Linden, J.V., Rezuke, W.N., O'Brien, J.E., Smith, L., Watters, F. and Sunderman, F.W., Jr (1987) Increased nickel concentrations in body fluids of patients with chronic alcoholism during disulfiram therapy. *Res. Commun. Chem. Pathol. Pharmacol.*, **55**, 101–9.

Horak, E., Sunderman, F.W., Jr and Sarkar, B. (1976) Comparison of antidotal efficiency of chelating drugs upon acute toxicity on Ni(II) in rats. *Res. Commun. Chem. Pathol. Pharmacol.*, **14**, 153–65.

Hörding, M., Götzsche, P.C., Bygbjerg, I.C., Christensen, L.D. and Faber, V. (1990) Lack of immunostimulating effect of disulfiram on HIV positive patients. *Int. J. Immunopharmacol.*, **12**, 145–7.

Hoshino, T., Ohta, Y. and Ishiguro, I. (1985) The effect of sulfhydryl compounds on the catalytic activity of Cu, Zn-superoxide dismutase purified form rat liver. *Experientia*, **41**, 1416–9.

Hotson, J.R. and Langston, J.W. (1976) Disulfiram-induced encephalopathy. *Arch. Neurol.*, **33**, 141–2.

Howell, J.M. (1964) Effect of sodium diethyldithiocarbamate on blood copper-levels and pregnancy in the rabbit. *Nature*, **201**, 83–4.

Howell, J.M. and Edington, N. (1968) The neurotoxicology of sodium diethyldithiocarbamate in the hen. *J. Neuropath. Exp. Neurol.*, **27**, 464–72.

Hsu, L.C., Tani, K., Fujiyoshi, T., Kurachi, K. and Yoshida, A. (1985) Cloning of cDNAs for human aldehyde dehydrogenases 1 and 2. *Proc. Natl. Acad. Sci. USA*, **82**, 3771–5.

Hulanicki, A. (1967) Complexation reactions of dithiocarbamates. *Talanta*, **14**, 1371–92.

Hunt, E.C., McNally, W.A. and Smith, A.F. (1973) A modified field test for the determination of carbon disulphide vapour in air. *Analyst*, **98**, 585–92.

Hunt, G.M. and Azrin, N.H. (1973) A community-reinforcement approach to alcoholism. *Behav. Res. Ther.*, **11**, 91–104.

Hunter, A.L. and Neal, R.A. (1975) Inhibition of hepatic mixed-function oxidase activity *in vitro* and *in vivo* by various thiono-sulfur-containing compounds. *Biochem. Pharmacol.*, **24**, 2199–205.

Hunter, F.E, and Lowry, O.H. (1956) The effects of drugs on enzyme systems. *Pharmacol. Rev.*, **8**, 89–135.

Hunter, J., Burnham, W.R., Chasseaud, L.F. and Down, W. (1974) Changes in D-glucaric acid excretion in relationship to alterations in the rate of antipyrine metabolism in man. *Biochem. Pharmacol.*, **23**, 2480–3.

Iber, F.L. and Chowdhury, B. (1977) The persistence of the alcohol-disulfiram reaction after discontinuation of drug in patients with and without liver disease. *Alcohol. Clin. Exp. Res.*, **1**, 365–70.

Iber, F.L., Dutta, S., Shamszad, M. and Krause, S. (1977) Excretion of radioactivity following the administration of ^{35}sulfur-labeled disulfiram in man. *Alcohol. Clin. Exp. Res.*, **1**, 359–64.

Iber, F.L., Lee, K., Lacoursiere, R. and Fuller, R. (1987) Liver toxicity encountered in the Veterans Administration trial of disulfiram in alcoholics. *Alcohol. Clin. Exp. Res.*, **11**, 301–4.

Impraim, C., Wang, G. and Yoshida, A. (1982) Structural mutation in a major aldehyde dehydrogenase gene results in loss of enzyme activity. *Am. J. Hum. Genet.*, **34**, 837–41.

Innes, J.R.M., Ulland, B.M., Valerio, M.G. *et al.* (1969) Bioassay of pesticides and industrial chemicals for tumorgenicity in mice: a preliminary note. *J. Natl. Cancer Inst.*, **42**, 1101–14.

Inoue, K., Ohbora, Y. and Yamasawa, K. (1978) Metabolism of acetaldehyde by human erythrocytes. *Life Sci.*, **23**, 179–84.

Inoue, K., Nishimukai, H. and Yamasawa, K. (1979) Purification and partial characterization of aldehyde dehydrogenase from human erythrocytes. *Bioch. Biophys. Acta*, **569**, 117–23.

Inoue, K., Kera, Y., Kiriyama, T. and Komura, S. (1985) Suppression of acetaldehyde accumulation by 4-methylpyrazole in alcohol-hypersensitive Japanese. *Jap. J. Pharmacol.*, **38**, 43–8.

Ioannides, C. and Parke, D.V. (1987) The cytochromes P-448 - A unique family of enzymes involved in chemical toxicology and carcinogenesis. *Biochem. Pharmacol.*, **36**, 4197–207.

Irth, H., De Jong, G.J., Brinkman, U.A.Th. and Frei, R.W. (1986) Metallic copper-containing post-column reactor for the detection of thiram and disulfiram in liquid chromatography. *J. Chromatogr.*, **370**, 439–47.

Irth, H., De Jong, G.J., Brinkman, U.A.Th. and Frei, R.W. (1988) Determination of disulfiram and two of its metabolites in urine by reversed-phase chromatography and spectrophotometric detection after post-column complexation. *J. Chromatogr.*, **424**, 95–102.

Jacobsen, D., Sebastian, C.S., Blomstrand, R. and McMartin, K.E. (1988) 4-Methylpyrazole: A controlled study of safety in healthy human subjects after single, ascending doses. *Alcohol. Clin. Exp. Res.*, **12**, 516–522.

Jacobsen, E. and Larsen, V. (1949) Site of the formation of acetaldehyde after ingestion of Antabuse (tetraethylthiuramdisulphide) and alcohol. *Acta Pharmacol.*, **5**, 285–91.

Jacobsen, E. and Martensen-Larsen, O. (1949) Treatment of alcoholism with tetraethylthiuram disulfide (Antabus). *J. Am. Med. Assoc.*, **139**, 918–22.

Jacobsen, E. (1952) Deaths of alcoholic patients treated with disulfiram (tetraethylthiuram disulfide) in Denmark. *Q. J. Stud. Alcohol*, **13**, 16–26.

Jacobsen, E. (1987) The road to Antabuse. Dumex, Copenhagen, 5 pp.

Jakubowski, M. and Gessner, T. (1972) S-methylation of dithiocarbamates derived from amino acids. *Biochem. Pharmacol.*, **21**, 3073–6.

James, W.O. (1953) The use of respiratory inhibitors. *Rev. Plant. Physiol.*, **4**, 59–90.

Jamieson, D. and van den Brenk, H.A.S. (1964) The effects of antioxidants on high pressure oxygen toxicity. *Biochem. Pharmacol.*, **13**, 159–64.

Jasim, S. and Tjälve, H. (1984) Effect of thiuram sulphides on the uptake and distribution of nickel in pregnant and non-pregnant mice. *Toxicology*, **32**, 297–313.

Jasim, S., Danielsson, B.R.G., Tjälve, H. and Dencker, L. (1985) Distribution of ^{64}Cu in foetal and adult tissues in mice: Influence of sodium diethyldithiocarbamate treatment. *Acta Pharmacol. Toxicol.*, **57**, 262–70.

Jasim, S. and Tjälve, H. (1986) Mobilization of nickel by potassium ethylxanthate in mice: comparison with sodium diethyldithiocarbamate and effect of intravenous versus oral administration. *Toxicol. Lett.*, **31**, 249–55.

Jensen, J.C. and Faiman, M.D. (1980) Determination of disulfiram and metabolites from biological fluids by high-performance liquid chromatography. *J. Chromatogr.*, **181**, 407–16.

Jensen, J.C., Faiman, M.D. and Hurwitz, A. (1982) Elimination characteristics of disulfiram over time in five alcoholic volunteers: A preliminary study. *Am. J. Psychiatry*, **139**, 1596–8.

Jensen, J.C. (1984) Pharmacokinetics and pharmacodynamics of the disulfiram-ethanol reaction. PhD Thesis, University of Kansas.

Jensen, J.C. and Faiman, M.D. (1984) Hypothermia as an index of the disulfiram-ethanol reaction in the rat. *Alcohol*, **1**, 97–100.

Jensen, J.C. and Faiman, M.D. (1986) Disulfiram-ethanol reaction in the rat. 1. Blood alcohol, acetaldehyde, and liver aldehyde dehydrogenase relationships. *Alcohol. Clin. Exp. Res.*, **10**, 45–9.

Jocelyn, P.C. (1972) *Biochemistry of the SH Group*, Academic Press, London, pp. 95–6.

Johansson, B. and Stankiewicz, Z. (1985) Bis-(diethyldithiocarbamato) copper complex: a new metabolite of disulfiram?. *Biochem. Pharmacol.*, **34**, 2989–91.

Johansson, B. (1986) Rapid and sensitive on-line precolumn purification and high-performance liquid chromatographic assay for disulfiram and its metabolites. *J. Chromatogr.*, **378**, 419–29.

Johansson, B. (1988) Stabilization and quantitative determination of disulfiram in human plasma samples. *Clin. Chim. Acta*, **177**, 55–64.

Johansson, B. (1989a) Pharmacological studies on disulfiram (Antabuse) in relation to its metabolism, inhibitory action, and elimination kinetics, with special reference to the metabolite diethylthiocarbamic acid methyl ester. Doctoral Dissertation, Lund University, Malmo, 118 pp.

Johansson, B. (1989b) Carbonyl sulfide: copper chelating metabolite of disulfiram. *Drug Metab. Disp.*, **17**, 351–3.

Johansson, B. (1989c) Diethylthiocarbamic acid methyl ester: A suicide inhibitor of liver aldehyde dehydrogenase? *Pharmacol. Toxicol.*, **64**, 471–4.

Johansson, B. and Stankiewicz, Z. (1989) Inhibition of erythrocyte aldehyde dehydrogenase activity and elimination kinetics of diethyldithiocarbamic acid methyl ester and its monothio analogue after administration of single and repeated doses of disulfiram to man. *Europ. J. Clin. Pharmacol.*, **37**, 133–8.

Johansson, B., Petersen, E.N. and Arnold, E. (1989) Diethylthiocarbamic acid methyl ester: A potent inhibitor of aldehyde dehydrogenase found in rats treated with disulfiram or diethyldithiocarbamic acid methyl ester. *Biochem. Pharmacol.*, **38**, 1053–9.

Johansson, B. (1990a) Distribution of disulfiram and its chief metabolites over erythrocyte cell membranes and inactivation of erythrocyte aldehyde dehydrogenase activity. *Pharmacol. Toxicol.*, **66**, 104–8.

Johansson, B. (1990b) Plasma protein binding of disulfiram and its metabolite diethyldithiocarbamic acid methyl ester. *J. Pharm. Pharmacol.*, **42**, 806–7.

Johansson, B., Angelo, H.R., Christensen, J.K., Moller, I.W. and Rønsted, P. (1991) Dose-effect relationship of disulfiram in human volunteers. II. A study of the relation between the disulfiram-ethanol reaction and plasma concentrations of acetaldehyde, diethyldithiocarbamic acid methyl ester, and erythrocyte aldehyde dehydrogenase activity. *Pharmacol. Toxicol.*, **68**, 166–70.

Johansson, J., von Bahr-Lindström, H., Jeck, R., Woenckhaus, C. and Jörnvall, H. (1988) Mitochondrial aldehyde dehydrogenase from horse liver: Correlations of the same species variants for both the cytosolic and the mitochondrial forms of an enzyme. *Eur. J. Biochem.*, **172**, 527–33.

Johnsen, J., Stowell, A., Stensrud, T., Ripel, and Mørland, J. (1990) A double-blind placebo controlled study of healthy volunteers given a subcutaneous disulfiram implant. *Pharmacol. Toxicol.*, **66**, 227–30.

Johnson, G.A., Boukma, S.J. and Kim, E.G. (1969) Inhibition of dopamine β-hydroxylase by aromatic and alkyl thioureas. *J. Pharmacol. Exp. Ther.*, **168**, 229–34.

Johnson, G.A., Boukma, S.J. and Kim, E.G. (1970) *In vivo* inhibition of dopamine β-hydroxylase by 1-phenyl-3(2-thiazolyl)-2-thiourea (U-14,624). *J. Pharmacol. Exp. Ther.*, **171**, 80–7.

Johnson, G.A., Kim, E.G. and Boukma, S.J. (1972) 5-Hydroxyindole levels in rat brain after inhibition of dopamine β-hydroxylase. *J. Pharmacol. Exp. Ther.*, **180**, 539–46.

Johnston, C.D. and Prickett, C.S. (1952) The production of carbon disulfide from tetraethylthiuram disulfide (Antabuse) by rat liver. *Biochim. Biophys. Acta*, **9**, 219–220.

Johnston, C.D. (1953) The *in vitro* reaction between tetraethylthiuram disulfide (Antabuse) and glutathione. *Arch. Bioch. Biophys.*, **44**, 249–51.

Jones, D.E., Jr, Brennan, M.D., Hempel, J. and Lindahl, R. (1988) Cloning and complete nucleotide sequence of a full-length cDNA encoding a catalytically functional tumor-associated aldehyde dehydrogenase. *Proc. Natl. Acad. Sci. USA*, **85**, 1782–6.

Jones, D.G. (1967) Human liver aldehyde oxidase: Differential inhibition of oxidation of charged and uncharged substrates. *J. Clin. Inv.*, **46**, 1492–505.

Jones, M.M., Basinger, M.A., Mitchell, W.M. and Bradley, C.A. (1986) Inhibition of *cis*-diamminedichloroplatinum(II)-induced renal toxicity in the rat. *Cancer Chemother. Pharmacol.*, **17**, 38–42.

Jones, M.M., Gale, G.R., Singh, P.K. and Smith, A.B. (1989) The rate of the *in vivo* dithiocarbamate-induced mobilization of hepatic and renal cadmium deposits. *Toxicology*, **58**, 313–23.

Jones, R.O. (1949) Death following ingestion of alcohol in an Antabuse treated patient. *Can. Med. Assoc. J.*, **60**, 609–12.

Jones, S.G. and Jones, M.M. (1984) Structure-activity relationships among dithiocarbamate antidotes for acute cadmium chloride intoxication. *Envir. Health Perspect.*, **54**, 285–90.

Jonsson, J., Grobecker, H. and Gunne, L.-M. (1967) Phenylethyldithiocarbamate: a new dopamine-β-hydroxylase inhibitor. *J. Pharm. Pharmacol.*, **19**, 201–3.

Jørgensen, L. and Johansen, T. (1983) Affinity of drugs for cytochrome P-450 determined by inhibition of *p*-nitrophenetole *O*-deethylation by rat liver microsomes. *Acta Pharmacol. Toxicol.*, **53**, 70–7.

Kaaber, K., Menne, T., Tjell, J.C. and Veien, N. (1979) Antabuse treatment of nickel dermatitis. Chelation – a new principle in the treatment of nickel dermatitis. *Contact Dermatitis*, **5**, 221–8.

Kaaber, K., Manne, T., Veien, N.K. and Baadsgaard, O. (1987) Some adverse effects of disulfiram in the treatment of nickel-allergic patients. *Dermatosen*, **35**, 209–11.

Kachru, D.N and Tandon, S.K. (1986) Chelation in metal intoxication. XX: Effect of pre-treatment with chelators on the distribution of mercury. *Res. Commun. Chem. Pathol. Pharmacol.*, **52**, 399–402.

Kahn, S., Farnum, J.B. and Thomas, E. (1990) Disulfiram-induced hepatitis. *South. Med. J.*, **83**, 833–6.

Kamerbeek, H.H., Rauws, A.G., ten Ham, M. and van Heijst, A.N.P. (1971) Dangerous redistribution of thallium by treatment with sodium diethyldithiocarbamate. *Acta Med. Scand.*, **189**, 149–54.

Kane, F.J. (1970) Carbon disulfide intoxication from overdosage of disulfiram. *Am. J. Psychiatry*, **127**, 690–4.

Kaplan, C.S., Petersen, E.A., Yocum, D. and Hersh, E.M. (1989) A randomized, controlled dose response study of intravenous diethyldithiocarbamate in patients with advanced human immunodeficiency virus infection. *Life Sci.*, **45**, iii–ix.

Karlsson, K. and Marklund, S.L. (1987) Heparin-induced release of extracellular superoxide dismutase to human blood plasma. *Biochem. J.*, **242**, 55–9.

Karlsson, K. and Marklund, S.L. (1988a) Plasma clearance of human extracellular-superoxide dismutase C in rabbits. *J. Clin. Inv.*, **82**, 762–6.

Karlsson, K. and Marklund, S.L. (1988b) Heparin-, dextran sulfate-, and protamine-induced release of extracellular-superoxide dismutase to plasma in pigs. *Biochim. Biophys. Acta*, **967**, 110–4.

Karlsson, K. and Marklund, S.L. (1989) Binding of human extracellular-superoxide dismutase C to cultured cell lines and to blood cells. *Lab. Invest.*, **60**, 659–66.

Kaslander, J. (1963) Formation of an *S*-glucuronide from tetraethylthiuram disulfide (Antabuse) in man. *Biochim. Biophys. Acta*, **71**, 730–2.

Keeffe, E.B. and Smith, F.W. (1974) Disulfiram hypersensitivity hepatitis. *J. Am. Med. Assoc.*, **230**, 435–6.

Keilin, D. and Hartree, E.F. (1940) Succinic dehydrogenase-cytochrome system of cells. Intracellular respiratory system catalyzing aerobic oxidation of succinic acid. *Proc. R. Soc., Lond.*, **B129**, 277–306.

Kelner, M.J. and Alexander, N.M. (1986) Inhibition of erythrocyte superoxide dismutase by diethyldithiocarbamate also results in oxyhemoglobin-catalyzed glutathione depletion and methemoglobin production. *J. Biol. Chem.*, **261**, 1636–41.

Kent, C.R.H. and Blekkenhorst, G.H. (1988) *In vivo* radiosensitization by diethyldithiocarbamate. *Radiat. Res.*, **116**, 539–46.

Khandekar, J.D. (1983) Improved therapeutic index of *cis*-diammine dichloro platinum by diethyldithiocarbamate in rodents. *Res. Commun. Chem. Pathol. Pharmacol.*, **40**, 55–66.

Khandelwal, S., Kachru, D.N. and Tandon, S.K. (1987) Influence of metal chelators on metalloenzymes. *Toxicol. Lett.*, **37**, 213–9.

Kiørboe, E. (1966) Phenytoin intoxication during treatment with Antabuse (disulfiram). *Epilepsia*, **7**, 246–9.

Kirchmayer, S., Cichocki, T., Bogdał, J. *et al.* (1979) Experimental studies on hepatotoxicity of disulfiram. *Materia Med. Polona*, **11**, 40–6.

Kitson, T.M. (1975) The effect of disulfiram on the aldehyde dehydrogenases of sheep liver. *Biochem. J.*, **151**, 407–12.

Kitson, T.M. (1976) The effect of some analogues of disulfiram on the aldehyde dehydrogenases of sheep liver. *Biochem. J.*, **155**, 445–8.

Kitson, T.M. (1977) The disulfiram-ethanol reaction: a review. *J. Stud. Alcohol*, **38**, 96–113.

Kitson, T.M. (1978) Studies on the interaction between disulfiram and sheep liver cytoplasmic aldehyde dehydrogenase. *Biochem. J.*, **175**, 83–90.

Kitson, T.M. (1979) 2,2-Dithiodipyridine activates aldehyde dehydrogenase and protects enzyme against inactivation by disulfiram. *Biochem. J.*, **183**, 751–3.

Kitson, T.M. (1982) Further studies of the action of disulfiram and 2,2-dithiodipyridine on the dehydrogenase and esterase activities of sheep liver cytoplasmic aldehyde dehydrogenase. *Biochem. J.*, **203**, 743–54.

Kitson, T.M. (1983) Mechanism of inactivation of sheep liver cytoplasmic aldehyde dehydrogenase by disulfiram. *Biochem. J.*, **213**, 551–4.

Kitson, T.M. and Loomes, K.M. (1984) The reaction of cytoplasmic aldehyde dehydrogenase, with various thiol-modifying reagents. *Prog. Clin. Biol. Res.*, 43–56.

Kitson, T.M. and Loomes, K.M. (1985) Modification of thiol groups in cytoplasmic aldehyde dehydrogenase. *Alcohol*, **2**, 97–101.

Kitson, T.M. (1987) Effect of disulfiram on the pre-steady-state burst in the reactions of sheep liver cytoplasmic aldehyde dehydrogenase. *Biochem. J.*, **248**, 989–91.

Kitson, T.M. (1988) Disulfide interchange reactions: An enzymic case study. *J. Chem. Ed.*, **9**, 829–32.

Kitson, T.M. (1989) Reaction between sheep liver mitochondrial aldehyde dehydrogenase and various thiol-modifying reagents. *Biochem. J.*, **261**, 281–4.

Kiyozumi, M., Nouchi, T., Honda, T., Kojima, S. and Tsuruoka, M. (1990) Comparison of effectiveness of 3 dithiocarbamates on excretion and distribution of cadmium in rats and mice. *Toxicology*, **60**, 275–85.

Kjeldgaard, N.E. (1949) Inhibition of aldehyde oxidase from liver by tetraethyl-thiuramdisulphide (Antabuse). *Acta Pharmacol.*, **5**, 397–403.

Klaassen, C.D., Waalkes, M.P. and Cantilena, L.R., Jr (1984) Alteration of tissue disposition of cadmium by chelating agents. *Environ. Health Perspect.*, **54**, 233–42.

Klebanskii, A.L. and Fomina, L.P. (1960) Radical and ionic reactions of tetraethyl-thiuram disulfide. *J. Gen. Chem. (USSR)*, **30**, 794.

Knee, S.T. and Razani, J. (1974) Acute organic brain syndrome: A complication of disulfiram therapy. *Am. J. Psychiatry*, **131**, 1281–2.

Kofoed, L.L. (1987) Chemical monitoring of disulfiram compliance: A study of alcoholic outpatients. *Alcohol. Clin. Exp. Res.*, **11**, 481–5.

Kohn, F.R., Landkamer, G.J., Manthey, C.L., Ramsay, N.K.C. and Sladek, N.E. (1987) Effect of aldehyde dehydrogenase inhibitors on the *ex vivo* sensitivity of human multipotent and committed hematopoietic progenitor cells and malignant blood cells to oxazaphosphorines. *Cancer Res.*, **47**, 3180–5.

Kolthoff, I.M. and Tan, B.H. (1965) Reactivity of sulfhydryl and disulfide in proteins. VI. Effect of heat denaturation of bovine serum albumin (BSA) on sulfhydryl and reactive disulfide content. *J. Am. Chem. Soc.*, **87**, 2717–20.

Kono, Y. and Fridovich, I. (1982) Superoxide radical inhibits catalase. *J. Biol. Chem.*, **257**, 5751–4.

Korhonen, A., Hemminiki, K. and Vainio, H. (1983) Embryotoxicity of industrial chemicals on the chicken embryo: dithiocarbamates. *Teratogen. Carcinogen. Mutagen.*, **3**, 163–75.

Koutenský, J., Eybl, V., Koutenská, M., Sýkora, J. and Mertl, F. (1971) Influence of sodium diethyldithiocarbamate on the toxicity and distribution of copper in mice. *Europ. J. Pharmacol.*, **14**, 389–92.

Kraemer, R.J. and Deitrich, R.A. (1968) Isolation and characterization of human liver aldehyde dehydrogenase. *J. Biol. Chem.*, **243**, 6402–8.

Kraml, M. (1973) A rapid test for Antabuse ingestion. *Cand. Med. Ass. J.*, **109**, 578.

Kristensen, M.E. (1981) Toxic hepatitis induced by disulfiram in a non-alcoholic. *Acta Med. Scand.*, **209**, 335–6.

Krivchenkova, R.S. and Safronov, A.P. (1964) K voprosu o primenenii dietilditiokarbamate natriya pri porazhenii poloniem (The use of sodium diethyldithiocarbamate in animals affected by polonium). In *Polonii Meditsina*, Moscow pp. 245–9 (*Biol. Abstr.*, **47**, 10458, 1966).

Kromhout, J., McClain, C.J., Zieve, L., Doizaki, W.M. and Gilberstadt, S. (1980) Blood mercaptan and ammonia concentrations in cirrhotics after a protein load. *Am. J. Gastroenterol.*, **74**, 507–11.

Kumar, K.S., Sancho, A.M. and Weiss, J.F. (1986) A novel interaction of diethyldithiocarbamate with glutathione/glutathione peroxidase system. *Int. J. Rad. Oncol.*, **12**, 1463–7.

Kupari, M., Lindros, K., Hillbom, M., Heikkilä, J. and Ylikahri, R. (1983) Cardiovascular effects of acetaldehyde accumulation after ethanol ingestion: Their modification by β-adrenergic blockade and alcohol dehydrogenase inhibition. *Alcohol. Clin. Exp. Res.*, **7**, 283–8.

Kurys, G., Ambroziak, W. and Pietruszko, R. (1989) Human aldehyde dehydrogenase: Purification and characterization of a third isozyme with low K_m for γ-aminobutyraldehyde. *J. Biol. Chem.*, **264**, 4715–21.

Kwentus, J. and Major, L.F. (1979) Disulfiram in the treatment of alcoholism. *J. Stud. Alcohol*, **40**, 428–46.

Lake, C.R., Major, L.F., Ziegler, M.G. and Kopin, I.J. (1977) Increased sympathetic nervous system activity in alcoholic patients treated with disulfiram. *Am. J. Psychiatry*, **134**, 1411–4.

Lake, C.R., Ziegler, M.G., Major, F.L., Brown, G.L. and Ebert, M.H. (1980) The effects of disulfiram on peripheral and central norepinephrine metabolism and blood pressure. In *Phenomenology and Treatment of Alcoholism*, (eds W.E. Fann, I. Karacan, A.C. Pokorny and R.L. Williams), Spectrum, New York, pp. 229–40.

Lakomaa, E.L., Sato, S., Goldberg, A.M. and Frazier, J.M. (1982) The effect of sodium diethyldithiocarbamate treatment on copper and zinc concentrations in rat brain. *Toxicol. App. Pharmacol.*, **65**, 286–90.

Lam, C-W. and DiStefano, V. (1986) Characterization of carbon disulfide binding in blood and to other biological substances. *Toxicol. App. Pharmacol.*, **86**, 235–42.

Lam, C-W., DiStefano, V. and Morken, D.A. (1986) The role of the red blood cell in the transport of carbon disulfide. *J. App. Toxicol.*, **6**, 81–6.

Lamboeuf, Y., de Saint-Blanquat, G. and Derache, R. (1974) Effects of disulfiram and three related compounds on the activity of alcohol dehydrogenase and aldehyde dehydrogenase in rat liver and gastric mucosa. *Clin. Exp. Pharmacol. Physiol.*, **1**, 361–8.

Landauer, M.R., Davis, H.D., Dominitz, J.A. and Weiss, J.F. (1988) Comparative behavioral toxicity of four sulfhydryl radioprotective compounds in mice: WR-

2721, cysteamine, diethyldithiocarbamate, and *N*-acetylcysteine. *Pharmacol. Ther.*, **39**, 97-100.

Lang, J.M., Oberling, F., Aleksijevic, A., Falkenrodt, A. and Mayer, S. (1985) Immunomodulation with diethyldithiocarbamate in patients with AIDS-related complex. *Lancet,* **ii**, 1066.

Lang, J.M., Aleksijevic, A., Falkenrodt, A., Mayer, S. and Oberling, F. (1986) Immunomodulation with sodium diethyldithiocarbamate (DTC) (Imuthiol) in patients with HIV-related illness. *Immunobiol.*, **173**, 412–3.

Lang, J.M., Oberling, F., Aleksijevic, A., Falkenrodt, A. and Mayer, S. (1987) Immunomodulation with diethyldithiocarbamate (DTC) (Imuthiol) in patients with HIV-related illness. In *Clinical Immunology* (eds W. Puzanski and M. Seligman), Elsevier, Amsterdam, pp. 205–8.

Lang, J.M., Falkenrodt, A., Colombat, P., Renoux, M. and Renoux, G. (1988a) Traitement par l'Imuthiol du complexe symptomatique associé au syndrome d'immunodéficit acquis: Premiers resultats a 2-3 ans. *Presse Med.*, **17**, 186–7.

Lang, J.M., Trepo, C., Kirstetter, M. *et al.* (1988b) Randomised, double-blind placebo-controlled trial of ditiocarb sodium ('Imuthiol') in human immunodeficiency virus infection. *Lancet,* **2**, 702–706.

Lang, J.M., Kirstetter, M., Touraine, J.L. and Livrozet, J.M. for the AIDS-Imuthiol French Study Group (1988c) Clinical and immunological effects of one-year treatment with Imuthiol in HIV⁺ infected homosexuals. *Fourth International Conference on AIDS*, Abstract volume I, Stockholm, p. 233, Abstract 3055.

Lang, M., Marselos, M. and Törrönen, R. (1976) Modification of drug metabolism by disulfiram and diethyldithiocarbamate. I. Mixed-function oxygenase. *Chem. Biol. Interact.*, **15**, 267–76.

Larseille, J., Younes, M. and Siegers, C.P. (1982) Influence of (+)-catechin and dithiocarb on the urinary excretion of D-glucaric acid in man. *IRCS-Biochem.*, **10**, 437.

Larsen, V. (1948) The effect on experimental animals of Antabuse (tetraethylthiuramdisulphide) in combination with alcohol. *Acta Pharmacol.*, **4**, 321–32.

Laskin J.D. and Piccini, L.A. (1986) Tyrosine isozyme heterogeneity in differentiating B16/C3 melanoma. *J. Biol. Chem.*, **261**, 16626–33.

Lear, J. and Navarro, D. (1987) Autoradiographic comparison of thallium-210 diethyldithiocarbamate, isopropyliodoamphetamine and iodoantipyrine as cerebral blood flow tracers. *J. Nucl. Med.*, **28**, 481–6.

Lear, J.L. (1988) Quantitative local cerebral blood flow measurements with technetium-99m HM-PAO: Evaluation using multiple radionuclide digital quantitative autoradiography. *J. Nucl. Med.*, **29**, 1387–92.

Lehr, H.A., Zimmer, J.P., Hubner, C. *et al.* (1989) Decreased plasma membrane fluidity of peripheral blood lymphocytes after diethyldithiocarbamate (DTC) therapy in HIV-infected patients. *Europ. J. Clin. Pharmacol.*, **37**, 521–3.

Lemarie, E., Lemarie, B. Saudeau, D., Lavandier, M., Renoux, M. and Renoux, G. (1986) Disseminated aspergillosis in a patient with bronchiectasis: A 15-month clinical and immunological follow-up. *Respiration,* **49**, 235–40.

Lemere, F. (1953) Disulfiram as a sedative in alcoholics. *Q. J. Stud. Alc.,* **14**,197–9.

Leo, M.A., Kim, C.-I., Lowe, N. and Lieber, C.S. (1989) Increased hepatic retinal dehydrogenase activity after phenobarbital and ethanol administration. *Biochem. Pharmacol.*, **38**, 97–103.

Lerner, A.B., Fitzpatrick, T.B., Calkins, E. and Summerson, W.H. (1950) Mammalian tyrosinase: The relationship of copper to enzymatic activity. *J. Biol. Chem.*, **187**, 793–802.

Lesourd, B.M., Vincent-Falquet, J.C., Deslandes, D., Musset, M. and Moulias, R. (1988) Influenza vaccination in the elderly: improved antibody response with imuthiol (Na diethyldithiocarbamate) adjuvant therapy. *Int. J. Immunopharmacol.*, **10**, 135–43.

Lester, D., Conway, E.J. and Mann, N.M. (1952) Evaluation of antidotes for the alcohol reaction syndrome in patients treated with disulfiram (tetraethylthiuram disulfide). *Q. J. Stud. Alcohol*, **13**, 1–8.

Levinson, W., Mikelens, P., Oppermann, H. and Jackson, J. (1978) Effect of Antabuse (disulfiram) on Rous sarcoma virus and on eukarotic cells. *Bioch. Biophys. Acta*, **519**, 65–75.

Levy, M.S., Livingstone, B.L. and Collins, D.M. (1967) A clinical comparison of disulfiram and calcium carbimide. *Am. J. Psychiatry*, **123**, 1018–22.

Lewis, M.J., Bland, R.C. and Baile, W. (1975) Disulfiram implantation for alcoholism. *Can. Psychiat. Ass. J.*, **20**, 283–6.

Li, T.-K. and Vallee, B.L. (1969) Alcohol dehydrogenase and ethanol metabolism. *Surg. Clin. North Am.*, **49**, 577–82.

Liddon, S.C. and Satran, R. (1967) Disulfiram (Antabuse) psychosis. *Am. J. Psychiatry*, **123**, 1284–9.

Liebson, I. and Faillace, L.A. (1971) The pharmacological reinforcement of disulfiram maintenance in chronic alcoholism. *Committee Report of the 33rd Annual Scientific Meeting of the Committee on Drug Dependence*, Toronto, pp. 1262–72.

Liebson, I. and Bigelow, G. (1972) A behavioural-pharmacological treatment of dually addicted patients. *Behav. Res. Ther.*, **10**, 403–5.

Liebson, I., Bigelow, G. and Flamer, R. (1973) Alcoholism among methadone patients: A specific treatment method. *Am. J. Psychiatry* **130**, 483–5.

Liebson, I.A., Tommasello, A. and Bigelow, G. (1978) A behavioral treatment of alcoholic methadone patients. *Ann. Intern. Med.*, **89**, 342–4.

Lieder, P.H. and Borch, R.F. (1985) Triethyloxonium tetrafuoroborate derivatization and HPLC analysis of diethyldithiocarbamate in plasma. *Anal. Lett.*, **18**, 57–66.

Lin, P.S., Kwock, L. and Butterfield, C.E. (1979) Diethyldithiocarbamate enhancement of radiation and hyperthermic effects on Chinese hamster cells *in vitro*. *Radiat. Res.*, **77**, 501–11.

Lin, P.S., Quamo, S., Ho, K.-L. and Baur, K. (1985) The diethyldithiocarbamate concentration effects and interactions with other cytotoxic agents on chinese hamster cells (V79). *Radiat. Res.*, **102**, 271–82.

Lindahl, R. and Evces, S. (1984a) Rat liver aldehyde dehydrogenase. I. Isolation 40 and characterization of four high K_m normal liver isozymes. *J. Biol. Chem.*, **259**, 11986–90.

Lindahl, R. and Evces, S. (1984b) Rat liver aldehyde dehydrogenase. II. Isolation and characterization of four inducible isozymes. *J. Biol. Chem.*, **259**, 11991–6.

Lindahl, R. and Evces, S. (1984c) Comparative subcellular distribution of aldehyde dehydrogenase in rat, mouse and rabbit liver. *Bioch. Pharmacol.*, **33**, 3383–9.

Linderholm, H. and Berg, K. (1951) A method for the determination of tetraethylthiuram disulphide (Antabus, Abstinyl) and diethyldithiocarbamate in blood and urine: Some studies on the metabolism of tetraethylthiuram disulphide. *Scand. J. Clin. Lab. Invest.*, **3**, 96–102.

Lindros, K.O., Vihma, R. and Forsander, O.A. (1972) Utilization and metabolic effects of acetaldehyde and ethanol in the perfused rat liver. *Biochem. J.*, **126**, 945–52.

Lindros, K.O., Stowell, A., Pekkarainen, P. and Salaspuro, M. (1981) The disulfiram (Antabuse)-alcohol reaction in male alcoholics: Its efficient management by 4-methylpyrazole. *Alcohol. Clin. Exp. Res.*, **5**, 528–30.

Lippmann, W. and Lloyd, K. (1969) Dopamine-β-hydroxylase inhibition by dimethyldithiocarbamate and related compounds. *Biochem. Pharmacol.*, **18**, 2507–16.

Liskow, B.I. and Goodwin, D.W. (1987) Pharmacological treatment of alcohol intoxication, withdrawal and dependence: a critical review. *J. Stud. Alcohol*, **48**, 356–70.

Loft, S., Sonne, J., Pilsgaard, H., Døssing, M. and Poulsen, E. (1986) Inhibition of antipyrine elimination by disulfiram and cimetidine: the effect of concomitant administration. *Br. J. Clin. Pharmacol.*, **21**, 75–7.

Loi, C.-M., Day, J.D., Jue, S.G., Bush, E.D., Costello, P., Dewey, L.V. and Vestal, R.E. (1989) Dose-dependent inhibition of theophylline metabolism by disulfiram in recovering alcoholics. *Clin. Pharmacol. Ther.*, **45**, 476–86.

Loiseau, P., Brachet, A., Henry, P. and Cenraud, P. (1975) Intoxication par la diphénylhydantoïne lors d'une cure de disulfirame. *Nouv. Pres. Med.*, **4**, 504.

Lubetkin, B.S., Rivers, P.C. and Rosenberg, C.M. (1971) Difficulties of disulfiram therapy with alcoholics. *Q. J. Stud. Alcohol*, **32**, 168–71.

Ludwig, A.M., Levine, J. and Stark, L.H. (1970) *LSD and Alcoholism: A Study of Treatment Efficiency.* Charles Thomas, Springfield, IL, USA.

Ludwig, R.A. and Thorn, G.D. (1960) Chemistry and mode of action of dithiocarbamate fungicides. *Adv. Pest Control Res.*, **3**, 219–52.

Lundwall, L. and Baekeland, F. (1971) Disulfiram treatment of alcoholism: A review. *J. Nerv. Ment. Dis.*, **153**, 381–94.

Luzy, T., Creach, O. and Fontanges, R. (1983) Efficacité de la vaccination par voie buccale contre *Salmonella typhimurium* chez la souris préalablement soumise à un traitement immunostimulant. *C.R. Soc. Biol.*, **177**, 616–25.

Mach, T. (1986) Effect of disulfiram on function of the liver of rats with galactosamine-induced hepatitis. *Pol. J. Pharmacol. Pharm.*, **38**, 235–41.

MacKerell, A.D., Jr, Vallari, R.C. and Pietruszko, R. (1985) Human mitochondrial aldehyde dehydrogenase inhibition by diethyldithiocarbamic acid methanethiol mixed disulfide: a derivative of disulfiram. *FEBS Lett.*, **179**, 77–81.

MacKerell, A.D., Jr, Blatter, E.E. and Pietruszko, R. (1986) Human aldehyde dehydrogenase: Kinetic identification of the isozyme for which biogenic aldehydes and acetaldehyde compete. *Alcohol. Clin. Exp. Res.*, **10**, 266–70.

MacLeod, S.M., Sellers, E.M., Giles, H.G. *et al.* (1978) Interaction of disulfiram with benzodiazepines. *Clin. Pharmacol. Ther.*, **24**, 583–9.

Magos, L. and Jarvis, J.A.E. (1970) The effect of carbon disulfide exposure on brain catecholamines in rats. *Br. J. Pharmacol.*, **39**, 26–33.

Mains, R.E., Park, L.P. and Eipper, B.A. (1986) Inhibition of peptide amidation by disulfiram and diethyldithiocarbamate. *J. Biol. Chem.*, **261**, 11938–41.

Maj, J. and Vetulani, J. (1969) Effect of some *N,N*-disubstituted dithiocarbamates on catecholamines level in rat brain. *Biochem. Pharmacol.*, **18**, 2045–7.

Maj, J. and Vetulani, J. (1970) Some pharmacological properties of *N,N*-disubstituted dithiocarbamates and their effects on the brain catecholamine levels. *Europ. J. Pharmacol.*, **9**, 183–9.

Major, L.F., Ziegler, M.G., Lake, C.R. and Brown, G.L. (1977a) The effects of disulfiram on plasma norepinephrine in male alcoholics. In *Currents in Alcoholism,* Vol. 1 (ed. F.A. Seixas), Grune and Stratton, New York, pp. 197–208.

Major, L.F., Ballenger, J.C., Goodwin, F.K. and Brown, G.L. (1977b) Cerebrospinal fluid homovanillic acid in male alcoholics: Effects of disulfiram. *Biol. Psychiatry*, **12**, 635–42.

Major, L.F. and Goyer, P.F. (1978) Effects of disulfiram and pyridoxine on serum cholesterol. *Ann. Intern. Med.*, **88**, 53–6.

Major, L.F., Lerner, P., Ballenger, J.C., Brown, G.L., Goodwin, F.K. and Lovenberg, W (1979a) Dopamine-β-hydroxylase in the cerebrospinal fluid: Relationship to disulfiram-induced psychosis. *Biol. Psychiatry*, **14**, 337–44.

Major, L.F., Murphy, D.L., Gershon, E.S. and Brown, G.L. (1979b) The role of plasma amine oxidase, platelet monoamine oxidase, and red cell catechol-O-methyl transferase in severe behavioral reactions to disulfiram. *Am. J. Psychiatry*, **136**, 679–84.

Major, L.F., Lerner, P., Dendel, P.S., Glaser, L. and Post, R.M. (1982) Effects of prolonged disulfiram treatment on plasma dopamine-β-hydroxylase activity in rhesus monkeys. *J. Stud. Alcohol*, **43**, 146–52.

Maners, A.W., Walker, E.M., Jr, Baker, M. and Pappas, A. (1985) Diethyldithiocarbamate as a radiation modifier. *Ann. Clin. Lab. Sci.*, **15**, 343–4.

Mannervik, B. (1985) The isoenzymes of glutathione transferase. *Adv. Enzymol.*, **57**, 357–417.

Mansner, R., Mattila, M.J. and Idänpään-Heikkilä, J.E. (1968) Lack of responses to 5-hydroxytryptamine of the ileum of the disulfiram-treated rat. *Ann. Med. Exp. Fenn.*, **46**, 385–9.

Mansour, H., Levacher, M., Gougerot-Pocidalo, M.A., Rouveix, B. and Pocidalo, J. (1986) Diethyldithiocarbamate provides partial protection against pulmonary and lymphoid oxygen toxicity. *J. Pharmacol. Exp. Ther.*, **236**, 476–80.

Manthey, C.L., Landkamer, G.J. and Sladek, N.E. (1990) Identification of the mouse aldehyde dehydrogenases important in aldophosphamide detoxication. *Cancer Res.*, **50**, 4991–5002.

Marchand, J.E., Hershman, K., Kumar, M.S.A., Thompson, M.L. and Kream, R.M. (1990) Disulfiram administration affects substance P-like immunoreactive and monoaminergic neural systems in rodent brain. *J. Biol. Chem.*, **265**, 264–73.

Marchner, H. and Tottmar, O. (1978) A comparative study on the effects of disulfiram, cyanamide and 1-aminocyclopropanol on the acetaldehyde metabolism in rats. *Acta Pharmacol. Toxicol.*, **43**, 219–32.

Marconi, J., Solari, G. and Gaete, S. (1961) Comparative clinical study of the effects of disulfiram and calcium carbimide. II. Reaction to alcohol. *Q. J. Stud. Alcohol*, **22**, 46–51.

Mardini, H.A., Bartlett, K. and Record, C.O. (1984) Blood and brain catecholamine concentrations of mercaptans in hepatic and methanethiol induced coma. *Gut*, **25**, 284–90.

Marie, C. (1955) A propos d'un nouveau mode de traitement de l'alcoolisme chronique par implantation de disulfure de tétra-éthyle-thio-urame. Thèse, Paris, 51 pp.

Mariman, E.C.M. (1986) The AIDS combat: A survey. *Biomed. Pharmacother.*, **40**, 399-407.

Markham, J.D. and Hoff, E.C. (1953) Toxic manifestations in the Antabuse-alcohol reaction: A study of electrocardiographic changes. *J. Am. Med. Assoc.*, **152**, 1597–600.

Marklund, S.L. (1980) Distribution of CuZn superoxide dismutase and Mn superoxide dismutase in human tissues and extracellular fluid. *Acta Physiol. Scand.*, **Suppl. 429**, 19–23.

Marklund, S.L. and Westman, G. (1980) Copper-zinc superoxide dismutase and the radiation sensitivity of Chinese hamster cells. In *Biological and Clinical Aspects of Superoxide and Superoxide Dismutase*, (eds W.H. Bannister and J.V. Bannister), Elsevier Biomedical, Amsterdam, pp. 318–26.

Marklund, S.L. (1984) Properties of extracellular superoxide dismutase from human lung. *Biochem. J.*, **220**, 269–72.

Marquart, D.W. (1964) NLIN: Least-squares estimation of nonlinear parameters. IBM Share General Program Library, No. 3094.

Marselos, M., Lang, M. and Torronen, R. (1976) Modifications of drug metabolism by disulfiram and diethyldithiocarbamate. II. Glucuronic acid pathway. *Chem. Biol. Interact.*, **15**, 277–87.

Martensen-Larsen, O. (1948) Treatment of alcoholism with a sensitizing drug. *Lancet*, **255**, 1004–5.

Martensen-Larsen, O. (1950) Antabusdosering til alkoholpavirkede. *Nord. Med.*, **43**, 805.

Martensen-Larsen, O. (1951) Psychotic phenomena provoked by tetraethylthiuram disulfide. *Q. J. Stud. Alcohol*, **12**, 206–16.

Masso, P.D. and Kramer, P.A. (1981) Simultaneous determination of disulfiram and two of its dithiocarbamate metabolites in human plasma by reversed-phase liquid chromatography. *J. Chromatogr.*, **224**, 457–64.

Masuda, Y., Yasoshima, M. and Nakayama, N. (1986) Early, selective and reversible suppression of cytochrome P-450-dependent monooxygenase of liver microsomes following administration of low doses of carbon disulfide in mice. *Biochem. Pharmacol.*, **35**, 3941–7.

Masuda, Y. (1988) Oxidation of diethyldithiocarbamate to disulfiram by liver microsomes in the presence of NADPH and subsequent loss of microsomal enzyme activity *in vitro*. *Res. Commun. Chem. Pathol. Pharmacol.*, **62**, 251–66.

Masuda, Y., Yasoshima, M. and Shibata, K. (1988) Effects of carbon disulfide, diethyldithiocarbamate, and disulfiram on drug metabolism in the perfused rat liver. *Res. Commun. Chem. Pathol. Pharmacol.*, **61**, 65–82.

Masuda, Y. and Nakamura, Y. (1989) Oxidation of diethyldithiocarbamate to disulfiram by liver microsomal cytochrome P-450 containing monooxygenase system. *Res. Commun. Chem. Pathol. Pharmacol.*, **66**, 57–67.

Mathews, A.P. and Walker, S. (1909) The action of metals and strong salt solutions on the spontaneous oxidation of cystein. *J. Biol. Chem.*, **6**, 299–312.

Matkovics, B., Barabás, K., Varga, S.I., Szabó, L. and Berencsi, G. (1982) Some new data to the toxicological effects of paraquat and the therapy. *Gen. Pharmacol.*, **13**, 333–41.

Mazumder, R., Das, T.K. and Biswas, N.M. (1985) Spermatogenesis of rat: Effect of central norepinephrine synthesis inhibition by diethyldithiocarbamate. *Andrologia*, **17**, 400–5.

McClain, C.J., Zieve, L., Doizaki, W.M., Gilberstadt, S. and Onstad, G.R. (1980) Blood methanethiol in alcoholic liver disease with and without hepatic encephalopathy. *Gut*, **21**, 318–23.

McConchie, R.D., Panitz, D.R., Sauber, S.R. and Shapiro, S. (1983) Disulfiram-induced *de novo* seizures in the absence of ethanol challenge. *J. Stud. Alcohol*, **44**, 739–43.

McKee, R.W. (1941) A quantitative microchemical colorimetric determination of carbon disulfide in air, water and biological fluids. *J. Ind. Hyg. Toxicol.*, **23**, 151–8.

McKenna, M.J. and DiStefano, V. (1977a) Carbon disulfide I. The metabolism of inhaled carbon disulfide in the rat. *J. Pharmacol. Exp. Ther.*, **202**, 245–52.

McKenna, M.J. and DiStefano, V. (1977b) Carbon disulfide II. A proposed mechanism for the action of carbon disulfide on dopamine beta-hydroxylase. *J. Pharmacol. Exp. Ther.*, **202**, 253–66.

McNichol, R.W., Ewing, J.A. and Faiman, M.D. (1987) *Disulfiram (Antabuse), a Unique Medical Aid to Sobriety: History, Pharmacology, Research, Clinical Use.* Charles C. Thomas, Springfield, IL, 101 pp.

Medical Letter (1980) Disulfiram (Antabuse) *Med. Lett. Drugs Ther.*, **22**, (1) 1–2.

Meister, A. and Anderson, M.E. (1983) Glutathione. *Annu. Rev. Biochem.*, **52**, 711–60.

Mello, N.K. and Mendelson, J.H. (1972) Drinking patterns during work-contingent and noncontingent alcohol acquisition. *Psychosom. Med.*, **34**, 139–64.

Menné, T., Kaaber, K. and Tjell, J.C. (1980) Treatment of nickel dermatitis: The influence of tetraethylthiuramdisulfide (Antabuse) on nickel metabolism. *Ann. Clin. Lab. Sci.*, **10**, 160–4.

Menné, T. and Hjorth, N. (1982) Reactions from systemic exposure to contact allergens. *Some. Dermatol.*, **1**, 15–24.

Menon, C.R. and Nieboer, E. (1986) Uptake of nickel(II) by human peripheral mononuclear leukocytes. *J. Inorg. Biochem.*, **28**, 217–25.

Merck Index (1968) *The Merck Index, An Encyclopedia of Chemical and Drugs* (ed. P.G. Stecher), 8th edn., Merck, Rahway, NJ, p. 958.

Merck Index (1987) *The Merck Index, An Encyclopedia of Chemical, Drugs and Biologicals* (ed. S. Budavari), 11th edn., Merck, Rahway, NJ, p. 533.

Mercurio, F. (1952) Antabuse-alcohol reaction following use of after-shave lotion. *J. Am. Med. Assoc.*, **149**, 82.

Merlevede, E. and Casier, H. (1961) Teneur en sulfure de carbone de l'air expiré chez des personnes normales ou sous l'influence de l'alcool éthylique au cours du traitement par l'Antabuse (disulfiram) et le diéthyldithiocarbamate de soude (1). *Arch. Int. Pharmacodyn. Ther.*, **82**, 427–53.

Meshnick, S., Febbraio, M., Edwards, S., Abosch, A., Fairfield, A. and Eaton, J. (1986) The antimalaria activity of DDC-treated superoxide dismutase. In *Superoxide and Superoxide Dismutase in Chemistry, Biology and Medicine* (ed. G. Rotilio), Elsevier, Amsterdam, pp. 562–4.

Meshnick, S.R., Scott, M.D., Lubin, B., Ranz, A. and Eaton, J.W. (1990) Antimalarial activity of diethyldithiocarbamate: Potentiation by copper. *Biochem. Pharmacol.*, **40**, 213–6.

Metcalf, D. (1984) *The Hemopoietic Colony Stimulating Factors.* Elsevier, Amsterdam, pp. 124–8.

Michiels, C. and Remacle, J. (1988) Use of inhibition of enzymatic antioxidant systems in order to evaluate their physiological importance. *Eur. J. Biochem.*, **177**, 435–41.

Milandri, M., Poulsen, H.E., Ranek, L. and Andreasen, P.B. (1980) Effect of long-term disulfiram administration on rat liver. *Pharmacology*, **21**, 76–80.

Milas, L., Hunter, N., Ito, H. and Peters, L.J. (1984) *In vivo* radioprotective activities of diethyldithiocarbamate (DDC). *Int. J. Rad. Oncol.*, **10**, 2335–43.

Milich, D.R. and Gershwin, M.E. (1977) T cell differentiation and the congenitally athymic (nude) mice. *Develop. Comp. Immunol.*, **1**, 289–98.

Miller, G.E., Zemaitis, M.A. and Greene, F.E. (1983) Mechanism of diethyldithiocarbamate-induced loss of cytochrome P-450 from the liver. *Biochem. Pharmacol.*, **32**, 2433–42.

Mills, C.F. and Fell, B.F. (1960) Demyelination in lambs born of ewes maintained on high intakes of sulphate and molybdate. *Nature*, 185, 20–2.

Minegishi, A., Fukumori, R., Satoh, T., Kitagawa, H. and Yanura, S. (1979) Changes in serotonin turnover and the brain sensitivity to barbiturates by disulfiram treatment in rats. *Res. Commun. Chem. Pathol. Pharmacol.*, 24, 273–87.

Misra, H.P. (1979) Reaction of copper-zinc superoxide dismutase with diethyldithiocarbamate. *J. Biol. Chem.*, 254, 11623–8.

Mitchell, C.L., Barnes, M.I. and Grimes, L.M. (1990) Diethyldithiocarbamate and dithizone augment the toxicity of kainic acid. *Brain Res.*, 506, 327–30.

Mitchell, J., Horak, E. and Sunderman, F.J., Jr (1978) Antidotal efficacy of chelating drugs upon acute toxicity of nickel carbonyl inhalation in rats. *Clin. Toxicol.*, 12, 606–7.

Miura, T., Ogawa, N. and Ogiso, T. (1978) Involvement of superoxide radicals in the formation of methemoglobin from oxyhemoglobin: Inhibition of superoxide dismutase by diethyldithiocarbamate. *Chem. Pharm. Bull. (Tokyo)*, 26, 1261–6.

Mizoi, Y., Ijiri, I., Tatsuno, Y. *et al.* (1979) Relationship between facial flushing and blood acetaldehyde levels after alcohol intake. *Pharm. Biochem. Behav.*, 10, 303–11.

Mizoi, Y., Adachi, J., Kogame, M. and Fukunaga, T. (1982) Polymorphism of aldehyde dehydrogenase and catecholamine metabolism. *Prog. Clin. Biol. Res.*, 114, 363–77.

Mizoi, Y., Tatauno, Y., Adachi, J. *et al.* (1983) Alcohol sensitivity related to polymorphism of alcohol-metabolizing enzymes in Japanese. *Pharmacol. Biochem. Behav.*, 18, Suppl. 1, 127–33.

Mizoi, Y., Kogame, M., Fukunaga, T. *et al.* (1988) Profile of ethanol metabolism: Aldehyde dehydrogenase deficiency and its significance. In *Biomedical Aspects of Alcohol and Alcoholism* (eds T. Kamada, K. Kuriyama and H. Suwaki), Gendaikikakushitsu Publishing, Tokyo, pp. 31–45.

Moddel, G., Bilbao, J.M., Payne, D. and Ashby, P. (1978) Disulfiram neuropathy. *Arch. Neurol.*, 35, 658–60.

Mokri, B., Ohnishi, A. and Dyck, P.J. (1981) Disulfiram neuropathy. *Neurology*, 31, 730–5.

Moldowan, M.J. and Acholonu, W., Jr (1982) Effect of ascorbic acid or thiamine on acetaldehyde, disulfiram-ethanol- or disulfiram-acetaldehyde induced mortality. *Agents Actions*, 12, 731–6.

Mondovì, B., Rotilio, G., Costa, M.T. Finazzi-Agrò, A., Chiarcone, E., Hanson, R.E. and Beinert, H. (1967) Diamine oxidase from pig kidney: Improved purification and properties. *J. Biol. Chem.*, 242, 1160–7.

Montine, T.J. and Borch, R.F. (1988) Quiescent LLC-PK$_1$ cells as a model for cis-diamminedichloroplatinum(II) nephrotoxicity and modulation by thiol rescue agents. *Cancer Res.*, 48, 6017–24.

Moore, K.E. (1969) Effects of disulfiram and diethyldithiocarbamate on spontaneous locomotor activity and brain catecholamine levels in mice. *Biochem. Pharmacol.*, 18, 1627–34.

Morell, A.G. and Scheinberg, L.H. (1958) Preparation of an apoprotein from ceruloplasmin by reversible dissociation of copper. *Science*, 127, 588–90.

Mori, T., Watanabe, M., Horikawa, M., Nikaido, P., Kimuri, H., Aoyama, T. and Sugahara, T. (1983) WR-2721, its derivatives and their radioprotective effects on mammalian cells in culture. *Int. J. Radiat. Biol.*, 44, 41–53.

Mörland, J., Johnsen, J., Bache-Wiig, J.E., Ripel, A., Stensrud, T. and Stowell, A. (1984) Implanted disulfiram: Pharmacological and clinical studies in man. In *Pharmaco-*

logical Treatment of Alcoholism: Withdrawal and Aversion Therapy, Socialstyrelsens Lakemedelsavdelning, 75125 Uppsala, Sweden, 1985/2 pp. 89–98.

Morpurgo, L., Desideri, A., Rigo, A., Viglino, P. and Rotilio, G. (1983) Reaction of *N,N*-diethyldithiocarbamate and other bidentate ligands with Zn, Co, and Cu bovine carbonic anhydrases: Inhibition of the enzyme activity and evidence for stable ternary enzyme-metal-ligand complexes. *Biochim. Biophys. Acta*, **746**, 168–75.

Morpurgo, L., Agostinelli, E., Befani, O. and Mondovì, B. (1987a) Reactions of bovine serum amine oxidase with *N,N*-diethyldithiocarbamate: Selective removal of one copper ion. *Biochem. J.*, **248**, 865–70.

Morpurgo, L., Savini, I., Mondovi, B. and Avigliano, L. (1987b) Removal of type 2 Cu from ascorbate oxidase and laccase by reaction with *N,N*-diethyldithiocarbamate. *J. Inorg. Chem.*, **29**, 25–31.

Morpurgo, L., Savini, I., Gatti, G., Bolognesi, M. and Avigliano, L. (1988) Reassessment of copper stoichiometry in ascorbate oxidase. *Biochem. Biophys. Res. Commun.*, **152**, 623–8.

Morris, S.J., Kanner, R., Chiprut, R.O. and Schiff, E.R. (1978) Disulfiram hepatitis. *Gastroenterology*, **75**, 100–2.

Mossalayi, M.D., Descombe, J.J., Musset, M., Tanzer, J. and Goube de Laforest, P. (1986) *In vitro* effects of sodium diethyldithiocarbamate (Imuthiol) on human T lymphocytes. *Int. J. Immunopharmacol.*, **8**, 841–4.

Mozdzierz, G.J., Goetz, D.J., Semyck, R., DeVito, R. and Davis, W.E. (1981) Coffee consumption among alcoholics as a function of time hospitalized. *Int. J. Addict.*, **16**, 253–62.

Mullin, M.J. and Ferko, A.P. (1981) Ethanol and functional tolerance: Interactions with pimozide and clonidine. *J. Pharmacol. Exp. Ther.*, **216**, 459–64.

Mür, J. (1964) Analytische Reagenzstoffe im neuropathologischen Versuch: Demyelinisation durch Chelat bildende Stoffe. *Confin. Neurol.*, **24**, 235–56.

Murthy, M.S., Rao, L.N., Khandekar, J.D. and Sanilon, E.F. (1987) Enhanced therapeutic efficacy of cisplatin by combination with diethyldithiocarbamate and hyperthermia in a mouse model. *Cancer Res.*, **47**, 774–9.

Musacchio, J., Kopin, I.J. and Snyder, S. (1964) Effects of disulfiram on tissue norepinephrine content and subcellular distribution of dopamine, tyramine and their β-hydroxylated metabolites. *Life Sci.*, **3**, 769–75.

Musacchio, J.M., Goldstein, M., Anagnoste, B., Poch, G. and Kopin, I.J. (1966a) Inhibition of dopamine-β-hydroxylase by disulfiram *in vivo*. *J. Pharmacol. Exp. Ther.*, **152**, 56–61.

Musacchio, J.M., Bhagat, C. Jackson, C.J. and Kopin, I.J. (1966b) The effect of disulfiram on the restoration of the response to tyramine by dopamine and α-methyldopa in the reserpine-treated cat. *J. Pharmacol. Exp. Ther.*, **152**, 293–7.

Nagatsu, T., Levitt, M. and Udenfriend, S. (1964) Tyrosine hydroxylase: The initial step in norepinephrine synthesis. *J. Biol. Chem.*, **239**, 2910–7.

Nakano, J., Holloway, J.E. and Schackford, J.S. (1969) Effect of disulfiram on the cardiovascular responses to ethanol in dogs and guinea pigs. *Toxicol. App. Pharmacol.*, **14**, 439–46.

Nakayama, N. and Masuda, Y. (1985) Suppression of phenacetin-induced methemoglobinemia by diethyldithiocarbamate and carbon disulfide and its relation to phenacetin metabolism in mice. *J. Pharmacobio-Dyn.*, **8**, 868–76.

Nakano, J., Gin, A.C. and Nakano, S.K. (1974) Effects of disulfiram on cardiovascular responses to acetaldehyde and ethanol in dogs. *Q. J. Stud. Alcohol*, **35**, 620–34.

Nakazawa, M., Tsuchiya, M., Hayasaka, S. and Mizuno, K. (1985) Tyrosinase activity in the uveal tissue of the adult bovine eye. *Exp. Eye. Res.*, 41, 249–58.

Nash, N.G. and Daley, R.D. (1975) Disulfiram. *Anal. Profiles Drug Subs.*, 4, 168–91.

Nasrallah, H.V. (1979) Vulnerability to disulfiram psychoses. *West J. Med.*, 130, 575–7.

Nässberger, L. (1984a) Disulfiram-induced hepatitis–report of a case and review of the literature. *Postgrad. Med. J.*, 60, 639–41.

Nässberger, L. (1984b) Hepatotoxicity due to disulfiram. *J. Toxicol. Clin. Toxicol.*, 22, 403–8.

National Cancer Institute (1979) Bioassay of sodium diethyldithiocarbamate for possible carcinogenicity. *Carcinogenesis Technical Report Series*, 172, 35 pp.

Neiderhiser, D.H., Fuller, R.K., Hejduk, L.J. and Roth, H.P. (1976) Method for the detection of diethylamine, a metabolite of disulfiram, in urine. *J. Chromatog.*, 117, 187–92.

Neiderhiser, D.H. and Fuller, R.K. (1980) The metabolism of ^{14}C-disulfiram by the rat. *Alcohol. Clin. Exp. Res.*, 4, 277–81.

Neiderhiser, D.H., Wych, G. and Fuller, R.K. (1983) The metabolic fate of double-labeled disulfiram. *Alcohol. Clin. Exp. Res.*, 7, 199–202.

Neims, A.H., Coffey, D.S. and Hellerman, L. (1966a) A sensitive radioassay for sulfhydryl groups with tetraethylthiuram disulfide. *J. Biol. Chem.*, 241, 3036–40.

Neims, A.H., Coffey, D.S. and Hellerman, L. (1966b) Interaction between tetraethylthiuram disulfide and the sulfhydryl groups of D-amino acid oxidase and of hemoglobin. *J. Biol. Chem.*, 241, 5941–8.

Netter, K.J., Honjo, T. and Magnussen, M.P. (1970) Influence of disulfiram on oxidative drug demethylation. *Humangenetik*, 9, 275–7.

Neveu, P.J. (1978) The effects of thiol moiety of levamisole on both cellular and humoral immunity during the early response to a hapten-carrier complex. *Clin. Exp. Immunol.*, 32, 419–22.

Neveu, P.J., Buscot, N. and Thierry, D. (1980) Effect of sodium diethyl dithiocarbamate on mitogen induced lympho-proliferation *in vitro*. *Biomedicine*, 33, 247–8.

Neveu, P.J., Perdoux, D. and Lafleur, L. (1982) *In vivo* enhancement of mitogen-induced lymphocyte DNA synthesis by sodium diethyl-dithiocarbamate (DTC). *Int. J. Immunopharmacol.*, 4, 9–13.

Neveu, P.J. and Vincendeau, P. (1983) Sodium diethyl dithiocarbamate and the mononuclear phagocytic system in guinea pigs. *Int Arch. Allergy Appl. Immunol.*, 71, 276–8.

Neveu, P.J., Taghzouti, K., Dantzer, R., Simon, H. and Le Moal, M. (1986a) Modulation of mitogen-induced lymphoproliferation by cerebral neocortex. *Life Sci.*, 38, 1907–13.

Neveu, P.J., Barneoud, S., Vitiello, S. and Le Moal, M. (1986b) Immunomodulatory roles of the cerebral neocortex. *Can. J. Neurol. Sci.*, 13, 379.

Neveu, P.J. (1988) Cerebral neocortex modulation of immune functions. *Life Sci.*, 42, 1917–23.

Newman, R.A., Lu, E.M. and Paredes, J. (1988) Cisplatin and flurouracil with and without sodium diethyldithiocarbamate rescue. *J. Clin. Oncol.*, 6, 1786–7.

Niblo, G., Nowinski, W.W. and Roark, D. (1951) Effects of ascorbic acid in Antabuse-alcohol reactions. *Dis. Nerv. Syst.*, 12, 340–3.

Nieboer, E., Stafford, A.R., Evans, S.L. and Dolovich, J. (1984) Cellular binding and/or uptake of nickel(II) ions. *IARC Sci. Publ.*, 53, 321–31.

Nilsson, G.E., Tottmar, O and Wahlström, G. (1987) Effects of aldehyde dehydrogenase inhibitors on hexobarbital sensitivity and neuroamine metabolism in rat brain. *Brain Res.*, **409**, 265–74.

Nilsson, G.E. and Wahlström, G. (1989) Inhibition of acute CNS-tolerance to hexobarbital anaesthesia by disulfiram treatment in rats. *Pharmacol. Toxicol.*, **64**, 137–43.

NIOSH (1985) *NIOSH Pocket Guide to Chemical Hazards*, Department of Health Education and Welfare, Washington, DC.

Nirenberg, T.D., Sobell, L.C., Ersner-Hershfield, S. and Cellucci, A.J. (1983) Can disulfiram use precipitate urges to drink alcohol? *Addict. Behav.*, **8**, 311–13.

Nishigaki, R., Utsugi, K., Maeda, K. *et al.* (1985) Effects of diethyldithiocarbamate, a metabolite of disulfiram, on the pharmacokinetics of alcohol and acetaldehyde in the rat. *J. Pharmacobio-Dyn.*, **8**, 847–52.

Nogué, S., Mas, A., Parés, A. *et al.* (1983) Acute thallium poisoning: An evaluation of different forms of treatment. *J. Toxicol. Clin Toxicol.*, **19**, 1015–21.

Nomenclature of Mammalian Aldehyde Dehydrogenases (1988) *Prog. Clin. Biol. Res.*, **290**, xix–xxi.

Norseth, T. (1974) The effect of diethyldithiocarbamate on biliary transport, excretion and organ distribution of mercury in the rat after exposure to methyl mercuric chloride. *Acta Pharmacol. Toxicol.*, **34**, 76–87.

Nousiainen, U. and Törrönen, R. (1984) Differentiation of microsomal and cytosolic carboxylesterases in the rat liver by *in vivo* and *in vitro* inhibition. *Gen. Pharmacol.*, **15**, 223–8.

Obrebska, M.J., Kentish, P. and Parke, D.V. (1980) The effects of carbon disulphide on rat liver microsomal mixed-function oxidases, *in vivo* and *in vitro. Biochem. J.*, **188**, 107–12.

O'Callaghan, J.P. and Miller, D.B. (1986) Diethyldithiocarbamate increases distribution of cadmium to brain but prevents cadmium-induced neurotoxicity. *Brain Res.*, **370**, 354–8.

Ogishima, T., Deguchi, S. and Okuda, K. (1987) Purification and characterization of cholesterol 7α-hydroxylase from rat liver microsomes. *J. Biol. Chem.*, **262**, 7646–50.

Ohman, M. and Marklund, S. (1986) Plasma extracellular superoxide dismutase and erythrocyte Cu,Zn-containing superoxide dismutase in alcoholics treated with disulfiram. *Clin. Sci.*, **70**, 356–69.

Öjehagen, A. and Berglund, M. (1986) To keep the alcoholic in out-patient treatment: A differentiated approach through treatment contracts. *Acta Psychiatr. Scand.*, **73**, 68–75.

Öjehagen, A., Skjaeris, A. and Berglund, M. (1988) Prediction of posttreatment drinking outcome in a 2-year out-patient alcoholic treatment program: A follow-up study. *Alcohol. Clin. Exp. Res.*, **12**, 46–51.

Olesen, O.V. (1966) Disulfiramum (Antabuse) as inhibitor of phenytoin metabolism. *Acta Pharmacol. Toxicol.*, **24**, 317–22.

Olesen, O.V. (1967) The influence of disulfiram and calcium carbimide on the serum diphenylhydantoin: Excretion of HPPH in the urine. *Arch. Neurol.*, **16**, 642–4.

Olney, R.K. and Miller, R.G. (1980) Peripheral neuropathy associated with disulfiram administration. *Muscle Nerve*, **3**, 172–5.

Ooms, P.C.A., Brinkman, U.A. Th. and Das, H.A. (1977) Radiometric determination of the conditional extraction of some metal diethyl-dithiocarbamates in the system chloroform/water. *Radiochem. Radioanal. Lett.*, **31**, 317–22.

O'Reilly, R.A. (1971) Potentiation of anticoagulant effect by disulfiram. *Clin. Res.*, **19**, 180.

O'Reilly, R.A. (1973) Interaction of sodium warfarin and disulfiram (Antabuse) in man. *Ann. Intern. Med.*, **78**, 73–6.

Orrego, H., Carmichael, F.J., Saldivia, V., Giles, H.G., Sandrin, S. and Israel, Y. (1988) Ethanol-induced increase in portal blood flow: role of adenosine. *Am. J. Physiol.*, **254**, G495–G501.

Oskarsson, A. and Tjälve, H. (1980) Effects of diethyldithiocarbamate and penicillamine on the tissue distribution of ^{63}NiCl$_2$ in mice. *Arch. Toxicol.*, **45**, 45–52.

Oskarsson, A. (1983) Redistribution and increased brain uptake of lead in rats after treatment with diethyldithiocarbamate. *Arch. Toxicol.*, **Suppl. 6**, 279–84.

Oskarsson, A. (1984) Dithiocarbamate-induced redistribution and increased brain uptake of lead in rats. *Neurotoxicology*, **5**, 283–94.

Oskarsson, A. and Lind, B. (1985) Increased lead levels in brain after long-term treatment with lead and dithiocarbamate or thiuram derivatives in rats. *Acta Pharmacol. Toxicol.*, **56**, 309–15.

Oskarsson, A., Olson, L., Palmer, M.R., Lind, B., Björklund, H. and Hoffer, B. (1986a) Increased lead concentrations in brain and potentiation of lead-induced neuronal depression in rats after combined treatment with lead and disulfiram. *Environ. Res.*, **41**, 623–32.

Oskarsson, A., Ljungberg, T., Stähle, L., Tossman, U. and Ungerstedt, U. (1986b) Behavioral and neurochemical effects after combined perinatal treatment of rats with lead and disulfiram. *Neurobehav. Toxicol. Teratol.*, **8**, 591–9.

Oskarsson, A. (1987a) Effect of disulfiram on milk transfer and tissue distribution of lead in the neonatal rat. *Toxicol. Lett.*, **36**, 73–9.

Oskarsson, A. (1987b) Comparative effects of ten dithiocarbamates and thiuram compounds on tissue distribution and excretion of lead in rats. *Environ. Res.*, **44**, 82–93.

Oskarsson, A. and Johansson, A. (1987) Lead-induced inclusion bodies in rat kidney after perinatal treatment with lead and disulfiram. *Toxicology*, **44**, 61–72.

Oskarsson, A. and Hellström-Lindahl, E. (1988) Increased lead uptake and inhibition of ALAD-activity in isolated rat hepatocytes incubated with lead-diethyldithiocarbamate complex. *Chem. Biol. Interact.*, **67**, 59–70.

Oskarsson, A. (1989) Effects of perinatal treatment with lead and disulfiram on ALAD activity in blood, liver and kidney and urinary ALA excretion in rats. *Pharmacol. Toxicol.*, **64**, 344–8.

Palliyath, S.K. and Schwartz, B.D. (1988) Disulfiram neuropathy: electrophysiological study. *Electromyogr. Clin. Neurophysiol.*, **28**, 245–7.

Palliyath, S.K., Schwartz, B.D. and Gant, L. (1990) Peripheral nerve functions in chronic alcoholic patients on disulfiram: A six month follow up. *J. Neurol. Neurosurg. Psychiatry*, **53**, 227–30.

Palmer, G. (1962) The purification and properties of aldehyde oxidase. *Biochim. Biophys. Acta*, **56**, 444–59.

Pannacciulli, I.M., Lerza, R.A., Bogliolo, G.V., Mencoboni, M.P. and Saviane, A.G. (1989) Effect of diethyldithiocarbamate on toxicity of doxorubicin, cyclophosphamide and *cis*-diamminedichloroplatinum (II) on mice haemopoietic progenitor cells. *Br. J. Canc.*, **59**, 371–4.

Papp, J.P., Gay, P.C., Dodson, V.N. and Pollard, H.M. (1969) Potassium chloride treatment of thallotoxicosis. *Ann. Intern. Med.*, **71**, 119–23.

Paredes, J., Hang, W.K., Felder, T.B. *et al.* (1988) Prospective randomized trial of high-dose cisplatin and fluorouracil infusion with and without sodium diethyldithiocarbamate in recurrent and/or metastatic squamous cell carcinoma of the head and neck. *J. Clin. Oncol.*, 6, 955–62.

Parrilla, R., Ohkawa, K., Lindros, K.O., Zimmerman, U.-J. P., Kobayashi, K. and Williamson, J.R. (1974) Functional compartmentation of acetaldehyde oxidation in rat liver. *J. Biol. Chem.*, 249, 4926–33.

Paulson, S.M., Krause, S. and Iber, F.L. (1977) Development and evaluation of a compliance test for patients taking disulfiram. *Johns Hopkins Med. J.*, 141, 119–25.

PDR (1991) *Physicians' Desk Reference*, 45th edn., Medical Economics Data, Oradell, NJ, pp. 2358–9.

Peachey, J.E. and Sellers, E.M. (1981) The disulfiram and calcium carbimide acetaldehyde-mediated ethanol reactions. *Pharmacol. Ther.*, 15, 89–97.

Peachey, J.E., Maglana, S., Robinson, G.M., Hemy, M. and Brien, J.F. (1981a) Cardiovascular changes during the calcium carbimide-ethanol interaction. *Clin. Pharmacol. Ther.*, 29, 40–6.

Peachey, J.E., Brien, J.F., Roach, C.A. and Loomis, C.W. (1981b) A comparative review of the pharmacological and toxicological properties of disulfiram and calcium carbimide. *J. Clin. Psychopharmacol.*, 1, 21–6.

Peachey, J.E., Zlim, D.H. and Cappell, H. (1981c) 'Burning off the Antabuse': fact or fiction? *Lancet*, i, 943–4.

Peachey, J.E. and Naranjo, C.A. (1983) The use of disulfiram and other alcohol-sensitizing drugs in the treatment of alcoholism. *Res. Adv. Alc. Drug Prob.*, 7, 397–431.

Peachey, J.E., Zlim, D.H., Robinson, G.M., Jacob, M. and Cappell, H. (1983) A placebo-controlled double-blind comparative clinical study of the disulfiram- and calcium carbimide-acetaldehyde mediated ethanol reactions in social drinkers. *Alcohol. Clin. Exp. Res.*, 7, 180–7.

Peachey, J.E. and Annis, H. (1984) Pharmacologic treatment of chronic alcoholism. *Psychiatr. Clin. North Am.*, 7, 745–56.

Peachey, J.E. and Annis, H. (1985) New strategies for using the alcohol-sensitizing drugs. In *Research Advances in New Psychopharmacological Treatments for Alcoholism* (eds C.A. Naranjo and E.M. Sellers), Elsevier, Amsterdam, pp. 199–216.

Pedersen, S.B. (1980) Analysis and preliminary pharmacokinetics of disulfiram. *Arch. Pharm. Chem. Sci. Ed.*, 8, 65–82.

Peeke, S.C., Prael, A.R., Herning, R.I., Rogers, W., Benowitz, N.L. and Jones, R.T. (1979) Effect of disulfiram on cognition, subjective response, and cortical-event-related potentials of nonalcoholic subjects. *Alcohol. Clin. Exp. Res.*, 3, 223–9.

Pérez-Clausell, J. and Danscher, G. (1985) Intravascular localization of zinc in rat telencephalic butons: A histochemical study. *Brain Res.*, 337, 91–8.

Perman, E.S. (1962a) Studies on the Antabuse-alcohol reaction in rabbits. *Acta Physiol. Scand.*, 55, Suppl. 190, 1–46.

Perman, E.S. (1962b) Antabuse-alcohol reaction in rabbits. *Experientia*, 18, 516–7.

Petersen, E.A., Hersh, E.M., Yocum, D.E., Gorman, R.S. and Darragh, J.M. (1988) Dose response study of diethyldithiocarbamate (DTC) in patients (PTS) with ARC/AIDS. *Fourth International Conference on AIDS*, Abstract volume I, Stockholm, p. 230, Abstract 3041.

Petersen, E.N. (1989) Pharmacological effects of diethylthiocarbamic acid methyl ester, the active metabolite of disulfiram? *Europ. J. Pharmacol.*, 166, 419–25.

Peterson, C.M. and Polizzi, C.M. (1987) Improved method for acetaldehyde in plasma and hemoglobin-associated acetaldehyde: results in teetotalers and alcoholics reporting for treatment. *Alcohol*, 4, 477–80.

Peterson, C.M., Jovanovic-Petersen, L. and Schmid-Formby, F. (1988) Rapid association of acetaldehyde with hemoglobin in human volunteers after low dose ethanol. *Alcohol*, **5**, 371–4.

Pettersson, H. and Tottmar, O. (1982) Inhibition of aldehyde dehydrogenases in rat brain and liver by disulfiram and coprine. *J. Neurochem.*, **39**, 628–34.

Phillips, M. and Gresser, J.D. (1984) Sustained-release characteristics of a new implantable formulation of disulfiram. *J. Pharm. Sci.*, **73**, 1718–20.

Phillips, M., Agarwal, R.P., Brodeur, R.J., Garagusi, V.F. and Mossman, K.L. (1985) Stability of an injectable disulfiram formulation sterilized by gamma irradiation. *Am. J. Hosp. Pharm.*, **42**, 343–5.

Phillips, M., Greenberg, J. and Martinez, V. (1986) Measurement of breath carbon disulfide during disulfiram therapy by gas chromatography with flame photometric detection. *J. Chromatogr.*, **381**, 164–7.

Phillips, M. (1988) Persistent sensitivity to ethanol following a single dose of parenteral sustained-release disulfiram. *Adv. Alcohol Subst. Abuse*, **7**, 51–61.

Pietruszko, R., Crawford, K. and Lester, D. (1973) Comparison of substrate specificity of alcohol dehydrogenases from human liver, horse liver, and yeast towards saturated and 2-enoic alcohols and aldehydes. *Arch. Bioch. Biophys.*, **159**, 50–60.

Pietruszko, R. and Vallari, R.C. (1978) Aldehyde dehydrogenase of human blood. *FEBS Lett.*, **92**, 89–91.

Pietruszko, R. (1983) Aldehyde dehydrogenase isozymes. *Isozymes*, **8**, 195–217.

Pietruszko, R. and MacKerell, A.D. (1986) Stoichiometry of chemical modification of human aldehyde dehydrogenase: Evidence for 'quarter of the sites' reactivity. *Prog. Clin. Biol. Res.*, **232**, 37–52.

Pietruszko, R., Ryzlak, M.T. and Forte-McRobbie, C.M. (1987) Multiplicity and identity of human aldehyde dehydrogenases. *Alcohol Alcohol.*, **Suppl. 1**, 175–179.

Pietruszko, R. (1989) Aldehyde dehydrogenase (EC 1.2.1.3). In *Biochemistry and Physiology of Substance Abuse* Vol. 1 (ed. R. Watson), CRC Press Inc., Boca Raton, FL, pp. 89–127.

Pimentel, E. (1990) Colony-stimulating factors. *Ann. Clin. Lab. Sci.*, **20**, 36–55.

Plant, M.A. (1983) Probation linked disulfiram treatment. *Br. Med. J.*, **287**, 1795.

Plouvier, B., Lemoine, X., De Coninck, P., Baclet, J.L. and François, M. (1982) Effet antabuse lors de l'application d'un topique à base de monosulfirame. *Nouv. Presse Med.*, **11**, 3209.

Pomerantz, S.H. (1963) Separation, purification, and properties of two tyrosinases from hamster melanoma. *J. Biol. Chem.*, **238**, 2351–7.

Pomerantz, S.H. (1966) The tyrosine hydroxylase activity of mammalian tyrosinase. *J. Biol. Chem.*, **241**, 161–8.

Pompidou, A., Mace, B., Esnous, D. and Michel, P. (1980) The nuclear refringence test: A new method for the evaluation of blood lymphocytes nuclei response *in vitro* to lectins and immunomodulators in man. In *International Symposium on New Trends in Human Immunology and Cancer Immunotherapy* (eds B. Serrou and C. Rosenfeld), Doin, Paris, pp. 696–703.

Pompidou, A., Renoux, M., Guillaumin, J.M. *et al.* (1984a) Kinetics of the histological changes in lymphoid organs and of the T-cell inducing capacity of serum in mice treated with Imuthiol (sodium diethyldithiocarbamate). *Int. Arch. Allergy Appl. Immun.*, **74**, 172–7.

Pompidou, A., Rousset, S., Mace, B., Michel, P., Esnous, D. and Renard, N (1984b) Chromatin structure and nucleic acid synthesis in human lymphocyte activation by phytohemagglutinin. *Exp. Cell. Res.*, **150**, 213–25.

Pompidou, A. Delsaux, M.C., Telvi, L. *et al.* (1985a) Isoprinosine and imuthiol, two potentially active compounds in patients with AIDS-related complex symptoms. *Cancer Res.*, **45**, 4671s–4673s.

Pompidou, A., Duchet, N., Cooper, M.D. *et al.* (1985b) The generation and regulation of human T lymphocytes by imuthiol. Evidence from an *in vitro* differentiation induction system. *Int. J. Immunopharmacol.*, **4**, 561–6.

Pompidou, A., Zagury, D., Gallo, R.C., Sun, D., Thornton, A. and Sarin, P.S. (1985c) *In-vitro* inhibition of Lav/HTLV-III infected lymphocytes by dithiocarb and inosine pranobex. *Lancet*, **ii**, 1423.

Pompidou, A., Lang, J.M., Telvi, L., Delsaux, M.C. and Sarin, P. (1986) Influence of immunomodulators on T lymphocyte differentiation in ARC patients and resistance to LAV/HTLV III infection. *Comp. Immun. Microbiol. Infect. Dis.*, **9**, 263–67.

Potchoo, Y., Braguer, D., Peyrot, V., Chauvet-Monges, A.M., Sari, J.C. and Crevat, A. (1986) *In vitro* inhibition of microtubule assembly by disulfiram. *Intern. J. Clin. Pharmacol. Ther. Toxicol.*, **24**, 499–504.

Poulsen, L.L., Hyslop, R.M. and Ziegler, D.M. (1979) *S*-Oxygenation of *N*-substituted thioureas catalyzed by the pig liver microsomal FAD-containing monooxygenase. *Arch. Bioch. Biophys.*, **198**, 78–88.

Price, T.R.P and Silberfarb, P.M. (1976) Disulfiram-induced convulsion without challenge by alcohol. *J. Stud. Alcohol*, **37**, 980–2.

Prickett, C.S. and Johnston, C.D. (1953) The *in vivo* production of carbon disulfide from tetraethylthiuramdisulfide (Antabuse). *Biochim. Biophys. Acta*, **12**, 542–6.

Pristach, C.A. and Smith, C.M. (1990) Medication compliance and substance abuse among schizophrenic patients. *Hosp. Comm. Psychiat.*, **41**, 1345–8.

Prohaska, J.R. and Ganther, H.E. (1977) Glutathione peroxidase activity of glutathione-*S*-transferases purified from rat liver. *Biochem. Biophys. Res. Commun.*, **76**, 437–45.

Puglia, C.D and Loeb, G.A. (1984) Influence of rat brain superoxide dismutase inhibition by diethyldithiocarbamate upon rate and development of central nervous system oxygen toxicity. *Toxicol. App. Pharmacol.*, **75**, 258–64.

Qazi, R., Chang, A.Y.C., Borch, R.F., Montine, T., Dedon, P., Loughner, J. and Bennett, J.M. (1988) Phase I clinical and pharmacokinetic study of diethyldithiocarbamate as a chemoprotector from toxic effects of cisplatin. *J. Nat. Canc. Inst.*, **80**, 1486–8.

Raby, K. (1952) Potassium concentration in blood during Antabuse-alcohol reaction. *Acta Pharmacol. Toxicol.*, **8**, 85–100.

Raby, K. (1953a) Investigations on the disulfiram-alcohol reaction: Clinical observations. *Q. J. Stud. Alcohol*, **14**, 545–56.

Raby, K. (1953b) Electrocardiographic changes following the ingestion of disulfiram and alcohol. *Q. J. Stud. Alcohol*, **14**, 557–67.

Raby, K. (1954a) Relation of blood acetaldehyde level to clinical symptoms in the disulfiram-alcohol reaction. *Q. J. Stud. Alcohol*, **15**, 21–32.

Raby, K. (1954b) Effect of alcohol on respiration before and after treatment with disulfiram. *Q. J. Stud. Alcohol*, **15**, 33–42.

Raby, K. (1954c) Investigations of the acid-base balance of the blood during the disulfiram-alcohol reaction. *Q. J. Stud. Alcohol*, **15**, 207–19.

Raby, K. (1956) The antabus-alcohol reaction: Summary of clinical and experimental investigations. *Dan. Med. Bull.*, **3**, 168–71.

Radojičić, R., Spasić, M., Milić, B., Saičić, Z. and Petrović, M.V. (1987) Age related differences in the effect of diethyldithiocarbamate and cycloheximide on the liver copper-zinc containing superoxide dismutase in the rat. *Iugo. Phys. Pharm. Acta*, **23**, 227–32.

Rainey, J.M. (1977) Disulfiram toxicity and carbon disulfide poisoning. *Am. J. Psychiatry*, **134**, 371–78.

Ramsey, A.J., Hill, J.P. and Dickinson, F.M. (1989) Some comparison of pig and sheep liver cytosolic aldehyde dehydrogenases. *Comp. Bioch. Physiol.*, **93B**, 77–83.

Ranek, L. and Andreasen, P.B. (1977) Disulfiram hepatotoxicity. *Br. Med. J.*, **2**, 94–6.

Rannug, A. and Rannug, U. (1984) Enzyme inhibition as a possible mechanism of the mutagenicity of dithiocarbamic acid derivatives in *Salomonella typhimurium*. *Chem. Biol. Interact.*, **49**, 329–40.

Rannug, A., Rannug, U. and Ramel, C. (1984) Genotoxic effects of additives in synthetic elastomers with special consideration of the mechanism of action of thiurames and dithiocarbamates. *Prog. Clin. Biol. Res.*, **141**, 407–19.

Ranz, A. and Meshnick, S.R. (1989) *Plasmodium falciparum*: Inhibitor sensitivity of the endogenous superoxide dismutase. *Exp. Parasitol.*, **69**, 125–8.

Rasul, A.R. and Howell, J.M. (1973a) A comparison of the effect of sodium diethyldithiocarbamate on the central nervous system of young and adult domestic fowl. *Acta Neuropath.*, **24**, 68–75.

Rasul, A.R. and Howell, J.M. (1973b) Further observations on the response of the peripheral and central nervous system of the rabbit to sodium diethyldithiocarbamate. *Acta Neuropath.*, **24**, 161–73.

Rasul, A.R. and Howell, J.M. (1974) The toxicity of some dithiocarbamate compounds in young and adult domestic fowl. *Toxicol. Appl. Pharmacol.*, **30**, 63–78.

Rauws, A.G., Ten Ham, M. and Kamerbeek, H.H. (1969) Influence of the antidote dithiocarb on distribution and toxicity of thallium in the rat. *Arch. Int. Pharmacodyn. Ther.*, **182**, 425–26.

Rawles, J.W., Rhodes, D.L., Potter, J.J. and Mezey, E. (1987) Characterization of human erythrocyte aldehyde dehydrogenase. *Biochem. Pharmacol.*, **36**, 3715–22.

Register, U.D., Tordecilla, A.G., Ask, M.N., Beierle, G. and Hubbard, R.W. (1990) Effect of disulfiram on the urinary excretion of 5-hydroxytryptophol in human subjects consuming serotonin rich foods. *FASEB J.*, **4**, A365.

Reisinger, E.C., Kern, P., Ernst, M, Bock, P. Flad, H.D., Dietrich, M. and the German DTC study group (1990) Inhibition of HIV progression by dithiocarb. *Lancet*, **i**, 679–82.

Rejas, M.T., Rojo, J.M., Ojeda, G. and Barasoain, I. (1988) Sodium diethyldithiocarbamate restores T lymphocyte proliferation, interleukin-2 production and NK activity in cyclophosphamide-immunosuppressed animals. *Immunopharmacology*, **16**, 191–7.

Renoux, G. and Renoux, M. (1974) Immunopotentiation par les thiols et disulfures. *C.R. Acad. Sc. (III)*, **278 D**, 1139–41.

Renoux, G. and Renoux, M. (1977a) Thymus-like activities of sulphur derivatives on T-cell differentiation. *J. Exp. Med.*, **145**, 466–71.

Renoux, G. and Renoux, M. (1977b) Roles of the imidazole or thiol moiety on the immunostimulant action of levamisole. In *Control of Neoplasia by Modulation of the Immune System* (ed. M.A. Chirigos), Raven Press, New York, pp. 67–80.

Renoux, G., Renoux, M. and Guillaumin, J.M. (1977) Le diéthyldithiocarbamate de sodium est un stimulant de l'immunité. *C.R. Soc. Biol. (Paris)*, **171**, 313–8.

Renoux, G. and Renoux, M. (1979) Immunopotentiation and anabolism induced by sodium diethyldithiocarbamate. *J. Immunopharmacol.*, **1**, 247–67.

Renoux, G., Renoux, M., Guillaumin, J.M. and Gouzien, C. (1979) Differentiation and regulation of lymphocyte populations: evidence for immunopotentiator-induced T cell recruitment. *J. Immunopharmacol.*, **1**, 415–22.

Renoux, G. (1980) Differentiation of the T-cell lineage by sodium diethyldithiocarbamate (DTC): Influence of the neocortex. In *International Symposium on New Trends in Human Immunology and Cancer Immunotherapy* (eds B. Serrou and C. Rosenfeld), Doin, Paris, pp. 986–94.

Renoux, G. and Renoux, M. (1980a) The effects of sodium diethyldithiocarbamate, azathioprine, cyclophosphamide, or hydrocortisone acetate administered alone or in association for 4 weeks on the immune responses of BALB/c mice. *Clin. Immunol. Immunopathol.*, **15**, 23–32.

Renoux, G. and Renoux, M. (1980b) Administration of DTC gives evidence of a role of the thymus in the control and regulation of factors inducing thymocyte differentiation in the mouse. *Thymus*, **2**, 139–46.

Renoux, G., Touraine, J.L. and Renoux, M. (1980a) Induction of differentiation of human null cells into T lymphocytes under the influence of serum of mice treated with sodium diethyldithiocarbamate. *J. Immunopharmacol.*, **2**, 49–59.

Renoux, G., Renoux, M., Greco, J., Bawdoin, J., Lavandier, M. and Lemarie, E. (1980b) Phase I-II studies of sodium diethyldithiocarbamate (DTC). In *International Symposium on New Trends in Human Immunology and Cancer Immunotherapy* (eds B. Serrou and C. Rosenfeld), Doin, Paris, pp. 974–85.

Renoux, G. (1981) Levamisole and sodium diethyldithiocarbamate. *Trends Pharmacol. Sci.*, **2**, 248–49.

Renoux, G. and Renoux, M. (1981) Immunological activity of DTC: Potential for cancer therapy. In *Augmenting Agents in Cancer Therapy* (eds E.M. Hersh *et al.*), Raven Press, New York, pp. 427–40.

Renoux, G. (1982) Immunopharmacologie et pharmacologie du diethyldithiocarbamate (DTC). *J. Pharmacol. (Paris)*, **13, Suppl. 1**, 95–134.

Renoux, G., Renoux, M. and Guillaumin, J.M. (1982a) Hepatosin. *Int. J. Immunopharmacol.*, **4**, 300.

Renoux, G., Bardos, P., Degenne, D. and Musset, M. (1982b) Sodium diethyldithiocarbamate (DTC)-induced modifications of NK activity in the mouse. In *NK Cells and Other Natural Effector Cells* (ed. R.B. Herberman), Academic Press, New York, pp. 443–8.

Renoux, G., Biziere, K., Bardos, P., Degenne, D. and Renoux, M. (1982c) NK activity in mice is controlled by the brain neocortex. In *NK Cells and Other Natural Effector Cells* (ed. R.B. Herberman), Academic Press, New York, pp. 639–43.

Renoux, G. and Renoux, M. (1983) DTC, a T-cell-specific agent in *nu/nu* mice. In *Current Drugs and Methods of Cancer Treatment* (eds G. Mathe, E. Mihich and P. Reizerstein), Masson, New York, pp. 171–3.

Renoux, G., Biziere, K., Renoux, M. and Guillaumin, J.M. (1983a) The production of T-cell-inducing factors in mice is controlled by the brain neocortex. *Scand. J. Immunol.*, **17**, 45–50.

Renoux, G., Renoux, M., Lemarie, E. *et al.* (1983b) Sodium diethyldithiocarbamate and cancer. *Adv. Exp. Med.*, **166**, 223–39.

Renoux, G., Biziere, K., Renoux, M. and Guillaumin, J.M. (1983c) A balanced brain asymmetry modulates T cell mediated events. *J. Neuroimmunol.*, **5**, 227–238.

Renoux, G. (1984) The mode of action of imuthiol (sodium diethyldithiocarbamate): A new role for the brain neocortex and the endocrine liver in the regulation of the T-cell linage. In *Immune Modulation Agents and their*

Mechanism (eds R.L. Fenichel and M.A. Chirigos), Marcel Dekker, New York, pp. 607–24.

Renoux, G. and Renoux, M. (1984) Diethyldithiocarbamate (DTC): A biological augmenting agent specific for T cells. In *Immune Modulation Agents and their Mechanism* (eds R.L. Fenichel and M.A. Chirigos), Marcel Dekker, New York, pp. 7–20.

Renoux, G., Renoux, M., Biziere, K., Guillaumin, J.M., Bardos, P. and Degenne, D. (1984) Involvement of brain neocortex and liver in the regulation of T cells: The mode of action of sodium diethyldithiocarbamate (Imuthiol). *Immunopharmacology*, **7**, 89–100.

Renoux, G. (1985a) Modulation of immunity by levamisole and DTC. In *The Modulation of Immunity* (ed. M.S. Mitchell), *Int. Encyc. Pharmacol. Ther*, Section 115, Pergamon Press, New York, pp. 393–410.

Renoux, G. (1985b) Immunomodulatory agents. In *Immunotoxicology and Immunopharmacology* (eds J.H. Dean, M.I. Laster, A.E. Munson and H. Amos), Raven Press, New York, pp. 193–205.

Renoux, G., Guillaumin, J.M. and Renoux, M. (1985) Favorable influences of Imuthiol on mouse reproduction and immune system of offspring. *Am. J. Reprod. Immunol. Microbiol.*, **8**, 101–6.

Renoux, G. and Biziere, K. (1987) Asymmetrical involvement of the cerebral neocortex on the response to an immunopotentiator, sodium diethyldithiocarbamate. *J. Neurosci. Res.*, **18**, 230–8.

Renoux, G., Biziere, K., Renoux, M., Bardos, P. and Degenne, D. (1987) Consequences of bilateral brain neocortical ablation on Imuthiol-induced immunostimulation in mice. *Ann. NY Acad. Sci.*, **496**, 346–53.

Renoux, G. (1988) The cortex regulates the immune system and the activities of a T-cell specific immunopotentiator. *Int. J. Neurosci.*, **39**, 177–87.

Renoux, G., Renoux, M. and Biziere, K. (1988a) Brain neocortex and Imuthiol regulate the expression of MHC antigens on mouse T lymphocytes. *Immunopharm. Immunotoxicol.*, **10**, 219–29.

Renoux, G., Renoux, M., Guillaumin, J.-M. (1988b) Immunopharmacology and immunotoxicity of zinc diethyldithiocarbamate. *Int. J. Immunopharmacol.*, **10**, 489–93.

Renoux, M., Giroud, J.P., Florentin, I., Guillaumin, J.M., Degenne, D. and Renoux, G. (1986) Early changes in immune parameters induced by an acute nonantigenic inflammation in the mouse: influence of Imuthiol. *Int. J. Immunopharmacol.*, **8**, 107–17.

Rieders, F. and Cordova, V.F. (1965) Effect of sodium diethyldithiocarbamate (NaDEDTC) on urinary thallium excretion in man. *Pharmacologist*, **7**, 162.

Rigas, D.A., Eginitis-Rigas, C. and Head, C. (1979) Biphasic toxicity of diethyldithiocarbamate, a metal chelator, to T lymphocytes and polymorphonuclear granulocytes: Reversal by zinc and copper. *Biochem. Biophys. Res. Commun.*, **88**, 373–9.

Rigas, D.A., Eginitis-Rigas, C., Bigley, R.H., Stankova, L. and Head, C. (1980) Biphasic radiosensitization of human lymphocytes by diethyldithiocarbamate: possible involvement of superoxide dismutase. *Int. J. Rad. Biol.*, **38**, 257–66.

Rinaldi, A., Giartosio, A., Floris, G., Medda, R. and Agro, A.F. (1984) Lentil seedlings amine oxidase: Preparation and properties of the copper-free enzyme. *Biochem. Biophys. Res. Commun.*, **120**, 242–9.

Robens, J.F. (1969) Teratologic studies of carbaryl, diazinon, norea, disulfiram and thiram in small laboratory animals. *Toxicol. App. Pharmacol.*, **15**, 152–63.

Roberfroid, M.B., Malaveille, C., Hautefeuille, A., Brun, G., Vo, T.K.-O. and Bartsch, H. (1983) Interrelationships in mice of antipyrine half-life, hepatic monooxygenase activities and liver S9-mediated mutagenicity of aflatoxin B₁, benzo[a]pyrene-7,8-dihydrodiol, 2-acetylaminofluorene and N-nitrosomorpholine. *Chem. Biol. Interact.*, **47**, 175–94.

Robichaud, C., Strickler, D., Bigelow, D. and Liebson, I. (1979) Disulfiram maintenance employee alcoholism treatment: A three-phase evaluation. *Behav. Res. Ther.*, **17**, 618–21.

Robins, A.H. and Barron, J.L. (1983) The effect of disulfiram on the urinary excretion of catecholamine metabolites in alcoholic males. *S. Afr. Med. J.*, **63**, 41–2.

Rogers, E.L. and Naseem, S.M. (1981) Disulfiram-associated hypercholesterolemia. *Alcohol. Clin. Exp. Res.*, **5**, 75–7.

Rogers, W.K., Wilson, K.M. and Becker, C.E. (1978) Methods for detecting disulfiram in biologic fluids: Application in studies of compliance and effect of divalent cations on bioavailability. *Alcohol. Clin. Exp. Res.*, **2**, 375–80.

Rogers, W.K., Benowitz, N.L., Wilson, K.M. and Abbott, J.A. (1979) Effect of disulfiram on adrenergic function. *Clin. Pharmacol. Ther.*, **25**, 469–77.

Roitt, I., Brostoff, J. and Male, D. (1989) *Immunology*, 2nd eds, C.V. Mosby, St. Louis, pp. 2.8-2.9.

Romelsjö, A. (1987) Decline in alcohol-related in-patient care and mortality in Stockholm county. *Br. J. Addict.*, **82**, 653–63.

Rothenberg, M.L., Ostchega, Y., Steinberg, S.M., Young, R.C., Hummel, S. and Ozols, R.F. (1988) High-dose carboplatin with diethyldithiocarbamate chemoprotection in treatment of women with relapsed ovarian cancer. *J. Natl. Cancer Inst.*, **80**, 1488–92.

Rothstein, E. (1968) Warfarin effect enhanced by disulfiram. *J. Am. Med. Assoc.*, **206**, 1574–5.

Rothstein, E. and Clancy, D.D. (1969a) Toxicity of disulfiram combined with metronidazole. *N. Engl. J. Med.*, **280**, 1006–7.

Rothstein, E. and Clancy, D.D. (1969b) Disulfiram-metronidazole (continued). *N. Engl. J. Med.*, **281**, 331.

Rothstein, E. (1972a) Safety of disulfiram (Antabuse). *N. Engl. J. Med.*, **286**, 162.

Rothstein, E. (1972b) Warfarin effect enhanced by disulfiram (Antabuse). *J. Am. Med. Assoc.*, **229**, 1052–3.

Ruiz de Elvira, M.-C., Sinha, A.K. and Ekins, R.P. (1987) Development of an enzyme assay for the measurement of calmodulin-dependent phosphatase in brain tissue. *Biochem. Soc. Trans.*, **16**, 297–8.

Russo, J.E., Hilton, J. and Colvin, O.M. (1988) The role of acetaldehyde dehydrogenase isozymes in cellular resistance to the alkylating agent cyclophosphamide. *Prog. Clin. Biol. Res.*, **290**, 65–79.

Rychtarik, R.G., Smith, P.O., Jones, S.L., Doerfler, L., Hale, R. and Prue, D.M. (1983) Assessing disulfiram compliance: Validation study of an abbreviated breath test procedure. *Addict. Behav.*, **8**, 361–8.

Ryle, P.R., Chakraborty, J. and Thomson, A.D. (1985) The roles of the hepatocellular redox state and the hepatic acetaldehyde concentration in determining the ethanol elimination rate in fasted rats. *Biochem. Pharmacol.*, **34**, 3577–83.

Ryzlak, M.T. (1986) Purification and characterization of aldehyde dehydrogenases from human brain. PhD Thesis, Rutgers, The State University of New Jersey, New Brunswick, NJ.

Ryzlak, M.T. and Pietruszko, R. (1987) Purification and characterization of aldehyde dehydrogenase from human brain. *Arch. Bioch. Biophys.*, **255**, 409–18.

Ryzlak, M.T. and Pietruszko, R. (1988) Human brain 'high K_m' aldehyde dehydrogenase: Purification, characterization, and identification as NAD$^+$-dependent succinic semialdehyde dehydrogenase. *Arch. Bioch. Biophys.*, **266**, 386–96.

Ryzlak, M.T. and Pietruszko, R. (1989) Human brain glyceraldehyde-3-phosphate dehydrogenase, succinic semialdehyde dehydrogenase and aldehyde dehydrogenase isozymes: Substrate specificity and sensitivity to disulfiram. *Alcohol. Clin. Exp. Res.*, **13**, 755–61.

Sabréus, E., Bejerot, N. and Jonasson, L. (1982) En dobbelt-blind cross-over jamforeise med aveseende pa bivirningar mellan kalciumkarbimid, disulfiram och pacebo, udford pa friska, frivillige forsokspersoner. *Acta Soc. Med. Svec. Hyg.*, **91**, 183.

Salgo, M.P. and Oster, G. (1974) Fetal resorption induced by disulfiram in rats. *J. Reprod. Fertil*, **39**, 375–7.

Samitz, M.H. and Pomerantz, H. (1958) Studies of the effects on the skin of nickel and chromium salts. *A.M.A. Archiv. Ind. Health*, **18**, 473–9.

Sanhadji, K., Touraine, J.L., Othmane, O. and Musset M. (1985) Imuthiol (DTC), an agent inducing T cell characteristics onto human prothymocytes. *Int. J. Immunopharmacol.*, **7**, 616.

Sanny, C.G. (1985) Canine liver aldehyde dehydrogenases: distribution, isolation, and partial characterization. *Alcohol. Clin. Exp. Res.*, **9**, 255–62.

Sanny, C.G. and Weiner, H. (1987) Inactivation of horse liver mitochondrial aldehyde dehydrogenase by disulfiram: Evidence that disulfiram is not an active-site-directed reagent. *Biochem. J.*, **242**, 499–503.

Sanny, C.G., Mahoney, A.J., Kilmore, M.A. and Rymas, K. (1988) Effect of disulfiram on canine liver aldehyde dehydrogenase activity: *In vivo* inactivation in a nonrodent animal model. *Alcohol. Clin. Exp. Res.*, **12**, 622–4.

Sauter, A.M., Wiegrebe, W. and von Wartburg, J.P. (1976) Determination of disulfiram and its metabolites in human blood. *Arzneimittelforschung*, **26**, 173–7.

Sauter, A.M. and von Wartburg, J.P. (1977) Quantitative analysis of disulfiram and its metabolites in human blood by gas-liquid chromatography. *J. Chromatogr.*, **133**, 167–72.

Sauter, A.M., Boss, D. and von Wartburg, J.-P. (1977) Reevaluation of the disulfiram-alcohol reaction in man. *J. Stud. Alcohol*, **38**, 1680–95.

Savolainen, K., Hervonen, H., Lehto, V.-P. and Mattila, M.J. (1984) Neurotoxic effects of disulfiram on autonomic nervous system in rat. *Acta Pharmacol. Toxicol.*, **55**, 339–44.

Schade, R.R., Gray, J.A., Dekker, A., Varma, R.R., Shaffer, R.D. and Van Thiel, D.H. (1983) Fulminant hepatitis associated with disulfiram: Report of a case. *Arch. Intern. Med.*, **143**, 1271–3.

Scheibel, L.W., Adler, A. and Trager, W. (1979) Tetraethylthiuram disulfide (Antabuse) inhibits the human malaria parasite *Plasmodium falciparum*. *Proc. Natl. Acad. Sci. USA*, **76**, 5303–7.

Scheid, M.P., Goldstein, G. and Boyse, E.A. (1978) The generation and regulation of lymphocyte populations. Evidence for differentiative induction systems in vitro. *J. Exp. Med.*, **147**, 1727.

Schlesinger, K., Kakihana, R. and Bennett, E.L. (1966) Effects of tetraethylthiuramdisulfide (Antabuse) on the metabolism and consumption of ethanol in mice. *Psychos. Med.*, **28**, 514–20.

Schlick, E., Hartung, K., Piccoli, M., Bartucci, A. and Chirigos, M.A. (1984) The *in vitro* induction of colony-stimulating factor, prostaglandin E, and interferon in macrophages and tumor cells by biological response modifiers. In *Immune*

Modulation Agents and Their Mechanisms (eds R.L. Fenichel and M.A. Chirigos) Dekker, New York, pp. 513–29.

Schmalbach, T.K. and Borch, R.F. (1989a) Myeloprotective effects of diethyldithio-carbamate treatment following 1,3-bis(2-chloroethyl)-1-nitrosourea, adriamycin, or mytomycin C in mice. *Cancer Res.*, **49**, 2574–7.

Schmalbach, T.K. and Borch, R.F. (1989b) Diethyldithiocarbamate modulation of murine bone marrow toxicity induced by *cis*-diammine(cyclobutanedicar-boxylato)platinum(II). *Cancer Res.*, **49**, 6629–33.

Schmalbach, T.K. and Borch, R.F. (1990) Mechanism of diethyldithio-carbamate modulation of murine bone marrow toxicity. *Cancer Res.*, **50**, 6218–21.

Schmidt, H. (1979) Phenol- und Peroxidaseakivität in Gegenwart verschiedener Effektoren. *Acta Histochem.*, **64**, 194–205.

Schmidt, H. (1988) Phenol oxidase (EC 1.14.18.1) a marker enzyme for defense cells. *Prog. Histochem. Cyctochem.*, **17**, 1–187.

Scholler, J., Brown, D.E. and Timmens, E.K. (1961) Toxicological and pathological studies with diethyldithiocarbamate (DDC). *Pharmacologist*, **3**, 62.

Schönenberger, H. and Lippert, P. (1972) Antimikrobielle und tumorhemmende Eigenschaften von Dithiourethanen und Untersuchungen zum Wirkungs-mechanismus. *Pharmazie*, **27**, 139–45. .

Schröder, H.D., Fjerdingstad, E., Danscher, G. and Fjerdingstad, E.J. (1978) Heavy metals in the spinal cord of normal rats and of animals treated with chelating agents: A quantitative (zinc, copper, and lead) and histochemical study. *Histochemistry*, **56**, 1–12.

Schuckit, M.A. (1985) A one-year follow-up of men alcoholics given disulfiram. *J. Stud. Alcohol*, **46**, 191–5.

Schütz, H.J., Busse, O. and Vuia, O. (1983) Polyneuropathie nach Disulfiram-Intoxikation. *Arch. Psychiat. Nervenkr.*, **233**, 1–8.

Schwarcz, M.N. and Stoppani, A.O.M. (1960) The effect of metal-binding agents on aldehyde dehydrogenases. *Bioch. Biophys. Acta*, **39**, 383–4.

Schwetz, B.A., O'Neil, P.V., Voelker, F.A and Jacobs, D.W. (1967) Effect of diphenyl-thiocarbazone and diethyldithiocarbamate on the excretion of thallium in rats. *Toxicol. App. Pharmacol.*, **10**, 79–88.

Searle, A.J.F. and Tomasi, A. (1982) Hydroxyl free radical production in iron-cysteine solutions and protection by zinc. *J. Inorg. Bioch.*, **17**, 161–6.

Sellers, E.M., Giles, H.G., Greenblatt, D.J. and Naranjo, C.A. (1980) Differential effects on benzodiazepine disposition by disulfiram and ethanol. *Arzneimittelforschung*, **30**, 882–6.

Sellers, E.M., Naranjo, C.A. and Peachey, J.E. (1981) Drugs to decrease alcohol consumption. *N. Engl. J. Med.*, **305**, 1255–62.

Sereny, G., Sharma, V., Holt, J. and Gordis, E. (1986) Mandatory supervised Antabuse therapy in an outpatient alcoholism program: a pilot study. *Alcohol. Clin. Exp. Res.*, **10**, 290–2.

Sharkawi, M. and Cianflone, D. (1978) Disulfiram-induced hypothermia in the normal rat: Its attenuation by pimozide. *Neuropharmacology*, **17**, 401–4.

Sharkawi, M. and Caillé, G. (1979) Disulfiram enhances ethanol pharmacological activity and impairs its elimination. *Toxicol. Lett.*, **4**, 485–91.

Sharkawi, M. (1980) Inhibition of alcohol dehydrogenase by disulfiram: possible relation to the disulfiram-ethanol reaction. *Life Sci.*, **27**, 1939–45.

Shaw, I.A. (1951) The treatment of alcoholism with tetraethylthiuram disulfide in a state mental hospital; A clinical study based on 43 cases. *Q. J. Stud. Alcohol*, **12**, 567–86.

Shimada, H., Kawagoe, M., Kiyozumi, M. and Kojima, S. (1990) Comparative effects of three dithiocarbamates on tissue distribution and excretion of cadmium in mice. *Res. Commun. Chem. Pathol. Pharmacol.*, **69**, 49–58.

Shinobu, L.A., Jones, M.M., Basinger, M.A., Mitchell, W.M., Wendel, D. and Razzuk, A. (1983a) In vivo screening of potential antidotes for chronic cadmium intoxication. *J. Toxicol. Envirn. Health*, **12**, 757–65.

Shinobu, L.A., Jones, S.G. and Jones, M.M. (1983b) Mobilization of aged cadmium deposits by dithiocarbamates. *Arch. Toxicol.*, **54**, 235–42.

Sidhu, R.S. and Blair, A.H. (1975) The action of chelating agents on human aldehyde dehydrogenase. *Biochem. J.*, **151**, 443–5.

Siegers, C.-P., Larseille, J. and Younes M. (1982) Effects of dithiocarb and (+)-catechin on microsomal enzyme activities of rat liver. *Res. Commun. Chem. Pathol. Pharmacol.*, **236**, 61–73.

Siew, C., Deitrich, R.A. and Erwin, V.G. (1976) Localization and characteristics of rat liver mitochondrial aldehyde dehydrogenases. *Arch. Bioch. Biophys.*, **176**, 638–49.

Silver, D.F., Ewing, J.A., Rouse, B.A. and Mueller, R.A. (1979) Responses to disulfiram in healthy young men: a double-blind study. *J. Stud. Alcohol*, **40**, 1003–13.

Simmons, T.W. and Jamall, I.S. (1988) Significance of alterations in hepatic anti-oxidant enzymes: Primacy of glutathione peroxidase. *Biochem. J.*, **251**, 913–7.

Singh, P.K., Jones, S.G., Gale, G.R., Jones, M.M., Smith, A.B. and Atkins, L.M. (1990) Selective removal of cadmium from aged hepatic and renal deposits: *N*-substituted talooctamine dithiocarbamates as cadmium mobilizing agents. *Chem. Biol. Interact.*, **74**, 79–91.

Sisson, R.W. and Azrin, N.H. (1986) Family-member involvement to initiate and promote treatment of problem drinkers. *J. Behav. Ther. Exp. Psychiatry*, **17**, 15–21.

Sladek, N.E. and Landkamer, G.J. (1985) Restoration of sensitivity to oxazaphosphorines by inhibitors of aldehyde dehydrogenase activity in cultured oxazaphosphorine-resistant L1210 and cross-linking agent-resistant P338 cell lines. *Cancer Res.*, **45**, 1549–55.

Sladek, N.E. (1988) Metabolism of oxazaphosphorines. *Pharmacol. Ther.*, **37**, 301–55.

Sladek, N.E., Manthey, C.L., Maki, P.A., Zhang, Z. and Landkamer, G.J. (1989) Xenobiotic oxidation catalyzed by aldehyde dehydrogenases. *Drug Metab. Rev.*, **20**, 697–720.

Snyderwine, E.G. and Hunter, A. (1987) Metabolism and distribution of ^{14}C- and ^{35}S-labeled carbon disulfide in immature rats of different ages. *J. Pharmacol. Exp. Ther.*, **15**, 289–94.

Snyderwine, E.G., Kroll, R. and Rubin, R.J. (1988) The possible role of the ethanol-inducible isozyme of cytochrome P_{450} in the metabolism and distribution of carbon disulfide. *Toxicol. Appl. Pharmacol.*, **93**, 11–21.

Socialstyrelsen (1984) English version: Opinions and recommendations from group. In *Pharmacological Treatment of Alcoholism: Withdrawal and Aversion Therapy.* Socialstyrelsens Lakemedelsavdelning, 75125 Uppsala, Sweden, 1985/2 pp. 131–7.

Sorensen, J.A. and Andersen, O. (1989) Effects of diethyldithiocarbamate and tetraethylthiuram disulfide on zinc metabolism in mice. *Pharmacol. Toxicol.*, **65**, 209–13.

Spath, A. and Tempel, K. (1987) Diethyldithiocarbamate inhibits scheduled and unscheduled DNA synthesis of rat thymocytes *in vitro* and *in vivo*: Dose-effect relationships and mechanisms of action. *Chem. Biol. Interact.*, **64**, 151–66.

Sprince, H., Parker, C.M., Smith, G.G., and Gonzales, L.J. (1974) Protection against acetaldehyde toxicity in the rat by L-cysteine, thiamin and L-2-methylthiazoline-4-carboxylic acid. *Agents Actions*, 4, 125–30.

Sprince, H., Parker, C.M., Smith, G.G. and Gonzales, L.J. (1975) Protective action of ascorbic acid and sulfur compounds against acetaldehyde toxicity: Implications in alcoholism and smoking. *Agents Actions*, 5, 164–73.

Sprince, H., Parker, C.M. and Smith, G.G. (1979) Comparison of protection by L-ascorbic acid, L-cysteine and adrenergic-blocking agents against acetaldehyde, acreoline, and formaldehyde toxicity: Implications in smoking. *Agents Actions*, 9, 407–14.

Srivastava, S.K. and Beutler, E. (1969) The transport of oxidized glutathione from human erythrocytes. *J. Biol. Chem.*, 244, 9–16.

Stacey, N.H. and Craig, G.K. (1989) Role of thiols in human peripheral blood natural killer and killer lymphocyte activities. *Experientia*, 45, 180–1.

Stanton, T.H., Calkins, C.E., Jandinski, J. *et al.* (1978) The Qa-1 antigenic system: relation of Qa-1 phenotypes to lymphocytes sets, mitogen response, and immune functions. *J. Exp. Med.*, 148, 963–73.

Starý, J. and Kratzer, K. (1968) Determination of extractions of metal diethyl-dithiocarbamates. *Anal. Chim. Acta*, 40, 93–100.

Stavinoha, W.B., Emerson, G.A. and Nash, J.B. (1959) The effects of some sulfur compounds on thallotoxicosis in mice. *Toxicol. Appl. Pharmacol.*, 1, 638–46.

Steckler, P.P. and Harris, L. (1951) A preliminary report on Antabuse therapy for alcoholism. *Psychiatr. Q.*, 25, 91–6.

Sternberg, D.E., van Kammen, D.P., Lerner, P. *et al.* (1983) CSF dopamine-β-hydroxylase in schizophrenia: Low activity associated with good prognosis and good response to neuroleptic treatment. *Arch. Gen. Psychiatry*, 40, 743–7.

Stewart, D.J., Verma, S. and Maroun, J.A. (1987) Phase I study of the combination of disulfiram and cisplatin. *Am. J. Clin. Oncol.*, 10, 517–9.

Stites, D.P., Stobo, J.D. and Wells, J.V. (1987) *Basic and Clinical Immunology*, 6th ed, Appleton and Lange, Norwalk, CN, USA, pp. 128–32.

Stohs, S.J. and Wu, C.L.J. (1982) Effect of various xenobiotics and steroids on aryl hydrocarbon hydroxylase activity of intestinal and hepatic microsomes from male rats. *Pharmacology*, 25, 237–49.

Stoppani, A.O.M., Schwarcz, M.N. and Freda, C.E. (1966) Action of zinc-complexing agents on nicotinamide adenine dinucleotide-linked aldehyde dehydrogenase from yeast and liver. *Arch. Biochem. Biophys.*, 113, 464–77.

Storm, J.E., Millington, W.R. and Fechter, L.D. (1984) Diethyldithiocarbamate depresses the acute startle response in rats. *Psychopharmacology*, 82, 68–72.

Stripp, B., Greene, F.E. and Gillette, J.R. (1969) Disulfiram impairment of drug metabolism by rat liver microsomes. *J. Pharmacol. Exp. Ther.*, 170, 347–54.

Strömme, J.H. (1963a) Inhibition of hexokinase by disulfiram and diethyldithiocarbamate. *Biochem. Pharmacol.*, 12, 157–66.

Strömme, J.H. (1963b) Effects of diethydithiocarbamate and disulfiram on glucose metabolism and glutathione content of human erythrocytes. *Biochem. Pharmacol.*, 12, 705–15.

Strömme, J.H. (1965a) Interactions of disulfiram and diethyldithiocarbamate with serum proteins studied by means of a gel-filtration technique. *Biochem. Pharmacol.*, 14, 381–91.

Strömme, J.H. (1965b) Metabolism of disulfiram and diethyldithiocarbamate in rats with demonstration of an *in vivo* ethanol-induced inhibition of the glucuronic acid conjugation of the thiol. *Biochem. Pharmacol.*, 14, 393–410.

Strömme, J.H. and Eldjarn, L. (1966) Distribution and chemical forms of diethyl-dithiocarbamate and tetraethylthiuram disulphide (disulfiram) in mice in relation to radioprotection. *Biochem. Pharmacol.*, **15**, 287–97.

Sugimoto, E., Takahashi, N., Kitagawa, Y. and Chiba, H. (1976) Intracellular localiz-ation and characterization of beef liver aldehyde dehydrogenase isozymes. *Agr. Biol. Chem.*, **40**, 2063–70.

Sunderman, F.W. and Sunderman, F.W., Jr (1958) Nickel poisoning. VIII. Dithiocarb: A new therapeutic agent for persons exposed to nickel carbonyl. *Am. J. Med. Sci.*, **236**, 26–31.

Sunderman, F.W. (1964) Nickel and copper mobilization by sodium diethyl-dithiocarbamate. *J. New Drugs*, **4**, 154–61.

Sunderman, F.W., Paynter, O.E. and George, R.B. (1967) The effects of the protrac-ted administration of the chelating agent, sodium diethyldithiocarbamate (dithiocarb). *Am. J. Med. Sci.*, **254**, 24–33.

Sunderman, F.W., Jr (1967) Diethyldithiocarbamate therapy of thallotoxicosis. *Am J. Med. Sci.* **253**, 209–20.

Sunderman, F.W., Jr. Reid, M.C., Bibeau, L.M. and Linden, J.V. (1983a) Nickel induction of microsomal heme oxygenase activity in rodents. *Toxicol. Appl. Pharmacol.*, **68**, 87–95.

Sunderman, F.W., Jr, Bibeau, L.M. and Reid, M.C. (1983b) Synergistic induction of microsomal heme oxygenase activity in rat liver and kidney by diethyldithiocar-bamate and nickel chloride. *Toxicol. Appl. Pharmacol.*, **71**, 436–44.

Sunderman, F.W., Sr (1971) The treatment of acute nickel carbonyl poisoning with sodium diethyldithiocarbamate. *Ann. Clin. Res.*, **3**, 182–5.

Sunderman, F.W., Sr (1981) Chelation therapy in nickel poisoning. *Ann. Clin. Lab. Sci.*, **11**, 1–8.

Sunderman, F.W., Sr, Schneider, H.P. and Lumb, G. (1984) Sodium diethyldithiocar-bamate administration in nickel-induced malignant tumors. *Ann. Clin. Lab. Sci.*, **14**, 1–9.

Sunderman, F.W., Sr (1990) Use of sodium diethyldithiocarbamate in the treatment of nickel carbamyl poisoning. *Ann. Clin. Lab. Sci.*, **20**, 12–21.

Suokas, A., Kupari, M., Pettersson, J. and Lindros, K. (1985) The nitrefazole-ethanol interaction in man: cardiovascular responses and the accumulation of acetaldehyde and catecholamines. *Alcohol. Clin. Exp. Res.*, **9**, 221–7.

Symchowicz, S., Korduba, C.A., Veals, J. and Tabachnick, I.I.A. (1966) Duration of the effect of disulfiram on incorporation and metabolism of dopamine-^{14}C in hypertensive rat. *Biochem. Pharmacol.*, **15**, 1607–10.

Syvertsen, C. and McKinley-McKee, J.S. (1984) Binding of ligands to the catalytic zinc ion in horse liver alcohol dehydrogenase. *Arch. Biochem. Biophys.*, **228**, 159–69.

Szendzikowski, S., Stetkiewicz, J., Wronska-Nofer, T. *et al.* (1974) Pathomorphology of the experimental lesion of the peripheral nervous system in white rats chronically exposed to carbon disulfide. In *Structure and Function of Normal and Diseased Muscle and Peripheral Nerve* (eds I. Hausmanowa-Petrusewicz and H. Jedrizejowska), Polish Medical Publishers, Warsaw, pp. 310–26.

Szerdahelyi, P. and Kasa, P. (1987a) Partial depletion and altered distribution of synaptic zinc in the rat hippocampus after treatment with sodium diethyl-dithiocarbamate. *Brain Res.*, **422**, 287–94.

Szerdahelyi, P. and Kasa, P. (1987b) Regional differences in the uptake of exogenous copper into rat brain after acute treatment with sodium diethyl-dithiocarbamate: A histochemical and atomic absorption spectrometric study. *Histochemistry*, **86**, 627–32.

Taelman, H., Sprecher, S., Teirlynck, O., Bogaerts, M., Gigase, P. and Piot, P. (1987) Suramin–Imuthiol combination therapy of patients with AIDS-related complex (ARC): Results in 6 cases. *Third International Conference on AIDS*, Abstract volume, National Institute of Health, Bethesda, MD, p. 201, Abstract THP. 227.

Tahsildar, H.I. Biaglow, J.E., Kligerman, M.M. and Varnes, M.E. (1988) Factors influencing the oxidation of the radioprotector WR-1065. *Radiat. Res.*, **113**, 243–51.

Takagi, Y., Shikita, M., Terasima, T. and Akaboshi, S. (1974) Specificity of radio-protective and cytotoxic effects of cysteamine in HeLa S_3: Generation of peroxide as the mechanism of paradoxical toxicity. *Radiat. Res.*, **60**, 292–301.

Takahashi, N., Kitabatake, N., Sasaki, R. and Chiba, H. (1979) Enzymatic improve-ment of food flavor. I. Purification and characterization of bovine liver mitochon-drial aldehyde dehydrogenase. *Agric. Biol. Chem.*, **43**, 1873–82.

Tandon, S.K., Behari, R. and Ashquin, M. (1983) Effect of thiol chelators on trace metal levels. *Res. Commun. Chem. Pathol. Pharmacol.*, **42**, 501–4.

Tandon, S.K., Flora, S.J.S. and Singh, S. (1985) Chelation in metal intoxication. XIV. Comparative effect of thiol and amino chelators on lead-poisoned rats with normal or damaged kidneys. *Toxicol. Appl. Pharmacol.*, **79**, 204–10.

Taylor, R.D., Maners, A.W., Salari, H., Baker, M. and Walker, E.M., Jr (1986) Disulfiram as a radiation modifier. *Ann. Clin. Lab. Sci.*, **16**, 443–9.

Tempel, K., Schmerold, I. and Goette, A. (1985) The cytotoxic action of diethyl-dithiocarbamate *in vitro*: Different inhibitions of scheduled and unscheduled DNA synthesis of rat thymic and splenic cells *Arzneimittelforschung*, **35**, 1052–4.

Teng, Y.S. (1981) Human liver aldehyde dehydrogenase in Chinese and Asiatic Indians: gene deletion and its possible implications in alcohol metabolism. *Biochem. Genet.*, **19**, 107–14.

Thoenen, H., Haefely, W., Gey, K.F. and Hürlimann, A. (1965) Diminished effects of sympathetic stimulation in cats pretreated with disulfiram; Liberation of dopamine as sympathetic transmitter. *Life Sci.*, **4**, 2033–8.

Thoenen, H., Haefely, W., Gey, K.F. and Hürlimann, A. (1967) Quantitative aspects of the replacement of norepinephrine by dopamine as a sympathetic transmitter after inhibition of dopamine-β-hydroxylase by disulfiram. *J. Pharmacol. Exp. Ther.*, **156**, 246–51.

Thorn, G.D. and Ludwig, R.A. (1962) *The Dithiocarbamates and Related Com-pounds*, Elsevier, New York, 297 pp.

Till, J.E. and McCulloch, E.A. (1961) A direct measurement of the radiation sensitivity of normal mouse bone marrow cells. *Radiat. Res.*, **14**, 213–22.

Tjälve, H., Jasim, S. and Oskarsson, A. (1984) Nickel mobilization by sodium diethyldithiocarbamate in nickel-carbonyl-treated mice. *IARC Sci. Publ.*, **53**, 311–20.

Tompsett, S.L. (1964) The determination of disulfiram (Antabus, tetraethylthiuram-disulphide) in blood and urine. *Acta Pharmacol. Toxicol.*, **21**, 20–2.

Torronen, R. (1985) Isolation and characterization of rat liver cytosolic aldehyde dehydrogenases induced by phenanthrene or benzo[*a*]pyrene. *Int. J. Biochem.*, **17**, 101–6.

Tottmar, S.O.C., Pettersson, H. and Kiessling, K.-H. (1973) The subcellular distribu-tion and properties of aldehyde dehydrogenases in rat liver. *Biochem. J.*, **135**, 577–86.

Tottmar, O. and Marchner, H. (1976) Disulfiram as a tool in the studies on the metabolism of acetaldehyde in rats. *Acta Pharmacol. Toxicol.*, **38**, 366–75.

Tottmar, O. and Hellström, E. (1979) Blood pressure response to ethanol in relation to acetaldehyde levels and dopamine-beta-hydroxylase activity in rats pretreated with disulfiram, cyanamide and coprine. *Acta Pharmacol. Toxicol.*, **45**, 272–81.

Tottmar, O. and Hellström, E (1983) Aldehyde dehydrogenase in blood: sensitive assay and inhibition by disulfiram. *Pharm. Biochem. Behav.*, **18, Suppl. 1**, 103–7.

Towell, J.F., Cho, J.-K., Roh, B.L. and Wang, R.I.H. (1983a) Disulfiram and erythrocyte aldehyde dehydrogenase inhibition. *Clin. Pharmacol. Ther.*, **33**, 517–21.

Towell, J.F., Cho, J.-K., Roh, B.L. and Wang, R.I.H. (1983b) Aldehyde dehydrogenase and alcoholism. *Lancet*, **1**, 364–5.

Traiger, G.J., Vyas, K.P. and Hanzlick, R.P. (1984) Effect of thiocarbonyl compounds on α-naphthylisothiocyanate-induced hepatotoxicity and urinary excretion of ^{35}S α-naphthylisothiocyanate in the rat. *Toxicol. Appl. Pharmacol.*, **72**, 504–12.

Traiger, G.J., Vyas, K.P. and Hanzlick, R.P. (1985) Effect of inhibitors of α-naphthylisothiocyanate-induced hepatotoxicity on the *in vitro* metabolism of α-naphthylisothiocyanate. *Chem. Biol. Interact.*, **52**, 335–45.

Trombetta, L.D., Toulon, M. and Jamall I.S. (1988) Protective effects of glutathione on diethyldithiocarbamate (DDC) cytotoxicity: a possible mechanism. *Toxicol. App. Pharmacol.*, **93**, 154–64.

Truitt, E.B., Jr (1970) Ethanol-induced release of acetaldehyde from blood and its effect on the determination of acetaldehyde. *Q. J. Stud. Alcohol*, **31**, 1–12.

Truitt, E.B., Jr and Walsh, M.J. (1971) The role of acetaldehyde in the actions of ethanol. In *The Biology of Alcoholism* Vol. 1. *Biochemistry* (eds B. Kissin and H. Begleiter), Plenum, New York, pp. 161–87.

Udenfriend, S., Zaltzman-Nirenberg, P., Gordon, R. and Spector, S. (1966) Evaluation of the biochemical effects produced *in vivo* by inhibitors of the three enzymes involved in norepinephrine biosynthesis. *Mol. Pharmacol.*, **2**, 95–105.

USAN (1990) *USAN and the USP dictionary of drug names* (ed. W.M. Heller), Rockville, MD, United States Pharmacopeial Convention, p. 196.

Valeriote, F. and Grates, H.E. (1986) Potentiation of nitrogen mustard cytotoxicity to leukemia cells by sulfur-containing compounds administered *in vivo*. *Int. J. Rad. Oncol. Biol. Phys.*, **12**, 1165–69.

Valeriote, F. and Grates, H.E. (1989) Potentiation of nitrogen mustard cytotoxicity by disulfiram, diethyldithiocarbamic acid, and diethylamine in mice. *Cancer Res.*, **49**, 6658–61.

Vallari, R.C. and Pietruszko, R. (1982) Human aldehyde dehydrogenase: Mechanism of inhibition by disulfiram. *Science*, **216**, 637–9.

Vallari, R.C. and Pietruszko, R. (1983) Interaction of human cytoplasmic aldehyde dehydrogenase E_1 with disulfiram. *Pharm. Biochem. Behav.*, **18, Suppl. 1**, 97–102.

Van Bekkum, D.W. (1956) The protective action of dithiocarbamates against the lethal effects of X-irradiation in mice. *Acta Physiol. Pharmacol. Neerl.*, **4**, 508–23.

Van Doorn, R., Delbressine, L.P.C., Leijdekkers, C.M., Vertin, P.G. and Henderson, P. Th. (1981) Identification and determination of 2-thiothiazolidine-4-carboxylic acid in urine of workers exposed to carbon disulfide. *Arch. Toxicol.*, **47**, 51–8.

Van Doorn, R., Leijdekkers, C.M., Nossent, S.M. and Henderson, P. Th. (1982) Excretion of TTCA in human urine after administration of disulfiram. *Toxicol. Lett.*, **12**, 59–64.

Van Driessche, E., Beeckmans, S., Dejaegere, R. and Kanarek, L. (1984) Thiourea: The antioxidant of choice for the purification of proteins from phenol-rich plant tissues. *Anal. Biochem.*, **141**, 184–8.

van Royen, E.A. (1987) Thallium-201 DDC, an alternative radiopharmaceutical for rCBF. *Nucl. Med. Comm.*, **8**, 603–10.

van Royen, E.A., de Bruine, J.F., Hill, T.C. *et al.* (1987) Cerebral blood flow imaging with thallium-201 diethyldithiocarbamate SPECT. *J. Nucl. Med.*, **28**, 178–83.

Van Thiel, D.H., Gavaler, J.S., Paul, G.M. and Smith, W.I., Jr (1979) Disulfiram-induced disturbances in hypothalamic-pituitary function. *Alcohol. Clin. Exp. Res.*, **3**, 230–4.

Vergroesen, A.J., Budke, L. and Vos, O. (1967) Protection against X-irradiation by sulphydryl compounds. II. Studies on the relation between chemical structure and protective activity for tissue culture cells. *Int. J. Radiat. Biol.*, **13**, 77–92.

Verma, S., Stewart, D.J., Maroun, J.A. and Nair, R.C. (1990) A randomized phase II study of cisplatin alone versus cisplatin plus disulfiram. *Am. J. Clin. Oncol.*, **13**, 119–24.

Vesell, E.S., Passananti, G.T. and Lee, C.H. (1971) Impairment of drug metabolism by disulfiram in man. *Clin. Pharmacol. Ther.*, **12**, 785–92.

Vesell, E.S., Passananti, G.T. and Glenwright, P.A. (1975) Anomalous results of studies on drug interaction in man. *Pharmacology*, **13**, 481–91.

Volicer, L. and Nelson, K.L. (1984) Development of reversible hypertension during disulfiram therapy. *Arch. Intern. Med.*, **144**, 1294–6.

von Bahr-Lindström, H., Hempel, J. and Jörnvall, H. (1984) The cytoplasmic isoenzyme of horse liver aldehyde dehydrogenase: Relationship to the corresponding human isoenzyme. *Eur. J. Biochem.*, **141**, 37–42.

von Bahr-Lindström, H., Jeck, R., Woenckhaus, C., Sohn, S., Hempel, J. and Jörnvall, H. (1985) Characterization of the coenzyme binding site of liver aldehyde dehydrogenase: Differential reactivity of coenzyme analogues. *Biochemistry*, **24**, 5847–51.

Wagner, H., Jr, Parkinson, D.R., Madoc-Jones, H., Sternick, E.S., Vrusho, K. and Krasin, F. (1984) Combined effect of diethyldithiocarbamate (DDC) and modest hypothermia on Chinese hamster (V79) cell survival and DNA strand break repair following photon irradiation. *Int. J. Radiat. Oncol. Biol. Phys.*, **10**, 1575–9.

Walker, E.M., Jr and Gale, G.R. (1981) Methods of reduction of cisplatin nephrotoxicity. *Ann. Clin. Lab. Sci.*, **11**, 397–410.

Walker, E.M., Jr, Gale, G.R., Greene, W.B. *et al.* (1984) Effects of substituted dithiocarbamates on the testicular toxicity of cadmium. *Res. Commun. Chem. Pathol. Pharmacol.*, **46**, 449–67.

Walker, E.M., Jr, Gale, G.R., Fody, E.P., Atkins, L.M., Smith, A.B. and Jones, M.M. (1986) Comparative antidotal effects of diethyldithiocarbamate, dimercaptosuccinate, and diethylenetriaminepentaacetate against cadmium-induced testicular toxicity in mice. *Res. Commun. Chem. Pathol. Pharmacol.*, **51**, 231–44.

Wallerstein, R.S. (1956) Comparative study of treatment methods for chronic alcoholism: The alcoholism research project at Winter VA Hospital. *Am. J. Psychiatry*, **113**, 228–33.

Wallerstein, R.S., Chotlos, J.W., Friend, M.B., Hammersley, D.W., Perlswig, E.A. and Winship, G.M. (1957) *Hospital Treatment of Alcoholism: A Comparative Experimental Study*. Basic Books, New York, 212 pp.

Wallerstein, R.S. (1958) Psychologic factors in chronic alcoholism. *Ann. Intern. Med.*, **48**, 114–22.

Waxman, D.J. (1986) Rat hepatic cholesterol 7 α-hydroxylase: Biochemical properties and comparison to constitutive and xenobiotic-inducible cytochrome P-450 enzymes. *Arch. Bioch. Biophys.*, **247**, 335–45.

Waxman, D.J. (1988) Interactions of hepatic cytochromes P-450 with steroid hormones: Regioselectivity and stereospecificity of steroid metabolism and hormonal regulation of rat P-450 enzyme expression. *Biochem. Pharmacol.*, 37, 71–84.

Weddington, W.W., Marks, R.C. and Verghese, J.P. (1980) Disulfiram encephalopathy as a cause of the catatonia syndrome. *Am. J. Psychiatry*, 137, 1217–19.

Weiner, H., Simpson, C.W., Thurman, J.A. and Myers, R.D. (1978) Disulfiram alters dopamine metabolism at sites in rat's forebrain as detected by push-pull perfusions. *Brain Res. Bull.*, 3, 541–8.

Weiner, H. and Ardelt, B. (1984) Distribution and properties of aldehyde dehydrogenase in regions of rat brain. *J. Neurochem.*, 42, 109–15.

Weiner, H. (1987) Subcellular localization of acetaldehyde oxidation in liver. *Ann. N.Y. Acad. Sci.*, 492, 25–33.

Weisiger, R.A. and Jakoby, W.B. (1979) Thiol S-methyltransferase from rat liver. *Arch. Bioch. Biophys.*, 196, 631–7.

Weisiger, R.A. and Jakoby, W.B. (1980) S-Methylation: Thiol S-methyltransferase. In *Enzymatic Basis of Detoxication* Vol. 2 (ed W.B. Jakoby), Academic Press, New York, pp. 131–40.

Weiss, B., Cory-Slechta, D.A. and Cox, C. (1990) Modification of lead distribution by diethyldithiocarbamate. *Fund. Appl. Toxicol.*, 15, 791–9.

Wells, J. and Koves, E. (1974) Detection of carbon disulphide (a disulfiram metabolite) in expired air by gas chromatography. *J. Chromatogr.*, 92, 442–4.

West, B. and Sunderman, F.W. (1958) Nickel poisoning. VII. The therapeutic effectiveness of alkyl dithiocarbamates in experimental animals exposed to nickel carbonyl. *Am. J. Med. Sci.*, 236, 15–25.

Westman, G. and Marklund, S.L. (1980) Diethyldithiocarbamate, a superoxide dismutase inhibitor, decreases the radioresistance of Chinese hamster cells. *Radiat. Res.*, 83, 303–1.

Westman, G. and Midander, J. (1984) Post-irradiation diethyldithiocarbamate-inhibition of CuZn superoxide dismutase reduces clonogenic survival of Chinese hamster V-79 cells. *Int. J. Rad. Biol.*, 45, 11–20.

Whittington, H.G. and Grey, L. (1969) Possible interaction between disulfiram and isoniazid. *Am. J. Psychiatry*, 125, 1725–9.

Williams, E.E. (1937) Effects of alcohol on workers with carbon disulfide. *J. Am. Med. Assoc.*, 109, 1472.

Williams, R.J.P. (1981) Physico-chemical aspects of inorganic element transfer through membranes. *Philos. Trans. R. Soc., Lond.*, B 294, 57–74.

Willson, R.A., Hart, F.E. and Hew, J.T. (1979) Breath analysis of $^{14}CO_2$ production from aminopyrine in the normal rat. *Res. Commun. Chem. Pathol. Pharmacol.*, 23, 505–21.

Willson, R.L. (1987) Vitamin, selenium, zinc and copper interactions in free radical protection against ill-placed iron. *Proc. Nutr. Soc.*, 46, 27–34.

Wilson, A., Davidson, W.J. and Blanchard, R. (1980) Disulfiram implantation: A trial using placebo implants and two types of controls. *J. Stud. Alcohol*, 41, 429–36.

Wise, J.D. (1981) Disulfiram toxicity - a review of the literature. *J. Arkansas Med. Soc.*, 78, 87–92.

Wittenberg, C. and Triplett, E.L. (1985) A detergent-activated tyrosinase from *Xenopus laevis*. I. Purification and partial characterization. *J. Biol. Chem.*, 260, 12535–40.

Wokittel, E. (1960) Vergiftung mit Antabus bei einem 10 jäahrigen Mädchen. *Arch. Kinderheilk.*, **161**, 145–9.

Worner, T.M. (1982) Peripheral neuropathy after disulfiram administration: Reversibility despite continued therapy. *Drug Alcohol Dep.*, **10**, 199–201.

Wratten, C.C. and Cleland, W.W. (1963) Product inhibition studies on yeast and liver alcohol dehydrogenases. *Biochemistry*, **2**, 935–41.

Wright, C. (1989) Disulfiram treatment of alcoholism. *Ann. Intern. Med.*, **111**, 943–45.

Wright, C. and Moore, R.D. (1990) Disulfiram treatment of alcoholism. *Am. J. Med.*, **88**, 647–55.

Wysor, M.S., Zwelling, L.A., Sanders, J.E. and Grenan, M.M. (1982) Cure of mice infected with *Trypanosoma rhodesiense* by *cis*-diamminedichloroplatinum (II) and disulfiram rescue. *Science*, **217**, 454–6.

Yeh, S.J., Lo, J.M. and Shen, L.H. 1980 Determination of extraction constants for metal diethyldithiocarbamates and chloride-mixed metal diethyldithiocarbamates by substoichiometric extraction. *Anal. Chem.*, **52**, 528–31.

Yin, S.-J., Cheng, T.-C., Chang, C.-P. *et al.* (1988) Human stomach alcohol and aldehyde dehydrogenases (ALDH): A genetic model proposed for ALDH III isozymes. *Biochem. Genet.*, **26**, 343–60.

Yoshida, A., Huang, I-Y. and Ikawa, M. (1984) Molecular abnormality of an inactive aldehyde dehydrogenase variant commonly found in Orientals. *Proc. Nat. Acad. Sci. USA*, **81**, 258–61.

Yoshida, A. and Davé, V. (1985) Enzymatic activity of atypical Oriental types of aldehyde dehydrogenases. *Biochem. Genet.*, **23**, 585–90.

Yoshida, A., Ikawa, M., Hsu, L.C. and Tani, K. (1985) Molecular abnormality and cDNA cloning of human aldehyde dehydrogenases. *Alcohol*, **2**, 103–6.

Yoshimoto, T., Yamamoto, K. and Tsuru, D. (1985) Extracellular tyrosinase from *Streptomyces* sp. KY-453: Purification and some enzymatic properties. *J. Biochem.*, **97**, 1747–54.

Yourick, J.J. and Faiman, M.D. (1987) Diethyldithiocarbamic acid-methyl ester: A metabolite of disulfiram and its alcohol sensitizing properties in the disulfiram-ethanol reaction. *Alcohol*, **4**, 463–7.

Yourick, J.J. and Faiman, M.D. (1989) Comparative aspects of disulfiram and its metabolites in the disulfiram-ethanol reaction in the rat. *Biochem. Pharmacol.*, **38**, 413–21.

Zanocco, A.L., Pavez, R., Videla, L.A. and Lissi, E.A. (1989) Antioxidant capacity of diethyldithiocarbamate in metal independent lipid peroxidative process. *Free Rad. Biol. Med.*, **7**, 151–6.

Zemaitis, M.A. and Green, F.E. (1976a) Impairment of hepatic microsomal and plasma esterases of the rat by disulfiram and diethyldithiocarbamate. *Biochem. Pharmacol.*, **25**, 453–9.

Zemaitis, M.A. and Green, F.E. (1976b) Impairment of hepatic microsomal drug metabolism in the rat during daily disulfiram administration. *Biochem. Pharmacol.*, **25**, 1355–60.

Zemaitis, M.A. and Green, F.E. (1979) *In vivo* and *in vitro* effects of thiuram disulfides and dithiocarbamates on hepatic microsomal drug metabolism in the rat. *Toxicol. Appl. Pharmacol.*, **48**, 343–50.

Ziegler, D.M. (1980) Microsomal flavin-containing monooxygenase: Oxygenation of nucleophilic nitrogen and sulfur compounds. In *Enzymatic Basis of Detoxication* Vol. 1 (ed W.B. Jakoby), Academic Press, New York, pp. 201–27.

Author and citation index

Journal or book page and volume of articles being cited are given in parentheses, the volume number in **bold**. Pages on which citations occur in this book are in *italics*. Titles of publications are listed in a contracted form; full book titles and conventional journal abbreviations are to be found in References.

Aarnio M
  86 Prog Clin Biol Res (**232**, 103) - *138*
Aaseth J
  79 Acta Pharm Tox (**45**, 41) - *72, 87*
  81 Arch Toxicol (**48**, 29) - *66, 72, 88*
Adachi J
  90 Alc Clin Exp Res (**13**, 601) - *177*
Adachi T
  89 J Biol Chem (**264**, 8537) - *133*
Agarwal DP
  86 Experientia (**42**, 1148) - *6*
  87 Isozymes (**16**, 21) - *6*
  89 Alcohol (**6**, 517) - *6, 144*
  89 Enzyme (**42**, 47) - *139, 158*
Agarwal RP
  83 Res Comm C P P (**42**, 293) - *14, 16, 17, 22-24*
  86 Bioch Pharm (**235**, 3341) - *7, 8, 10, 14, 16, 22, 30, 31*
Akabane JS
  64 Jap J Pharmacol (**14**, 295) - *193*
Akerboom TPM
  81 Method Enzymol (**77**, 373) - *32*
Åkerström S
  56 Acta Chem Scand (**10**, 699) - *8*
Alderman JL
  74 J Pharm Exp Ther (**190**, 334) - *304*
Alexander P
  55 Rad Res (**2**, 392) - *306*
Allain P
  91 Life Sci (**48**, 291) - *87*
Allalunis-Turner J
  84 Int J Rad Oncol (**10**, 1569) - *308, 326*
Allerberg F

91 Arzn-Forsch (**41**, 443) - *5*
Altura BM
  78 Eur J Pharm (**52**, 73) - *196*
Amaral D
  66 Methods Enzym (**9**, 87) - *97*
Andersen MP
  91 Alc Alcoholism (**26**, 233) - *58, 59, 170, 227*
Andersen O
  84 Environ Health Persp (**54**, 249) - *66*
  88 Toxicology (**52**, 331) - *74, 76*
  89 Pharm Tox (**64**, 239) - *76*
  89 Toxicology (**55**, 1) - *76*
Andersson S
  84 Bioch Pharm (**33**, 2930) - *98, 104, 116*
Ansbacher LE
  82 Neurology (**32**, 424) - *238, 244, 341*
Anzil AP
  78 J Neuropath Exp Neur (**37**, 585) - *341*
  80 Adv Neurotoxicol (359) - *341*
  85 Neurotoxicology (535) - *341*
Armor DJ
  76 Alcoholism Treatment (70) - *209*
  76 Alcoholism Treatment (120) - *220*
Armstrong JD
  57 Cand Med Ass J (**77**, 228) - *170*
Arthur JR
  87 Biochem J (**248**, 539) - *133*
Asmussen E
  48 Acta Pharm (**4**, 297) - *169, 172, 174*
  48 Acta Pharm (**4**, 311) - *178, 188, 195*
Aspila KI
  75 Anal Chem (**47**, 945) - *8*

Azrin NH
76 Behav Res Ther (**14**, 339) - *210, 214-216*
82 J Behav Ther (**13**, 105) - *206, 207, 211, 212, 215-217, 223, 224*

Bach JF
77 Nature (**266**, 55) - *265*
Bacq ZM
53 Arch Int Physiol (**61**, 433) - *306*
Baekeland F
75 Res Adv Alc Drug Prob (**2**, 247) - *105*
77 Biology Alcoholism (**5**,161) - *105*
Bakish D
86 J Clin Psychopharm (**6**, 178) - *236*
Bandow GT
77 Arch Int Pharm (**230**, 120) - *194, 195*
Bannister JV
87 Methods Bioch Anal (**32**, 279) - *126*
87 CRC Crit R Bioch (**22**, 111) - *126*
Bannister SJ
79 J Chromat (**173**, 333) - *91*
Bardos P
81 Scand J Imm (**13**, 609) - *258*
85 Int J Immunopharm (**7**, 335) - *258*
Bardsley WG
74 Biochem J (**139**, 169) - *101*
Barneoud P
87 Physiol Behav (**41**, 525) - *256*
Barth R
87 Dig Dis Sci (**32**, 1059) - *240*
Bartkowiak A
83 Int J Biochem (**5**, 763) - *129*
Bartle WR
85 Dig Dis Sci (**30**, 834) - *238, 240*
Baselt RC
77 Res Comm C P P (**18**, 677) - *84*
Basinger MA
89 Tox App Pharm (**97**, 279) - *91*
Bass M
63 J Am Osteopath Ass (**63**, 229) - *68, 70*
Beach CA
86 Clin Pharm Ther (**39**, 265) - *105, 107*
Beauchamp RO
83 CRC Crit Rev Tox (**11**, 169) - *5, 37, 38, 42, 115, 241, 244*
Beck O
86 Drug Alcohol Dep (**16**, 303) - *164*

Becker MC
52 J Am Med Ass (**149**, 568) - *164, 175, 176*
Beedham C
87 Prog Med Chem (**24**, 85) - *166*
Bell RG
49 Cand Med Ass J (**60**, 286) - *169*
Belliveau JF
85 Ann Clin Lab Sci (**15**, 349) - *82*
Bennett AE
51 J Am Med Ass (**145**, 483) - *235*
Benson AM
85 Cancer Res (**45**, 4219) - *135*
Berger D
77 Bioch Pharm (**26**, 741) - *162*
Bergouignan FX
88 J Neurol (**238**, 382) - *341*
Bergström B
82 Lancet (**1**, 49) - *245*
Berlin RG
89 Alc Alcoholism (**24**, 241) - *238*
Berry JM
90 J Clin Oncol (**8**, 1585) - *329-331, 333*
Bertram B
85 J Cancer Res (**109**, 9) - *135*
88 Comb Effec Chem (**193**) - *5, 103, 344*
Beyeler C
85 Alc Clin Exp Res (**9**, 118) - *104, 106, 170, 174, 177, 179-182, 187, 203, 227, 228*
87 Schweiz Med Wschr (**117**, 52) - *104, 170, 173, 174, 177, 181, 182, 187, 227, 228*
Bhagat B
66 Nature (**210**, 823) - *123*
Biaglow JE
84 Rad Res (**100**, 298) - *300*
Bigelow G
76 Behav Res Ther (**14**, 378) - *210, 212, 221*
Bihari B
88 Ultrastruct Pathol (**7**, 295) - *275, 288*
Bilbao JM
84 Ultrastruct Pathol (**7**, 295) - *238, 342*
Black JL
85 J Clin Psychiatry (**46**, 67) - *238*
Black SD
89 Adv Enzymol (**60**, 35) - *102, 117*
Bláha K

85 Toxicol Xenobioch (**1985**, 183) - *79*
88 Toxicol Lett (**42**, 207) - *79*
Blair AH
69 Cand J Biochem (**47**, 265) - *150, 155*
Blanc D
90 Lancet (**335**, 1290) - *232*
Blaustein JD
86 Neuroendocrinology (**43**, 143) - *124*
Bliding A
81 Acta Soc Med Svec(**90**, 278) - *234*
Bloom AS
77 Neuropharm (**16**, 411) - *126*
Blum J
83 Arch Bioch Bioph (**222**, 35) - *134*
85 Arch Bioch Bioph (**240**, 500) - *133, 134*
Bode H
54 Z Anal Chem (**142**, 414) - *8, 9*
Bodenner DL
86 Cancer Res (**46**, 2745) - *45, 46, 61, 92*
86 Cancer Res (**46**, 2751) - *60, 92, 100, 318, 319, 320, 324, 338*
Bond EJ
69 Br J Ind Med (**26**, 335) - *241*
Borch RF
79 P Nat Acad S USA (**76**, 6611) - *317-319*
80 P Nat Acad S USA (**77**, 5441) - *317, 318, 324*
83 Platinum Coordinatio (154) - *319*
86 Chem Abstr (**105**, 30097r) - *328*
86 Chem Abstr (**105**, 35630u) - *328*
87 Platinum Other Metal (216) - *330*
89 Pharm Ther (**41**, 371) - *314*
Borg S
84 Socialstyr (**1985/2**, 65) - *246*
Borrett D
85 Ann Neurol (**17**, 396) - *238, 344*
Bosron WF
86 Hepatology (**6**, 502) - *144*
Bourne PG
66 Q J Stud Alc (**27**, 42) - *222, 231*
Bowman KM
51 Am J Psychi (**107**, 832) - *172*
Branchey L
87 Am J Psychi (**144**, 1310) - *235*
Brewer C
83 Br Med J (**287**, 1282) - *223, 229, 231*

83 Br Med J (**287**, 1795) - *222*
84 Br J Psychi (**144**, 200) - *104, 170, 228*
86 Alc Alcoholism (**21**, 385) - *214, 229*
87 J Am Med Ass (**257**, 926) - *220*
Brewton GW
87 3 C AIDS (Abstract TP218) - *285*
89 Life Sci (**45**, 2509) - *200, 285*
Brieger H
47 Ind Med (**16**, 473) - *338*
Brien JF
83 Alc Clin Exp Res (**7**, 256) - *5, 21, 27*
83 Cand J Physiol Pharm (**61**, 1) - *6, 194*
83 Drug Metab Rev (**14**, 113) - *5*
85 Cand J Physiol Pharm (**63**, 438) - *145*
85 Trends Pharm Sci (**6**, 477) - *6*
Brown CT
51 US Arm Forces Med J (**2**, 191) - *169*
Brown MW
74 J Pharm Pharmacol (**26 S**, 95P) - *25*
Brown ZW
83 Alc Clin Exp Res (**7**, 276) - *192, 193, 226, 227, 229*
Brubaker RG
87 Addict Behav (**12**, 43) - *224, 233*
Brugere S
86 Alcohol (**3**, 317) - *194, 198*
Bruley-Rosset
86 Int J Immunopharm (**8**, 287) - *257, 259, 260*
Burgess I
90 Lancet (**336**, 873) - *232*
Bus JS
85 Neurotoxicology (**6**, 73) - *244*
Buskowicz C
62 Neurol Neuroch Psych (**12**, 293) - *341*
Busse S
78 Disulfiram Treatment (346) - *6*
Byczkowski JZ
88 Int J Biochem (**20**, 569) - *126*

Canellakis ES
53 Arch Bioch Bioph (**42**, 446) - *41*
Cantilena LR
81 Tox App Pharm (**58**, 452) - *74, 76-78, 338*
82 Tox App Pharm (**63**, 338) - *77*

Cao Q
  89 Bioch Pharm (**38**, 77) - *141*
Cardwell M
  87 J Am Med Ass (**257**, 926) - *219*
Carey-Smith
  88 J Stud Alc (**49**, 571) - *246*
Carfagna PF
  90 Fund Appl Tox (**14**, 706) - *316, 317, 319, 320*
Carlsson A
  66 J Pharm Pharmacol (**18**, 60) - *122, 123*
  67 J Pharm Pharmacol (**19**, 481) - *124*
Carmichael FJ
  87 Bioch Pharm (**36**, 2673) - *190, 191*
  88 Am J Physiol (**255**, G417) - *190*
Carper WR
  87 Clin Chem (**33**, 1906) - *99, 100*
Carrara M
  88 Pharm Res Comm (**20**, 611) - *339*
Casagrande G
  89 Blut (**59**, 231) - *242*
Catignani GL
  75 Bioch Biophys R C (**65**, 629) - *117*
Cavanagh JB
  73 CRC Crit Rev Tox (**2**, 365) - *6*
Cederbaum AI
  79 Arch Bioch Bioph (**193**, 551) - *192*
  81 Bioch Pharm (**30**, 3079) - *192*
Centers for Disease Control
  86 Morb Mort W R (**35**, 334) - *281, 285*
Cerutti I
  83 Infect Immun (**42**, 728) - *274*
Cha Y-N
  82 Drug Met Disp (**10**, 434) - *99*
  83 Drug Nutr Interact (**2**, 35) - *109, 135*
Chabal J
  87 Press Med (**16**, 1244) - *290*
Champault G
  83 Med Chir Dig (**12**, 537) - *261, 290*
Chengelis CP
  79 Bioch Biophys R C (**90**, 993) - *38*
Chevens LCF
  53 Br Med J (**1**, 1450) - *229*
Child GP
  50 Fed Proc (**9**, 22) - *202*
  51 Am J Psychi (**107**, 774) - *170, 172, 174, 188, 339*
  52 Acta Pharm Tox (**8**, 305) - *337, 338,*

  340
  52 Q J Stud Alc (**13**, 571) - *184, 185*
Choo LY
  87 Cand J Physiol Pharm (**65**, 2503) - *99*
Christensen JK
  73 Ugeskr Laeger (**135**, 1457) - *234*
  84 Acta Psychiatr Scand (**69**, 265) - *233*
  91 Pharm Tox (**68**, 163) - *170, 227, 228*
Christensen OB
  82 Contact Dermatitis (**8**, 59) - *83*
Chung V
  85 J Immunopharmacol (**7**, 335) - *267, 273*
Ciarulo DA
  85 Am J Psychi (**142**, 1373) - *107*
Cikrt M
  84 Res Comm C P P (**43**, 497) - *78*
  86 J Tox Envir Health (**17**, 419) - *78*
  86 J Tox Envir Health (**17**, 429) - *76, 77*
Cobby J
  77 J Pharm Exp Ther (**202**, 724) - *22, 23, 26, 27*
  77 Life Sci (**21**, 937) - *38, 155*
  78 J Pharmacokin (**6**, 369) - *27, 38, 44, 45, 50, 51, 54, 57, 59, 61, 62*
Cocco D
  81 Biochem J (**199**, 675) - *97, 100, 129*
  81 J Biol Chem (**256**, 8983) - *97, 129, 130*
Cochran AJ
  72 Br Med J (**4**, 67) - *291*
Collins GGS
  65 J Pharm Pharmacol (**17**, 526) - *123*
Conkling P
  82 Infec Immun (**38**, 114) - *298, 299*
  85 Inflammation (**9**, 149) - *132, 298, 299*
Coogan TP
  86 Adv Exp Med Biol (**197**, 284) - *132, 298, 299*
Cooper AJL
  83 Annu Rev Bioch (**52**, 187) - *42*
Corke CF
  84 Int J Immunopharm (**6**, 245) - *255, 273*
  84 Int J Immunopharm (**6**, 535) - *273*
  86 Int J Immunotherap (**2**, 163) - *290*
Council on Pharmacy and Chemistry
  52 J Am Med Ass (**149**, 275) - *170*
Cox PJ

76 Cancer Treat Rep (**60**, 321) - *316*
Crabtree GR
  89 Science (**243**, 355) - *276*
Cramer JA
  89 J Am Med Ass (**261**, 3273) - *206*
Cronholm T
  85 Biochem J (**229**, 315) - *192*
Crow KE
  74 Bioch Biophys Acta (**350**, 121) - *141*
  77 Alc Clin Exp Res (**1**, 43) - *192*
Currie WD
  73 Aerosp Med (**44**, 996) - *304*

Dalvi RR
  74 Life Sci (**14**, 1785) - *117, 241*
  75 Chem Biol Interact (**10**, 347) - *241*
Danielsson BRG
  84 Arch Toxicol (**55**, 27) - *80*
  84 Arch Toxicol (**55**, 161) - *88, 89*
Danscher G
  73 Exp Brain Res (**16**, 521) - *72*
  75 Brain Res (**85**, 522) - *72*
Davidson WJ
  79 J Stud Alc (**40**, 1073) - *23, 24, 56, 57*
Dawson AG
  81 Bioch Pharm (**30**, 2349) - *192*
  83 Bioch Pharm (**32**, 2157) - *192*
de Bruïne JF
  85 J Nucl Med (**26**, 925) - *67, 69*
  88 Brain SPECT with Tl - *69*
  90 Europ J Nucl Med (**17**, 248) - *70*
Dedon PC
  87 Bioch Pharm (**36**, 1955) - *91, 92*
DeGregorio MW
  89 Canc Chemoth Ph (**23**, 276) - *329, 330, 333*
Deitrich RA
  66 Bioch Pharmacol (**15**, 1911) - *144*
  71 Mol Pharm (**7**, 301) - *145, 147, 154*
De La Bastide B
  86 Chem Abstr (**105**, 85204d) - *248*
Delepine N
  85 Lancet (**2**, 1246) - *291*
De Matteis F
  73 Chem Biol Interact (**7**, 375) - *116, 117, 241*
  74 Mol Pharm (**10**, 849) - *117*

Deneke SM
  79 J Pharm Exp Ther (**208**, 377) - *127, 128, 302, 303, 305*
  80 Bioch Pharm (**29**, 1367) - *302, 306*
Derr RF
  83 Res Comm C P P (**39**, 503) - *41*
  84 Res Comm C P P (**46**, 363) - *41*
Diaz JH
  79 Anesthesiology (**51**, 366) - *241*
Dible SE
  87 Eur J Cancer (**23**, 813) - *316, 318, 320, 324*
Dickinson FM
  79 Biochem J (**179**, 709) - *140, 150*
  81 Biochem J (**199**, 573) - *140, 151*
Dierickx PJ
  84 Pharm Res Comm (**16**, 135) - *135*
Diquet B
  90 Eur J Clin Pharm (**38**, 157) - *107, 108*
Divatia KJ
  52 J Lab Clin Med (**39**, 974) - *14, 17, 22-24*
Djurić D
  73 Arch Environ Health (**26**, 287) - *342*
Domar G
  49 Acta Clin Scand (**3**, 1441) - *24*
Domingo JL
  85 Toxicol Lett (**26**, 95) - *338*
Donelli MG
  76 Cancer Treat Rep (**60**, 395) - *328*
Donner M
  83 Scand J Work Envir (**9 S2**, 27) - *344*
Dössing M
  84 Br J Ind Med (**41**, 142) - *241*
Doucette SR
  80 US Navy Med (**71**, 6) - *105*
Drum DE
  69 Biochemistry (**8**, 3783) - *97, 100*
  69 Biochemistry (**8**, 3792) - *97, 100*
  70 Biochemistry (**9**, 4078) - *97, 100*
Dry J
  73 Therapie (**28**, 799) - *104*
Dunlap CE
  85 Neuropharm (**8**, 797) - *202*
Duritz G
  64 Q J Stud Alc (**25**, 498) - *177*
Dutton GJ
  72 Biochem J (**129**, 539) - *34, 36*

Eade NR
59 J Pharm Exp Ther (**127**, 29) - *193*
Eckert G
57 Z Anal Chem (**155**, 22) - *11*
Eckfeldt J
76 J Biol Chem (**251**, 236) - *140, 150, 159*
Edington N
69 Acta Neuropath (**12**, 339) - *341*
Edwards BS
84 J Immunol (**132**, 2868) - *260*
Egle JL
73 Tox App Pharm (**24**, 636) - *193, 194, 198*
Eisen HJ
75 Ann Int Med (**83**, 673) - *240*
Eldjarn L
50 Scand J Clin Lab (**2**, 198) - *45, 48, 53*
50 Scand J Clin Lab (**2**, 202) - *46, 49, 53*
Ellis CN
79 Arch Dermatol (**115**, 1367) - *232*
Eneanya DI
81 Annu Rev Pharmacol (**21**, 575) - *5*
83 Res Comm C P P (**41**, 441) - *34*
Eriksson CJP
77 Anal Biochem (**80**, 116) - *177*
82 Anal Biochem (**125**, 259) - *177*
83 Pharm Bioch Beh (**18 S1**, 141) - *177*
85 Bioch Pharm (**34**, 3979) - *166, 177*
Escaich S
88 4 C AIDS (Abstract 3155) - *288*
Etzioni A
73 Technological Shortc - *6*
Evans RG
82 Cancer Res (**42**, 3074) - *310, 311*
83 Int J Rad Oncol (**9**, 1635) - *307-309, 312, 326*
83 Rad Res (**93**, 319) - *132, 311, 312*
84 Cancer Res (**44**, 3686) - *315, 321, 322, 326*
85 Int J Rad Oncol (**11**, 1163) - *307, 309*
Ewing SP
80 J Am Chem Soc (**102**, 3072) - *41*
Eybl Y
88 Arch Toxicol (**S12**, 438) - *78*
Ezrielev GI
73 Zhurn Nevropat Psik (**73**, 238) - *202*

Fackler JP
68 J Am Chem Soc (**90**, 2707) - *91*
Faiman MD
71 Bioch Pharm (**20**, 3059) - *303-305*
71 Life Sci Part II (**10**, 21) - *303, 305*
77 Res Comm C P P (**17**, 481) - *23, 24, 26, 27, 46, 56, 57, 59, 155*
78 Alc Clin Exp Res (**2**, 366) - *23, 24, 56*
78 Res Comm C P P (**21**, 543) - *39, 56*
79 Biochem Pharm Ethanol (**2**, 325) - *5*
80 Alc Clin Exp Res (**4**, 412) - *45, 48, 52, 55, 56*
83 Alc Clin Exp Res (**7**, 307) - *27, 39, 46, 48, 62, 157, 339*
84 Clin Pharm Ther (**36**, 520) - *34, 37, 47, 49, 52, 53, 55-59, 101, 243, 244*
Fairfield AS
83 Science (**221**, 764) - *131*
Farrés J
88 Biochem J (**256**, 461) - *149, 165*
89 Eur J Bioch (**180**, 67) - *142*
Feldman RI
72 J Biol Chem (**247**, 267) - *151*
Ferencz-Biro K
84 Bioch Biophys R C (**118**, 97) - *144*
Ferguson JKW
49 Cand Med Ass J (**60**, 295) - *169*
Fiala ES
81 Inhibition Tumor Ind (**23**) - *5, 103, 344*
Fisher CM
89 Arch Neurol (**46**, 798) - *236*
Flohe L
82 Free Rad Biol(**5**, 223) - *133*
Flood JF
86 Pharm Bioch Beh (**24**, 631) - *126*
Florentin I
88 Int J Immunotherap (**4**, 5) - *257, 260*
89 Immunopharm Imm (**11**, 645) - *257, 258*
Ford DB
88 Bioch Biophys R C (**153**, 149) - *118*
Forman HJ
80 J Pharm Exp Ther (**212**, 452) - *127, 128, 303*
Forte-McRobbie CM
85 Alcohol (**2**, 375) - *143, 144*

86 J Biol Chem (**261**, 2154) - *138, 139, 165*

Fournier E
67 Thérapie (**22**, 559) - *341*

Fox R
58 NY State J Med (**58**, 1540) - *209*

Frank L
78 Bioch Pharm (**27**, 251) - *127, 302, 339*

Frederickson RE
90 Behav Brain Res (**38**, 25) - *72, 73*

Freireich EJ
66 Canc Chemother (**50**, 219) - *329*

Freund G
73 Life Sci (**13**, 345) - *188*

Freundt KJ
78 Int J Clin Pharm (**16**, 323) - *104, 107*

Fridovich I
83 Annu Rev Pharmacol (**23**, 239) - *126*
89 J Biol Chem (**264**, 7761) - *126*

Fried R
80 Sub Alc Act/Mis (**1**, 5) - *245*

Friedman H
79 Cardiovasc Res (**13**, 477) - *195, 196*

Friedman S
65 J Biol Chem (**240**, 4763) - *125*

Frisoni GB
89 Alc Alcoholism (**24**, 429) - *237, 239*

Fukumori R
79 Life Sci (**25**, 123) - *164*

Fuller RK
79 Ann Int Med (**90**, 901) - *211, 218, 219, 231*
80 Alc Clin Exp Res (**4**, 298) - *218*
81 J Stud Alc (**42**, 202) - *37, 244*
83 J Chron Dis (**36**, 161) - *211, 212, 218, 219, 245*
86 J Am Med Ass (**256**, 1449) - *212, 218, 219, 224, 235, 245*

Furusawa S
88 J Pharmacobio Dyn (**11**, 284) - *316*

Gale GR
81 Ann Clin Lab Sci (**11**, 476) - *74, 78, 339*
81 Drugs of the Future (**6**, 225) - *6*
82 Ann Clin Lab Sci (**12**, 345) - *317, 319, 324, 329*

82 Ann Clin Lab Sci (**12**, 463) - *76, 77*
83 Ann Clin Lab Sci (**13**, 33) - *76, 77*
83 Ann Clin Lab Sci (**13**, 207) - *76, 77*
83 Ann Clin Lab Sci (**13**, 474) - *76, 77*
83 Res Comm C P P (**41**, 293) - *79*
84 Ann Clin Lab Sci (**14**, 137) - *78*
84 Life Sci (**35**, 2571) - *78*
84 Res Comm C P P (**45**, 119) - *90*
85 Res Comm C P P (**47**, 107) - *76, 77*
85 Res Comm C P P (**49**, 423) - *76*
86 Res Comm C P P (**52**, 29) - *80*
86 Res Comm C P P (**53**, 129) - *76, 77*
87 Res Comm C P P (**58**, 371) - *78*
88 Toxicol Let (**44**, 77) - *78*
89 Res Comm C P P (**63**, 395) - *77*
89 Toxicol Let (**48**, 105) - *79*

Gallagher CH
76 Aust J Exp Biol (**54**, 593) - *102*

Gandara DR
88 J Clin Oncol (**6**, 1785) - *331*
88 P Am Soc Clin OncOL (**7**, 69) - *329*
89 P Am Ass Canc Res (**30**, 241) - *329, 331, 333*
90 Crit Rev Oncol (**10**, 353) - *314, 329, 331, 333*

Gardner-Thorpe C
71 J Neurol Neuros Psych (**34**, 253) - *237*

Gendre F
83 CR Acad Sc (III)(**296**, 15) - *264*

Gerrein JR
73 Arch Gen Psychi (**28**, 798) - *221, 223*

Gerschman R
58 Am J Physiol (**192**, 563) - *303*

Gessner PK
73 P 1st Annu Alc C Nat (**79**) - *185*
74 Drug Interactions (**349**) - *185*
87 J Pharm Sci (**76**, 319) - *19*
88 J Am Coll Tox (**7**, 987) - *184, 185, 189, 191*

Gessner T
72 Bioch Pharm (**21**, 219) - *34, 38, 39, 41, 45, 48, 62, 120, 155*

Gigon PL
68 Bioch Biophys R Cm (**31**, 558) - *114*

Giles HG
82 J Liq Chromat (**5**, 945) - *23, 26, 28, 46, 57, 58*

Gleerup G

90 Haemostasis (**20**, 215) - *243*
Glud E
    49 Q J Stud Alc (**10**, 185) - *169*
Goedde HW
    79 Hum Genet (**51**, 331) - *144*
    86 Am J Hum Genet (**38**, 395) - *144*
    90 Pharm Ther (**45**, 345) - *6, 144*
Goering PL
    85 Tox App Pharm (**80**, 467) - *76*
Gold S
    66 Lancet (**2**, 1417) - *232*
Goldstein BD
    79 Bioch Pharm (**28**, 27) - *134, 135,
        265, 304, 306*
Goldstein G
    74 Nature (**147**, 11) - *265*
Goldstein M
    64 Life Sci (**3**, 763) - *8, 121, 125, 193*
    65 J Biol Chem (**240**, 2066) - *125*
    66 Life Sci (**5**, 1133) - *124*
    67 J Pharm Exp Ther (**157**, 96) - *122,
        124*
Gonias SL
    84 Cancer Res (**44**, 5764) - *92*
Goodchild M
    69 J Pharm Pharmacol (**21**, 54) - *126*
Gordis E
    77 Alc Clin Exp Res (**1**, 213) - *37, 244*
Gosselin RE
    84 Clin Tox Commer Prod (III 159) - *6*
Goyer PF
    79 J Stud Alc (**40**, 133) - *240, 343*
    84 J Stud Alc (**45**, 209) - *234, 235*
Grafström R
    80 Bioch Pharm (**29**, 1517) - *108, 109,
        119*
    80 Toxicol Lett (**7**, 79) - *119*
Graham WD
    51 J Pharm Pharmacol (**3**, 160) - *166*
Grandjean P
    90 Ann Clin Lab Sci (**20**, 28) - *72, 86*
Graveleau J
    80 Nouv Presse Med (**9**, 2905) - *238*
Green AL
    64 Bioch Bioph Acta (**81**, 394) - *125*
Greenblatt DJ
    83 Clin Pharm Ther (**33**, 253) - *108*
Greenfield NJ
    77 Bioch Bioph Acta (**483**, 35) - *139,*

    140, 149, 150
Griffiths DE
    61 J Biol Chem (**236**, 1850) - *102*
Gringeri A
    88 Cancer Res (**48**, 5708) - *320-323,
        325, 326*
Guan KL
    88 Alc Clin Exp Res (**12**, 713) - *140*
Guarnieri C
    81 Bioch Pharm (**30**, 2174) - *127, 128*
Guillaumin JM
    84 Reprod Nutr Develop (**24**, 208) - *251*
    86 Int J Immunopharmac (**8**, 859) - *38,
        63, 276*
Gylys JA
    79 Res Comm C P P (**23**, 61) - *319*

Habs M
    84 Arzn-Forsch (**34**, 792) - *316, 328*
Hacker MP
    82 Cancer Res (**42**, 4490) - *328*
    82 Res Comm C P P (**35**, 145) - *328*
Hadden JW
    89 Int J Immunopharm (**11**, 13) - *262*
Haddock NF
    82 Arch Dermatol (**118**, 157) - *232*
Hald J
    48 Acta Pharm (**4**, 285) - *169, 171, 172,
        174, 224*
    48 Acta Pharm (**4**, 305) - *169, 171, 172,
        177-180, 226*
    48 Lancet (**2**, 1001) - *169, 171, 172,
        174, 178*
    49 Acta Pharm (**5**, 179) - *169, 192*
    49 Acta Pharm (**5**, 292) - *169*
    49 Acta Pharm (**5**, 298) - *169, 178*
    52 Acta Pharm Tox (**8**, 329) - *232, 338*
Hald JG
    53 Chem Abstr (**48**, 8257i) - *170, 226*
Haley TJ
    79 Drug Metab Rev (**9**, 319) - *5, 202*
Hallaway M
    59 Bioch Biophys Acta (**36**, 538) - *8, 9*
Halls DJ
    69 Mikrochim Acta (**1969**, 62) - *5*
Halpern MD
    90 Clin Imm Imm (**55**, 242) - *270, 274*
    91 Clin Imm Imm (**58**, 69) - *270, 274*

Hanes CS
72 Cand J Biochem (**50**, 1385) - *192*
Harada S
80 Life Sci (**26**, 1773) - *138, 139*
82 Sub Alc Act/Mis (**3**, 107) - *142, 144, 155*
Harari PM
89 Biochem J (**260**, 487) - *301*
Häring N
80 Talanta (**27**, 873) - *10, 67*
Harrington MC
88 Biochem Soc Trans (**16**, 239) - *192*
Hart BW
90 Alcohol (**7**, 165) - *41, 154, 155, 157, 191, 201*
Haycock JW
77 Behavior Biol (**20**, 281) - *73*
Haynes SN
73 J Behav Ther (**4**, 31) - *222*
Hazard R
57 Arch Int Pharm (**112**, 36) - *338*
Heath RG
65 Dis Nerv System (**26**, 99) - *235*
Heikkila RE
76 J Biol Chem (**252**, 2182) - *127-129*
Helander A
86 Alc Clin Exp Res (**10**, 71) - *160, 161*
87 Bioch Pharmacol (**36**, 1077) - *160*
87 Bioch Pharmacol (**36**, 3981) - *160*
88 Bioch Pharm (**37**, 3360) - *159, 160, 161, 226*
88 Pharm Tox (**63**, 262) - *160*
89 Bioch Pharm (**38**, 2195) - *160*
90 Alc Clin Exp Res (**14**, 48) - *161, 226*
Held KD
87 Rad Res (**112**, 544) - *299, 300, 310, 312*
Hellström E
80 Pharm Bioch Beh (**13: S1**, 73) - *245*
82 Bioch Pharm (**31**, 3899) - *162, 165*
82 Pharm Bioch Beh (**17**, 1103) - *186-188, 190, 191, 195*
83 Alc Clin Exp Res (**7**, 231) - *147*
Hellström-Lindahl E
89 Toxicol Lett (**49**, 87) - *88, 89*
89 Toxicology (**56**, 9) - *76*
Hempel JD
81 J Biol Chem (**256**, 10889) - *152*
82 Biochemistry (**21**, 6834) - *152*

84 Eur J Bioch (**141**, 21) - *139, 151*
85 Eur J Bioch (**153**, 13) - *139, 150, 152*
86 Prog Clin Biol Res (**232**, 1) - *152*
89 Biochemistry (**28**, 1160) - *142, 143, 152*
Henehan GTM
85 Alcohol (**2**, 107) - *146*
Hepner GW
74 N Engl J Med (**291**, 1384) - *106*
Hersh EM
87 3 C AIDS (Abstract MP225) - *285*
88 4 C AIDS (Abstract 3035) - *273*
91 J Am Med Ass (**265**, 1538) - *261, 280, 286, 287*
Heubusch P
78 Tox App Pharmacol (**46**, 143) - *126*
Hidaka H
73 Mol Pharm (**9**, 172) - *125*
Hilton J
84 Bioch Pharm (**33**, 1867) - *327*
84 Cancer Res (**44**, 5156) - *327*
Hine CH
50 J Pharm Exp Ther (**98**, 13) - *170*
52 J Clin Invest (**31**, 317) - *171-174, 176, 177-181*
Hirschberg M
87 Eur Neurol (**26**, 222) - *340*
Ho BT
85 Metal Ions (139) - *86*
Ho SB
88 Alc Clin Exp Res (**12**, 705) - *202*
Hoeldtke R
78 Bioch Pharm (**27**, 2499) - *125*
Hoeldtke RD
80 J Clin Endocr (**51**, 810) - *124, 125, 162, 199*
Honjo T
69 Bioch Pharm (**18**, 2681) - *109, 115, 116*
Hoon DSB
87 Cancer Res (**47**, 1529) - *291*
Hopfer SM
87 Res Comm C P P (**55**, 101) - *82, 243*
Horak E
76 Res Comm C P P (**14**, 153) - *81*
Hörding M
90 Int J Immunopharm (**12**, 145) - *289*
Hoshino T

85 Experientia (**41**, 1416) - *129*
Hotson JR
  76 Arch Neurol (**33**, 141) - *236*
Howell JM
  64 Nature (**201**, 83) - *345*
  68 J Neuropath Exp Neur (**27**, 464) - *341*
Hsu LC
  85 P Nat Acad S USA (**82**, 3771) - *139*
Hulanicki A
  67 Talanta (**14**, 1371) - *5, 8*
Hunt EC
  73 Analyst (**98**, 585) - *244*
Hunt GM
  73 Behav Res Ther (**11**, 91) - *215*
Hunter AL
  75 Bioch Pharm (**24**, 2199) - *109, 111, 115, 116, 241, 343*
Hunter FE
  56 Pharmacol Rev (**8**, 89) - *96*
Hunter J
  74 Bioch Pharm (**23**, 2480) - *104*

Iber FL
  77 Alc Clin Exp Res (**1**, 359) - *49, 53-55, 243*
  77 Alc Clin Exp Res (**1**, 365) - *225*
Impraim C
  82 Am J Hum Genet (**34**, 837) - *139*
Innes JRM
  69 J Natl Canc Inst (**42**, 1101) - *344*
Inoue K
  78 Life Sci (**23**, 179) - *149, 158*
  79 Bioch Biophys Acta (**569**, 117) - *139, 158, 159*
  85 Jap J Pharmacol (**38**, 43) - *181*
Ioannides C
  87 Bioch Pharm (**36**, 4197) - *115*
Irth H
  86 J Chromat (**370**, 439) - *24, 25*
  88 J Chromat (**424**, 95) - *24, 25*

Jacobsen D
  88 Alc Clin Exp Res (**12**, 516) - *201*
Jacobsen E
  49 Acta Pharm (**5**, 285) - *169*
  49 J Am Med Ass (**139**, 918) - *169, 171*
  52 Q J Stud Alc (**13**, 16) - *170*

87 The road to Antabuse - *169, 170*
Jakubowski M
  72 Bioch Pharm (**21**, 3073) - *38*
James WO
  53 Rev Plant Physiol (**4**, 59) - *96*
Jamieson D
  64 Bioch Pharm (**13**, 159) - *304*
Jasim S
  84 Toxicology (**32**, 297) - *82*
  85 Acta Pharm Tox (**57**,262) - *87*
  86 Toxicol Lett (**31**, 249) - *82*
Jensen JC
  80 J Chromat (**181**, 407) - *23, 24, 26, 27, 38*
  82 Am J Psychi (**139**, 1596) - *56, 57*
  84 Alcohol (**1**, 97) - *186, 188*
  84 Thesis, Univ of Kansas - *28, 39, 46, 49, 50, 53, 61, 62, 157*
  86 Alc Clin Exp Res (**10**, 45) - *186, 188, 189, 191*
Jocelyn PC
  72 Bioch SH Group (**95**) - *299*
Johansson B
  85 Bioch Pharm (**34**, 2989) - *12, 14, 15, 18, 22, 24, 26, 34, 67*
  86 J Chromat (**378**, 419) - *22-26, 47, 56-58*
  88 Clin Chim Acta (**177**, 55) - *13, 19, 22, 26, 56, 98*
  89 Bioch Pharm (**38**, 1053) - *25, 26, 39-41, 147, 155, 157-159, 186, 187, 189, 200*
  89 Drug Metab Disp (**17**, 351) - *36, 37, 120*
  89 Eur J Clin Pharm (**37**, 133) - *40, 47, 58, 156-159*
  89 Pharm Tox (**64**, 471) - *41, 157*
  89 Thesis, Lund Univ - *101, 120, 157*
  90 J Pharm Pharmacol (**42**, 806) - *7, 40*
  90 Pharm Tox (**66**, 104) - *18, 19, 160*
  91 Pharm Tox (**68**, 166) - *58, 156, 158, 170, 227*
Johansson J
  88 Eur J Bioch (**172**, 527) - *142*
Johnsen J
  90 Pharm Tox (**66**, 227) - *246*
Johnson GA
  69 J Pharm Exp Ther (**168**, 229) - *125*
  70 J Pharm Exp Ther (**171**, 80) - *124*

72 J Pharm Exp Ther (**180**, 539) - *164*
Johnston CD
  52 Bioch Bioph Acta (**9**, 219) - *36*
  53 Arch Bioch Bioph (**44**, 249) - *8, 15, 32*
Jones DE
  88 P Nat Acad S USA (**85**, 1782) - *142*
Jones DG
  67 J Clin Inv (**46**, 1492) - *166*
Jones MM
  86 Canc Chemoth Ph (**17**, 38) - *91*
  89 Toxicology (**58**, 313) - *79*
Jones RO
  49 Cand Med Ass J (**60**, 609) - *170, 175, 176*
Jones SG
  84 Environ Health Persp (**54**, 285) - *78*
Jonsson J
  67 J Pharm Pharmacol (**19**, 201) - *124*
Jørgensen L
  83 Acta Pharm Tox (**53**, 70) - *115*

Kaaber K
  79 Contact Dermatitis (**5**, 221) - *83*
  87 Dermatosen (**35**, 209) - *83*
Kachru DN
  86 Res Comm C P P (**52**, 399) - *88*
Kahn S
  90 South Med J (**83**, 833) - *238*
Kamerbeek HH
  71 Acta Med Scand (**189**, 149) - *69, 71*
Kane FJ
  70 Am J Psychi (**127**, 690) - *244*
Kaplan CS
  89 Life Sci (**45**, iii) - *285*
Karlsson K
  87 Biochem J (**242**, 55) - *133*
  88 Bioch Bioph Acta (**967**, 110) - *133*
  88 J Clin Inv (**82**, 762) - *133*
  89 Lab Invest (**60**, 659) - *133*
Kaslander J
  63 Bioch Bioph Acta (**71**, 730) - *34, 53*
Keeffe EB
  74 J Am Med Ass (**230**, 435) - *240*
Keilin D
  40 Proc R Soc Lond (**B129**, 277) - *8*
Kelner MJ
  86 J Biol Chem (**261**, 1636) - *30, 33, 300*

Kent CRH
  88 Rad Res (**116**, 539) - *309*
Khandekar JD
  83 Res Comm C P P (**40**, 55) - *316, 324*
Khandelwal S
  87 Toxicol Lett (**37**, 213) - *135*
Kiørboe E
  66 Epilepsia (**7**, 246) - *104*
Kirchmayer S
  79 Materia Med Polona (**11**, 40) - *343*
Kitson TM
  75 Biochem J (**151**, 407) - *7, 140, 150, 152, 155*
  76 Biochem J (**155**, 445) - *39, 156*
  77 J Stud Alc (**38**, 96) - *5, 193*
  78 Biochem J (**175**, 83) - *150, 159*
  79 Biochem J (**183**, 751) - *153*
  82 Biochem J (**203**, 743) - *150, 151, 153, 155, 160*
  83 Biochem J (**213**, 551) - *140, 151*
  84 Prog Clin Biol Res (**174**, 43) - *153, 154*
  85 Alcohol (**2**, 97) - *153, 154*
  87 Biochem J (**248**, 989) - *151, 152*
  88 J Chem Ed (**9**, 829) - *6, 98, 153, 154*
  89 Biochem J (**261**, 281) - *156*
Kiyozumi M
  90 Toxicology (**60**, 275) - *78*
Kjeldgaard NE
  49 Acta Pharm (**5**, 397) - *166, 178*
Klaassen CD
  84 Environ Health Persp (**54**, 233) - 77
Klebanskii AL
  60 J Gen Chem (USSR) (**30**, 794) - *8*
Knee ST
  74 Am J Psychi (**131**, 1281) - *236*
Kofoed LL
  87 Alc Clin Exp Res (**11**, 481) - *223*
Kohn FR
  87 Cancer Res (**47**, 3180) - *328*
Kolthoff IM
  65 J Am Chem Soc (**87**, 2717) - *30*
Kono Y
  82 J Biol Chem (**257**, 5751) - *135*
Korhonen A
  83 Terat Carcin Mutag (**3**, 163) - *345*
Koutenský J
  71 Eur J Pharm (**14**, 389) - *86, 87*
Kraemer RJ

68 J Biol Chem (**243**, 6402) - *150*
Kraml M
    73 Cand Med Ass J (**109**, 578) - *243, 244*
Kristensen ME
    81 Acta Med Scand (**209**, 335) - *83, 238*
Krivchenkova RS
    64 Polonii Meditsina Moscow (245) - *93*
Kromhout J
    80 Am J Gastroenterol (**74**, 507) - *42, 152*
Kumar KS
    86 Int J Rad Oncol (**12**, 1463) - *134, 301*
Kupari M
    83 Alc Clin Exp Res (**7**, 283) - *183, 201*
Kurys G
    89 J Biol Chem (**264**, 4715) - *138, 140*
Kwentus J
    79 J Stud Alc (**40**, 428) - *6*

Lake CR
    77 Am J Psychi (**134**, 1411) - *125*
    80 Phenomenology Treat (229) - *125*
Lakomaa EL
    82 Tox App Pharm (**65**, 286) - *73, 87*
Lam C
    86 J App Toxicol (**6**, 81) - *24*
    86 Tox App Pharm (**86**, 235) - *24*
Lamboeuf Y
    74 Clin Exp Pharm Physiol (**1**, 361) - *192*
Landauer MR
    88 Pharm Ther (**39**, 97) - *307*
Lang JM
    85 Lancet (**2**, 1066) - *261, 271, 280*
    86 Immunobiol (**173**, 412) - *261, 271, 281*
    87 Clin Immunol (205) - *261, 271, 281*
    88 4 C AIDS (Abstract 3055) - *261, 284*
    88 Lancet (**2**, 702) - *261, 281, 284, 286, 288*
    88 Presse Med (**17**, 186) - *261, 281*
Lang M
    76 Chem Biol Interact (**15**, 267) - *109*
Larseille J
    82 IRCS-Biochem (**10**, 437) - *104, 107*
Larsen V
    48 Acta Pharm (**4**, 321) - *169*
Laskin JD
    86 J Biol Chem (**261**, 16626) - *101*

Lear J
    87 J Nucl Med (**28**, 481) - *69, 70*
Lear JL
    88 J Nucl Med (**29**, 1387) - *70*
Lehr HA
    89 Eur J Clin Pharm (**37**, 521) - *276*
Lemarie E
    86 Respiration (**49**, 235) - *290*
Lemere F
    53 Q J Stud Alc (**14**, 197) - *235*
Leo MA
    89 Bioch Pharm (**38**, 97) - *99*
Lerner AB
    50 J Biol Chem (**187**, 793) - *101*
Lesourd BM
    88 Int J Immunopharm (**10**, 135) - *292*
Lester D
    52 Q J Stud Alc (**13**, 1) - *198, 202*
Levinson W
    78 Bioch Biophys Acta (**519**, 65) - *344*
Levy MS
    67 Am J Psychi (**123**, 1018) - *175*
Lewis MJ
    75 Cand Psychiat Ass J (**20**, 283) - *245*
Li T-K
    69 Surg Clin N Am (**49**, 577) - *155*
Liddon SC
    67 Am J Psychi (**123**, 1284) - *235, 236*
Liebson I
    71 Annu Sci M Drug Dep (1262) - *105*
    72 Behav Res Ther (**10**, 403) - *221*
    73 Am J Psychi (**130**, 483) - *210, 221*
Liebson IA
    78 Ann Int Med (**89**, 342) - *211, 221, 231*
Lieder PH
    85 Anal Lett (**18**, 57) - *26, 28, 46, 61*
Lin PS
    79 Rad Res (**77**, 501) - *132, 310, 311*
    85 Rad Res (**102**, 271) - *295, 296, 297, 298, 311*
Lindahl R
    84 Bioch Pharmacol (**33**, 3383) - *145*
    84 J Biol Chem (**259**, 11986) - *141*
    84 J Biol Chem (**259**, 11991) - *141*
Linderholm H
    51 Scand J Clin Lab (**3**, 96) - *24, 46, 49, 52*
Lindros KO

72 Biochem J (**126**, 945) - *192*
81 Alc Clin Exp Res (**5**, 528) - *181, 183, 201*
Lippmann W
69 Bioch Pharm (**18**, 2507) - *122*
Liskow BI
87 J Stud Alc (**48**, 356) - *6, 229*
Loft S
86 Br J Clin Pharm (**21**, 75) - *106, 108*
Loi C-M
89 Clin Pharm Ther (**45**, 476) - *107*
Loiseau P
75 Nouv Pres Med (**4**, 504) - *104, 105*
Lubetkin BS
71 Q J Stud Alc (**32**, 168) - *223, 224, 233*
Ludwig AM
70 LSD Alcoholism - *223*
Ludwig RA
60 Adv Pest Control Res (**3**, 219) - *96*
Lundwall L
71 J Nerv Ment Dis (**153**, 381) - *6*
Luzy T
83 CR Soc Biol (**177**, 616) - *275*

Mach T
86 Pol J Pharmac Pharm (**38**, 235) - *343*
MacKerell AD
85 FEBS Lett (**179**, 77) - *32, 42, 152, 153*
86 Alc Clin Exp Res (**10**, 266) - *138, 149, 165*
MacLeod SM
78 Clin Pharm Ther (**24**, 583) - *105, 106*
Magos L
70 Br J Pharmacol (**39**, 26) - *126*
Mains RE
86 J Biol Chem (**261**, 11938) - *102*
Maj J
69 Bioch Pharm (**18**, 2045) - *124*
70 Eur J Pharm (**9**, 183) - *124, 338*
Major LF
77 Biol Psychi (**12**, 635) - *164*
77 Currents Alcoholism (**1**, 197) - *125*
78 Ann Int Med (**88**, 53) - *104, 107, 242*
79 Am J Psychi (**136**, 679) - *236, 237*
79 Biol Psychi (**14**, 337) - *125, 236, 237*
82 J Stud Alc (**43**, 146) - *124*
Maners AW

85 Ann Clin Lab Sci (**15**, 343) - *295, 297*
Mannervik B
85 Adv Enzymol (**57**, 357) - *133*
Mansner R
68 Ann Med Exp Fenn (**46**, 385) - *341*
Mansour H
86 J Pharm Exp Ther (**236**, 476) - *253, 302, 303, 305, 306*
Manthey CL
90 Cancer Res (**50**, 4991) - *328*
Marchand JE
90 J Biol Chem (**265**, 264) - *164*
Marchner H
78 Acta Pharm Tox (**43**, 219) - *145, 148*
Marconi J
61 Q J Stud Alc (**22**, 46) - *171, 172*
Mardini HA
84 Gut (**25**, 284) - *42*
Marie C
55 Thesis, Univ of Paris - *245*
Mariman ECM
86 Biomed Pharmacother (**40**, 399) - *288*
Markham JD
53 J Am Med Ass (**152**, 1597) - *198, 202, 203*
Marklund SL
80 Acta Physiol Scand (**S429**, 19) - *126*
80 Biol Clin Aspects Sup (**318**) - *102, 127*
84 Biochem J (**220**, 269) - *130*
Marquart DW
64 IBM Share Prog 3094 - *44*
Marselos M
76 Chem Biol Interact (**15**, 277) - *99, 118, 119*
Martensen-Larsen O
48 Lancet (**255**, 1004) - *169*
50 Nord Med (**43**, 805) - *170, 226*
51 Q J Stud Alc (**12**, 206) - *235*
Masso PD
81 J Chromat (**224**, 457) - *22-24, 56*
Masuda Y
86 Bichem Pharmacol (**35**, 3941) - *113, 117*
88 Res Comm C P P (**62**, 251) - *33, 115, 116*
88 Res Comm C P P (**61**, 65) - *34, 116, 192*
89 Res Comm C P P (**66**, 57) - *33, 115,*

116

Mathews AP
    09 J Biol Chem (6, 299) - *300*
Matkovics B
    82 Gen Pharmacol (13, 333) - *304*
Mazumder R
    85 Andrologia (17, 400) - *124*
McClain CJ
    80 Gut (21, 318) - *42*
McConchie RD
    83 J Stud Alc (44, 739) - *236*
McKee RW
    41 J Ind Hyg Toxicol (23, 151) - *244*
McKenna MJ
    77 J Pharm Exp Ther (202, 245) - *24*
    77 J Pharm Exp Ther (202, 253) - *24*
McNichol RW
    87 Disulfiram (Antabuse) (1) - *6*
Medical Letter
    80 Med Lett (22/1, 1) - *6*
Meister A
    83 Annu Rev Bioch (52, 711) - *32, 165*
Mello NK
    72 Psychosom Med (34, 139) - *209*
Menné T
    80 Ann Clin Lab Sci (10, 160) - *82, 83*
    82 Some Dermatol (1, 15) - *83*
Menon CR
    86 J Inorg Bioch (28, 217) - *82*
Merck Index
    68 8th Edition (958) - *1*
    87 11th Edition (323) - *1*
Mercurio F
    52 J Am Med Ass (149, 82) - *232*
Merlevede E
    61 Arch Int Pharm (82, 427) - *36, 47, 49,*
        54, 55, 60, 243
Meshnick S
    86 Superoxide Superoxid (562) - *131*
Meshnick SR
    90 Bioch Pharm (40, 213) - *86, 131*
Metcalf D
    84 Hemopoietic Colony S (124) - *327*
Michiels C
    88 Eur J Bioch (177, 435) - *134, 135*
Milandri M
    80 Pharmacology (21, 76) - *343*
Milas L
    84 Int J Rad Oncol (10, 2335) - *307-309*

Milich DR
    77 Develop Comp Imm (1, 289) - *252*
Miller GE
    83 Bioch Pharm (32, 2433) - *84, 110,*
        111, 114, 116, 117
Mills CF
    60 Nature (185, 20) - *342*
Minegishi A
    79 Res Comm C P P (24, 273) - *164*
Misra HP
    79 J Biol Chem (254, 11623) - *129*
Mitchell CL
    90 Brain Res (506, 327) - *73*
Mitchell J
    78 Clin Toxicol (12, 606) - *84*
Miura T
    78 Chem Pharm Bull (26, 1261) - *127,*
        135
Mizoi Y
    79 Pharm Bioch Beh (10, 303) - *181*
    82 Prog Clin Biol Res (114, 363) - *196*
    83 Pharm Bioch Beh (S1 18, 127) - *144,*
        181
    88 Biomed Aspects A (31) - *144, 181,*
        182, 187, 196
Moddel G
    78 Arch Neurol (35, 658) - *237*
Mokri B
    81 Neurology (31, 730) - *237, 238*
Moldowan MJ
    82 Agents Actions (12, 731) - *184*
Mondovì B
    67 J Biol Chem (242, 1160) - *101*
Montine TJ
    88 Cancer Res (48, 6017) - *91, 93*
Moore KE
    69 Bioch Pharm (18, 1627) - *124, 128*
Morell AG
    58 Science (127, 588) - *97, 129*
Mori T
    83 Int J Radiat Biol (44, 41) - *299*
Mörland J
    84 Socialstyr (1985/2, 89) - *245*
Morpurgo L
    83 Bioch Bioph Acta (746, 168) - *15, 67,*
        97, 100
    87 Biochem J (248, 865) - *99*
    87 J Inorg Chem (29, 25) - *99*
    88 Bioch Biophys R C (152, 623) - *99*

Morris SJ
78 Gastroenterology (**75**, 100) - *238*
Mossalayi MD
86 Int J Immunopharm (**8**, 841) - *254, 267, 272, 276*
Mozdzierz GJ
81 Int J Addict (**16**, 253) - *105*
Mullin MJ
81 J Pharm Exp Ther (**216**, 459) - *189*
Mür J
64 Confin Neurol (**24**, 235) - *341*
Murthy MS
87 Cancer Res (**47**, 774) - *316, 317*
Musacchio J
64 Life Sci (**3**, 769) - *121, 123*
Musacchio JM
66 J Pharm Exp Ther (**152**, 56) - *122, 123*
66 J Pharm Exp Ther (**152**, 293) - *123*

Nagatsu T
64 J Biol Chem (**239**, 2910) - *126*
Nakano J
69 Tox App Pharm (**14**, 439) - *186, 187, 196*
74 Q J Stud Alc (**35**, 620) - *186, 187, 194-196*
Nakayama and Masuda
85 J Pharmacobio-Dyn (**8**, 868) - *117*
Nakazawa M
85 Exp Eye Res (**41**, 249) - *101*
Nash NG
75 Anal Profil Drug Sub (**4**, 168) - *5*
Nasrallah HV
79 West J Med (**130**, 575) - *235*
Nässberger L
84 Postgrad Med J (**60**, 639) - *238*
84 J Tox Clin Tox (**22**, 403) - *240*
National Cancer Institute
79 Carcinog Tech Rep Ser (**172**) - *344*
Neiderhiser DH
76 J Chromatog (**117**, 187) - *37, 244*
80 Alc Clin Exp Res (**4**, 277) - *37, 46, 48, 52, 54*
83 Alc Clin Exp Res (**7**, 199) - *36, 46, 48, 52*
Neims AH
66 J Biol Chem (**241**, 3036) - *15, 32*

66 J Biol Chem (**241**, 5941) - *8, 16, 30-32, 98*
Netter KJ
70 Humangenetik (**9**, 275) - *109*
Neveu PJ
78 Clin Exp Immunol (**32**, 419) - *261*
80 Biomedicine (**33**, 247) - *254, 255, 272*
82 Int J Immunopharm (**4**, 9) - *252*
83 Int Arch All Appl Imm (**71**, 276) - *272, 273*
86 Cand J Neurol Sci (**13**, 379) - *256*
86 Life Sci (**38**, 1907) - *256*
88 Life Sci (**42**, 1917) - *256*
Newman RA
88 J Clin Oncol (**6**, 1786) - *330*
Niblo G
51 Dis Nerv System (**12**, 340) - *202*
Nieboer E
84 IARC Sci Publ (**53**, 321) - *82*
Nilsson GE
87 Brain Res (**409**, 265) - *164*
89 Pharm Tox (**64**, 137) - *109, 164*
NIOSH
85 Guide Chemical Hazard - *244*
Nirenberg TD
83 Addict Behav (**8**, 311) - *229, 230*
Nishigaki R
85 J Pharmacobio-Dyn (**8**, 847) - *192*
Nogué S
83 J Tox Clin Tox (**19**, 1015) - *69, 71*
Nomencl Mammal Aldehyde Dehydrogenases
88 Prog Clin Biol Res (**290**, xix) - *139, 142*
Norseth T
74 Acta Pharm Tox (**34**, 76) - *90*
Nousiainen U
84 Gen Pharmacol (**15**, 223) - *99*

Obrebska MJ
80 Biochem J (**188**, 107) - *113, 117*
O'Callaghan JP
86 Brain Res (**370**, 354) - *78*
Ogishima T
87 J Biol Chem (**262**, 7646) - *116*
Ohman M
86 Clin Sci (**70**, 356) - *126, 128, 243*

Öjehagen A
  86 Acta Psychiatr Scand (**73**, 68) - *224*
  88 Alc Clin Exp Res (**12**, 46) - *209*
Olesen OV
  66 Acta Pharm Tox (**24**, 317) - *104-106*
  67 Arch Neurol (**16**, 642) - *106*
Olney RK
  80 Muscle Nerve (**3**, 172) - *237*
Ooms PCA
  77 Radioch Radioanal Lett (**31**, 317) - *11*
O'Reilly RA
  71 Clin Res (**19**, 180) - *105*
  73 Ann Int Med (**78**, 73) - *105, 106*
Orrego H
  88 Am J Physiol (**254**, G495) - *190*
Oskarsson A
  80 Arch Toxicol (**45**, 45) - *82*
  83 Arch Toxicol (**S6**, 279) - *66, 80*
  85 Acta Pharm Tox (**56**, 309) - *80*
  86 Environ Res (**41**, 623) - *81*
  86 Neurobehav Tox Terat (**8**, 591) - *81*
  87 Environ Res (**44**, 82) - *68, 80*
  87 Toxicol Lett (**36**, 73) - *81*
  87 Toxicology (**44**, 61) - *81*
  88 Chem Biol Interact (**67**, 59) - *80*
  89 Pharm Tox (**64**, 344) - *81*
Palliyath SK
  88 Electromy Clin Neuro (**28**, 245) - *242*
  90 J Neur Neurosurg Psych (**53**, 227) - *242*
Palmer G
  62 Bioch Bioph Acta (**56**, 444) - *166*
Pannacciulli IM
  89 Br J Cancer (**59**, 371) - *323, 325, 326*
Papp JP
  69 Ann Int Med (**71**, 119) - *71*
Paredes J
  88 J Clin Oncol (**6**, 955) - *329-331, 333, 334*
Parrilla R
  74 J Biol Chem (**249**, 4926) - *144*
Paulson SM
  77 Johns Hopk M J (**141**, 119) - *243, 244*
Physicians' Desk Reference
  91 45th edition (2358) - *202, 203*
Peachey JE
  81 Clin Pharm Ther (**29**, 40) - *176*
  81 J Clin Psychopharm (**1**, 21) - *6*
  81 Lancet (**1**, 943) - *230*

  81 Pharm Ther (**15**, 89) - *5*
  83 Alc Clin Exp Res (**7**, 180) - *177, 180, 181, 227, 230, 231*
  83 Res Adv Alc Drug Prob (**7**, 397) - *6*
  84 Psychiatr Clin N Am (**7**, 745) - *226*
  85 Res Adv New Psychoph (199) - *226*
Pedersen SB
  80 Arch Pharm Chem Sci (**8**, 65) - *17, 18, 22, 23, 46-48, 52, 56-58*
Peeke SC
  79 Alc Clin Exp Res (**3**, 223) - *234*
Pérez-Clausell J
  85 Brain Res (**337**, 91) - *72*
Perman ES
  62 Acta Physiol Scand (**55 S190**, 1) - *178, 186, 187, 193, 195, 197*
  62 Experientia (**18**, 516) - *186*
Petersen EA
  88 4 C AIDS (Abstract 3041) - *285*
Petersen EN
  89 Eur J Pharm (**166**, 419) - *186-189, 191, 200, 201*
Peterson CM
  87 Alcohol (**4**, 477) - *177*
  88 Alcohol (**5**, 371) - *177*
Pettersson H
  82 J Neurochem (**39**, 628) - *161*
Phillips M
  84 J Pharm Sci (**73**, 1718) - *340*
  85 Am J Hosp Pharm (**42**, 343) - *246, 340*
  86 J Chromat (**381**, 164) - *244*
  88 Adv Alc Sub Abu (**7**, 51) - *246, 340*
Pietruszko R
  73 Arch Bioch Bioph (**159**, 50) - *192*
  78 FEBS Lett (**92**, 89) - *158*
  83 Isozymes (**8**, 195) - *6, 138, 143, 144*
  86 Prog Clin Biol Res (**232**, 37) - *152*
  87 Alc Alcoholism (**S1**, 175) - *139*
  89 Bioch Physiol Subs (**1**, 89) - *6*
Pimentel E
  90 Ann Clin Lab Sci (**20**, 36) - *327*
Plant MA
  83 Br Med J (**287**, 1795) - *222*
Plouvier B
  82 Nouv Presse Med (**11**, 3209) - *232*
Pomerantz SH
  63 J Biol Chem (**238**, 2351) - *101*
  66 J Biol Chem (**241**, 161) - *101*

Pompidou A
80 New Trend Hum Imm (696) - *267*
84 Exp Cell Res (**150**, 213) - *267*
84 Int Arch Allerg A Imm (**74**, 172) -
263, 264
85 Cancer Res (**45**, 4671s) - *261, 266,
267, 276, 288*
85 Int J Immunopharm (**4**, 561) - *265,
266, 272*
85 Lancet (**2**, 1423) - *288*
86 Comp Imm Microbio (**9**, 263) - *267,
266, 271, 276, 288*
Potchoo Y
86 Int J Clin Pharm Ther (**24**, 499) - *342*
Poulsen LL
79 Arch Bioch Bioph (**198**, 78) - *33*
Price TRP
76 J Stud Alc (**37**, 980) - *236*
Prickett CS
53 Bioch Bioph Acta (**12**, 542) - *24-26,
36, 45, 48, 55, 57, 62*
Pristach CA
90 Hosp Comm Psychiat (**41**, 1345) -
206
Prohaska JR
77 Bioch Biophys R C (**76**, 437) - *133*
Puglia CD
84 Tox App Pharm (**75**, 258) - *127, 128,
134, 304*

Qazi R
88 J Natl Canc Inst (**80**, 1486) - *47, 50,
61, 100, 328-333*

Raby K
52 Acta Pharm Tox (**8**, 85) - *174, 188*
53 Q J Stud Alc (**14**, 545) - *171-174, 179*
53 Q J Stud Alc (**14**, 557) - *174, 188*
54 Q J Stud Alc (**15**, 21) - *177, 179, 180*
54 Q J Stud Alc (**15**, 33) - *172, 173*
54 Q J Stud Alc (**15**, 207) - *172*
56 Dan Med Bull (**3**, 168) - *179, 193*
Radojičić R
87 Iugo Phys Pharm Acta (**23**, 227) - *128*
Rainey JM
77 Am J Psychi (**134**, 371) - *6, 244, 342*
Ramsey AJ

89 Comp Bioch Physiol (**93B**, 77) - *140*
Ranek L
77 Br Med J (**2**, 94) - *238, 240*
Rannug A
84 Chem Biol Interact (**49**, 329) - *344*
84 Prog Clin Biol Res (**141**, 407) - *344*
Ranz A
89 Exp Parasitol (**69**, 125) - *131*
Rasul AR
73 Acta Neuropath (**24**, 68) - *341*
73 Acta Neuropath (**24**, 161) - *341*
74 Toxicol Appl Pharmacol (**30**, 63) -
341
Rauws AG
69 Arch Int Pharm (**182**, 425) - *69, 339*
Rawles JW
87 Bioch Pharm (**36**, 3715) - *158, 159*
Register UD
90 FASEB J (**4**, A365) - *229*
Reisinger EC
90 Lancet (**1**, 679) - *286, 289*
Rejas MT
88 Immunopharmacology (**16**, 191) - *274*
Renoux G
74 CR Acad Sc (III) (**278 D**, 1139) - *249*
77 J Exp Med (**145**, 466) - *250, 251 262*
77 Contr Neopl Mo (**67**) - *249, 250, 251*
77 CR Soc Biol (**171**, 313) - *249, 251*
79 J Immunopharm (**1**, 247) - *249, 250,
251, 261, 273-275*
79 J Immunopharm (**1**, 415) - *248, 250,
262, 263*
80 Clin Imm Immunop (**15**, 23) - *251,
252, 254, 274*
80 J Immunopharm (**2**, 49) - *262*
80 New Trend Hum Imm (974) - *291*
80 New Trend Hum Imm (986) - *250,
256, 262, 263*
80 Thymus (**2**, 139) - *262-264*
81 Augm Agent Ca (427) - *248, 250-252,
262, 291*
81 Trends Pharm Sci (**2**, 248) - *248*
82 Int J Immunopharm (**4**, 300) - *264,
265*
82 J Pharmacol (**13 S1**, 95) - *250-252,
260, 262, 275, 337, 338*
82 NK Cells (443) - *258, 259*
82 NK Cells (639) - *256, 259, 260*
83 Adv Exp Med (**166**, 223) - *248, 253-*

255, 258, 259, 261, 271, 292
83 Current Drugs Meth (171) - *251, 252*
83 J Neuroimm (**5**, 227) - *256*
83 Scand J Imm (**17**, 45) - *263, 264*
84 Imm Modul Ag (7) - *250, 252, 253, 264, 265*
84 Imm Modul Ag (607) - *250-252, 265, 275*
84 Immunopharm (**7**, 89) - *251, 252, 256, 260, 264, 265*
85 Am J Reprod Immunol (**8**, 101) - *254*
85 Immunotox Immunoph (193) - *266*
85 Modul Imm (393) - *254*
87 Ann NY Ac Sci (**496**, 346) - *250, 260*
87 J Neurosci Res (**18**, 230) - *251-253, 256, 259, 260, 268-270*
88 Immunopharm Immunot (**10**, 219) - *270, 277*
88 Int J Immunopharm (**10**, 489) - *252, 276*
88 Int J Neurosci (**39**, 177) - *256*
Renoux M
86 Int J Immunopharm (**8**, 107) - *251-253, 258, 259, 268, 270, 275, 277*
Rieders F
65 Pharmacologist (**7**, 162) - *69*
Rigas DA
79 Bioch Biophys R C (**88**, 373) - *295-298, 300*
80 Int J Radiat Biol (**38**, 257) - *296, 310*
Rinaldi A
84 Bioch Biophys R C (**120**, 242) - *101*
Robens JF
69 Tox App Pharm (**15**, 152) - *345*
Roberfroid MB
83 Chem Biol Interact (**47**, 175) - *109*
Robichaud C
79 Behav Res Ther (**17**, 618) - *211, 221*
Robins AH
83 S Afr Med J (**63**, 41) - *198*
Rogers EL
81 Alc Clin Exp Res (**5**, 75) - *242*
Rogers WK
78 Alc Clin Exp Res (**2**, 375) - *37, 47, 49, 54, 55, 243, 244*
79 Clin Pharm Ther (**25**, 469) - *125, 197-199*
Roitt I
89 Immunology - *254*

Romelsjö A
87 Br J Addict (**82**, 653) - *224*
Rothenberg ML
88 J Natl Canc Inst (**80**, 1488) - *100, 329, 330, 332, 334*
Rothstein E
68 J Am Med Ass (**206**, 1574) - *105*
69 N Engl J Med (**281**, 331) - *233*
69 N Engl J Med (**280**, 1006) - *233*
72 N Engl J Med (**286**, 162) - *170, 175*
72 J Am Med Ass (**229**, 1052) - *105*
Ruiz de Elvira M-C
87 Biochem Soc Trans (**16**, 297) - *101*
Russo JE
88 Prog Clin Biol Res (**290**, 65) - *328*
Rychtarik RG
83 Addict Behav (**8**, 361) - *243, 244*
Ryle PR
85 Bioch Pharm (**34**, 3577) - *192*
Ryzlak MT
86 Thesis, Rutgers Univ - *149*
87 Arch Bioch Bioph (**255**, 409) - *139, 142, 149, 150*
88 Arch Bioch Bioph (**266**, 386) - *149*
89 Alc Clin Exp Res (**13**, 755) - *138, 139, 142, 149, 150, 165*

Sabréus E
82 Acta Soc Med Svec (**91**, 183) - *234*
Salgo MP
74 J Reprod Fertil (**39**, 375) - *345*
Samitz MH
58 AMA Arch Ind Health (**18**, 473) - *83*
Sanhadji K
85 Int J Immunopharm (**7**, 616) - *266*
Sanny CG
85 Alc Clin Exp Res (**9**, 255) - *140*
87 Biochem J (**242**, 499) - *152*
88 Alc Clin Exp Res (**12**, 622) - *146*
Sauter AM
76 Arzn-Forsch (**26**, 173) - *14, 23-25, 27, 68*
77 J Chromat (**133**, 167) - *22, 23, 25*
77 J Stud Alc (**38**, 1680) - *56, 170, 172, 173, 175, 177, 179, 180, 188, 193*
Savolainen K
84 Acta Pharm Tox (**55**, 339) - *341*
Schade RR

83 Arch Intern Med (**143**, 1271) - *240*
Scheibel LW
  79 P Nat Acad S USA (**76**, 5303) - *131*
Scheid MP
  78 J Exp Med (**147**, 1727) - *265*
Schlesinger K
  66 Psychosom Med (**28**, 514) - *192*
Schlick E
  84 Immune Modulat Ag (513) - *272*
Schmalbach TK
  89 Cancer Res (**49**, 2574) - *323, 325,
    326*
  89 Cancer Res (**49**, 6629) - *322*
  90 Cancer Res (**50**, 6218) - *327*
Schmidt H
  79 Acta Histochem (**64**, 194) - *101*
  88 Prog Histochem Cycto (**17**, 1) - *101*
Scholler J
  61 Pharmacologist (**3**, 62) - *338, 339*
Schönenberger H
  72 Pharmazie (**27**, 139) - *338*
Schrøder HD
  78 Histochemistry (**56**, 1) - *72*
Schuckit MA
  85 J Stud Alc (**46**, 191) - *212*
Schütz HJ
  83 Arch Psychi Nervenkr (**233**, 1) - *340*
Schwarcz MN
  60 Bioch Biophys Acta (**39**, 383) - *155*
Schwetz BA
  67 Tox App Pharm (**10**, 79) - *69*
Searle AJF
  82 J Inorg Bioch (**17**, 161) - *300*
Sellers EM
  80 Arzn-Forsch (**30**, 882) - *105, 106, 119*
  81 N Engl J Med (**305**, 1255) - *6*
Sereny G
  86 Alc Clin Exp Res (**10**, 290) - *214,
    220, 221*
Sharkawi M
  78 Neuropharm (**17**, 401) - *188, 189*
  79 Toxicol Lett (**4**, 485) - *192*
  80 Life Sci (**27**, 1939) - *99*
Shaw IA
  51 Q J Stud Alc (**12**, 567) - *169, 170,
    175, 176*
Shimada H
  90 Res Comm C P P (**69**, 49) - *78*
Shinobu LA

83 Arch Toxicol (**54**, 235) - *77*
83 J Tox Envir Health (**12**, 757) - *76*
Sidhu RS
  75 Biochem J (**151**, 443) - *155*
Siegers C-P
  82 Res Comm C P P (**236**, 61) - *112*
Siew C
  76 Arch Bioch Bioph (**176**, 638) - *141*
Silver DF
  79 J Stud Alc (**40**, 1003) - *234*
Simmons TW
  88 Biochem J (**251**, 913) - *133*
Singh PK
  90 Chem Biol Interact (**74**, 79) - *79*
Sisson RW
  86 J Behav Ther (**17**, 15) - *207, 214,
    217, 224*
Sladek NE
  85 Cancer Res (**45**, 1549) - *327*
  88 Pharm Ther (**37**, 301) - *327*
  89 Drug Metab Rev (**20**, 697) - *327*
Snyderwine EG
  87 J Pharm Exp Ther (**15**, 289) - *37*
  88 Tox App Pharm (**93**, 11) - *115*
Socialstyrelsen
  84 Socialstyr (**1985/2**, 131) - *213, 220,
    234*
Sorensen JA
  89 Pharm Tox (**65**, 209) - *72*
Spath A
  87 Chem Biol Interact (**64**, 151) - *298,
    299*
Sprince H
  74 Agents Actions (**4**, 125) - *198, 202*
  75 Agents Actions (**5**, 164) - *202*
  79 Agents Actions (**9**, 407) - *202*
Srivastava SK
  69 J Biol Chem (**244**, 9) - *32*
Stacey NH
  89 Experientia (**45**, 180) - *298, 299*
Stanton TH
  78 J Exp Med (**148**, 963) - *251*
Starý J
  68 Anal Chim Acta (**40**, 93) - *8, 9, 11*
Stavinoha WB
  59 Tox App Pharm (**1**, 638) - *69*
Steckler PP
  51 Psychiatr Q (**25**, 91) - *170, 175, 176*
Sternberg DE

83 Arch Gen Psychiatry (**40**, 743) - *237*
Stewart DJ
  87 Am J Clin Oncol (**10**, 517) - *329*
Stites DP
  87 Basic Clin Immunolog (128) - *290*
Stohs SJ
  82 Pharmacology (**25**, 237) - *115, 119*
Stoppani AOM
  66 Arch Bioch Bioph (**113**, 464) - *155*
Storm JE
  84 Psychopharmacology (**82**, 68) - *124*
Stripp B
  69 J Pharm Exp Ther (**170**, 347) -
    108-110, 114
Strömme JH
  63 Bioch Pharm (**12**, 157) - *2, 97, 102,
    301*
  63 Bioch Pharm (**12**, 705) - *32*
  65 Bioch Pharm (**14**, 381) - *7, 8, 10, 14,
    15-17, 22, 23, 25-27, 30-33*
  65 Bioch Pharm (**14**, 393) - *18, 23, 25,
    26. 32-34, 36, 39, 45, 48, 50, 52,
    53, 55-62*
  66 Bioch Pharm (**15**, 287) - *45, 306*
Sugimoto E
  76 Agr Biol Chem (**40**, 2063) - *140, 150*
Sunderman FW
  58 Am J Med Sci (**236**, 26) - *1*
  64 J New Drugs (**4**, 154) - *67, 68, 82, 86,
    87*
  67 Am J Med Sci (**254**, 24) - *86, 342*
Sunderman FW Jr
  67 Am J Med Sci (**253**, 209) - *70, 71*
  83 Toxicol Appl Pharmacol (**68**, 87) - *84*
  83 Toxicol Appl Pharmacol (**71**, 436) -
    84
Sunderman FW Sr
  71 Ann Clin Res (**3**, 182) - *85*
  81 Ann Clin Lab Sci (**11**, 1) - *84*
  84 Ann Clin Lab Sci (**14**, 1) - *84*
  90 Ann Clin Lab Sci (**20**, 12) - *84*
Suokas A
  85 Alc Clin Exp Res (**9**, 221) - *177, 183,
    201*
Symchowicz S
  66 Bioch Pharm (**15**, 1607) - *122*
Syvertsen C
  84 Arch Bioch Bioph (**228**, 159) - *97*
Szendzikowski S

74 Structure Function (310) - *238*
Szerdahelyi P
  87 Brain Res (**422**, 287) - *73*
  87 Histochemistry (**86**, 627) - *87*

Taelman H
  87 3 C AIDS (Abstract THP227) - *288*
Tahsildar HI
  88 Rad Res (**113**, 243) - *299*
Takagi Y
  74 Rad Res (**60**, 292) - *299, 300*
Takahashi N
  79 Agric Biol Chem (**43**, 1873) - *140*
Tandon SK
  83 Res Comm C P P (**42**, 501) - *72*
  85 Toxicol Appl Pharmacol (**79**, 204) -
    81
Taylor RD
  86 Ann Clin Lab Sci (**16**, 443) - *295, 297*
Tempel K
  85 Arzn-Forsch (**35**, 1052) - *298, 299*
Teng YS
  81 Biochem Genet (**19**, 107) - *144*
Thoenen H
  65 Life Sci (**4**, 2033) - *121*
  67 J Pharm Exp Ther (**156**, 246) - *121*
Thorn GD
  62 Dithiocarbamates Rel - *5, 8, 96*
Till JE
  61 Rad Res (**14**, 213) - *307*
Tjälve H
  84 IARC Sci Publ (**53**, 311) - *85*
Tompsett SL
  64 Acta Pharm Tox (**21**, 20) - *24*
Torronen R
  85 Int J Biochem (**17**, 101) - *141*
Tottmar O
  76 Acta Pharm Tox (**38**, 366) - *146, 192*
  79 Acta Pharm Tox (**45**, 272) - *197*
  83 Pharm Bioch Beh (**18 S1**, 103) - *145,
    147, 159, 161*
Tottmar SOC
  73 Biochem J (**135**, 577) - *143, 146*
Towell JF
  83 Clin Pharm Ther (**33**, 517) - *147, 158,
    159*
  83 Lancet (**1**, 364) - *159*
Traiger GJ

84 Tox App Pharm (**72**, 504) - *118*
85 Chem Biol Interact (**52**, 335) - *118*
Trombetta LD
88 Tox App Pharm (**93**, 154) - *132*
Truitt EB
70 Q J Stud Alc (**31**, 1) - *177*
71 Biology Alcoholism (**1**, 161) - *5, 185, 193, 194*

Udenfriend S
66 Mol Pharm (**2**, 95) - *120*
USAN
90 Dictionary Drug Names (196) - *1*

Valeriote F
86 Int J Rad Oncol (**12**, 1165) - *324, 325*
89 Cancer Res (**49**, 6658) - *323, 325*
Vallari RC
82 Science (**216**, 637) - *149, 150, 159*
83 Pharm Bioch Beh (**18 S1**, 97) - *149, 150, 159*
Van Bekkum DW
56 Acta Physiol Pharm (**4**, 508) - *307*
Van Doorn R
81 Arch Toxicol (**47**, 51) - *38*
82 Toxicol Lett (**12**, 59) - *38*
Van Driessche E
84 Anal Biochem (**141**, 184) - *101*
van Royen EA
87 J Nucl Med (**28**, 178) - *69*
87 Nucl Med Comm (**8**, 603) - *70*
Van Thiel DH
79 Alc Clin Exp Res (**3**, 230) - *243*
Vergroesen AJ
67 Int J Radiat Biol (**13**, 77) - *299*
Verma S
90 Am J Clin Oncol (**13**, 119) - *329*
Vesell ES
71 Clin Pharm Ther (**12**, 785) - *104, 106, 198*
75 Pharmacology (**13**, 481) - *104, 106*
Volicer L
84 Arch Intern Med (**144**, 1294) - *241*
von Bahr-Lindström H
84 Eur J Bioch (**141**, 37) - *142*
85 Biochemistry (**24**, 5847) - *152*

Wagner H
84 Int J Rad Oncol (**10**, 1575) - *311*
Walker EM
81 Ann Clin Lab Sci (**11**, 397) - *90*
84 Res Comm C P P (**46**, 449) - *78*
86 Res Comm C P P (**51**, 231) - *78*
Wallerstein RS
56 Am J Psychi (**113**, 228) - *226*
57 Hospital Treatment A - *226*
58 Ann Int Med (**48**, 114) - *226*
Waxman DJ
86 Arch Bioch Bioph (**247**, 335) - *104, 116*
88 Bioch Pharm (**37**, 71) - *102*
Weddington WW
80 Am J Psychi (**137**, 1217) - *236*
Weiner H
78 Brain Res Bull (**3**, 541) - *162*
84 J Neurochem (**42**, 109) - *147, 165*
87 Ann NY Ac Sci (**492**, 25) - *144*
Weisiger RA
79 Arch Bioch Bioph (**196**, 631) - *38*
80 Enzym Basis Detox (**2**, 131) - *38, 39*
Weiss B
90 Fund Appl Tox (**15**, 791) - *80, 81*
Wells J
74 J Chromat (**92**, 442) - *244*
West B
58 Am J Med Sci (**236**, 15) - *1, 82, 84, 85, 338, 339*
Westman G
80 Rad Res (**83**, 303) - *127, 131, 132, 310*
84 Int J Radiat Biol (**45**, 11) - *295, 297, 310, 311*
Whittington HG
69 Am J Psychi (**125**, 1725) - *105*
Williams EE
37 J Am Med Ass (**109**, 1472) - *168*
Williams RJP
81 Philos Trans R Soc(**B 294**, 57) - *66*
Willson RA
79 Res Comm C P P (**23**, 505) - *108*
Willson RL
87 Proc Nutr Soc (**46**, 27) - *300*
Wilson A
80 J Stud Alc (**41**, 429) - *246*
Wise JD

81 J Arkansas Med Soc (**78**, 87) - *6*
Wittenberg C
  85 J Biol Chem (**260**, 12535) - *101*
Wokittel E
  60 Arch Kinderheilk (**161**, 145) - *341*
Worner TM
  82 Drug Alcohol Dep (**10**, 199) - *238*
Wratten CC
  63 Biochemistry (**2**, 935) - *192*
Wright C
  89 Ann Int Med (**111**, 943) - *6*
  90 Am J Med (**88**, 647) - *6*
Wysor MS
  82 Science (**217**, 454) - *319*

Yeh SJ
  80 Anal Chem (**52**, 528) - *8, 10, 11*
Yin S-J
  88 Biochem Genet (**26**, 343) - *139*
Yoshida A
  84 P Nat Acad Sci USA (**81**, 258) - *144*
  85 Biochem Genet (**23**, 585) - *144*
  85 Alcohol (**2**, 103) - *144*
Yoshimoto T
  85 J Biochem (**97**, 1747) - *101*
Yourick JJ
  87 Alcohol (**4**, 463) - *39, 156, 200*
  89 Bioch Pharm (**38**, 413) - *39, 148,*
    154-156, 186-189, 191, 200

Zanocco AL
  89 Free Rad Biol Med (**7**, 151) - *305*
Zemaitis MA
  76 Bioch Pharm (**25**, 453) - *109*
  76 Bioch Pharm (**25**, 1355) - *108, 109,*
    114-116
  79 Tox App Pharm (**48**, 343) - *115, 116*
Ziegler DM
  80 Enzym Basis Deto (**1**, 201) - *33*

Subject index

Acetaldehyde
see also Disulfiram-ethanol reaction
assays 165-6, 177
blood levels, animal
  endogenous 165
  post-ethanol 40, 185, 187, 189-93,
    195, 200-1
blood levels, human post-ethanol
  artefactual, ex vivo 177, 179, 193
  in E_2-deficient 144, 181-2, 196
  normal 137, 177
  post-disulfiram 138, 177-9, 180-3, 193,
    201-2, 227, 351
blood pressure 193-4, 196, 199
  dopamine β-hydroxylase inhibition
    197
  post-disulfiram pretreatment 197
cardiac output 194, 196, 199
ethanol elimination rate 192-3, 229
heart rate 193-6
metabolism 137-8, 144, 165-6, 226, 245
  alcohol dehydrogenase 98-9, 137
  aldehyde dehydrogenase 6, 137, 226
  inhibitors 150, 154-6, 199-201, 232
norepinephrine release 193, 197-8, 202
peripheral resistance 191, 194, 196,
    198-9
substrate for aldehyde dehydrogenases
    138, 148-50
  high-K_m 142-3, 148-9
  isozyme detection 138, 145-8, 161,
    164-5
  low-K_m 142-3, 148-9
toxicity 198, 202
Acquired immune deficiency syndrome
    (AIDS) 275, 279-81, 283, 285-8
see also HIV infection
Adenosine triphosphate (ATP) 343
Adriamycin, see Doxorubicin
AIDS related complex (ARC) 275, 285
Albumin 10, 15-7, 24, 30-2, 34, 131
Alcohol dehydrogenase (ADH) 137, 192
  diethyldithiocarbamate 96-7, 100

disulfiram 96, 98-100, 192
ethanol metabolism 98-9, 137, 189, 192,
    201
inhibition by
  acetaldehyde 98-9, 192-3, 229
  cadmium diethyldithiocarbamate 76
  mercury diethyldithiocarbamate 88-9
  4-methylpyrazole 181, 189, 201
Alcoholism, disulfiram therapy of
abdominal discomfort 234-5, 335
acceptance by patients 223-4
after-shaves 231, 232
behavioral therapy 207, 215, 217
compliance 206-8, 219, 245
  assured 207, 210-5, 217, 220-1
  failure 214-5, 222-3
  monitoring 9, 37, 208, 211-2, 214,
    218-9, 223-4, 244-5
contingency, motivating 210-3, 219-21
craving for alcohol 206, 209, 220,
    229-30
dosage 226-9
drinking-days 206-13, 218, 221
drowsiness 234-6
duration of
  action 224-6
  therapy 209
effectiveness 206-23
euphoria 208, 229
goals 209
implants 245-6
libido 233-4
side-effects 6, 224, 232-42
tolerance 230-1
treatment paradigms 4, 169-70, 208,
    214-23
untoward effects
  encephalopathy 233, 235-7
  hepatotoxicity 233, 238, 240-1, 336,
    343
  peripheral neuropathy 6, 233, 237-9,
    242, 336, 341
Aldehyde dehydrogenase (ALDH) 4, 6, 96

Aldehyde dehydrogenase *(continued)*
  assays 138-49, 161
    substrate, role 145
  distribution
    cytoplasmic 139-40, 159
    cytosolic activity 96, 139-41, 145-7,
      159
    erythrocytes 147, 149, 158-60
    leukocytes 160-1, 226
    microsomal activity 141, 145-6
    mitochondrial activity 139-41, 145-7
    species 140-3, 145-7
    tissues 139, 142, 147, 149, 158, 161,
      164-5
  esterase activity 151
  genetic polymorphism of E_2 144, 181-2,
    187, 196, 231
  high-K_m activity 138-9, 142-51
  inhibition by
    diethyldithiocarbamate, *in vitro* 155,
      160
    diethyldithiocarbamate, *in vivo* 97,
      148, 154, 200
    diethyldithiocarbamate methyl ester
      39, 148, 155-7, 200
    N,N-diethyldithiocarbamyl-*S*-methyl
      disulfide 32, 42, 152-3
    diethylmonothiocarbamate methyl
      ester 41, 157-8, 200-1
    disulfiram, *in vitro* 32, 97-9, 140-1,
      149-54, 158-61
    disulfiram, *in vivo* 97, 104, 125,
      145-8, 152, 158-61, 197, 205, 226,
      328
    S-methyl diethylmonothiocarbamate
      sulfoxide 42
  isozymes 6, 138-44
    Class 1 39, 98, 139, 142-3, 150-153,
      155-6, 160, 164
    Class 2 41, 139, 142-4, 150-57, 199
    Class 3 142-3
    E_1 96, 98, 138-40, 142-4, 149-52, 155,
      158, 165, 328
    E_2 32, 138-140, 142-4, 149-50, 152-3,
      155, 160, 165, 181-2, 196, 205,
      226-7
    E_3 138-9, 140
    E_4 138-9, 165
    F1 140, 142-3

  F2 140, 142-3
    terminology 138-9, 142-4
  low-K_m activity 138-9, 142-51, 156-7,
    205, 226
  mechanism of inhibition 96, 151, 153-4
    mixed disulfides 152
    stearic hinderance 152
    vicinal thiol groups 96, 151
  metabolism of
    acetaldehyde 137-9, 144-50, 154, 156,
      164-5, 168, 182, 196-7, 201, 226
    aldophosphamide 327-8
    biogenic amine aldehydes 125, 161-4
    cyclophosphamide 327-8
  reactivation by
    cysteine 149
    dithiothreitol 147
    glutathione 149
    2-mercaptoethanol 147-52, 158-9
  sensitivity to disulfiram *in vitro*
    Class 1 isozyme 140-1, 150
    Class 2 isozyme 32, 140, 149-50, 152
  specific
    glyceraldehyde-3-phosphate dehydro-
      genase 96, 149, 164-5
    inhibition by disulfiram 149, 164-6
    1-pyrroline-5-carboxylate dehydroge-
      nase 139, 149, 165
    succinic semialdehyde dehydrogenase
      149, 164-5
  stoichiometry of inhibition 98, 140-1,
    149-50, 152
  time course of *in vivo* inhibition
    erythrocytes 158-9
    functional 224-6
    leukocytes 161
    liver 145, 148, 197
Aldehyde oxidase 96, 166
Aldehyde reductase (AR) 163
Alkaline phosphatase (AP) 92, 96, 240,
  343
Alloantigens 247, 249, 255-6
Alprazolam 107-8
Amine oxidase of serum 96, 99
D-Amino acid dehydrogenase 98
Amino acid dithiocarbamates 35
  formation from carbon disulfide 38
  metabolism to methyl esters 38
δ-Aminolevulinic acid (ALA) 80-1

δ-Aminolevulinic acid dehydratase (ALAD) 80-1
Aminopyrine 106, 108-9, 111-3, 118
Amylase 96
Antibody
  see also Immunoglobulin
  autoimmune disease 274, 290
  titers post-influenza vaccination 280, 292
Antibody-dependent cell cytotoxicity (ADCC) 249, 257, 260, 298-9
Antipyrine 104, 106
Arginine 81
Ascorbate oxidase from zucchini 99
Ascorbic acid 8, 202
Aspartate aminotransferase (AST) 240
Athymic (nude) mice 248, 250-2, 254, 257-8, 262-5
Atomic sulfur 37, 84, 117-8, 120, 241, 343
ATPases 92
Atropine 176-7, 194, 198, 203
Autoimmune disease 4, 270, 274, 279, 280, 290-1
Azathioprine 274
Azidothymidine (AZT) 288

Bicarbonate, protection of
  oral diethyldithiocarbamate 70, 85
  urinary diethyldithiocarbamate 52
Biliary excretion of
  cadmium 77
  mercury 90
  platinum 91
Bilirubin 343
Bioavailability of
  cadmium 76
  heavy metals 66
  zinc 72
1,3-Bis(2-chloroethyl)-1-nitrosourea (BCNU) 323
Bleomycin 298-299
Blood/plasma levels of
  copper 67, 86
  mercury 89
  nickel 82-3
  zinc 71
Blood urea nitrogen (BUN) 317-9
Body burdens of
  cadmium 77-8
  copper 67, 86
  heavy metals 66
  lead 81
  nickel 67, 82-3
  polonium 93
  zinc 72
Bone lead levels 80
Brain levels of
  cadmium 77-8
  copper 67, 86-7
  heavy metals 65, 67
  lead 80-1
  mercury 88-90
  nickel 82, 85
  platinum 91
  polonium 93
  thallium 69-70
  zinc 67, 71-3
Brucella melitensis 274

Cadmium 11, 67, 73-9
  biliary excretion 77
  bioavailability 73
  body burdens 77-8
  fecal excretion 77
  metallothionein levels 76, 79
  mortality 73-5
  neurotoxicity 78
  tissue levels 67, 76-8
  toxicity 67, 73-5, 345
  uptake by cell cultures 76
  urinary excretion 76
Cadmium diethyldithiocarbamate [Cd(DS)$_2$] 11, 66-7, 76-8
  dissociation *in vivo* 78
  extraction constant 11
  glutathione reductase inhibition 76
  succinic dehydrogenase inhibition 76
  toxicity 78
  uptake by hepatocytes 76
Caffeine 105, 107
Calcium 276
Calcium carbimide (cyanamide) 6, 197, 227
Calcium carbimide-ethanol reaction (CCER) 176, 182-184, 188, 201
Candida 261

Carbon dioxide 35, 37, 42
Carbon disulfide (CS$_2$) 5, 6, 157, 208, 240
  aldehyde dehydrogenase 155
  assays 9, 24-6, 244
  blood 24, 36, 47
  breath 9, 36-7, 39, 45, 47-9, 51, 54-5,
      243-4
  compliance marker 9, 36, 244
  cytochrome P-450 37, 83-4, 103, 111,
      113, 115-7
    see also Hepatic monooxygenases
  desulfuration 30, 37, 84, 117, 120
  diethylamine assay 27
  diethyldithiocarbamate assay 25-6
  diethyldithiocarbamate-derived 8-9, 30,
      35-7, 45-9, 52, 60, 87, 342
    in stomach 30, 60, 68, 71, 87, 109,
      111, 336
  disulfiram-derived 35-7, 45-9, 54, 56, 243
    implants 245
    liver homogenates 36
  erythrocytes 24
  metabolism 35, 37-8
    amino acid dithiocarbamates 24, 35,
      37, 103, 244, 342
    anaerobic 38
    atomic sulfur 37, 84, 117, 120, 241,
      343
  toxicity 37, 243, 336, 343
    hepatotoxicity 83-4, 115, 241, 343
    neurotoxicity 238, 244, 342
Carbon monoxide 33, 102, 111, 114
Carbon tetrachloride 27, 33
Carbonic anhydrase 15, 38, 97, 100
Carbonyl sulfide (COS) 41
  carbon disulfide-derived 29, 30, 35, 37,
      84, 117
  cytochrome P-450 117, 120
  diethyldithiocarbamate-derived 35, 343
  disulfiram-derived 35, 37, 120, 241
    alcoholics 37, 120
  metabolism by carbonic anhydrase 37-8
  metabolism to
    carbon dioxide 35, 37-8, 42
    sulfate 37, 42
Carboplatin chemotherapy (clinical)
  myelosuppression 332-4
  tumoricidal action 334
Carboplatin toxicology (preclinical)

diethyldithiocarbamate rescue
  mechanism 325-7
  timing 316, 321-2
  mortality 316
  myelotoxicity 314, 320-3
  tumoricidal action 323-4
Carboxyesterase
  microsomal 99, 108-9
  plasma 108-9
Carcinogens 5, 84, 103
Cardiac output 197, 199
  acetaldehyde 194, 196
    disulfiram-treated animals 197
  disulfiram-ethanol reaction 174
  4-methylpyrazole-treated 183
  sympathetic stimulation 196-7
Catalase 97, 133, 135, 299-300
Catechol-*O*-methyltransferase (COMT) 163
Cell cultures 5, 127, 131, 134, 264, 295-8
  bone marrow 320-1, 323, 325-7
  exponential phase 295-6, 301, 310-2
  H9 leukemic CD4$^+$ 288
  L1210 murine leukemic 327
  LLC-PK$_1$ porcine kidney 90, 93
  long-term bone marrow (LTBMC) 327
  lymphocyte 296, 310, 312
    T-lymphocyte 267
  P388 leukemic 327
  peripheral blood leukocyte (PBL) 255,
      260
  peripheral blood mononuclear cell
      (PBMC) 248-9, 254-5, 265-7,
      271-2, 276, 288-9, 291-92, 296
  plateau phase 310-2
  primary hepatocyte 80, 88-90,
  Raji lymphoid 255
  spleen 251-4
Cell-surface antigens
  CD2 267
  CD3 248, 255, 266, 271, 280, 292
  CD4 248, 255, 256, 266, 271, 276,
      279-90, 292
  CD8 255, 266, 271, 276, 280, 289, 290,
      292
  CR 262
  HLA-DR 266
  HTLA 262, 265
  I-A 269-70
  I-E 269-70

Cell-surface antigens *(continued)*
  K 269-70
  Mac 271, 273
  sIg 268
  Thy-1 251-2, 262, 264-5, 268, 271
Centers for Disease Control (CDC) 281,
    284-6
Ceruloplasmin 97, 129
Chicken red blood cells (CRBC) 260
Chlordiazepoxide 105-6
Cholesterol 7α-hydroxylase 98, 104, 116,
    242
Cholesterol serum levels 104, 107, 242
Cholinesterase, plasma 108-9
Chromatin dispersion 247, 266-7, 276, 288
Cisplatin chemotherapy (clinical)
  diethyldithiocarbamate rescue 2, 5, 100,
    328-34
    dose conversion, animal-human 329
    infusion side-effects 329-31
  disulfiram 329
  myelosuppression 333-4
  nausea and vomiting 331-2
  nephrotoxicity 90, 331, 334
  neuropathy 333
  pharmacokinetics 333
  tumoricidal action 333-4
Cisplatin toxicology (preclinical)
  adducts, nucleoside 92
  diethyldithiocarbamate rescue
    mechanism 91-93, 325-7
    timing 314, 317-319, 321-2
  disulfiram 324-5
  gastrointestinal toxicity 319-20
  LD$_{50}$ 91
  mortality 315-6
  myelotoxicity 314, 320-2
  nephrotoxicity 90-1, 314, 317-9
  structure 90
  tumoricidal action 92-3, 323-4
Colony forming units (CFU) 321-6
  granulocyte-macrophage (GM-CFC) 321,
    323, 325-327
Colony stimulating factors (CSF) 236, 272,
    320-1, 327
  granulocyte/monocyte (GM-CSF) 272
Community-Reinforcement Behavioral
    Therapy (CRBT) 215, 217
Concanavalin A (Con A) 248, 251-6, 267,

    269, 271, 274, 276, 292, 303
  see also Mitogen-induced lymphopro-
    liferation
Copper
  brain levels 67, 86-7
  dopamine β-hydroxylase 86, 125, 236
  hippocampal levels 87
  metabolic balance of 86
  superoxide dismutase 97, 99, 100, 126,
    129-32
  tissue levels 86-7
  toxicity 86, 342
  uptake in cell culture 131
Copper diethyldithiocarbamate [Cu(DS)$_2$]
  assays 9, 22-4, 26, 67, 244
  assays for carbon disulfide 9, 26, 244
  assays for disulfiram 14, 22-6
  extraction constant 9-11
  formation from disulfiram 31, 35
    in blood 4, 8, 12-4, 18-9, 22, 34, 85
  stability in blood 14, 18-9
  ternary complexes with proteins 15
Copper-zinc superoxide dismutase (CuZn-
    SOD) 100, 126-31, 133-4
Coprine 197
Cutaneous vasodilation 174, 184
  flush, facial 169-71, 181-3, 186, 202,
    227, 231, 329
  heat sensation 171, 228, 329
  skin temperature rise 171-2, 181, 183,
    186, 202, 225
Cyanamide, *see* Calcium carbimide
Cyclophosphamide 274, 314, 316, 323,
    327-8
Cysteamine 98, 299-300
Cysteine
  reactivation of enzymes 96, 98, 129, 165
  reduction of disulfiram 32
  release of bound diethyldithiocarbamate
    16-7, 23, 30
  toxicity reversal 202, 260, 299-300
Cysteine residues
  aldehyde dehydrogenase 151-4
    Cys$_{302}$ 151-2
  cytochrome P-450 37, 83-4, 103, 117,
    120
    Cys$_{436}$ 103, 117
Cytochrome c 8, 33, 102, 114
Cytochrome oxidase 102

Cytochrome P-420 84, 103, 113, 117
Cytochrome P-450 115, 117, 166, 327
  see also Hepatic monooxygenases
  carbon disulfide metabolism 37, 83-4,
    242, 343
    phenobarbital effect 83, 115, 343
  cysteine residue 37, 83-4, 103, 117, 120
  diethyldithiocarbamate oxidation 33,
    120
  inactivation 37, 83-4, 109-11, 114-15,
    117, 159
  inhibition and
    drug metabolism 95, 97, 102-4,
      108-17, 159
    monooxygenase reactions 97-8, 102-4,
      108-17, 242
  intestinal 119
Cytochrome P-450 reductase 111, 114
Cytotoxic T lymphocytes (T$_C$) 249, 257

Deferoxamine 300
Delayed cutaneous hypersensitivity (DCH)
    261, 280-1, 284-6
Delayed-type hypersensitivity (DTH) 247,
    249, 261
Deoxyhemoglobin 31
Desipramine 107
Desulfuration of
  carbon disulfide 30, 37, 84, 117, 120
  diethyldithiocarbamate methyl ester 30,
    39, 41-2, 118
  α-naphthylisothiocyanate 118
Diamine oxidases 101
Diazepam 105-6
cis-Dichlorodiammineplatinum, *see* Cispla-
    tin
Diethylamine (Et$_2$NH) 42, 51, 155, 246,
    275
  assay 27, 244
  carbon disulfide trapping 9, 26-7
    in urine 37, 48-9, 52, 244
  diethyldithiocarbamate-derived 8, 30,
    35-7, 68, 71, 87, 109, 336
  disulfiram compliance 37, 244
Diethylcarbamate 41
Diethyldithiocarbamate (DSH)
  acid decomposition 8-9, 35-6, 68, 71, 87,
    275, 336

adjuvant effect 4, 292
aldehyde dehydrogenase inhibition
  in vitro 155, 160
  in vivo 97, 148, 154, 200
assays 14-7, 23-8
biotransformation to
  carbon disulfide 27, 35-7, 45, 47-49,
    60, 155
  diethylamine 30, 35-6, 52, 155
  diethyldithiocarbamate methyl ester
    30, 35, 38-9, 45, 49, 61-3, 276
  disulfiram 29-33, 134
  glucuronide conjugate 30, 34-6, 45,
    48, 62
blood/plasma level 57-8, 60-1, 100-1
  half-life 45-7, 57, 61
cancer chemotherapy modulation 313-4
carcinogenesis assessment 344-5
chelation of metalloenzymes
  cobalt 100
  copper 97, 99-102, 125, 129-31
  zinc 97, 100
chronic administration 80, 124
  enzyme activity 99, 118, 126, 135
  immune phenomena 252, 254, 257,
    259, 260, 262, 270-1, 281
clearance 61
cytotoxicity, in cell culture
  bimodal 295-7, 299-301, 310, 312, 344
  blood mononuclear cells 266
  Fe^{2+}-containing media 299-300, 310-2
  hydrogen peroxide 299-301, 310, 312
dose conversion, animal-humans 329
first pass metabolism 60, 317
formation from
  disulfiram 29-32, 35-6, 45-47, 49, 52,
    57-8
  mixed disulfides 23, 31-2, 35
forms
  anhydrous (Imuthiol®) 1, 8, 63, 200,
    248, 280, 337, 339
  gastroprotected (enterocoated) 248,
    287
  trihydrate 1, 8, 248, 280
glutathione peroxidase-like activity 134,
    301
infusion 46-7, 49, 50, 61, 331
  in combination cancer chemotherapy
    100, 329-32, 336

Diethyldithiocarbamate *(continued)*
   into hippocampus 72
   in HIV[+] patients 282, 285-6, 289
   side-effects 329-31
   in thallotoxicosis 69-71
   in Wilson's disease 87
   methylation by thiol-S-methyltransferase
      38
   mutagenicity assessment 344
   oxidation to disulfiram
      anaerobic 31
      hydrogen peroxide 30-1, 33, 301,
         310-1
      iron-catalyzed 30, 33, 260, 299, 300-1,
         310-1
      methemoglobin 31, 33
      oxyhemoglobin 31, 33
      superoxo-ferriheme P-450 complex 33
   plasma proteins binding 14-7, 25, 31-3
   radioprotection 306, 309-10
   radiosensitization, *in vitro* 296, 298,
      309-12
   trypsinization 310-2
  structure 8, 35
  teratogenicity assessment 345
  treatment of
      AIDS 275, 279-81, 283, 285-8
      autoimmune disease 4, 280, 290-1
      cisplatin nephrotoxicity 90-1, 314,
         317-9, 331, 334
      gastrointestinal surgery patients 261,
         280-1, 290
      HIV infection 2, 4, 200, 272, 280-89,
         292, 335
      nickel carbonyl intoxication 84-5
      rheumatoid arthritis 4, 280, 290-1
      systemic lupus erythematosus 280,
         291
      Wilson's disease 86-7
  toxicity
      hepatotoxicity assessment 343
      LD$_{50}$ 315, 336-9
  urinary excretion 49, 52
  volume of distribution 50
Diethyldithiocarbamate glucuronide (DSGa)
      30, 34-6
  assay 25, 27, 53
  bile 34
  half-life 45, 60, 62

  plasma 45, 59
  urine 34, 39, 48, 53, 60, 62
Diethyldithiocarbamate methyl ester
      (DSMe) 42, 35, 120
  aldehyde dehydrogenase inhibition
      39-40, 148, 155-7, 199-201
  assays 25-8
  blood/plasma 45-7, 49, 50, 58-9, 61-2
  clearance 62
  diethylmonothiocarbamate methyl ester
      40-1, 120, 157
  drug metabolism inhibition 118
  ethanol reaction *in vivo* 40, 189, 191
  half-life 45-7, 58-9, 61-2
  hypothermic effect 199, 201
  liver 39
  neocortex 38, 63, 276
  volume of distribution 50
Diethyldithiocarbamic acid ethyl ester
      (DSEt) 14, 25-6
Diethyldithiocarbamoyl-*S*-glucuronide, *see*
      Diethyldithiocarbamate glucuro-
      nide
N,N-Diethyldithiocarbamyl-*S*-methyl disul-
      fide (DSSMe) 31-2, 42, 152-154
Diethylenetriaminepentaacetic acid (DPTA)
      19, 22, 26, 56
Diethylmonothiocarbamate (DmSH) 35,
      41-2, 118, 189
Diethylmonothiocarbamic acid ethyl ester
      (DmSEt) 26
Diethylmonothiocarbamic acid methyl ester
      (DmSMe) 35, 40-2, 59, 118, 120
  aldehyde dehydrogenase 157-8, 160
  assay 26
  ethanol reaction *in vivo* 189, 199-201
  hypothermic effect 199, 201
Diglycyl L-histidine-*N*-methylamide 81
3,4-Dihydroxymandelic acid (DHMA) 163
3,4-Dihydroxymandelicaldehyde (DHMAL)
      162-3
3,4-Dihydroxyphenylacetaldehyde (DOPAL)
      161-3, 165
3,4-Dihydroxyphenylacetic acid (DOPAC)
      162-3
3,4-Dihydroxyphenylalanine (DOPA) 101,
      124
3,4-Dihydroxyphenylethanol (DOPET)
      162-3

3,4-Dihydroxyphenylglycol (DHPG)   163
2,3-Dimercaptopropanol (BAL)   76
Disulfides, mixed
  aldehyde dehydrogenase   152-4
  assay   25
  diethyldithiocarbamate release   23, 31-2,
    35
  formation   8, 14-17, 19, 22-3, 30-33, 35,
    42, 44, 96-98, 260, 312
Disulfiram (DSSD)   1, 5-6
  assays   21-23, 25, 27, 56
  biotransformation to
    carbon disulfide   35-6, 45, 47-49, 54-5
    carbonyl sulfide   35, 37
    diethylamine   35-6, 47, 49, 52, 57-8
    diethyldithiocarbamate   29-32, 35-6,
      45-47, 49, 52, 57-8
    diethyldithiocarbamate glucuronide
      34-5, 48-9, 53, 59-60
    diethyldithiocarbamate methyl ester
      38-9, 46-7, 58-9
    diethylmonothiocarbamate methyl
      ester   40-1, 47, 59
    S-methyl diethylmonothiocarbamate
      sulfoxide   42
    sulfate   45-6, 48, 53
  carcinogenicity assessment   344
  chelation of heavy metals   10, 66-68
  chemical properties   8
  chronic administration   37
    enzyme activity   99, 103, 108, 116,
      118-9, 226
    rate of metabolism   36, 53-4
  copper diethyldithiocarbamate formation
    8, 14, 18-9, 22-24, 34-5, 85
  diethyldithiocarbamate-derived via
    oxyhemoglobin   31, 33
    methemoglobin   31, 33
    superoxo-ferriheme P-450 complex   33
  erythrocytes uptake   17-9
  formulations
    effervescent   2, 59, 170, 227-8
    implants   208, 245-6
    microcrystalline   59, 170, 226-7, 351-2
  metabolism, induction of   36, 53-4
  mixed disulfide formation   35
    albumin   14-5
    glutathione   8
    hemoglobin   15

2-mercaptoethanol   8
  methanethiol   31-2, 42, 152
  protein sulfhydryls   8, 14-8, 22-3. 29,
    96-8
  mutagenicity assessment   343-4
  parenteral administration   68, 108, 337,
    340
  partition coefficient   7
  reaction with
    aldehyde dehydrogenase E_1 96
    protein sulfhydryls   96-8
    vicinal sulfhydryls   96
  reduction to diethyldithiocarbamate by
    albumin   30-2
    ascorbic acid   8
    cuprous ions   8
    cysteine   30, 32
    glutathione, reduced   8, 30-2
    hemoglobin   30-1
    2-mercaptoethanol   8
    methanethiol   31-2
    protein sulfhydryls   8, 29-31
  reproductive toxicity assessment   345
  solubility   7
  structure   7
  teratogenicity assessment   345
  toxicity, acute   340-1
    LD_{50}s   185, 336-8
    paralysis   340-1
    peripheral neuropathy   6, 233, 237-9,
      242, 336, 340-2
  treatment of
    AIDS patients   288-9
    alcoholics, *see* Alcoholism therapy
    nickel dermatitis   83-4
  untoward effects   5, 6, 341-3
    axonopathy   238, 244, 341-2
    encephalopathy   233, 235-7
    hepatotoxicity   83, 233, 238, 240-1,
      336, 343
    peripheral neuropathy   6, 233, 237-9,
      242, 336, 340-2
Disulfiram Assurance Program   213-5, 217
Disulfiram-ethanol interaction (animals)
  blood pressure   186, 187, 191, 195
  heart rate   187, 190, 195
  hypothermia   186, 188-9, 201
  isobologram   185
  mortality   185

Disulfiram-ethanol reaction (DER, humans)
1, 4, 6, 86, 97, 206, 218 233
analogous reactions
acetaldehyde infusion 178, 351
calcium carbimide-ethanol 182-4, 227
diethyldithiocarbamate-ethanol 200
diethyldithiocarbamate infusion 330-2
ethanol in E_2 deficient 144, 181-2,
187
monosulfiram-ethanol 232
nitrefazol-ethanol 182-4
after-shaves 231-2
aversive conditioning 169-70, 226
blood levels
acetaldehyde 138, 177-9, 180-3, 193,
201-2, 227, 351
diethyldithiocarbamate methyl ester
156
diethylmonothiocarbamate methyl
ester 157
blood pressure 169, 174, 176-8, 186,
202
diastolic 173-4, 179, 181-2, 187, 227
systolic 168, 173-4, 181-2, 184, 187,
203
cardiac output 174
discovery 167-70, 348, 349
disulfiram
dose 170, 172, 175-6, 180, 182, 226-8
implants 245-6
drinking through reaction 208, 230-1
electrocardiographic changes 174-5,
183, 188, 201
erythrocyte aldehyde dehydrogenase
158
ethanol dose 171, 175-6, 180-1, 191,
225-8, 349
ethanol elimination rate 192, 193, 229
hepatic status 225
high dose toxicity
cardiovascular collapse 175-7, 188,
198
treatment 183, 201-3
vagal reflex 176, 188, 198, 203
mechanism
acetaldehyde hypothesis 168, 178-9,
184-5
dopamine β-hydroxylase hypothesis
4-5, 168, 193-9

minute volume 172, 178, 188
peripheral resistance 174, 198-9, 203
plasma
pCO_2 172, 178, 181. 188
pH 171, 181, 188
pO_2 172, 188
potassium 174-5, 181, 188
signs and symptoms
acetaldehyde odor 169, 171-2, 179,
350
conjunctival injection 171
cough 171-2
cutaneous flushing 168, 170-1, 181,
183, 201-2, 227
dyspnea 170-2, 227-8
hyperesthesia 171-2
nausea and vomiting 171-2, 175-7,
181, 188, 202, 228
pallor 171, 176
palpitations 169, 171-2, 181, 202, 228
paresthesia 171-2
skin temperature rise 225
tachycardia 173-4, 178, 181-3, 187,
201
throbbing 171-2
ventilation 172-3
Disulfiram metabolite-ethanol interaction
40-2, 200-1
Dithiazone 73
Dithiocarbamates, novel 78-9
2,2'-Dithiopyridine (PSSP) 153-4
Dithiothreitol 98-9, 116, 147, 155, 159,
299, 300
DNA bifunctional cisplatin adducts 92-3
DNA synthesis 93, 251, 298-9, 322, 325
Dopa oxidase 101
Dopamine (DA) 120-5, 165, 189, 198-9
Dopamine β-hydroxylase (DBH) 233, 236
diethyldithiocarbamate 86, 122-3
disulfiram 5, 97, 121-5, 231, 241, 305,
330
catecholamine metabolite levels
162-164, 198-9
norepinephrine tissue stores 123, 193,
198, 330
sympathetic action 196-7
Dose modifying factor (DMF) 93, 307-8,
310, 321, 325
Doxorubicin toxicity 298-9, 323

Drug metabolism, disulfiram therapy and
    see also Hepatic monooxygenases
    alprazolam 101, 107
    aminopyrine 106
    antipyrine 104, 106
    caffeine 105, 107
    chlordiazepoxide 105-6
    cholesterol 104, 107
    desipramine 107
    diazepam 105-6
    imipramine 107
    lorazepam 105-6
    oxazepam 105-6
    phenytoin 104-6
    primidone 106
    theophylline 107
    warfarin 105, 107

Eagle's minimum essential medium (MEM)
        299, 311
Enzymes
    see also individual listings
    alcohol dehydrogenase 96-8, 100
    aldehyde dehydrogenase 4, 6, 32, 39,
        41-2, 96-9, 137-66, 168, 181-2,
        187, 196-7, 199-201, 205, 224-27,
        231, 327-8
    aldehyde oxidase 96, 166
    aldehyde reductase 163
    alkaline phosphatase 92, 96, 240, 343
    amine oxidase of serum 96, 99
    D-amino acid dehydrogenase 98
    δ-aminolevulinic acid dehydratase 80-1
    amylase 96
    ascorbate oxidase from zucchini 99
    aspartate aminotransferase (AST) 240
    carbonic anhydrase 15, 38, 97, 100
    carboxyesterase, microsomal 99, 108-9
    carboxyesterase, plasma 108-9
    catalase 97, 133, 135, 299-300
    catechol-*O*-methyltransferase 163
    ceruloplasmin 97, 129
    cholesterol 7α-hydroxylase 98, 104, 116,
        242
    cholinesterase, plasma 108-9
    copper-zinc superoxide dismutase 100,
        126-31, 133-4
    cytochrome *c* reductase 114

cytochrome oxidase 102
cytochrome P-450 monooxygenases
    see also Hepatic monooxygenases
cytochrome P-450 reductase 111, 114
diamine oxidases 101
dopa oxidase 101
dopamine β-hydroxylase 5, 86, 97,
        121-5, 162-4, 193, 196-9, 231, 233,
        236, 241, 304, 330
galactose oxidase 97
L-gluconate dehydrogenase 119
glucose-6-phosphate dehydrogenase 99,
        119, 306
β-glucuronidase 119
D-glucuronolactone dehydrogenase 119
glutamic γ-semialdehyde dehydrogenase
        139, 165
γ-glutamyltranspeptidase 92
glutathione peroxidase 97, 133-5, 301,
        306
glutathione reductase 76, 88-9, 306
glutathione-*S*-transferase 133, 135
D-glyceraldehyde-3-phosphate dehydroge-
        nase 96, 164-5
heme oxygenase 84, 114, 117
hexokinases 97-8
hydroxy β-methylglutaryl coenzyme A
        reductase 242
laccase, lacquer tree 99
lactate dehydrogenase 240, 343
leucine aminopeptidase 92
5-lipoxygenase 99
monoamine oxidase 96, 101, 162-4
peptidylglycine α-amidating monooxyge-
        nase 101
phenol oxidases 101
phosphatase, calmodulin-dependent 101
1-pyrroline-5-carboxylate dehydrogenase
        139, 165
retinal dehydrogenase 99
reverse transcriptase 288
serum glutamic oxaloacetic transaminase
        240, 343
succinic dehydrogenase 76, 96
succinic semialdehyde dehydrogenase
        164
superoxide dismutase 4, 97, 100,
        126-35, 243, 300, 305-6
    copper-zinc-containing 100, 126-1,

Enzymes *(continued)*
    133-4
    extracellular 126, 128, 130, 133
    iron-containing 126
    manganese-containing 126-7, 131
    thiol-*S*-methyltransferase 38
    tryptophan pyrrolase 96
    tyrosinases 101
    tyrosine hydroxylase 101, 126
    UDP-glucose dehydrogenase 119
    UDP-glucuronic acid pyrophosphatase
      119
    UDP-glucuronosyltransferase 36, 118
    xanthine oxidase 96, 166
Enzyme regeneration
    cysteamine 98
    cysteine 96, 98, 129
    dithiothreitol 98, 116
    glutathione; reduced 96, 98, 129, 134
    2-mercaptoethanol 98
    2-mercaptopropionylglycine 129
Epinephrine (E) 196, 198, 202
Ephedrine 203, 330
Erythrocyte levels of
    copper 86
    disulfiram 18
    lead 80
    mercury 89-90
    zinc 72
Erythrocyte-rosette forming cells (E-RFC)
    281
Erythrocyte sedimentation rate 291
Ethanol 1, 3, 4, 57, 147, 198, 221, 242-3,
    280, 325
    see also Disulfiram-ethanol reaction
    acetaldehyde appearance in blood
      E_2 deficient humans 144, 181-2
      non-enzymatic, *ex vivo* 177, 179
      post-calcium carbamide 183
      post-diethyldithiocarbamate methyl
        ester 156, 200
      post-diethylmonothiocarbamate methyl
        ester 200
      post-disulfiram (animals) 155, 187
      post-nitrefazol 156
    after-shave 232
    carbon disulfide, sensitization to 115
    cardiovascular effects in
      E_2 deficient humans 182, 196

      post-diethyldithiocarbamate methyl
        ester 40, 200
      post-diethylmonothiocarbamate methyl
        ester 41, 200-1
      post-disulfiram (animals) 186-91, 197
    challenge in disulfiram treated humans
      158, 169-70
    dose 157, 171-2, 174-6, 180, 182,
      225-31, 245-6
    consumption by alcoholics 207, 209,
      229
    craving 206, 209, 220, 229-30
    formation in gastrointestinal tract 165
    hypothermia post-disulfiram (animals)
      188-9
    LD_{50} 185
    metabolism to acetaldehyde 137, 150,
      169
      inhibition of 201
    rate of elimination
      acetaldehyde effect 98-9, 192-3, 229
      post-diethyldithiocarbamate 192
      post-disulfiram 98-9, 191-2
    skin-lotions 232
Ethofos (WR-2721) 299, 307, 312
Ethylenediaminetetraacetic acid (EDTA)
    10, 14-17, 24, 26, 31, 160
Extracellular superoxide dismutase (EC-
    SOD) 126, 128, 130, 133
Extraction constants 10-1, 67, 78, 91, 337

Facial flush, *see* Cutaneous vasodilation
Facteur Thymique Serique (FTS) 265
Fecal excretion of
    cadmium 77
    heavy metals 66
    lead 66, 68, 79
    mercury 66, 88, 90
    nickel 82
Fenton-type reaction 300, 305
Fetal calf serum (FCS) 260, 265, 267, 299,
    310-1
Fetal mercury levels 89
Fibrosarcoma 265
Fluorescein 265
Follicle-stimulating hormone (FSH) 243
Food and Drug Administration (FDA) 288
Formaldehyde 35, 102

Galactose oxidase 97
Gastrointestinal surgery 261, 280-1, 290
Gender specific effects 250, 254, 262
Gentamicin 265
D-Glucaric acid excretion 104, 107
L-Gluconate dehydrogenase 119
Glucose-6-phosphate dehydrogenase 99,
     119, 306
β-Glucuronidase 119
D-Glucuronolactone dehydrogenase 119
Glucuronosyltransferases, see UDP-Glucuro-
     nosyltransferase
Glutamic γ-semialdehyde dehydrogenase
     139, 165
Glutamine 265
γ-Glutamyltranspeptidase (GGTP) 92
Glutathione-glutathione reductase system
     32
Glutathione, oxidized (GSSG) 2, 31-2, 134
Glutathione peroxidase (GSHPx) 97, 133-5,
     301, 306
   selenium-containing (Se-GSHPx) 133-4
Glutathione, reduced (GSH) 2
   abundance 32, 165
   cytotoxicity, in vitro 299
   enzyme regeneration 96, 98, 129, 149,
     165
   generating system 32, 160
   microsomal membranes 116-7
   platinum complex 91
   reaction with carbon disulfide 35, 38
   reduction
     disulfiram 8, 15, 30-32, 301
     protein mixed disulfides 15-6, 23,
       32-3, 61
Glutathione reductase
   in vitro inhibition by
     cadmium diethyldithiocarbamate 76
     mercury diethyldithiocarbamate 88-9
   in vivo elevation by
     diethyldithiocarbamate 306
Glutathione-S-transferase (GST) 133, 135
D-Glyceraldehyde-3-phosphate dehydroge-
     nase 96, 164-5
Growth hormone, human (hGH) 243
Guinea pigs 104, 184, 252, 261, 272-3, 276

Hank's balanced salt solution (HBSS) 311

Hapten-carrier 261
Heart rate 57, 203
   acetaldehyde 178, 193-6
   disulfiram-ethanol reaction 173-4, 181-3,
     202, 231
   ethanol in
     disulfiram-implanted humans 245
     disulfiram-naive animals 186, 189
     disulfiram-treated animals 187, 190,
       195
     E_2-deficient 182, 187, 196, 231
     4-methylpyrazole-treated 182-3, 201
   sympathetic stimulation 196-7
Heat sensation, see Cutaneous vasodilation
Heme oxygenase 84, 114, 117
Hemoglobin 16, 24, 30-1, 33, 342
Hepatic levels of
   cadmium 76-7
   copper 87
   lead 80-1
   mercury 90
   platinum 91
   polonium 93
   zinc 72
Hepatic monooxygenases
   see also Drug metabolism
   and aldehyde dehydrogenase 104
   effect of pretreatment with
     3-methylcholanthrene 115, 119
     phenobarbital 115
   level of
     cytochrome P-420 103, 113, 117
     cytochrome P-450 103-4, 109-17
     monooxygenase activity 103-4, 109-18
     NADPH cytochrome c reductase 114
     NADPH cytochrome P-450 reductase
       114
   role of
     δ-aminolevulinic acid synthetase 114
     atomic sulfur 117-20
     carbon disulfide 103, 109-11, 113,
       115-7, 120
     carbonyl sulfide 117, 120
     cysteine Cys_{436} residue 103, 117
     diethyldithiocarbamate 103, 109-112,
       114-117
     diethyldithiocarbamic acid methyl
       ester 118-20
     disulfiram 103-4, 108-9, 111, 114-116

Hepatic monooxygenases *(continued)*
  heme iron 37, 117, 120
  heme oxygenase 84, 114, 117
  synergy with cimetidine inhibition 108
Hepatosin 249, 264-5
Hexokinases 97-8
Hippocampal levels of
  copper 87
  zinc 72-3
HIV infection 266-7
  animal models 273
  disulfiram 288-9
HIV infection, diethyldithiocarbamate
     treatment of 2, 4, 292
  concurrent therapy with
    suramin 288
    zidovudine 288
  decreased
    mortality 281-3, 286, 293
    opportunistic infection incidence
      286-7
    progression to AIDS 281-3, 286
    progression to AIDS related complex
      282, 285
    symptom incidence 281-2, 285-6
  dose
    intravenous 282-3, 285-6, 335-6
    oral 280-7, 289, 335
  increase in CD4$^+$ T cells
    absolute 271, 280-6
    relative to controls 282-3, 286
  increased
    delayed cutaneous hypersensitivity
      261, 280-1, 284-6
    IL-2R$^+$ monocytes 286
  long-term therapy 281
  phase I study 283, 285
    maximally tolerated dose 285, 289
  regression of
    lymphadenopathy 281-2, 284, 286
    splenomegaly 281-2
  side effects
    abdominal discomfort 281, 289
    chemical odor 281
    chemical taste 289
    disulfiram-like reaction to ethanol 200
  weight gain 281
Horse red blood cells 250
Hydrocortisone 274

Hydrogen peroxide 31, 33, 133, 305-6
  oxidation of diethyldithiocarbamate 8,
    30, 134, 299,
  product of thiol oxidation 299-301, 310,
    312, 344
Hydroxy β-methylglutaryl coenzyme A re-
    ductase 242
5-Hydroxyindoleacetaldehyde (5-HIAL)
    161, 164-5
5-Hydroxyindoleacetic acid (5-HIAA) 164
Hydroxyl free radicals 300, 304-5, 310, 312
7α-Hydroxylase, *see* Cholesterol
    7α-hydroxylase
5-Hydroxytryptamine (5-HT) 81, 162,
    164-5, 196, 341
5-Hydroxytryptophol (5-HTOL) 164
Hyperoxia toxicity 301-6
Hyperthermia toxicity 302, 311-2
Hypothermia 186, 188-9, 201
  see also Cutaneous vasodilation

Imipramine 107
Immunoglobulin G (IgG) blood titers 249
Immunoglobulin G-forming spleen B cells
  athymic mice 250, 262
  cell-surface antigens 270
  diethyldithiocarbamate effect on 248-50
    chronic 254
    in vitro 250
  hepatosin 265
  immunodepression 274
  neocortical lesions 256, 269-70
  pups, unweaned 264
  strain and gender dependence 250-2
Immunoglobulin M-forming spleen B cells
    249
  cell-surface antigens 270
  LP-BM5 retrovirus inoculation 273-4
  strain and gender dependence 250-1
Imuthiol® 1, 8, 63, 200, 248, 280, 337, 339
Indole-3-acetaldehyde (IAL) 145, 147, 161
Influenza vaccination 280, 292
Interaction isobolograms
  ethanol and disulfiram 185
  cisplatin and diethyldithiocarbamate 315
Interferon (IFN) 258, 274
Interleukin-1 (IL-1) 267, 272, 286
Interleukin-2 (IL-2) 258, 266-7, 272, 274,

Interleukin-2 *(continued)*
    276, 286
Interleukin-2 receptors (IL-2R) 266, 286
Interleukin-3 (IL-3) 327
^{14}C-Iodoantipyrine 70
Iron-containing superoxide dismutase (Fe-
    SOD) 126
^{123}I-Isopropyliodoamphetamine 70

Jejunum, radiation damage 308

K-cell, *see* Antibody-dependent cell
    cytotoxicity
Kainic acid toxicity 73

Laccase, lacquer tree 99
Lactate dehydrogenase (LDH) 240, 343
Lead
    body burdens 81
    excretion 66, 68, 79
    tissue levels 80-1
    toxicity 80-1
Lead diethyldithiocarbamate [Pb(DS)$_2$] 24,
    79-80
Lethal dose, 50% (LD$_{50}$)
    acetaldehyde 138, 198
    cisplatin 91, 315-6
    cisplatin-diethyldithiocarbamate 315-6
    ethanol 185
    ethanol-disulfiram 185
    disulfiram 185, 336-8
    metal diethyldithiocarbamates 67, 69,
        78, 84, 86, 91, 337, 339, 345
    radiation 308
Leucine aminopeptidase 92
Leukocytes 82, 99, 137, 160, 161, 226,
    268
Levamisole 251
Lipopolysaccharide of *E. Coli* (LPS) 252,
    267, 272
5-Lipoxygenase 99
Listeria 273
Local cerebral blood flow (LCBF) 70
Long-term bone marrow cultures (LTBMC)
    327
Lorazepam 105-6, 118

Luteinizing hormone (LH) 243
Lymph node hyperplasia 263
Lymphadenopathy 274, 281-2, 284, 286

α_2-Macroglobulin 92
Macrophages 82, 255, 267, 270, 272-3,
    291, 321, 326
Major histocompatibility complex (MHC)
    251, 255-258, 269-70, 276
Manganese-containing superoxide dismu-
    tase (Mn-SOD) 126-7, 131
Memory, spatial working 72
2-Mercaptoethanol (2-ME) 8, 14, 23, 25-6,
    98, 147-8, 150-2, 158-9, 165, 255,
    266
Mercuric acetate 88-90
Mercury
    excretion 66, 68, 90
    fetal levels 89
    tissue levels 88-90
    uptake by cell cultures 88-9
Mercury diethyldithiocarbamate [Hg(DS)$_2$]
    88-9, 91
    extraction constant 11
    hepatocyte uptake 88-9
    inhibition of
        alcohol dehydrogenase 88-9
        glutathione reductase 88-9
    platinum displacement of mercury 91
    serum protein binding 88
Metabolism of xenobiotics via
    see also Drug metabolism
    glucuronic acid pathway 103-4, 118-9
    glutathione pathway 103, 135
    hepatic monooxygenases 103-9, 111,
        114-6
    intestinal monooxygenases 103, 119
Metallothionein 76, 79
Metals, *see* Copper, Cadmium, Lead,
    Mercury, Nickel, Platinum,
    Polonium, Thallium, Tin, Zinc
Methadone 210-1, 221-2
Methanethiol (MeSH) 31-2, 35, 41-2, 152-3
Methemoglobin 31, 33, 160
N-(4-Methoxybenzyl)-*N*-dithiocarboxy-D-
    glucamine 79
3-Methoxy-4-hydroxyphenylacetic acid
    (HVA) 162-4, 198

3-Methoxy-4-hydroxyphenylglycol (MHPG) 162
Methyl mercury (MeHg) 65, 88-90
  tissue levels 90
3-Methylcholanthrene (MC) 34, 115, 119
4-Methylpyrazole 177, 181-4, 189-90, 201
Methyltransferase, *see* Thiol-*S*-methyltransferase
Mitogen-induced lymphoproliferation 248
  guinea pig spleen cells 252
  human blood mononuclear cells 254-5, 271, 291-2
  murine lymph node cells 253, 270
  murine spleen cells 251-2
    cell-surface antigens 251, 269-70
    immunodepression 274
    neocortical lesions 256, 259
    pretreatment time dependence 252-3
    pups 254
    strain dependence 252-3
    in vitro enhancement 254, 272
Mitomycin C 256, 257, 323
Mixed disulfides, *see* Disulfides, mixed
Mixed function oxygenases (MFO) 241
  see also Hepatic monooxygenases
Mixed lymphocyte culture (MLC) 255-6
Monoamine oxidase (MAO) 96, 162-4
  placental 101
Monocytes 248-9, 266-7, 272, 276, 286, 295, 297-8
Monothiocarbamates 41
Morning stiffness 291
Mossy fiber boutons 72-3
Mouse strains
  A/J 250
  B6-H-2^k 251
  B6TL 251
  BALB/c 250, 252-3, 257-60, 262, 270-2
  BDF$_1$ 91
  C3H/He 250, 252-3, 256, 258-60, 263-265, 268, 273
  C3H/HeJ 254, 260, 268, 270
  C57BL/6 109, 250, 253, 256, 258-9, 263, 265, 268, 270, 273
  DBA 109, 250
  nude (nu/nu; athymic) 248, 250-252, 254, 257-8, 262-5
  NZB 265, 270-1, 274
Multitest 261

Mutagenicity assessment 344
Myelosuppression 314, 332-4

NADH 146, 151-2, 158, 192
NADPH 32-3, 40, 102-3, 111, 114-9
NADPH cytochrome c reductase 114
NADPH cytochrome P-450 reductase 114
Nalmefene 202
α-Naphthylisothiocyanate 118
Natural killer cells (NK) 257-60, 266, 298-9
Neocortical lesions 256-8, 260, 263-4, 268-70
Neoplastic disease, immunostimulation 254-5, 271, 292
Nickel
  body burdens 67, 82-3
  excretion 82, 85
  tissue levels 82, 85
  toxicity 81
  uptake by cell cultures 82
Nickel carbonyl [Ni(CO)$_2$] 4, 65, 82, 84-5, 335
Nickel dermatitis, disulfiram therapy of 82, 83-4
Nickel subsulfide (Ni$_3$S$_2$) 65, 84
Nitrefazol-ethanol reaction (NER) 182-4, 201
Nitrogen mustard (HN$_2$) 323-5
NK-Cells, *see* Natural killer cells
Norepinephrine (NE) 4, 120-6, 162, 164-5, 193-4, 196-9, 202, 231, 236, 241, 330
Nuclear refringency, *see* Chromatin dispersion

Octopamine (OA) 121-2, 197
m-Octopamine 121
n-Octylamine 33
Oxazaphosphorine 314, 327-8
Oxazepam 105-6
Oxidative stress 5, 295, 301-2, 306
Oxyhemoglobin 31-3, 160, 300
Ozone 295, 301, 304, 306

Pain scores in rheumatoid arthritis 280, 291

Palpitations 169, 171-2, 181, 202, 228
Paraquat 295, 301, 304, 306
Partition coefficients 7, 69, 77, 82, 276
D-Penicillamine 81, 84, 291
Peptidylglycine α-amidating monooxyge-
        nase 101
Peripheral resistance
    acetaldehyde 191, 194, 196, 198-9
    counteracting lowered 183, 203
Phagocytotic clearance of colloids 272-3
Phenobarbital (PB) 33-4, 83, 115, 241, 343
Phenol oxidases 101
Phenytoin 104-6
Phosphatase, calmodulin-dependent 101
Phytohemagglutinin (PHA) 160, 248,
        251-2, 254-6, 267, 269, 271-2, 274,
        276, 292, 296
    see also Mitogen-induced lymphoprolife-
        ration
Plaque-forming cells (PFC) 249-2, 254,
        256, 262, 264, 269-70, 274-5
Plasminogen activator inhibitor (PAI-1) 243
Platelet Factor 4 (PF4) 243
Platinum, cisplatin-derived
    biliary excretion 91
    tissue levels 91
Platinum diethyldithiocarbamate [Pt(DS)₂]
    formation in cell culture 91
    physicochemical properties 67, 91
    toxicity 91
Pokeweed mitogen (PWM) 252
Polonium 93
Polymorphonuclear granulocytes (PMN)
        295-6
Prednisone 291
Primidone 106
Prolactin, human (hProl) 243
Propranolol 194, 265
Prostaglandin E₂ (PGE₂) 267, 272, 291
Proteus 261
1-Pyrroline-5-carboxylate dehydrogenase
        139, 165

Radiation toxicity 302
    in cell culture 296, 298, 310-2
    in vivo 306-9, 312, 325-6
Reactive oxygen species (ROS) 4, 97, 126,
        133, 135, 301, 304, 310-2

Receptors
    adenosine A₂ 190
    adrenergic 202
    dopamine 189
    interleukin-2 266, 286
Renal levels of
    cadmium 76-7
    copper 87
    heavy metals 65
    lead 80-1
    mercury 88
    nickel 82, 85
    platinum 91
    zinc 72
Reproductive toxicity 335, 345
Reserpine 123-4, 193
Retinal dehydrogenase 99
Reverse transcriptase expression 288
Rheumatoid arthritis 4
    articular index 280, 291
    CD4⁺/CD8⁺ ratio 280, 290
    pain scores 280, 291
Riboflavin (Vitamin B₂) 211-2, 218, 245
RNA synthesis 93, 296

S. typhimurium 275
Serotonin, *see* 5-Hydroxytryptamine
Serum factors 247, 256, 261
Serum glutamic oxaloacetic transaminase
        (SGOT) 240, 343
Sheep red blood cells (SRBC) 247-2, 254,
        256, 261-2, 269, 275, 302
Skin temperature, *see* Cutaneous vasodila-
        tion
Sodium metabisulfite 202
Spleen colony assay 307, 321
Spleen hyperplasia 263
Spleen levels of
    cadmium 76
    polonium 93
    zinc 72
Splenic lymphoproliferative response (S-
        LPR) 251-2, 254, 256, 269, 274,
        276
Splenomegaly 281-2
Stem cell proliferation 307-8, 312, 325-7
Streptococcus 261
Succinic dehydrogenase 76, 96

Succinic semialdehyde dehydrogenase
(SSA) 164
Sulfate
  assay 25, 27
  formation from
    carbonyl sulfide 37
    diethyldithiocarbamate 39, 48, 62
    diethyldithiocarbamate methyl ester
      30, 39, 41, 48, 62, 118
    disulfiram 33, 39, 42, 45-6, 48-9, 53
Sulfhydryl groups 58, 153, 260, 314
  albumin 15-6, 30
  enzymes 92
  disulfiram inhibition 96-8, 100, 116
  hemoglobin 16, 30
  ionization 19
  proteins
    binding of carbon disulfide by 24
    reduction of disulfiram by 8, 15, 16,
      22-3, 29-31, 33, 98, 260
  vicinal 29, 31, 96, 151, 153-4
Sulfur, atomic, *see* Atomic sulfur
Superoxide anion radical 97, 126, 301,
  305, 310
Superoxide dismutase (SOD) 4, 97, 126-33,
  300
  see also Copper-zinc superoxide dismu-
    tase
  diethyldithiocarbamate 127-30, 133, 305,
    310
    cell culture 131-2
    glutathione peroxidase 133-5, 306
  disulfiram 127-8, 243, 305
Superoxo-ferriheme 33
Suramin 288
Surviving fraction (SF) 309, 321-6
Synapsin I 78
Systemic lupus erythematosus
  juvenile 280, 291
  mouse model 274

T-Cell counts in patients with
  gastrointestinal surgery 290
  HIV infection 271, 280-9
  lung cancer 255, 271, 292
  rheumatoid arthritis 290
T Cell, cytotoxic (T_C) 247, 257-8
T-Cell differentiation

athymic mice *in vivo* 248, 261-4
bone marrow cultures
  human 266
  mouse 265
diethyldithiocarbamate-induced
  in vitro 248-9, 265-6, 272
  in vivo 248, 261-4, 271, 276
  hepatosin 249, 264-5
  humans *in vivo* 271, 276
  inducing factors in
    hepatocyte culture 264-5
    milk 264
    serum 262-4
  peripheral blood mononuclear cell cul-
    tures 249, 265-6, 272
    monocyte requirement 249, 266, 272
  spleen cultures from athymic mice
    262-5
Tachycardia, *see* Heart rate
Testicular
  levels of
    cadmium 77-8
    copper 87
    radiation damage 308
Tetanus toxoid 261
2,3,7,8-Tetrachlorodibenzo-p-dioxin (TCDD)
  142
Tetraplatin 316-20
Thallium 68-9, 337
  brain levels 69
  toxicity 68-71
  urinary excretion 69, 71
Thallium diethyldithiocarbamate [Tl(DS)]
  67, 69
  cerebral blood flow imaging 70
  computed tomography 65, 70
  dissociation 69
  extraction constant 11
  uptake into brain 69-70
Thallotoxicosis 68, 70-1
Theophylline 107
Thiamine 202
Thiazolidine-2-thione-4-carboxylic acid 35,
  38
Thiocyanate (SCN) 117
Thiol-disulfide exchange reactions 15, 30,
  42, 98, 152, 299
Thiol-S-methyltransferase 38
Thiolate ligand 37, 117

Thiols 58, 98-9, 299-300, 310, 312
  see also Sulfhydryl groups
2-Thiopyridylmethyl disulfide (PSSMe) 154
2-Thio-5-thiazolidinone 35, 38
Thiourea 35, 38
Thiuram disulfide 7, 96, 168
Thymidine 251, 255, 269
Thymus 38, 63, 250, 263-4, 270-1
Thyroid stimulating hormone, human
        (hTSH) 243
Thyrotropin-releasing factor (TRH) 243
Thyroxin (T_4) 243
Tin diethyldithiocarbamate
  extractability 11
  LD_{50} 339
Tomography 65, 70
Toxicity
  cadmium 67, 73-5, 78
  copper 86
  heavy metals 68
  lead 80-1
  nickel 81
  nickel carbonyl 84-5
  polonium 93
  platinum 91
  thallium 67, 69
Trichophyton 261
Triethylenetetramine 81
Triiodothyronine (T_3) 243
Tritiated water (THO) 124-5, 199
Trypsin 92, 311-2
Tryptophan pyrrolase 96
Tuberculin 261
Tumors 70, 92, 313-4, 333-4, 337, 344
  ADJ/PC6A tumor 328
  AKR leukemia 324
  human lung cancer 254-5, 271, 291
  human melanoma 291-2
  L1210 leukemia 260, 325, 327-8
  mammary carcinoma 324, 328
  murine allogeneic sarcoma 274
  murine fibrosarcoma 265
  nickel subsulfide-induced 84
  human ovarian cancer 332, 334
  P338 tumor 327
  180 TG Crocker 274
Tyramine (TA) 121-4, 197
m-Tyramine 121, 123
Tyrosinases 101

Tyrosine hydroxylase 101, 126

Ubiquitin 265
UDP-Glucose dehydrogenase 119
UDP-Glucuronic acid pyrophosphatase 119
UDP-Glucuronosyltransferase 36, 118
Uptake, in cell culture
  cadmium 76
  copper 131
  mercury 88-9
  nickel 82
Urinary excretion
  cadmium 76
  heavy metals 65
  lead 66, 79
  mercury 66, 88, 90
  nickel 82, 85
  thallium 69, 71

Vaccination 275, 280, 292

Warfarin 105-6
Wasting disease 274
Wilson's disease 67, 83, 86-7

Xanthine oxidase 96, 166

Zidovudine, *see* Azidothymidine
Zinc (Zn) 244, 252, 276, 345
  alcohol dehydrogenase 97, 100
  aldehyde dehydrogenase 155
  bioavailability 67, 71, 76
  carbonic anhydrase 99-100
  mossy fiber butons 72-3
  superoxide dismutase 100, 126, 129
  tissue levels 67, 71-3
Zinc diethyldithiocarbamate [$Zn(DS)_2$] 345
  extraction constant 10-1
  mitogen-induced lymphoproliferation
        252, 276